Lower Extremity Vascular Disease

Lower Extremity Vascular Disease

EDITED BY

Kenneth Ouriel, M.D.

Associate Professor of Surgery,
University of Rochester;
Attending Physician,
Strong Memorial Hospital
Rochester, New York

W. B. Saunders Company
A Division of Harcourt Brace & Company
PHILADELPHIA LONDON TORONTO MONTREAL SYDNEY TOKYO

W.B. SAUNDERS COMPANY

A Division of Harcourt Brace & Company

The Curtis Center
Independence Square West
Philadelphia, Pennsylvania 19106

Library of Congress Cataloging-in-Publication Data

Lower extremity vascular disease / [edited by] Kenneth Ouriel. — 1st
  ed.
    p.   cm.
  ISBN 0-7216-4749-9
  1. Leg—Blood-vessels—Diseases.   I. Ouriel, Kenneth.
  [DNLM: 1. Vascular Diseases. 2. Leg. WG 500 L917 1996]
RC694.L69 1996
616.1'31—dc20
DNLM/DLC   95-6842

LOWER EXTREMITY VASCULAR DISEASE   ISBN 0–7216–4749–9

Printed in The United States of America

Last digit is the print number: 9   8   7   6   5   4   3   2

This work is dedicated to my wife, Joy,
and my three children, David, Richard, and Elizabeth,
whose support and patience made this effort possible

Preface

Lower extremity arterial and venous diseases account for significant costs to society. Arterial disease can culminate in the loss of a limb, and patient mortality is frequent, usually the result of associated cardiac or cerebrovascular pathology. Venous disease is not normally associated with risks of limb loss, except in most unusual cases of phlegmasia. Chronic morbidity from venous valvular incompetence and patient mortality from massive pulmonary embolism are both major concerns, mandating the development of effective methods of prophylaxis and treatment.

As in any area of medical specialty, the most cost-effective method of addressing lower extremity vascular disease is prevention. With this in mind, the introductory chapters of this text have been directed at defining the pathogenesis and diagnosis of atherosclerotic and thrombotic disease. Once vascular pathology has become well established, the processes of arterial and venous thrombotic occlusion are strikingly similar. Only recently has the concept of intravascular, intrathrombus administration of thrombolytic agents been applied to the venous setting in a manner similar to that for arterial occlusions. Thus, the newer methods of thrombolysis as outlined in the chapters on arterial and venous lytic therapy are remarkably similar, whether the process involves the arterial or venous side of the circulation.

Chronic arterial occlusions are now well treated with open surgical techniques when the disease is diffuse and endovascular balloon angioplasty when the lesions are localized. The chapters on lower extremity revascularization and free tissue transfer outline the possibilities of extended limb salvage, albeit through a voracious consumption of hospital resources. The alternative to limb salvage, however, may be even more costly when one considers the long-term economic and psychological burden of amputation.

Recently, endovascular techniques have been applied to the treatment of aneurysms of the abdominal aorta. These modalities are experimental and have been used in selected centers with great technical expertise. Chapters authored by individuals involved in the development of these innovative devices outline the major and rapid advances that have been achieved during the first half of this decade. At the same time, their experience underscores the potential problems associated with any endovascular device and the reliance on open techniques for many, if not the majority, of abdominal aortic aneurysms.

The goal of this text is to provide a relatively compact, readable, and up-to-date source that provides comprehensive coverage of lower extremity vascular pathology. It is hoped that the text will serve this purpose for those engaged in developing a basic level of knowledge in vascular disease, as well as for those expanding or refreshing their knowledge in this area. If this goal is achieved, the ultimate beneficiaries will be our society at large. The dissemination of knowledge will result in improvements in the safe and efficacious treatment of lower extremity vascular disease, as well as a decrease in the overall incidence of these diseases from the widespread introduction of effective preventive strategies.

Acknowledgments

I would like to acknowledge the assistance of Ms. Allyson Shirtz and Ms. Marcia Mallory in the preparation of this text. I also wish to acknowledge the support of my mentors, Dr. Richard M. Green, Dr. James A. DeWeese, Dr. Seymour I. Schwartz, and Dr. Christopher K. Zarins, all of whom were instrumental in encouraging and shaping my growth and academic achievements.

K.O.

Contributing Authors

STEFANO BARTOLI, M.D.
Visiting Professor, Baylor College of Medicine,
Houston, Texas; Chief Assistant, Hospital CTO USL
RMC, Rome, Italy
Chapter 8. Thoracoabdominal Aortic Aneurysm

JOHN J. BERGAN, M.D., F.A.C.S.
Professor of Surgery, Loma Linda University Medical
School; Clinical Professor of Surgery, University of
California San Diego; Attending Surgeon, Scripps
Memorial Hospital, La Jolla, California
Chapter 27. Venous Stasis Disease

VICTOR M. BERNHARD, M.D.
Professor of Surgery, University of Arizona College of
Medicine, Tucson, Arizona; Vice President for
Medical Affairs, EndoVascular Technologies, Inc.
*Chapter 5. Prosthetic Vascular Grafts: Materials
and Their Properties*

KEITH D. CALLIGARO, M.D.
Associate Professor of Surgery, Thomas Jefferson
Medical College; Chief, Section of Vascular Surgery,
Pennsylvania Hospital, Philadelphia, Pennsylvania
Chapter 19. Infected Infrainguinal Grafts

ANTHONY J. COMEROTA, M.D.
Professor of Surgery, Temple University School of
Medicine; Chief of Vascular Surgery, Temple
University Hospital, Philadelphia, Pennsylvania
*Chapter 21. Thrombolytic Therapy in the
Management of Peripheral Arterial Occlusion*

JOHN P. COOKE, M.D., Ph.D.
Assistant Professor of Medicine, Director, Section of
Vascular Medicine, Stanford University School of
Medicine, Stanford, California
*Chapter 3. Medical Management of Peripheral
Arterial Occlusive Disease*

TIMOTHY A. M. CHUTER, M.D.
Assistant Professor of Surgery, Columbia University
College of Physicians and Surgeons; Assistant
Attending Surgeon, Columbia-Presbyterian Medical
Center, New York, New York
Chapter 10. Endovascular Aneurysm Repair

JACOB CYNAMON, M.D.
Department of Radiology, Montefiore Medical
Center, Bronx, New York
*Chapter 15. Interventional Angiographic
Techniques*

MICHAEL D. DAKE, M.D.
Assistant Professor of Radiology and Medicine,
Stanford University Medical Center; Chief,
Cardiovascular-Interventional Radiology, Stanford,
California
Chapter 22. Venous Thrombolysis

DOMINIC A. DeLAURENTIS, M.D.
Professor of Surgery, University of Pennsylvania
School of Medicine, Section of Vascular Surgery,
Pennsylvania Hospital, Philadelphia, Pennsylvania
Chapter 19. Infected Infrainguinal Grafts

JAMES A. DeWEESE, M.D.
Professor and Chairman Emeritus Vascular Surgery
and Cardiothoracic Surgery, University of Rochester,
Rochester, New York
Chapter 9. Popliteal and Femoral Artery Aneurysms

MAGRUDER C. DONALDSON, M.D.
Associate Professor of Surgery, Harvard Medical
School; Surgeon, Brigham and Women's Hospital,
Boston, Massachusetts
Chapter 4. The Hypercoagulable Syndromes

LUKE S. ERDOES, M.D.
Instructor in Surgery, University of Arizona College
of Medicine; Fellow in Vascular Surgery, Arizona
Health Sciences Center, Tucson, Arizona
*Chapter 5. Prosthetic Vascular Grafts: Materials
and Their Properties*

GIAN LUCA FAGGIOLI, M.D.
Vascular Fellow, SUNY at Buffalo, Buffalo, New
York; Research Physician in Vascular Surgery,
Cattedra de Chiruvgia Vascolare, Universita di
Bologna, Bologna, Italy
*Chapter 7. Juxtarenal, Pararenal and
Paraanastomic Aneurysms of the Abdominal
Aorta*

CHARLES W. FRANCIS, M.D.
Professor of Medicine, Hematology Unit, University
of Rochester School of Medicine and Dentistry;
Attending Physician, Strong Memorial Hospital,
Rochester, New York
*Chapter 24. Innovative Approaches to Fibrinolytic
Therapy*

KELLY R. GARDNER, M.D.
Chief of Interventional Radiology, Sunrise Hospital,
Las Vegas, Nevada
*Chapter 20. Techniques of Percutaneous
Intraarterial Thrombolysis (PIAT)*

ROBERT W. HOBSON II, M.D.
Professor of Surgery, Chief, Section of Vascular
Surgery, Department of Surgery, University of
Medicine and Dentistry of New Jersey—New Jersey
Medical School, Newark, New Jersey
Chapter 6. Infrarenal Aortic Aneurysms

RUSSELL D. HULL, M.B., B.S.
Professor of Medicine, University of Calgary;
Director, Clinical Trials Unit, Foothills Hospital,
Calgary, Alberta, Canada
*Chapter 28. Deep Vein Thrombosis and
Anticoagulation*

DONALD L. JACOBS, M.D.
Vascular Surgery Fellow, Department of Vascular
Surgery, Medical College of Wisconsin, Milwaukee,
Wisconsin
Chapter 12. Femoropopliteal Bypass

DOUGLAS L. JICHA, M.D.
Assistant Professor of Vascular Surgery, University of
Utah, Salt Lake City, Utah
Chapter 18. Infected Aortic Grafts

KRISHNA KANDARPA, M.D.
Associate Professor, Harvard Medical School;
Co-Director, Division of Cardiovascular and
Interventional Radiology, Brigham and Women's
Hospital, Boston, Massachusetts
*Chapter 25. Complications of Local Intraarterial
Thrombolysis for Lower Extremity Occlusions*

E. M. MICK KOLASSA, Ph.D.
Research Associate, University of Mississippi Research
Institute of Pharmaceutical Sciences, Jackson,
Mississippi
*Chapter 26. Cost-Effectiveness of Thrombolytic
Agents in Peripheral Arterial Occlusion*

ADRIAN O. MA, M.D.
Section of Vascular Medicine, Stanford University
School of Medicine, Stanford, California
*Chapter 3. Medical Management of Peripheral
Arterial Occlusive Disease*

MICHAEL L. MARIN, M.D.
Assistant Professor of Surgery, Albert Einstein College
of Medicine; Attending Surgeon, Montefiore Medical
Center, New York, New York
*Chapter 17. Endovascular Aortoiliac Reconstruction
for Occlusive Disease*

THOMAS O. McNAMARA, M.D.
Professor, UCLA Medical School, Interventional
Radiology Section, UCLA Medical Center, Los
Angeles, California
*Chapter 20. Techniques of Percutaneous
Intraarterial Thrombolysis (PIAT)*

JEFFREY W. OLIN, M.D.
Co-Director, Noninvasive Vascular Laboratory,
Department of Vascular Medicine, Cleveland Clinic
Foundation; Associate Professor of Medicine, Ohio
State University, Cleveland, Ohio
*Chapter 2. The Importance of Lipids and
Lipoproteins in the Progression and Regression of
Atherosclerosis*

KENNETH OURIEL, M.D.
Associate Professor of Surgery, University of
Rochester; Attending Physician, Strong Memorial
Hospital, Rochester, New York
*Chapter 14. Free-Tissue Transfer in Lower
Extremity Ischemia*
*Chapter 21. Thrombolytic Therapy in the
Management of Peripheral Arterial Occlusion*
*Chapter 26. Cost-Effectiveness of Thrombolytic
Agents in Peripheral Arterial Occlusion*

BRUCE A. PERLER, M.D.
Associate Professor of Surgery, The Johns Hopkins
University School of Medicine; Director of the
Vascular Noninvasive Laboratory and Vascular
Service, The Johns Hopkins Hospital, Baltimore,
Maryland
Chapter 11. Aortoiliac Reconstruction

GRAHAM F. PINEO, M.D.
Professor of Medicine, University of Calgary;
Director, Clinical Trials Unit, Calgary General
Hospital, Calgary, Alberta, Canada
*Chapter 28. Deep Vein Thrombosis and
Anticoagulation*

SESHADRI RAJU, M.D.
University of Mississippi Medical Center, Jackson,
Mississippi
*Chapter 30. Valvular Incompetence and Venous
Reconstructive Procedures*

JOHN J. RICOTTA, M.D.
Professor of Surgery, Chief, Division of Vascular
Surgery, SUNY at Buffalo; Chief of Surgery, Millard
Filmore Hospital, Buffalo, New York
*Chapter 7. Juxtarenal, Pararenal and
Paraanastomic Aneurysms of the Abdominal
Aorta*

HAZIM J. SAFI, M.D.
Associate Professor of Surgery, Baylor College of
Medicine; Associate Professor of Medicine, The
Methodist Hospital, Houston, Texas
Chapter 8. Thoracoabdominal Aortic Aneurysm

CHARLES P. SEMBA, M.D.
Assistant Professor of Radiology, Division of
Cardiovascular-Interventional Radiology, Standard
University Medical Center, Stanford, California
Chapter 22. Venous Thrombolysis

JOSEPH M. SERLETTI, M.D.
Associate Professor of Surgery, Division of Plastic
Surgery, University of Rochester School of Medicine
and Dentistry; Attending Surgeon, Strong Memorial
Hospital, Rochester, New York
*Chapter 14. Free-Tissue Transfer in Lower
Extremity Ischemia*

CYNTHIA K. SHORTELL, M.D.
Clinical Assistant Professor of Surgery, University of
Rochester School of Medicine and Dentistry;
Attending Surgeon, Rochester General Hospital,
Rochester, New York
*Chapter 29. Pulmonary Embolism and Vena Caval
Interruption*

MICHAEL B. SILVA, JR., M.D.
Assistant Professor of Surgery, Section of Vascular
Surgery, Department of Surgery, University of
Medicine and Dentistry of New Jersey—New Jersey
Medical School, Newark, New Jersey
Chapter 6. Infrarenal Aortic Aneurysms

RONALD J. STONEY, M.D.
Professor of Surgery, Emeritus, University of
California, San Francisco, California
Chapter 18. Infected Aortic Grafts

D. EUGENE STRANDNESS, JR., M.D.
Professor and Chief, Department of Surgery, Division
of Vascular Surgery, University of Washington
Medical Center, Seattle, Washington
Chapter 1. Arterial and Venous Hemodynamics

WILLIAM D. SUGGS, M.D.
Assistant Professor of Surgery, Albert Einstein College
of Medicine; Assistant Attending in Surgery,
Montefiore Medical Center, New York, New York
Chapter 13. Bypasses to the Infrapopliteal Arteries

JONATHAN B. TOWNE, M.D.
Professor of Surgery, Chief, Vascular Surgery, Medical
College of Wisconsin, Milwaukee, Wisconsin
Chapter 12. Femoropopliteal Bypass

FRANK J. VEITH, M.D.
Professor of Surgery, Albert Einstein College of
Medicine; Chief, Vascular Surgical Services,
Montefiore Medical Center, New York, New York
Chapter 13. Bypasses to the Infrapopliteal Arteries
Chapter 17. Endovascular Aortoiliac Reconstruction
   for Occlusive Disease
Chapter 19. Infected Infrainguinal Grafts

CHRISTOPHER J. WHITE, M.D.
Director, Invasive Cardiology, HCI International
Medical Center, Glasgow, Scotland, United Kingdom
Chapter 23. Comparison of Thrombolytic Agents

RODNEY A. WHITE, M.D.
Professor of Surgery, UCLA School of Medicine, Los
Angeles, California; Chief, Vascular Surgery, Associate
Chairman, Department of Surgery, Harbor-UCLA
Medical Center, Torrance, California
Chapter 16. Endovascular Imaging Techniques

ANTHONY D. WHITTEMORE, M.D.
Professor of Surgery, Harvard Medical School; Chief,
Division of Vascular Surgery, Brigham and Women's
Hospital, Boston, Massachusetts
Chapter 4. The Hypercoagulable Syndromes

Contents

PART I
General Principles

CHAPTER 1
Arterial and Venous Hemodynamics   *3*
D. EUGENE STRANDNESS JR.

CHAPTER 2
**The Importance of Lipids and Lipoproteins in the Progression
and Regression of Atherosclerosis**   *13*
JEFFREY W. OLIN

CHAPTER 3
Medical Management of Peripheral Arterial Occlusive Disease   *25*
JOHN P. COOKE
ADRIAN O. MA

CHAPTER 4
The Hypercoagulable Syndromes   *45*
MAGRUDER C. DONALDSON
ANTHONY D. WHITTEMORE

CHAPTER 5
Prosthetic Vascular Grafts: Materials and Their Properties   *53*
LUKE S. ERDOES
VICTOR M. BERNHARD

PART II
Aneurysmal Disease

CHAPTER 6
Infrarenal Aortic Aneurysms   *71*
MICHAEL B. SILVA, JR.
ROBERT W. HOBSON, II

CHAPTER 7
Juxtarenal, Pararenal, and Paraanastomotic Aneurysms
of the Abdominal Aorta   *87*
GIAN LUCA FAGGIOLI
JOHN J. RICOTTA

CHAPTER 8
Thoracoabdominal Aortic Aneurysms   *103*
HAZIM J. SAFI
STEFANO BARTOLI

CHAPTER 9
Popliteal and Femoral Artery Aneurysms   *121*
JAMES A. DeWEESE

CHAPTER 10
Endovascular Aneurysm Repair   *141*
TIMOTHY A. M. CHUTER

PART III
Lower Extremity Arterial Occlusive Disease

CHAPTER 11
Aortoiliac Reconstruction   *157*
BRUCE A. PERLER

CHAPTER 12
Femoropopliteal Bypass   *187*
DONALD L. JACOBS
JONATHAN B. TOWNE

CHAPTER 13
Bypasses to the Infrapopliteal Arteries   *195*
WILLIAM D. SUGGS
FRANK D. VEITH

CHAPTER 14
Free-Tissue Transfer in Lower Extremity Ischemia   *207*
JOSEPH M. SERLETTI
KENNETH OURIEL

CHAPTER 15
Interventional Angiographic Techniques   *219*
JACOB CYNAMON

CHAPTER 16
Endovascular Imaging Techniques   *223*
RODNEY A. WHITE

CHAPTER 17
Endovascular Aortoiliac Reconstruction for Occlusive Disease   *243*
MICHAEL L. MARIN
FRANK J. VEITH

CHAPTER 18
Infected Aortic Grafts   *253*
DOUGLAS L. JICHA
RONALD J. STONEY

CHAPTER 19
Infected Infrainguinal Grafts   *267*
KEITH D. CALLIGARO
DOMINIC A. DeLAURENTIS
FRANK J. VEITH

PART IV
Thrombolysis

CHAPTER 20
Techniques of Percutaneous Intraarterial Thrombolysis (PIAT)   *277*
THOMAS McNAMARA
KELLY R. GARDNER

CHAPTER 21
*Thrombolytic Therapy in the Management of Peripheral
Arterial Occlusion*   *295*
KENNETH OURIEL
ANTHONY J. COMEROTA

CHAPTER 22
Venous Thrombolysis   *321*
CHARLES P. SEMBA
MICHAEL D. DAKE

CHAPTER 23
Comparison of Thrombolytic Agents   *331*
CHRISTOPHER J. WHITE

CHAPTER 24
Innovative Approaches to Fibrinolytic Therapy   *337*
CHARLES W. FRANCIS

CHAPTER 25
Complications of Local Intraarterial Thrombolysis for Lower
Extremity Occlusions   *359*
KRISHNA KANDARPA

CHAPTER 26
Cost-Effectiveness of Thrombolytic Agents in Peripheral
Arterial Occlusion   *367*
KENNETH OURIEL
MICK KOLASSA

PART V
Lower Extremity Venous Disease

CHAPTER 27
Venous Stasis Disease   *375*
JOHN J. BERGAN

CHAPTER 28
Deep Venous Thrombosis and Anticoagulation   *385*
RUSSELL D. HULL
GRAHAM F. PINEO

CHAPTER 29
Pulmonary Embolism and Vena Caval Interruption   *409*
CYNTHIA K. SHORTELL

CHAPTER 30
Valvular Incompetence and Venous Reconstructive Procedures   *417*
SESHADRI RAJU

Index   *425*

General Principles

Arterial and Venous Hemodynamics

D. EUGENE STRANDNESS JR.

The long held practice of evaluating arterial and venous disorders by the standard history and physical examination followed by angiography has been greatly modified as we have come to understand the hemodynamics of vascular disorders and how they can be evaluated noninvasively.[1–3] Once it was realized that changes in the arterial inflow and venous outflow reflect the severity of the underlying disease, it was a matter of finding the most appropriate method to detect them. From a theoretical standpoint, information on pressure, volume flow, flow velocity, dimensions, and dimensional changes may be used to classify hemodynamic abnormalities. Obviously, this goal is not entirely achievable, but significant progress is being seen. From a practical standpoint, we need to determine the site, the degree of involvement with the vascular system, and how it affects function.

Most of the attention has been devoted to the arterial system, since this is where direct endovascular and surgical therapy can be applied with greatest success. The venous circulation, while equally important, has not yet lent itself to the same kind of direct therapeutic intervention. Also, the venous system is a much more complex system, making it more difficult to study.[4] It is important to remember that full appreciation of measurable physiologic changes requires some understanding of the underlying disease and its distribution. For example, an ankle systolic blood pressure of 30 mmHg requires a different interpretation if the underlying cause is atherosclerosis versus Buerger's disease. While the low pressure represents a reduction in perfusion, the distribution of disease that led to it is entirely different.

The discussion that follows will deal primarily with those hemodynamic parameters which can be measured and applied to patients as they are seen in everyday practice. The theoretical considerations will be noted only if they are important for an appreciation of the findings or if they currently are being studied and used in a practical manner.

THE ARTERIAL SYSTEM

The arterial system is provided with a cardiac output that has to be shared by all the organs in the body. These systems can be subdivided into those of low resistance (high metabolic activity), intermediate resistance (changes frequently throughout the day), and relatively high resistance (whose metabolic activity is relatively low and fairly constant).[5]

The low-resistance organs are the brain, liver, and kidney. These organs need high levels of blood flow at all times to function properly; viability is endangered with relatively short periods of ischemia. Intermediate-resistance areas include the small and large bowel and the musculoskeletal system. These regions of the circulation, if quiescent in terms of their metabolic activity, exhibit many aspects of a high-resistance system but frequently change to a low-resistance system for short periods of time.[6] For example, digestion for the gut and exercise for the limbs will transiently convert their vascular beds into low resistance circuits to meet the metabolic demands. The one organ system or tissue that is relatively high resistance most of the time is the skin, whose metabolic activity can remain at very low levels for prolonged periods of time without loss of viability.

The arteries serve as distributing conduits capable of handling wide variations in volume flow with very little expenditure of energy. For example, the mean pressure drop from the central aorta to the small unnamed arteries is about 10 mmHg, a reflection of the very low resistance under normal conditions. As will be noted, this dramatically changes as the arterial wall becomes diseased and areas of narrowing began to develop. Anatomically, it is necessary to define those arteries which are of particular interest from both a clinical and pathologic standpoint. Atherosclerosis is a disease of large and medium-sized (named) arteries. This disease largely affects branch points and bifurcations, with one important exception. For reasons which are poorly understood, atherosclerosis rarely involves the arteries of the arm distal to the origin of the subclavian artery. This is in contrast to Buerger's disease, which affects primarily the arteries below the knee and in one-half of patients affects the palmar and digital circulation of the hand.

One other factor that must be taken into account in assessing the hemodynamics of arterial flow is the presence of type II diabetes, which has profound effects on the arterial system as well as the nervous system, making evaluation and therapy much more difficult.[7] It also affects arterial hemodynamics in a manner that must be understood in order to accurately assess the effects of diabetes on function. Some of the important differences are

1. The distribution of disease is altered; i.e., there is a lower incidence of aortoiliac disease, a similar distribution in the femoropopliteal region, and a much higher incidence of involvement in the tibial and peroneal arteries.[8,9]
2. One of the hallmarks of diabetes is the development of medial calcification (Mönckeberg's sclerosis). This pathologic change affects only the media and does not bear any relationship to the atherosclerosis that develops in these same vessels.[10]
3. The development of a peripheral neuropathy occurs in up to 40 percent of diabetics seen with vascular disease.[8] This results in an autosympathectomy, which changes the microvasculature of the foot into a low-resistance system.

Pressure

The fact that the arterial system is normally a low-resistance set of conduits has led to the use of pressure measurement as an index of disease involvement. While it might be of theoretical interest to measure both systolic and diastolic pressures, the only one of clinical value that is also easy to assess is the systolic blood pressure.[11,12] Its use is made even more valuable by the fact that it is the first to change when areas of narrowing become significant enough to result in decreased blood flow. Normally, in the case of the lower limbs, there is an amplification of the systolic pressure as one proceeds from the central aorta to the pedal arteries. This must be accompanied, of course, by a fall in the mean blood pressure. Pressure measurements are used by clinicians in several ways to estimate the presence and severity of arterial occlusive disease.[13,14]

CLINICAL APPLICATION OF PRESSURE MEASUREMENTS

The assessment of blood pressure can be made at different times during the course of a patient evaluation. During each of these assessments, the questions asked are somewhat different and should be considered separately.

First Visit

At the time of the first visit and in the course of an examination, the most useful pressure measurement is the ankle/brachial systolic pressure index (ABI). The ABI is measured by use of a continuous wave (CW) Doppler device.[15] Both the arm and ankle pressures should be measured with the

CW Doppler to obtain the best and most consistent results. Normally, with the amplification of the systolic pressure, the ABI should be greater than 1.0.[5,10,16] Because of the variability in measurement, a cutoff value of 0.95 is used to separate normal individuals from those who have arterial disease. Hemodynamically, the clinician should use the absolute values of systolic pressure as well as the index in the initial evaluation. The guidelines used are as follows:

1. An ABI greater than 0.50 but less than 0.95 is generally associated with single segment disease.
2. An ABI of less than 0.50 is often associated with multisegment disease.
3. An absolute systolic pressure of greater than 50 mmHg is associated with good collateral function and is not often seen in patients with critical ischemia. It is also well known now that only one patent artery below the knee is needed to provide normal flow to the foot due to the excellent collateral circulation that exists in this area. When the pressure falls below 50 mmHg, it often can be associated with the appearance of rest pain and ulceration. It is also known that, in general, the lower the systolic pressure, the less likely it is that an ulceration will heal.[17]

If the patient is a type II diabetic, use of the ABI may not be appropriate because of the presence of medial calcification, which results in either incompressible arteries or a falsely high ABI. In this circumstance, the clinician must measure the toe systolic pressure index (TSPI). This will require a plethysmographic method (strain gauge or protocol). Normally, the TSPI should exceed 0.60. The variability in this measurement is ±17 percent. It also has been found useful for the prediction of healing of open lesions on the digits. If the pressure is greater than 30 mmHg, healing is likely to occur.[10,17]

It is important to understand that a normal ABI does not rule out the presence of arterial disease. This is due to the fact that some lesions, particularly those in the aortoiliac area, may not be hemodynamically significant under resting flow conditions.[12] The other circumstance which is very common is that of exercise-induced pain which is not due to arterial disease but to neuromuscular disease.[18] In both these scenarios, it becomes necessary to use exercise testing to uncover diagnostic hemodynamic changes. The important features from a hemodynamic standpoint are as follows:

1. A normal person can perform moderate exercise without a significant drop in ankle blood pressure. However, if one increases the workload in a progressive manner, there will be two changes worthy of note[19]:
   a. The arm systolic blood pressure will increase in response to the workload.
   b. The ankle systolic pressure will fall as the workload increases, but the recovery time will remain short.
2. If one is to use exercise to bring out the abnormality associated with arterial disease, the protocol should be standardized for each patient. For diagnostic purposes, we have found a load of 2 mi/h on a 12 percent grade to be satisfactory.[13] In addition, we limit the maximum walking time to 5 minutes (if the patient is able to do so). It is important for the technologist to closely monitor the time of onset of pain, its severity, and its location. The patient exercises with the ankle and arm cuffs in place so that these can be used immediately after exercise to assess the hemodynamic response.
3. The two most important hemodynamic parameters to assess are the magnitude of the fall in ankle systolic pressure and its recovery time.[12,13] The magnitude of the fall is determined by the amount of ischemia, with the recovery time (period of postexercise hyperemia) reflective of the collateral circulation available to repay the oxygen debt that has occurred.[20] While it is not possible to provide absolute values for each of these, generally, the following work well in practice:
   a. The ankle pressure fall should exceed 20 percent of the baseline to be abnormal.
   b. The recovery time should exceed 3 minutes to be abnormal. It is well known that with severe intermittent claudication, the fall in pressure will be well in excess of 20 percent and may even be unrecordable for several minutes. In addition, the recovery time will be much longer, ranging up to 20 to 30

minutes, in some patients. While it is common practice to express the postexercise pressure changes in terms of changes in the ABI, this is not necessary and should not be done.

4. With neuroclaudication in the absence of arterial disease, the ankle systolic blood pressure response to exercise will be normal. However, one fact about the walking pattern in these patients is worthy of consideration. The patient with leg discomfort due to spinal stenosis or degenerative joint disease will not be able to walk long on the treadmill. This becomes very important when one considers the patient who has both neurospinal and peripheral arterial disease. In this case, there may be a paradoxical relationship between the walking time and the ankle blood pressure response. For example, if a patient with arterial disease can walk only a minute or less before being stopped by pain, there will be a dramatic fall in ankle systolic blood pressure and a very prolonged recovery time. Conversely, if the short walking time is due to the neurospinal disease, the hemodynamic changes will be minimal, and this will be reflected in the ankle blood pressure fall and its recovery time.

At Time of Arteriography

It is not at all uncommon to discover lesions in the aortoiliac region whose hemodynamic significance is of great importance clinically. These can be assessed by duplex scanning but can be confirmed at the time of arteriography by measuring the systolic pressures as a catheter is slowly withdrawn across suspicious areas of narrowing.[21] Normally, one should not be able to measure a gradient across such a short segment as the iliac arteries. However, in practice, a gradient of 10 mmHg or less is considered normal. If the gradient under resting flow is greater than 10 mmHg, this is abnormal and may be associated with intermittent claudication when the ischemia of exercise increases the flow. If the gradient is 10 mmHg or less, it is possible to mimic the flow change with exercise by injecting a vasodilator such as papaverine (30 mg) and measuring the extent of the fall in the systolic pressure. If the pressure drop exceeds 15 mmHg, this is considered abnormal.

Follow-Up Use of Pressures

If the arterial lesion(s) have been totally corrected, the ABI should return to normal. If, on the other hand, only one of many lesions has been corrected, the ABI will increase to a degree commensurate with the resistance offered by existing collaterals.[14,22,23] In general terms, the ABI must change by ±0.15, which is the range of variability for the measurement.[10] The same applies to the use of the ABI as a method of follow-up for outcome with or without some form of intervention, be it endovascular or direct arterial surgery.

Volume Flow

While it would be desirable to measure volume flow to an organ, it is not as useful as one might think. This should not be surprising, since cardiac output values have never been found to be particularly helpful in assessing a patient's response to ischemic heart disease. This is due to the extremely wide range of normal values, which makes any single determination less than useful and perhaps even misleading. Also, the measurement of flow from an artery requires assessment not only of the true diameter of the vessel but also of the mean velocity in the vessel.

The only method which has potential utility is ultrasound. This method permits an estimation of diameter and also can assess peak systolic, end-diastolic, and mean velocity at any site within the arterial system.[5] However, the most critical value in measuring volume flow is the arterial diameter. Any error in measuring the diameter results in large errors in the calculation of volume flow. It is for this and the other reasons mentioned earlier that assessment of volume flow as a single parameter has very little, if any, clinical significance. Nonetheless, there may be circumstances where flow measurements might be of some value, particularly if they are done over time and show a trend. One area that needs to be explored in this regard is the saphenous vein graft, where sequential studies are done frequently in order to detect developing stenosis that can be corrected by repair before thrombosis occurs.[24,25]

CLINICAL APPLICATION TO VELOCITY DATA

The one parameter that is relatively simple to assess by both CW Doppler and pulsed Doppler is velocity. Surprisingly, in contrast to the limited value of volume flow estimations, velocity data are very useful.[5] These can be both qualitative and quantitative. Velocity data are used as follows:

1. Qualitative assessment of velocity information. As noted earlier, it is now known that vascular beds have resistance patterns that are unique and easily recognized.
   a. Low-resistance beds have end-diastolic velocities above zero without any reverse flow at any time in the pulse cycle;[5]
   b. The intermediate resistance beds such as the gut may have some reverse flow, but it is very small compared with that seen in the major arteries to the limbs. With ingestion of food, this reverse-flow component disappears very quickly as the flow increases and the end-diastolic velocity goes well above zero;[6]
   c. With the high-resistance circuits, there is *always* a very prominent reverse-flow component early diastole.[5]

These relationships can be assessed very easily and quickly by the use of a CW or pulsed Doppler.[26] Even simple inspection of the velocity waveform can provide diagnostic information as long as the site of the recording is known.[5] For example, the finding of a triphasic waveform (forward flow, reverse flow, forward flow) from any site in the arterial system of the lower limb nearly always rules out significant occlusive disease proximal to the recording site.[27] While I have seen restoration of a reverse-flow component distal to a severe stenosis, this is rare.

If one is interested not only in detecting a stenosis but also in quantitating the degree of narrowing, it is necessary to examine those aspects of the velocity patterns which can be recorded.[28]

Use of an absolute value for the recorded velocity requires a precise knowledge of the angle of the incident sound wave with the direction of the velocity vectors within the lumen.[29] In general, one assumes that flow in the normal arterial system is parabolic, with the velocity vectors being parallel to the wall. This is, of course, only true for certain locations and not others.[30] The only site within the arterial system where true laminar flow appears to be found regularly is in the superficial femoral artery, which is long, relatively straight, and has relatively few large branches until the crural arteries are reached. Nearly all other areas of clinical interest, such as the aortic bifurcation, the carotid bulb, the renal arteries, and the subclavian artery, will have "disturbed" flow secondary to boundary layer separation near the origin of the branches or within the bulb in the case of the carotid artery.[31] These unusual flow patterns make it more difficult to document with certainty the flow patterns and estimate the true velocity unless the examiner is certain of the site of interrogation. One need only examine the velocity patterns in the posterolateral aspect of the carotid bulb as compared with those recorded near the flow divider to see how geometry can affect the velocity patterns which are present.

Even given these limitations, there are circumstances in which absolute velocities can be used to both detect disease and estimate its severity. Two examples of how this can be done are seen in the carotid bulb and the renal artery. This is of sufficient importance to review in some detail:

1. *Carotid artery.* The normal carotid artery is recognized by the presence of boundary layer separation in the bulb.[31] However, if one measures the peak and end-diastolic velocities across an area of narrowing, it is possible to estimate in general terms the degree of stenosis. For example, if the peak systolic velocity is greater than 125 cm/s, the stenosis exceeds 50 percent in terms of diameter reduction.[32] If the end-diastolic velocity is greater than 145 cm/s, the stenosis has now exceeded 80 percent in terms of diameter reduction. This separation becomes important from a clinical standpoint because the higher-grade stenoses are most

often associated with the development of ischemic events.

2. In the renal artery, it is important not only to detect stenoses but also to determine if they are sufficient to activate the renin-angiotensin system. We have established that the normal range for peak systolic velocites in the renal artery is 100 ± 20 cm/s. In order to use the peak systolic velocity as a cutoff point to detect an area of narrowing, it is necessary to use a value that is not likely to lead to a large number of unnecessary arteriograms while not missing those lesions which are resposible for the development of hypertension. The level we found to be most satisfactory is 180 cm/s, which is about 2.5 standard deviations above what we consider the normal range.[33]

It is also possible to use ratios of the peak systolic velocities to estimate the degree of stenosis in an artery. The areas in which this has been done successfully are as follows:

1. In the carotid artery, it is well accepted now that lesions that narrow the artery by 70 percent or greater in patients with symptoms are best treated by endarterectomy. Most of the Doppler criteria that have been developed do not include this as a cutoff point. To address this problem, Edwards et al.,[34] in a study involving four separate vascular laboratories, showed that a greater than 70 percent diameter-reducing lesion can be recognized by calculating the ratio of peak systolic velocity within the stenosis divided by that found in the common carotid artery proximal to the lesion. When this ratio is greater than 4.0, there is a 90 percent chance that the patient has a greater than 70 percent diameter-reducing stenosis.

2. In the renal artery, I have come to accept a greater than 60 percent diameter-reducing stenosis as being necessary to promote the development of hypertension. For this degree of stenosis, I have found that the ratio of the peak systolic velocity in the stenosis divided by that from the aorta (RAR ratio) can be helpful. If this ratio is greater than 3.5, it is very likely that the patient has the degree of

stenosis sufficient to activate the renin-angiotension system.[33]

3. For the peripheral arteries, the rules that pertain to the detection of stenoses also can be applied. From a clinical standpoint, the only lesions that are of importance are those which result in a fall in pressure and flow. For an obstruction, flow is reduced, but with stenoses one has to define which lesions will result in a fall in flow and which will not. The "critical" stenosis for resting flow conditions is one that reduces the diameter by 50 percent or greater.[35] As noted earlier, some stenoses of less than 50 percent can become hemodynamically significant under the flow demands of exercise. Due to the variablility in the range of velocities found in the arterial system, ratios of the peak systolic velocity proximal to and in the area of narrowing have been determined to be the most predictive of the degree of narrowing. A ratio of the peak velocity from one segment of an artery to the next of greater than 100 percent has been found to be very predictive of finding a 50 percent diameter-reducing lesion.[36] Furthermore, it is clear that a therapeutic decision, be it angioplasty or surgery, can be based on this finding.[37]

The mesenteric circulation is an interesting circuit not just because of the degree of narrowing and subsequent changes in pressure and flow but also because of the prodigious collaterals that are available to supply the gut. For example, it is well known that for chronic mesenteric angina to develop there must be hemodynamically significant lesions of all three of the inputs to the gut—the celiac and the superior and inferior mesenteric arteries. Hemodynamically, in order to make the diagnosis, it is necessary to find significant lesions in all three vessels. In most cases, this is difficult, and an absolute level of velocity change which will rule out the problem with certainty has not been found. However, Moneta et al.[38] have established cutoff values for the celiac and superior mesenteric arteries that can be of value.[38] They are 200 cm/s for the celiac artery and 275 cm/s for the superior mesenteric artery. No such cutoff values have been established for the inferior mesenteric artery.

Hemodynamics of Disease Progression and Therapeutic Outcome

One of the major advantages of studying the hemodynamics of the arterial system is objective demonstration that the patient is in fact improved after intervention. On the other hand, if the patient's arterial reconstruction is failing, or if there is disease progression, there will be associated hemodynamic deterioration. The ground rules for using hemodynamic changes to document outcome are the same as those used for screening studies. The areas where such information has been most useful clinically are the carotid circulation, saphenous vein grafts, and more recently, the renal circulation. For these areas, follow-up hemodynamic changes can be used to dictate a change in therapy.[24,25,39–41]

THE VENOUS SYSTEM

The venous system is very complex from both anatomic and hemodynamic perspectives.[4] This is due to the fact that there are basically three sets of "tubes" that are important—the superficial system, the deep system, and the communicating veins. To complicate the situation even further, the veins have the capacity to change their dimensions dramatically to adapt to circulatory need. They are in fact often referred to as the *capacitance system*. The final factor that complicates the hemodynamics is that this is a low-pressure system that is continually being subjected to the pressures generated by changes in position and activation of the calf muscle pump. The venous system works efficiently only by the presence of valves which protect the limb from adverse volume and pressure changes. The distribution of valves in the deep system gives a glimpse of which areas are the most vulnerable. The greatest number of valves are found below the knee.[4] Most of the large communicating veins are also protected by a valve.

In the quiet state, venous flow is dominated largely by respiratory events.[42] As the diaphragm descends, there is an increase in intraabdominal pressure which will temporarily stop venous outflow from the limb. This is reversed during expiration. In assuming the upright position there are volume shifts, with blood being translocated to the deep veins of the lower leg that can be in amounts approaching 500 ml for each limb.

Activation of the calf muscle pump brings into play many of the features that distinguish the unique hemodynamics of the venous system. With each contraction, flow is directed in an antegrade direction, with the venous valves preventing translocation of blood into the distal venous segments. During the diastolic phase of muscle contraction, flow passes from the superficial to the deep system via the communicating veins.[43] With destruction of the venous valves, this situation often will be reversed, and it is these hemodynamic changes that set the groundwork for development of the post-thrombotic syndrome.

Interest in venous hemodynamics has come about as a result of increasing attention to the detection of acute deep vein thrombosis (DVT). This has led to a greater understanding of the pathophysiology of the post-thrombotic syndrome. The earliest studies focused on the measurement of maximum venous outflow (MVO). It was noted that as venous thrombi developed in the proximal venous segments (popliteal vein to the inferior vena cava), venous outflow was reduced as flow was diverted through high-resistance collateral channels.[44] As collaterals improved and the venous thrombi began to lyse, MVO often returned to normal levels.[45] The return of venous outflow to normal levels is associated with the resolution of edema that develops during the acute phase of DVT.

The more difficult problems to study are those changes in venous volume and flow which occur during the recovery phase after an episode of DVT. While it would be nice to measure not only the volume and flow changes but also pressure, this is not feasible. The latest method devised to study these changes is the air plethysmograph introduced by Nicolaides and Christopoulos.[46] This device permits evaluation of several parameters that bear relevance to the hemodynamic changes associated with chronic venous disease. It should be noted that the air plethysmograph is placed about the calf but can be used in both the supine and the upright positions to document the effects of gravity and the activation of the calf muscle pump:

1. When the legs are moved from an elevated position to promote maximal venous emptying to the upright position, it is used to measure the venous filling time and the venous volume.
2. Once the baseline venous volume has been reached, the patient can then do a single tiptoe to provide a value for ejection volume and ejection fraction, followed by 10 tiptoes to estimate what the residual venous volume is after this brief period of exercise.

From the preceding measurements, it is possible to do several calculations that reflect the current hemodynamic status of the deep and superficial venous system. For example, knowing the filling time to 90 percent of final level and the amount of the volume increase permits one to determine the venous filling index (VFI), which is expressed in milliliters per second. As one might expect, when the status of the venous system is stratified by level and extent of involvement, the VFI will become higher, with the most abnormal indices found in patients with advanced leg changes and popliteal reflux. One also might be able to separate those patients with chronic residual obstruction from those whose primary problem is reflux. In fact, the ejection fraction is lowest in patients with chronic obstruction. Unfortunately, there is considerable overlap between those patients whose primary problem is obstruction versus those in whom valvular incompetence appears to play a dominant role. It is most likely that there is a combination of obstruction and valvular incompetence present in most patients with chronic venous insufficiency.

One of the more difficult changes to assess has been the presence and distribution of valvular reflux in the lower limbs of patients with chronic venous insufficiency. From a clinical standpoint, these patients can be subdivided into those with primary varicose veins and those whose varicose veins are secondary to a previous episode of DVT. With primary varices, there is a strong family history, and with few exceptions, the valvular reflux is confined to the superficial system. With the secondary variety, which is responsible for the post-thrombotic syndrome, the involvement depends on the location and extent of the previous thrombosis and resulting damage.[47]

While global measures of reflux can be helpful clinically, it is much more useful to document the exact location and extent of the valvular insufficiency.[48,49] The major difficulties that have plagued the field relate to quantification of reflux. This is further complicated by the fact that in order to demonstrate reflux it is necessary to impose a transvalvular pressure gradient that will induce reverse flow. The easiest and most commonly used method is CW Doppler with the assistence of a Valsalva maneuver or limb compression proximal to the site of interrogation. This will be adequate if there is gross reflux and there are no competent valves cephalad to the examination site. For example, if one were examining the popliteal vein and there were one or more competent valves in the superficial femoral vein, the use of a Valsalva maneuver would be of little value.

Another question relates to the determination of normal time for valve closure. In order to determine this, the test employed must be standardized so that the values obtained will be constant from time to time in the same individual and from person to person. Van Bemmelen[50,51] developed a method that employed duplex scanning done in the upright position with pneumatic cuffs placed at the thigh, upper and lower calf, and foot. With this procedure, the pneumatic cuffs are rapidly inflated at pressure levels which are the same for each visit and each patient. The pressures used are 80 mmHg for the thigh, 100 mmHg for the calf, and 120 mmHg for the foot. To document reflux, the ultrasound transducer is placed within 5 cm of the upper end of the cuff over the vein of interest. As the cuff is inflated, the veins beneath the cuff are collapsed. With cuff release, blood can flow in a retrograde direction if there is valvular incompetence in that segment. The value which is the upper limit of normal for 95 percent of venous segments is 0.5 s.

The major questions with regard to hemodynamic studies of the venous circulation are how they should be used clinically and to what extent the information should influence clinical management. While there appears to be agreement as to the role of valvular incompetence, at least as the basic fault leading the abnormal pressure-flow changes, there is little appreciation of what will in the long term lead to complications and which hemodynamic changes are of little consequence.

One of the problems in this field is that up to one-half of patients who present with the post-thrombotic syndrome will not give a history of previous deep vein thrombosis. One has to surmise that in this case, the previous episode of DVT may have gone undetected, which is not unexpected given the vagaries of the clinical presentation and the difficulties in arriving at a diagnosis.[52,53] This is particularly true given the fact that the regular use of noninvasive testing to permit early and accurate detection of venous thrombi is a relatively recent innovation in medical practice.[52,54–56] Based on studies done in patients with a history of DVT versus those who did not have such a history, the location and extent of the valvular incompetence are very simlar.[47]

Other studies of the distribution of valvular incompetence in those with ulcers and those without has led to some interesting findings. For example, in patients with deep venus incompetence and stasis ulcers, there is also a very high prevalence of incompetence of the greater and lesser saphenous veins.[47] This was not seen in those patients who did not develop ulceration, even though the valves in the deep system were incompetent. The link between these findings and the final pathway to ulceration remains to be determined.

REFERENCES

1. Strandness DE Jr, Sumner DS: Hemodynamics for Surgeons. New York, Grune and Stratton, 1975.
2. vanRamshorst B, vanBemmelen PS, Hoeneveld H, Eikelboom BC: Thrombus regression in deep venous thrombosis: Quantification of spontaneous thrombolysis with duplex scanning. Circulation 1992;86:414.
3. Strandness DE Jr: Physiology of vascular system. In Fischer JE (ed): Surgical Basic Science. St. Louis, CV Mosby, 1993, pp 429–470.
4. Strandness DE Jr, Thiele BL: Selected Topics in Venous Disorders: Pathophysiology, Diagnosis and Treatment. Mt. Kisco, NY, Futura, 1981.
5. Strandness DE Jr: Hemodynamics of the normal arterial and venous system. In Strandness DE Jr (ed): Duplex Scanning in Vascular Disorders, 2d ed. New York, Raven Press, 1993, pp 45–79.
6. Strandness DE Jr: The mesenteric and portal circulation. In Strandness DE Jr (ed): Duplex Scanning in Vascular Disorders, 2d ed. New York, Raven Press, 1993, pp 217–229.
7. Beach KW, Bedford GR, Bergelin RO, et al: Progression of lower extremity arterial occlusive disease in type II diabetes. Diabetes Care 1988; 11:464.
8. Strandness DE Jr. Priest RR, Gibbons GE: A combined clinical and pathological study of nondiabetic and diabetic vascular disease. Diabetes 1964; 13:366.
9. Gensler SW, Haimovici H: Study of vascular lesions in diabetic, non-diabetic patients. Arch Surg 1965;91:617.
10. Orchard TJ, Strandness DE Jr: Assessment of peripheral vascular disease in diabetes. Circulation 1993;88:819.
11. Pokras R, Dyken M: Dramatic changes in the performance of endarterectomy for diseases of the extracranial arteries of the head. Stroke 1988;10:1289.
12. Carter SA: Response of ankle systolic pressure to leg exercise in mild or questionable arterial disease. N Engl J Med 1972;287:578.
13. Strandness DE Jr: Exercise testing in the evaluation of patients undergoing direct arterial surgery. J Cardiovasc Surg 1970;11:192.
14. Strandness DE Jr, Bell JW: Ankle blood pressure responses after reconstructive arterial surgery. Surgery 1966;59:514.
15. Marinelli MR, Beach KW, Glass MJ, et al: Noninvasive testing vs clinical evaluation of arterial disease: A prospective study. JAMA 1979; 241:2031.
16. McDonald DA: The pulsatile flow pattern in arteries. In McDonald DA (ed): Blood Flow in Arteries. Baltimore, Williams & Wilkins, 1960, pp 129–145.
17. Holstein P, Lassen N: Healing of ulcers on the feet correlated with distal blood pressure measurements in occlusive arterial disease. Acta Orthop Scand 1980;51:995.
18. Goodreau JJ, Greasy JK, Flanigan DP, et al: Rational approach to the differentiation of vascular and neurogenic claudication. Surgery 1978;84:749.
19. Stahler C, Strandness DE Jr: Ankle blood pressure response to graded treadmill exercise. Angiology 1967;18:237.
20. Sumner DS, Strandness DE Jr: The relationship between calf blood flow and ankle pressure in patients with intermittent claudication. Surgery 1969;65:763.
21. Thiele BL, Bandyk DW, Zierler RE: A systematic approach to the assessment of aortoiliac disease. Arch Surg 1983;18:477.
22. Strandness DE Jr, Bell JW: Peripheral vascular disease: Diagnosis and objective evaluation using a mercury strain gauge. Ann Surg 1965;161(suppl):1.
23. Strandness DE Jr, Carter SA: Outcome criteria in patients with peripheral arterial disease. Ann Vasc Surg 1993;7:491.
24. Bandyk DF, Schmitt DD, Seabrook GR, et al: Monitoring functional patency of in situ saphenous vein bypasses: the impact of a surveillance protocol and elective revision. J Vasc Surg 1989;9:286.

25. Bandyk DF: Postoperative surveillance of infrainguinal bypass. Surg Clin N Am 1990;70:71.
26. Strandness DE Jr, Schultz RA, Sumner DS, Rushmer RF: Ultrasonic flow detection: A useful technique in the evaluation of peripheral vascular disease. Am J Surg 1967;113:311.
27. Hatsukami TS, Primozich JP, Zierler RE, Strandness DE Jr: Color Doppler imaging of lower extremity arterial disease: A prospective validation study. J Vasc Surg 1992;16:527.
28. Phillips DJ, Powers JE, Eyer MK, et al: Detection of peripheral vascular disease using duplex scanner III. Ultrasound Med Biol 1980;6:205.
29. Beach KW: Physics and instrumentation for ultrasonic duplex scanning. In Strandness DE Jr (ed): Duplex Scanning in Vascular Disorders. New York, Raven Press, 1993, pp 273–317.
30. Phillips DJ, Beach KW, Primozich J, Strandness DE Jr: Should results of ultrasound Doppler studies be reported in units of frequency or velocity? Ultrasound Med Biol 1989;15:205.
31. Phillips DJ, Greene FM, Langlois Y, et al: Flow velocity patterns in the carotid bifurcations of young presumed normal subjects. Ultrasound Med Biol 1983;9:19.
32. Strandness DE Jr: Extracranial arterial disease. In Strandness DE Jr (ed): Duplex Scanning in Vascular Disorders, 2d ed. New York, Raven Press, 1993, pp 113–157.
33. Hoffman U, Edwards JM, Carter S, et al: Role of duplex scanning for the detection of athrosclerotic renal artery disease. Kidney Int 1991;39:1232.
34. Edwards JM, Moneta GL, Hatsukami T, et al: Duplex criteria for 70–99% internal carotid stenosis. In 19th International Joint Conference on Stroke and Cerebral Circulation, 1994. (Abstract).
35. May AG, VandeBerg L, DeWeese JA, et al: Critical arterial stenosis. Surgery 1963;54:250.
36. Jager KA, Phillips DJ, Martin R, et al: Noninvasive mapping of lower limb arterial lesions. Ultrasound Med Biol 1985;11:515.
37. Edwards JM, Coldwell DM, Goldman ML, Strandness DE Jr: The role of duplex scanning in the selection of patients for transluminal angioplasty. J Vasc Surg 1991;13:69.
38. Moneta GL, Lee RW, Caster JD, et al: Mesenteric duplex scanning: A blinded prospective study. J Vasc Surg 1993;17:79.
39. Guzman RP, Zierler RE, Isaacson JA, et al: Progressive renal atrophy with renal artery stenosis: A prospective evaluation with duplex ultrasound. Hypertension (in press).
40. Zierler RE, Bergelin RO, Isaacson JA, Strandness DE Jr: Natural history of renal artery stenosis: A prospective study with duplex ultrasound. J Vasc Surg (in press).
41. Zierler RE, Bandyk DF, Thiele BL, Strandness DE Jr: Carotid artery stenosis following carotid endarterectomy. Arch Surg 1982;117:1408.
42. Moneta GL, Bedford GR, Beach K, Strandness DE Jr: Duplex ultrasound assessment of venous diameters, peak velocities and flow patterns. J Vasc Surg 1988;8:286.
43. van Bemmelen PS, Bedford G, Beach KW, Strandness DE Jr: The mechanism of venous valve closure: its relationship to the velocity of reverse flow. Arch Surg 1990;125:617.
44. Wheeler HB, Pearson D, O'Connell D, Mullick SC: Impedance plethysmography: Techniques, interpretation and results. Arch Surg 1972;104:164.
45. Killewich LA, Martin R, Cramer M, et al: An objective assessment of the physiological changes in the post-thrombotic syndrome. Arch Surg 1985;120:424.
46. Nicolaides AN, Christopoulos D: Quantification of venous reflux and outflow obstruction with air plethysmography. In Bernstein EF (ed): Vascular Diagnosis. St. Louis, CV Mosby, 1993, pp 915–921.
47. van Bemmelen PS, Bedford G, Beach K, Strandness DE Jr: Status of the valves in superficial and deep venous system in chronic venous disease. Surgery 1991;109:730.
48. Markel A, Manzo RA, Bergelin RO, Strandness DE Jr: Valvular reflux after deep vein thrombosis: incidence and time of occurrence. J Vasc Surg 1992;15:377.
49. Meissner MH, Manzo RA, Bergelin RO, et al: Deep venous insufficiency: The relationship between lysis and subsequent reflux. J Vasc Surg 1993;18:596.
50. van Bemmelen PS, Bedford G, Beach K, Strandness DE Jr: Quantitative segmental evaluation of venous valvular reflux with ultrasonic duplex scanning. J Vasc Surg 1989;10:425.
51. van Bemmelen PS: Segmental evaluation of venous reflux. In Bernstein EF (ed): Vascular Diagnosis, 4th ed. St. Louis, CV Mosby, 1993.
52. Cranley JJ, Canos AJ, Sull WJ: The diagnosis of deep venous thrombosis: Fallability of clinical symptoms and signs. Arch Surg 1976;111:34.
53. Haeger K: Problems of acute venous thrombosis. I. The interpretation of symptoms and signs. Angiology 1969;20:219.
54. Killewich LA, Bedford GR, Beach KW, Strandness DE Jr: Diagnosis of deep venous thrombosis: A prospective study comparing duplex scanning to contrast venography. Circulation 1989;79:810.
55. Lensing AWA, Prandoni P, Brandjes D, et al: Detection of deep vein thrombosis by real time B-mode ultrasonography. N Engl J Med 1989;320:342.
56. Cogo A, Lensing AWA, Prandoni P, et al: Comparison of real-time B-mode ultrasonography and Doppler ultrasound with contrast venography in the diagnosis of venous thrombosis in symptomatic outpatients. Thromb Haemost 1993;70:404.

The Importance of Lipids and Lipoproteins in the Progression and Regression of Atherosclerosis

JEFFREY W. OLIN

EPIDEMIOLOGY OF LIPIDS AND CARDIOVASCULAR DISEASE

There are numerous well-defined cardiovascular risk factors that are important in the pathogenesis of coronary and peripheral vascular arterial disease. Some of these risk factors are immutable, such as age, gender, and genetics. However, most are changeable with lifestyle modification and/or drug therapy. While cigarette smoking, hypertension, central obesity, glucose intolerance, and diabetes mellitus are important in the pathogenesis of atherosclerosis, the focus of this chapter will be on the role that lipids play in the atherosclerotic process. It should be recognized that the cardiovascular risk factors mentioned above act synergistically with lipid abnormalities, thus accelerating the atherosclerotic process. In order to achieve the greatest reduction in cardiovascular disease, all cardiovascular risk factors should be modified[1] (Table 2-1). This is especially important if regression of atherosclerosis is the goal.

In the past, much of the focus on the prevention and treatment of coronary and peripheral vascular disease has been in men. In recent years, there has been increased recognition that atherosclerotic vascular disease is an important cause of morbidity and mortality in women also. Data from the American Heart Association have demonstrated that the leading cause of death in women is coronary heart disease; in fact, all other major causes of death combined do not cause as many deaths as heart disease.

The second adult treatment panel of the National Cholesterol Education Program (NCEP) Expert Panel on the Detection, Evaluation and Treatment of High Blood Cholesterol has now identified females 55 years of age and older or a female of any age with premature menopause without estrogen replacement as being at increased risk for the development of heart or vascular disease. For the first time, this report emphasizes the importance of vascular disease in women and recommends an aggressive approach in those who already have evidence of heart or vascular disease. Several studies have demonstrated that estrogen replacement therapy can have a major impact on reducing coronary heart disease in women[2] (Table 2-2).

Several epidemiologic studies have shown that increased serum total cholesterol level or low-density lipoprotein (LDL) cholesterol level and/or decreased high-density lipoprotein (HDL) cholesterol level are strongly associated with atherosclerotic coronary and peripheral vascular disease. The Framingham Study[3] demonstrated a strong association between total cholesterol levels and cardiovascular disease. The 8-year probability of developing cardiovascular disease was directly related to the total cholesterol level. If other cardiovascular risk factors also were present, the risk was substantially increased. The Framingham Study also has shown that HDL cholesterol is an important predictor of future cardiovascular events. There is a strong inverse

13

Table 2-1. Coronary Heart Disease Risk Factors

Positive
Age, years
   Men ≥ 45
   Women ≥ 55 or premature menopause without estro-
     gen replacement therapy
Family history of premature coronary heart disease
Smoking
Hypertension
HDL cholesterol < 35 mg/dl
Diabetes mellitus
Negative
HDL cholesterol ≥ 60 mg/dl

Source: From NCEP Guidelines II. JAMA 1993;269:3015.

Table 2-2. Prospective Studies of Postmenopausal Estrogen Use and Cardiovascular Disease

Study	Year	No. of Subjects	Age-Adjusted RR
Potocki	1971	158	0.31
Burch	1974	737	0.43
Hammond	1979	610	0.33
Nachtigall	1979	168	0.33
Lafferty	1985	124	0.17
Stampfer	1985	33,317	0.3
Wilson	1985	1,234	1.94
Bush	1987	2,270	0.34
Pettitti	1987	6,093	0.9
Hunt	1987	4,544	0.48
Criqui	1988	1,868	0.75
Henderson	1988	8,807	0.47
Avila	1990	24,900	0.7
Sullivan	1990	2,268	0.16
Stampfer	1991	48,470	0.56

Source: From Kuhn FE, Rackley CE: Coronary artery disease in women: Risk factors, evaluation, treatment, and prevention. Arch Intern Med 1993;153:2626, with permission.

relationship between the level of HDL cholesterol and the development of coro- nary heart disease[4] (Figure 2-1). Those with HDL cholesterol levels less than 35 mg/dl were at the greatest risk. While men generally have lower HDL cholesterol levels than women, women with HDL cholesterol levels less than 35 mg/dl appear to be at higher risk than their male counterparts.[4] It has been suggested that HDL cholesterol may be the most important lipoprotein fraction predicting future cardiovascular

mortality or morbidity. To date, there have been no trials to assess the role of raising HDL cholesterol as a sole therapeutic measure in preventing heart or vascular disease. There are no currently available drugs which selectively increase HDL cholesterol. Those agents which do increase HDL cholesterol (nicotinic acid, gemfibrozil, and to a lesser extent, HMG Co-A reductase inhibitors) also cause decreases in triglycerides and/or LDL cholesterol. There is evidence that lowering LDL cholesterol in association with raising HDL cholesterol causes a greater reduction in coronary heart disease mortality than lowering LDL cholesterol alone.[5] It also has been shown that significant regression of atherosclerosis may occur when the LDL cholesterol level is lowered in association with a raised HDL cholesterol level.[6,7]

The Multiple Risk Factor Intervention Trial (MRFIT) is one of the largest trials to date showing a correlation between total cholesterol level and cardiovascular disease[8] (Table 2-3). More than 350,000 middle-aged men with no prior history of cardiovascular disease were screened for this study. The follow-up period was 6 years. MRFIT showed that the risk of developing coronary heart disease was continuous and graded and based on the total cholesterol level (see Table 2-3). The lowest risk was present in patients with a total cholesterol level less than 181 mg/dl and increased as the total cholesterol level increased. In the group of patients with total cholesterol values of 245 mg/dl or

Table 2-3. Multiple Risk Factor Intervention Trial: Six-Year Coronary Mortality Rate

Quintile	Serum Cholesterol Level [mg/dl (mmol/liter)]	CHD Mortality		
		No. of Deaths	Rate per 1000	Relative Risk
1	≤ 181 (≤ 4.68)	196	3.2	1.00
2	182–202 (4.71–5.22)	288	4.2	1.29
3	203–220 (5.25–5.69)	395	5.6	1.73
4	221–244 (5.72–6.31)	533	7.1	2.21
5	≥ 245 (≥ 6.34)	846	11.1	3.42

Source: From Stamler J, Wentworth D, Neaton J: Is the relationship between serum cholesterol and risk of premature death from coronary heart disease continuous and graded? Findings in 356,222 primary screenees of the Multiple Risk Factor Intervention Trial (MRFIT). JAMA 1986;256:2823, with permission.

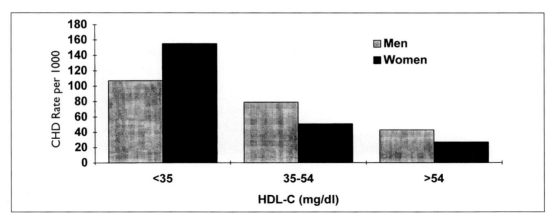

Figure 2-1. Risk of coronary heart disease based on HDL cholesterol and gender (The Framingham Study). (From Gordon T, Castelli WP, Hjortland MC, et al: High-density lipoprotein as a protective factor against coronary heart disease: The Framingham Study. Am J Med 1977;62:707 with permission.

greater, the relative risk of developing coronary heart disease was 3.42, or 11.1 cases per 1000. The development of stroke also was strongly associated with total cholesterol levels.[9]

These as well as other epidemiologic studies leave little doubt that cholesterol and various lipoproteins play an important role in cardiovascular morbidity and mortality. There are several epidemiologic reports with smaller numbers of patients that do show that cholesterol is an important predictor of cardiovascular morbidity and mortality in women as well.

Wong and associates[10] have shown that the total cholesterol level is also important in predicting reinfarction after a first myocardial infarction. This risk is more pronounced in women compared with men (Figure 2-2).

CARDIOVASCULAR RISK REDUCTION ASSOCIATED WITH CHOLESTEROL LOWERING

The Coronary Drug Project was conducted between 1966 and 1975 and assessed the efficacy of lipid-lowering drugs in 8341 men age 30 to 64 years with an electrocardiogram-documented previous myocardial infarction.[11,12] Thyroid hormone, clofibrate, and conjugated estrogens were not effective when compared with placebo in the secondary prevention of myocardial infarction.

Those patients treated with nicotinic acid demonstrated a decreased incidence of nonfatal recurrent myocardial infarction. All-cause mortality in the placebo group over a 15-year period of follow-up was 58.2 percent versus 52 percent in the group treated with niacin, representing an 11 percent lower mortality in the actively drug-treated group ($p = 0.0004$). This beneficial effect on nonfatal myocardial infarction and all-cause mortality was not present when the Coronary Drug Project formally ended after 6 years of active study. However, 9 years later, or 15 years after initiation of the study, a statistically significant benefit with niacin therapy was noted. The exact reasons for this late benefit are unclear, but it has been suggested that the drug either prevented mild, nonthreatening myocardial infarction early or reduced the progression of coronary atherosclerosis during the period of niacin administration.

While the Coronary Drug Project was a secondary prevention trial, several recently completed primary prevention trials have been reported.[5,13–15] The Lipid Research Clinics Coronary Primary Prevention Trial (LRC-CPPT)[13–15] was a randomized, placebo-controlled, double-blind multicenter trial testing the effectiveness of the bile acid sequestrant cholestyramine in preventing the development of coronary heart disease. All patients followed a low-cholesterol, low-saturated-fat diet and were randomized to placebo ($n = 1900$) or therapy with cholestyramine ($n = 1906$). Patients were followed from 7

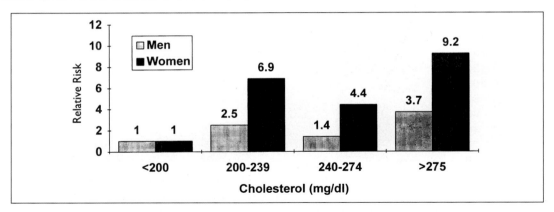

Figure 2-2. Long-term risk for reinfarction after myocardial infarction by cholesterol level using multivariate analysis. (From Wong ND, Wilson PWF, Kannel WB: Serum cholesterol as a prognostic factor after myocardial infarction: The Framingham Study. Ann Intern Med 1991;115:687 with permission.)

to 10 years, with a mean of 7.4 years. The primary endpoints of definite coronary heart disease, death and nonfatal myocardial infarction, were used. There was a 19 percent reduction in primary endpoints in the cholestyramine-treated group compared with the placebo group ($p < 0.05$). Coronary heart disease and nonfatal myocardial infarction were reduced by 24 and 19 percent, respectively, in the active drug group. Other secondary events such as a 25 percent reduction in the development of positive exercise tests, a 20 percent reduction in angina pectoris, a 21 percent reduction in coronary artery bypass surgery, and a 15 percent reduction in intermittent claudication also were apparent in the cholestyramine group compared with the placebo group. Despite these impressive changes, there was only a modest reduction in the total cholesterol level by today's standards from a mean of 280 to 257 mg/dl. Part of the reason for the absence of a more marked cholesterol-lowering effect is due to noncompliance in the patients treated with cholestyramine. There was, however, no significant difference in all-cause mortality between the two groups. This also has been noted in the Helsinki Heart Study trial.[5]

The Helsinki Heart Study design[5] was virtually identical to that of the LRC-CPPT. This randomized, double-blind, 5-year primary prevention trial compared placebo with gemfibrozil, a fibric acid derivative. A total of 4081 men aged 40 to 55

years were entered into the study. There was a 9 percent reduction in LDL cholesterol level. Again, the total cholesterol level reduction was modest, decreasing from a mean of 270 to 247 mg/dl. However, there was a 10 percent increase in HDL cholesterol. This differentiated the Helsinki Heart Study from the LRC-CPPT in that bile acid resins cause very little increase in HDL cholesterol. Triglyceride levels were reduced by approximately 35 percent in the gemfibrozil treated group. There was a 34 percent reduction in the incidence of fatal and nonfatal myocardial infarctions and cardiac deaths in patients treated with gemfibrozil compared with placebo. Coronary heart disease mortality was decreased by 26 percent. As in the LRC-CPPT, the overall mortality was no different between the two groups, and this was attributable to an increase in unexplained accidental and violent deaths occurring in the drug-treated patients.

REGRESSION OF ATHEROSCLEROSIS

There have been many animal studies over the last 30 to 40 years demonstrating that regression of atherosclerosis is possible with a low-cholesterol, low-saturated-fat diet. In the 1970s and early 1980s, several studies[16,17] showed that regression of atherosclerosis is possible in the human femoral artery with lipid-lowering therapy. The angiographic techniques used in these early regression studies were primitive when compared with the more sophisticated techniques available today.

Most of the recently reported regression studies use quantitative coronary angiography to measure progression and regression of coronary and peripheral atherosclerosis. DeFeyter and colleagues[18] have summarized the value, limitations, and implications of these quantitative angiographic techniques.

Brown et al.[19] have reviewed many of the important regression of atherosclerosis studies (Table 2-4). The cholesterol-lowering atherosclerosis study[6,7] and the familial atherosclerosis treatment study[23] used intensive drug therapy to lower the LDL cholesterol level and raise the HDL cholesterol level. In the Lifestyle Heart Study,[22] intensive lifestyle modification was employed as a means to lower lipid values and decrease coronary heart disease event rates. In the POSCH trial,[21] patients with a previous myocardial infarction were randomized to diet alone or to diet and partial ileal bypass as a means of lowering cholesterol values. There was a 35 percent coronary heart disease event reduction rate as well as more regression of atherosclerosis in the actively treated group compared with the control patients.

A detailed description of every regression study is beyond the scope of this review. However, several of the initial studies are so well performed that they merit a more detailed discussion.

Blankenhorn et al. showed in the Cholesterol Lowering Atherosclerosis Study[6] that regression was in fact possible with intensive lipid-lowering therapy. They reported on 162 nonsmoking, highly compliant men aged 40 to 59 years who had undergone previous coronary bypass surgery. Patients were randomized to receive a placebo or a combination of colestipol and nicotinic acid. Patients were studied angiographically at the initiation of the study and 2 years after treatment was instituted. There was a 26 percent reduction in total cholesterol level, a 43 percent reduction in LDL cholesterol level, and a 37 percent increase in HDL cholesterol level in patients receiving active drug. There was less progression of atherosclerosis ($p < 0.03$) and more regression of atherosclerosis ($p < 0.03$) in the native coronary arteries of those patients treated with colestipol

and niacin compared with those treated with placebo. In addition, in those patients undergoing coronary artery bypass grafting, there were fewer new lesions and less progression of atherosclerosis in patients receiving active drug compared with placebo ($p < 0.03$). At 2 years, regression of atherosclerosis occurred in 16.2 percent of the patients treated with colestipol-niacin as compared with 2.4 percent of the patients treated with placebo ($p < 0.002$). One-hundred and three of the original 162 subjects were treated for 4 years, and repeat arteriography was performed at that time.[7] A similar degree of lipid lowering was maintained over a 4-year period of time. There were significantly fewer patients in the drug treated group in whom new native coronary lesions developed (14 percent) compared with the placebo group (40 percent) ($p = 0.001$). There were fewer new lesions in the bypass grafts in drug-treated patients (16 percent) compared with those patients treated with placebo (38 percent) ($p < 0.006$). At 4 years, 18 percent of the patients treated with active drug demonstrated regression of native coronary artery lesions compared with only 6 percent in the placebo-treated group ($p < 0.04$).

As opposed to many of the later studies dealing with regression of atherosclerosis, the Blankenhorn et al. study utilized a panel of experts to visually interpret the coronary arteriograms. A consensus opinion was then formed. This method is probably less quantitative than some of the more recent studies using quantitative computer angiography. Nonetheless, the cholesterol-lowering atherosclerosis study was among the first detailed, well-studied cohort of patients demonstrating that regression is possible.

Brown et al.,[23] shortly thereafter, in one of the best studies published to date also showed that regression of coronary atherosclerosis is feasible with intensive lipid-lowering therapy. Computer-assisted quantitative coronary angiography was performed in 120 men with apolipoprotein B levels of 125 mg/dl or greater, and a family history positive for coronary heart disease. All patients received counseling regarding a low-cholesterol, low-saturated-fat diet and were then randomized to one of three groups: placebo (with the addition

Table 2-4. Lipid Lowering and Plaque Regression: Results of 9 Arteriographic Trials

Study	n	Control Regimen	Treatment Regimen	Treatment Response		Years	Control Patients		Treatment Patients		% Event Reduction
				LDL	HDL		Progression (5)	Regression (%)	Progression (%)	Regression (%)	
NHLBI[20]	143	Diet	D+R	−31%	+8%	5	49	7	32	7	33
CLAS I[6]	188	Diet	D+R+N	−43%	+37%	2	61	2	39	16	25
POSCH[21]	838	Diet	D+PIB+R	−42%	+5%	9.7	65	6	37	14	35
Lifestyle[22]	48	Ustal	D+M+E	−37%	−3%	1	32	32	14	41	0 vs. 1
FATS (N + C)[23]	146	Diet±R	D+R+N	−32%	+43%	2.5	46	11	25	39	80
FATS (L + C)[23]			D+R+L	−46%	+15%	2.5	46	11	22	32	70
CLAS II[7]	138	Diet	D+R+N	−40%	+37%	4	83	6	30	18	43
UC-SCOR[24]	97	Usual	D+R+N+L	−39%	+25%	2	41	13	20	33	1 vs. 0
STARS (D)[25]	90	Usual	D	−16%	0	3	46	4	15	38	69
STARS (D+R)[25]			D+R	−36%	−4%	3	46	4	12	33	89
SCRIP[26]	300	Usual	D+(R/N/L/F)+BP+E	−21%	+13%	4	—	10	—	21	50
Heidelberg[27]	113	Usual	D+E	−8%	+3%	11	42	4	20	30	27

Source: From Brown BG, Zhao X, Sacco DE, Albers JJ: Lipid lowering and plaque regression: New insights into prevention of plaque disruption and clinical events in coronary disease. Circulation 1993;87:1781, with permission.

of colestipol if needed) ($n = 46$), lovastatin and colestipol ($n = 38$), or nicotinic acid and colestipol ($n = 36$). Table 2-5 demonstrates the impressive reductions in LDL cholesterol levels, and the increases in HDL cholesterol levels that occurred in the actively treated groups. The LDL cholesterol level was reduced by 7 percent in the placebo-colestipol group, 46 percent in the lovastatin-colestipol group, and 32 percent in the niacin-colestipol group. The HDL cholesterol level was increased 5 percent in the placebo-colestipol group, 15 percent in the lovastatin-colestipol group, and 43 percent in the niacin-colestipol group. Apolipoprotein B levels decreased from 149 to 142 mg/dl in the conventional therapy group, from 159 to 103 mg/dl in the lovastatin-colestipol group, and from 155 to 111 mg/dl in the niacin-colestipol group. There was a marked increase in apolipoprotein A-I level from 132 to 151 mg/dl in the niacin-colestipol group. Regression of atherosclerosis occurred in 11 percent of the placebo group as compared with 32 percent of the lovastatin-colestipol group and 39 percent of the niacin-colestipol group. Both actively treated groups demonstrated significantly more regression ($p < 0.005$) compared with the placebo group. In

addition to arteriographic regression and lack of progression, cardiovascular events were fewer in both the lovastatin-colestipol group and the niacin-colestipol group ($p < 0.005$) compared with the placebo group.

Data from the Monitored Atherosclerosis Regression Study (MARS) were published in 1993.[28] This trial had several features which differentiated it from previously published trials. First, it used a single lipid-lowering therapy (lovastatin) to assess regression. Second, it is the only trial to prospectively evaluate coronary angiographic films by computed quantitative coronary angiographic system, with automated edge-detection algorithms as the primary endpoint methodology and panel-based reading as a secondary endpoint methodology. Lastly, B-mode ultrasound measurements of the distal common carotid artery far-wall intimal medial thickness (IMT) were an additional endpoint. For lesions greater than 50 percent stenotic at baseline, there was a mean decrease of -4.1 percent stenosis in the lovastatin group compared with the placebo group, which had an increase of 0.9 percent ($p = 0.005$). Progression occurred in fewer lovastatin subjects (29 percent) compared with placebo

Table 2-5. Familial Atherosclerosis Treatment Study (FATS)

	Placebo ± Colestipol ($n = 46$)	Lovastatin ± Colestipol ($n = 38$)	Niacin ± Colestipol ($n = 36$)
Total cholesterol (mg/dl)			
Baseline	262	275	270
During treatment	253	182*	209*
% change	−3%	−34%	−23%
LDL cholesterol			
Baseline	175	196	190
During treatment	162†	107*	129*
% change	−7%	−46%	−32%
HDL cholesterol			
Baseline	38	35	39
During treatment	40†	41‡	55
% change	+5%	+15%	+43%
Progression of atherosclerosis (no.)	21	8	9
Regression of atherosclerosis (no.)	5	12†	14†
Cardiovascular events (no.)	11	3†	2†

*$p < 0.001$.
†$p < 0.005$
‡$p < 0.01$.
Source: From Brown BG, Albers JJ, Fisher LD, et al: Regression of coronary artery disease as a result of intensive lipid-lowering therapy in men with high levels of apolipoprotein B. N Engl J Med 1990;323:1289, with permission.

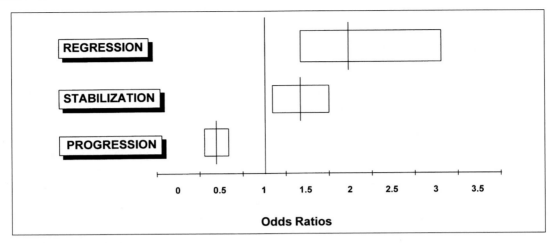

Figure 2-3. Graph showing odds ratios and 95 percent confidence limits for regression, stabilization, and progression comparing 688 treated subjects with 593 control subjects with entrance and exit angiograms derived from seven coronary angiographic trials. (From Blankenhorn DH, Hodis HN: Arterial imaging and atherosclerosis reversal. Artheroscler Thromb 1994;14:177 with permission.)

subjects (41 percent) ($p = 0.07$). Regression occurred twice as frequently in the lovastatin group compared with the placebo group ($p = 0.04$). The MARS trial was one of the few regression studies to have a large number of women. Subgroup analysis showed that the women had better lesion response to lipid-lowering therapy than the men, and estrogen replacement therapy enhanced the response to lipid-lowering therapy. These data are similar to data reported in the UCSF-SCOR study.[24]

Blankenhorn and Hodis[29] performed a meta-analysis using the data from NHLBI type II,[20] CLAS,[6,7] POSCH,[21] UCSF-SCOR,[24] FATS,[23] STARS,[25] and the Lifestyle Heart Trial[22] regarding lipid-lowering therapy in secondary prevention of coronary heart disease. They demonstrated that the odds ratio of achieving regression of atherosclerosis in the actively treated patients ($n = 688$) was 2.0 and progression of atherosclerosis was 0.4 when compared with control subjects ($n = 593$) (Fig. 2-3). Progression of atherosclerosis was much less frequent in the aggressively treated patients. They further analyzed 793 treated patients and 708 control patients from the same angiographic trials and showed that the odds ratios for cardiovascular disease events and revascularizations, cardiovascular disease events alone, and car-

diovascular disease deaths were significantly lower in the aggressively treated patients compared with those patients treated with placebo (Fig. 2-4). The odds ratio for all-cause mortality was reduced but fell short of the 95 percent confidence level.

This meta-analysis confirms what has been reported in individual studies, namely, that aggressive reduction in LDL cholesterol (and at times increases in HDL cholesterol) is an effective form of secondary prevention of coronary heart disease. Regression of atherosclerosis and event reduction have been demonstrated in many studies. The Adult Treatment Panel II of the NCEP now recommends an aggressive approach to the treatment of lipid disturbances in patients with coronary heart or other atherosclerotic vascular disease[1] (Table 2-6).

The exact mechanism by which regression occurs is unknown. It has been suggested that regression may mean a shrinkage of intimal plaque due to a reduction in the components of that plaque, such as lipid components, macrophages, smooth-muscle cells, and connective tissue. Certain components of the plaque, such as calcification and fibrous tissue,[30–32] may make regression less likely. Other possible mechanisms are well outlined by Brown and associates,[19] such as lysis of occlusive thrombi or mural thrombi, healing or

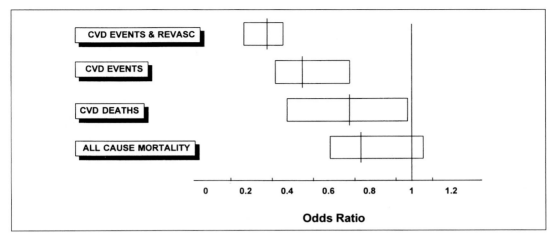

Figure 2-4. Graph showing odds ratios and 95 percent confidence limits for clinical coronary events and all-cause mortality, comparing all 793 treated with 708 control subjects from seven coronary angiographic trials. (From Blankenhorn DH, Hodis HN: Arterial imaging and atherosclerosis reversal. Artheroscler Thromb 1994;14:177 with permission.)

remodeling of an acutely disrupted plaque, physiologic remodeling independent of plaque size, relaxation of arterial vasomotor tone (vasodilator or vasoconstrictor responses), and the role that the endothelium plays in the function of the blood vessel itself. Arteriographically, it is impossible to determine what role each of these pathophysiologic mechanisms may play in the regression of atherosclerosis.

Several recent reports suggest that beneficial clinical effects may occur before actual regression occurs. Benzuly et al.[33] showed that functional improvement preceded structural regression of atherosclerosis. Adult male cynomolgus monkeys were fed an atherogenic diet for 2 years, followed by a normal diet (regression diet) for up to 12 months. The vasoconstrictor response to serotonin infusions returned to normal within several months of starting the normal diet, long before structural improvement occurred in the atherosclerotic vessels.

Gould and associates[34] showed, using dipyridamole positron emission tomographic scanning, that intensive cholesterol lowering over a 90-day period improved myocardial perfusion. This improvement in functional myocardial perfusion occurred before regression of atherosclerosis could be expected to occur.

Recently, there has been extensive literature on the use of noninvasive imaging (B-mode ultra-

sound) of the carotid and other peripheral arteries to serve as a marker of underlying atherosclerosis and to assess whether or not regression of atherosclerosis has occurred. There is epidemiologic evidence showing a strong association between intima-media thickness (IMT) measured by B-mode ultrasound and cardiovascular disease in men and women.[35,36] Data from the CLAS[37,38] have demonstrated that over a 48-month period of follow-up, patients receiving placebo actually showed an increase in intima-media wall thickness compared with a decrease in those patients receiving active drug. The

Table 2-6. Treatment Decisions Based on LDL Cholesterol Level

Patient Category	Initiation Level	LDL Goal
Dietary Therapy		
No CHD, <2 risk factors	≥160	<160
No CHD, >2 risk factors	≥130	<130
CHD	>100	≤100
Drug Therapy		
No CHD, <2 risk factors	≥190	<160
No CHD, >2 risk factors	≥160	<130
CHD	≥130	≤100

Source: From Expert Panel on Detection, Evaluation and Treatment of High Blood Cholesterol in Adults: Summary of the National Report of the National Cholesterol Education Program (NCEP): Expert Panel on Detection, Evaluation and Treatment of High Blood Cholesterol in Adults (Adult Treatment Panel II). JAMA 1993;269:3015, with permission.

intima-media wall thickness in the common carotid artery, as measured by B-mode ultrasound, correlated with the quantitative computed angiographic measurement of carotid atherosclerosis with an r value of 0.702 ($p < 0.001$).

In summary, there is irrefutable evidence that lipids play an important role in coronary heart and other vascular diseases. The Primary and Secondary Prevention Trials have definitively shown that cholesterol-lowering therapy decreases fatal and nonfatal coronary heart events. Over the last decade, a large body of literature has emerged demonstrating that regression of atherosclerosis and event reduction occur in patients who are aggressively treated. Recently, several trials have used noninvasive imaging such as B-mode ultrasound as a marker for underlying atherosclerosis and to determine whether or not early regression of atherosclerosis has occurred. These data should demonstrate to the clinician caring for the patient with coronary and peripheral vascular disease that an aggressive preventive approach is warranted.

REFERENCES

1. Expert Panel on Detection, Evaluation and Treatment of High Blood Cholesterol in Adults: Summary of the National Report of the National Cholesterol Education Program (NCEP). Expert Panel on Detection, Evaluation and Treatment of High Blood Cholesterol in Adults (Adult Treatment Panel II). JAMA 1993;269:3015.
2. Kuhn FE, Rackley CE: Coronary artery disease in women. Risk factors, evaluation, treatment, and prevention. Arch Intern Med 1993;153:2626.
3. Kannel WB, Castelli WP, Gordon T: Cholesterol in the prediction of atherosclerotic disease: New perspectives based on the Framingham Study. Ann Intern Med 1979;90:85.
4. Gordon T, Castelli WP, Hjortland MC, et al: High-density lipoprotein as a protective factor against coronary heart disease: The Framingham Study. Am J Med 1977;62:707.
5. Frick MH, Elo O, Haapa K, et al: Helsinki Heart Study: Primary Prevention Trial with gemfibrozil in middle-aged men with dyslipidemia. N Engl J Med 1987;317:1237.
6. Blankenhorn DH, Nessin SA, Johnson RO, et al: Beneficial effects of combined colestipol-niacin therapy on coronary atherosclerosis and coronary venous bypass grafts. JAMA 1987;257:3233.
7. Cashin-Hemphill L, Mack WJ, Pogoda JM, et al: Beneficial effects of colestipol-niacin on coronary atherosclerosis: A four-year follow-up. JAMA 1990; 264:3103.
8. Stamler J, Wentworth D, Neaton JD: Is the relationship between serum cholesterol and risk of premature death from coronary heart disease continuous and graded? Findings in 356,222 primary screenees of the Multiple Risk Factor Intervention Trial (MRFIT). JAMA 1986;256: 2823.
9. Iso H, Jacobs DR, Wentworth D, et al: Serum cholesterol levels in six-year mortality from stroke and 350,977 screenees for the Multiple Risk Factor Intervention Trial. N Engl J Med 1989;320: 904.
10. Wong ND, Wilson PWF, Kannel WB: Serum cholesterol as a prognostic factor after myocardial infarction: The Framingham Study. Ann Intern Med 1991;115:687.
11. Coronary Drug Project Group. Clofibrate and niacin in coronary heart disease. JAMA 1975;231:360.
12. Canner PL, Berge K, Wenger NK, et al: Fifteen-year mortality in Coronary Drug Project patients: Long-term benefit with niacin. J Am Coll Cardiol 1986;8:1245.
13. Lipid Research Clinics Program: Lipid Research Clinics Primary Prevention Trial results: I. Reduction in incidence of coronary heart disease. JAMA 1984; 251:355.
14. Lipid Research Clinics Primary Prevention Trial results: II. The relationship of reduction and incidence of coronary heart disease to cholesterol lowering. JAMA 1984;251:365.
15. Gordon DJ, Knoke J, Probstfield JL, et al: High-density lipoprotein cholesterol and coronary heart disease in hypercholesterolemic men: The Lipid Research Clinics Coronary Primary Prevention Trial. Circulation 1986;74:1217.
16. Duffield RGM, Lewis B, Miller NE, et al: Treatment of hyperlipidemia retards progression of symptomatic femoral atherosclerosis: A randomized, controlled trial. Lancet 1983;2:639.
17. Barndt R, Blankenhorn DH, Crawford DW, Brooks SH: Regression and progression of early femoral atherosclerosis in treated hyperlipoproteinemic patients. Ann Intern Med 1977;86:1139.
18. de Feyter PJ, Serruys PW, Davies MJ, et al: Quantitative coronary angiography to measure progression and regression of coronary atherosclerosis: Value, limitations and implications for future clinical trials. Circulation 1991;84:412.
19. Brown BG, Zhao X, Sacco DE, Albers JJ: Lipid lowering and plaque regression: New insights into prevention of plaque disruption and clinical events in coronary disease. Circulation 1993;87:1781.
20. Brensike JF, Levy RI, Kelsey SF, et al: Effects of therapy with cholestyramine on progression of coronary arteriosclerosis: Results of the NHLBI

Type II Coronary Intervention Study. Circulation 1984;69:313.

21. Buchwald H, Varco RL, Matts JP, et al: Effect of partial ileal bypass surgery on mortality and morbidity for coronary heart disease in patients with hypercholesterolemia: Report of the Program on Surgical Control of the Hyperlipidemias (POSCH). N Engl J Med 1990;323:946.

22. Ornish D, Brown SE, Scherwitz LW: Can lifestyle changes reverse coronary heart disease? The Lifestyle Heart Trial. Lancet 1990;336:129.

23. Brown BG, Albers JJ, Fisher LD, et al: Regression of coronary artery disease as a result of intensive lipid-lowering therapy in men with high levels of apolipoprotein B. N Engl J Med 1990; 323:1289.

24. Kane JP, Malloy MJ, Ports TA, et al: Regression of coronary atherosclerosis during treatment of familial hypercholesterolemia with combined drug regimens. JAMA 1990;264:3007.

25. Watts GF, Lewis B, Brunt JNH, et al: Effects on coronary artery disease of lipid-lowering diet or diet plus cholestyramine in the St. Thomas Atherosclerosis Regression Study (STARS). Lancet 1992; 339:563.

26. Alderman E, Haskell WL, Fain JM, et al: Beneficial angiographic and clinical response to multifactor modification in the Stanford Coronary Risk Intervention Project (SCRIP) (Abstract). Circulation 1991;84(suppl II):II-140.

27. Schuler G, Hambrecht R, Schlierf G, et al: Regular physical exercise and low-fat diet: Effects on progression of coronary artery disease. Circulation 1992;86:1.

28. Blankenhorn DH, Azen SP, Kramsch DM, et al: Coronary angiographic changes with lovastatin therapy: The Monitored Atherosclerosis Regression Study (MARS): Coronary angiographic changes with lovastatin therapy. Ann Intern Med 1993;119:969.

29. Blankenhorn DH, Hodis HN: Arterial imaging and atherosclerosis reversal. Arterioscler Thromb 1994;14:177.

30. Loscalzo J: Regression of coronary atherosclerosis. N Engl J Med 1990;323:1337.

31. Van Winkle M, Levy L: Further studies on the reversibility of serum sickness cholesterol-induced atherosclerosis. J Exp Med 1970;132:858.

32. Wagner WD, Clarkson TB, Foster J: Contrasting effects of ethane-1-hydroxy-1, 1-diphosphonate (EHDP) on the regression of two types of dietary-induced atherosclerosis. Atherosclerosis 1977; 27:419.

33. Benzuly KH, Padgett RC, Kaul S, et al: Functional improvement proceeds structural regression of atherosclerosis. Circulation 1994;89:1810.

34. Gould KL, Martucci JP, Goldberg DI, et al: Short-term cholesterol lowering decreases size and severity of perfusion abnormalities by positron emission tomography after dipyridamole in patients with coronary artery disease: A potential non-invasive marker of healing coronary endothelium. Circulation 1994;89:1530.

35. Salonen R, Salonen JT: Determinance of carotid intima-media thickness: A population-based ultrasonography study in Eastern Finnish men. J Intern Med 1991;229:225.

36. Bonithon-Kopp C, Scarbin PY, Taquet A, et al: Risk factors for early carotid atherosclerosis in middle-aged French women. Arterioscler Thromb 1991;11:966.

37. Blankenhorn DH, Selzer RH, Crawford DW, et al: Beneficial effects of colestipol-niacin therapy on the common carotid artery. Two- and year-reduction in intima-media thickness measured by ultrasound. Circulation 1993;88:20.

38. Mack WJ, Selzer RH, Hodis HN, et al: One-year reduction and longitudinal analysis of carotid intima-media thickness associated with colestipol/niacin therapy. Stroke 1993;24:1779.

Medical Management of Peripheral Arterial Occlusive Disease

JOHN P. COOKE
ADRIAN O. MA

Peripheral arterial occlusive disease (PAD) affecting the lower extremities is a common problem in the Western Hemisphere and is generally considered a disease of the elderly population, especially of those over age 65. This age group will comprise an increasing proportion of the population in the next four decades, and therefore, the impact of vascular disease affecting these individuals will impose a significant health problem in this country. About 12 percent of the current U.S. population is 65 years of age or older, and this figure will likely to increase to 22 percent by the year 2040.[1] Therefore, the challenge to the medical community is to develop a cost-effective strategy for early detection and management of PAD.

Several diagnostic criteria have been used to define the prevalence of chronic PAD in the general population. Traditionally, investigators used the symptom of intermittent claudication as an indicator of PAD. Using this criterion, the prevalence has been estimated to be approximately 2 percent in all individuals between 40 and 60 years of age and approximately 6 percent in those over age 70.[2,3] Prevalence rates are 1½ to 2 times higher in men than in women. However, the prevalence of the disease as defined by these surveys is almost certainly an underestimate. Approximately two-thirds of patients with angiographically documented stenosis report no symptoms on the Rose questionnaire commonly employed in these epidemiologic surveys. Therefore, use of the Rose questionnaire underestimates the prevalence of PAD. Using noninvasive testing as a "gold standard" for defining PAD, an abnormal posterior tibial pulse has been shown to be the single best discriminator for large-vessel disease affecting the lower extremity.[4] The prevalence of an abnormal posterior tibial pulse is estimated to be between four- and sevenfold higher than the prevalence of PAD estimated by the Rose questionnaire. An accurate predictor of PAD in the lower extremities is the presence of an abnormal ankle-brachial pressure index (ABI), which has been shown to have a sensitivity and specificity of 96 percent or higher when compared with angiography.[1] Based on a disease definition of ABI $\leq$ 0.9, the Edinburgh Artery Study reported a disease prevalence of 17 percent in a population aged between 55 and 74.[5] This figure increased to 25 percent when abnormal reactive hyperemic response also was included.

NATURAL HISTORY

In over 75 percent of patients, symptoms do not progress, and invasive intervention is not required. Medical therapy, including modification of risk factors and treatment of associated conditions, is the mainstay of therapy and is all that is necessary in most patients.[1,2,6–8] About 10 to 20 percent of patients with intermittent claudication will eventually require reconstructive surgery, and 3 to 6 percent will end up with amputation. In contrast, diabetes mellitus adversely affects the 5-year outcome of the claudicant and increases the amputation rate as much as sevenfold.[9] An adverse outcome (tissue loss or amputation) is also predicted by the severity of arterial disease, as determined by the ABI or arteriography at the time of presentation. In addition, patients with femoropopliteal or multilevel disease are at least twice as likely to end up with limb-threatening ischemia than those with isolated aortoiliac disease.

Generally, however, the great majority of patients with claudication will not have progression of their symptoms, tissue loss, or amputation. Although the natural history of PAD is relatively benign, the life expectancy of claudicants is markedly reduced. In fact, the symptom of intermittent claudication is associated with with a doubling of the age-specific risk of death, usually due to significant coronary artery or cerebrovascular disease.[1,6] Some studies have even suggested that intermittent claudication is an additional risk factor for coronary artery disease, independent of the standard risk factors of hypercholesterolemia, diabetes mellitus, tobacco use, and hypertension.[10] These individuals are at three- to sixfold higher risk of cardiovascular mortality when compared with those with similar risk factor profiles without PAD. Furthermore, in a recent prospective study of these patients, the presence of asymptomatic disease as defined by an abnormal ABI was a strong and independent predictor of all-cause and cardiovascular mortality over the ensuing 10 years.[10]

Unfortunately, only a minority of these patients receive appropriate medical care for their condition. Evidence of PAD should elicit a search for disease in other circulations (especially coronary, carotid, and aortic disease). These patients should receive aggressive risk factor modification and antiplatelet therapy to reduce the progression and complications of systemic arterial disease. Finally, an exercise rehabilitation program not only increases pain-free walking distance but also has beneficial effects on serum lipids, neurohormonal activation, blood fluidity, and cardiovascular conditioning.

PATHOPHYSIOLOGY OF PERIPHERAL VASCULAR DISEASE

Atherogenesis

An understanding of the underlying pathophysiology will be essential in the development of new therapeutic strategies for PAD. The most common etiology of PAD is atherosclerosis. The culprit lesion is the complex atheromatous plaque. The evolution of a lesion generally takes decades and is thought to be initiated as a "response to injury" of the endothelium.[11] The specific injuries that precipitate atherogenesis are not known, although risk factors have been identified. One of these is serum cholesterol, specifically the low-density lipoprotein (LDL) fraction. Elevated levels of LDL cholesterol (particularly oxidized LDL) perturb the cell membrane and may alter permeability, thereby facilitating passive entry of lipoprotein particles into the intima. Oxidized or modified LDL cholesterol also increases the adhesiveness of monocytes and endothelial cells, leading to the first observable event in atherogenesis: monocyte adhesion and infiltration into the intima.

Monocyte adhesion appears to be due to the expression by the endothelium of specific glycoprotein adhesion molecules (possibly members of the immunoglobulin superfamily, e.g., vascular cell adhesion molecule, or VCAM-1). The expression of these adhesion molecules may explain the observation that within several days of a high cholesterol diet, monocytes adhere to the endothelium, particularly at intercellular junctions.

Modified LDL cholesterol also induces the expression of monocyte chemotactic protein (MCP-1) and granulocyte colony stimulating factor (GCSF) in endothelial and vascular smooth muscle cells. These proteins are the major chemotactic factors elaborated by endothelial and vascular smooth muscle cells exposed to modified LDL cholesterol. In more advanced plaques with significant necrotic debris, the chemotactic stimulus also may be provided by peptide fragments resulting from the degradation of fibrin, fibronectin, elastin, and collagen.

Under the influence of these chemotactic factors, monocytes migrate into the subendothelial space, where they begin to accumulate lipid and develop into foam cells. Foam cell formation is accelerated by the unregulated uptake of oxidized or modified LDL cholesterol via the scavenger receptor of the macrophage. This receptor, unlike the native LDL receptor, is not down-regulated by the increasing accumulation of cholesterol within the macrophage. The unregulated uptake of modified LDL cholesterol by the scavenger receptor leads to the engorgement of the macrophage with lipid-filled vacuoles, which lends the foam cell its characteristic appearance. Collections of foam cells form the first grossly visible lesion of atherogenesis—the fatty streak. These activated macrophages release mitogens and chemoattractants (including tumor necrosis factor, interleukins, complement factor fragments, platelet-derived growth factor, and monocyte chemotactic protein) that recruit additional macrophages. The accumulation of monocytes in the lesion also may be facilitated by cytokines and lymphokines elaborated by T lymphocytes. A number of laboratories have now demonstrated the existence of T lymphocytes in atheroma; however, their role in atherogenesis is not yet defined. A complex interplay between T lymphocytes and monocytes has been demonstrated in other disease states, and it seems likely that in atherogenesis these cells may modulate monocyte chemotaxis, lipoprotein uptake, and elaboration of growth factors.

As the macrophages accumulate, the overlying endothelium becomes mechanically distorted and chemically altered by the oxidized lipid, oxygen-derived free radicals, and proteases released by the macrophages. Foam cells eventually erode through the endothelial surface, causing microulcerations. Platelets adhere to this thrombogenic surface. In some extreme cases, the thrombotic process initiated by these superficial ulcerations can lead to acute ischemic syndromes. In addition, growth factors and cytokines are elaborated in this milieu, including platelet-derived growth factor (PDGF), platelet activating factor (PAF), and interleukins. These paracrine factors contribute to the next step in atherogenesis—vascular smooth muscle cell proliferation and migration. In a non-diseased vessel of an adult, vascular smooth muscle cells have a "contractile" phenotype and a low index of mitotic activity. Under the influence of cytokines and growth factors released by platelets, macrophages, and injured endothelial cells (and possibly T lymphocytes), a phenotypic alteration from a mature to an immature ("secretory") form occurs. These altered cells proliferate in the media and then migrate to the intima, where they continue to proliferate as well as elaborate large quantities of extracellular matrix. The migration, proliferation, and secretion of these cells transform the lesion into a fibrous plaque. These smooth muscle cells also may accumulate lipid to form foam cells. The extracellular proteins elaborated by the synthetic vascular smooth muscle cells include collagen, elastin, glycoproteins, and glycosaminoglycans. Collagen is the major constituent of the extracellular matrix in an atherosclerotic plaque. Elastin and glycosaminoglycans bind lipoproteins and thereby contribute to lesion growth.

PDGF was the first growth factor to be implicated in the migration and proliferation of vascular smooth muscle cells in atherogenesis and restenosis. This basic protein contains two disulfide-linked polypeptide chains (A and/or B), and one or more of its various isoforms ($PDGF_{AA}$, $_{AB}$, or $_{BB}$) can be released by platelets, macrophages, endothelial cells, and vascular smooth muscle cells under certain conditions. Inhibition of its synthesis or release reduces intimal thickening in animal models of restenosis or atherogenesis. In addition to PDGF, other mitogenic factors produced by altered or infiltrating cells in the vessel wall include interleukins 1 and 6 (IL-1 and IL-6), transforming growth factor beta (TGF-B), fibroblast growth factor, thrombospondin, serotonin, thromboxane A_2, norepinephrine, endothelin, and angiotensin II.

These growth factors and chemotactic proteins lead to the recruitment of more cells, the elaboration of extracellular matrix, and the accumulation of lipid. As the lesion grows, it begins to limit blood flow. With moderate-sized lesions (i.e., occupying ≥ 50 percent of the cross-sectional area of the lumen), ischemia occurs only when the tissue supplied by the vessel requires more blood (i.e., exercise-induced skeletal ischemia, manifested by intermittent claudication). As the lesion enlarges (i.e., 80 to 90 percent of the cross-sectional area), it may limit basal blood flow, causing ischemia at rest (i.e., rest pain).

Macrophages in the enlarging lesion release oxidized lipid, free radicals, elastases, and collagenases that cause cell injury, death, and necrosis. As cellular debris and lipid accumulate, the lesion develops a necrotic core and is transformed into a complex plaque. This is an unstable lesion. The complex plaque is the major cause of acute cardiovascular events (i.e., unstable angina, myocardial infarction, embolic stroke, acute arterial occlusion). Hemorrhage into the plaque (secondary to spontaneous rupture of vasa vasorum supplying the lesion) can cause its rapid expansion to obstruct the lumen. Ulceration of the endothelium or fissuring of the plaque (i.e., due to hemodynamic forces or balloon angioplasty) exposes the highly thrombogenic necrotic core, leading to local thrombosis and/or distal embolization. Thrombus within the plaque fissure and adherent to the lesion may become organized over time and incorporated into the plaque, accelerating its growth. In the vicinity of the thrombus, there is increased local concentration of fibrinogen and thrombin, which contributes to propagation of the thrombus and induces further proliferation of vascular smooth muscle cells within the media and the intimal lesion.

The endothelium is the tissue that lines the intimal surface of the blood vessel. Although it is only one cell layer in thickness, it plays a major role in the regulation of vasomotor tone of the vascular system through the production of endothelium-derived relaxing and contracting factors. One of the earliest known endothelial dysfunctions induced by hypercholesterolemia is a reduction in the release of endothelium-dependent relaxing factor (EDRF).[12] EDRF is a potent endogenous vasodilator which is similar in its action to nitroglycerin. ERDF is now known to be nitric oxide (NO) derived from the enzymatic conversion (by NO synthase) of L-arginine to L-citrulline and NO. NO induces vascular smooth muscle relaxation and inhibits platelet and leukocyte adherence to the vessel wall. These actions appear to be due to the activation of soluble guanylate cyclase by NO, which leads to increased intracellular levels of cyclic GMP. The endothelium is induced to release NO by a wide variety of humoral and hemodynamic stimuli and plays a major role in modulating regional blood flow and systemic resistance.

It is widely recognized that hypercholesterolemia alters vascular reactivity in animal models and in humans; this is largely due to a reduced release of NO, although a contributing factor is altered sensitivity of the vascular smooth muscle to vasoactive substances. This disturbance of vasodilator function occurs long before any of the morphologic changes of atherosclerosis. For example, in young hypercholesterolemic subjects without clinical evidence of atherosclerosis, forearm blood flow in response to intraarterial methacholine (which stimulates the release of NO) is reduced. In addition to its vasodilating and platelet inhibiting properties, NO also serves to maintain balance between growth inhibitory and promoting influences on the vascular smooth muscle and prevents macrophage migration into vessel wall. In the vessel wall of hypercholesterolemic individuals, the activity of NO and prostacyclin is reduced. The consequence of this endothelial dysfunction is increased interaction of the vessel wall with circulating blood elements (platelets, monocytes) and increased proliferation and migration of vascular smooth muscle. Recent work from our laboratory indicates that restoration of NO activity can inhibit progression, and even induce regression, of vascular lesions in animal models of atherogenesis and restenosis.

CELLULAR ADAPTATION IN THE ISCHEMIC MUSCLE

As the arterial stenosis becomes hemodynamically significant, collateral vessel channels are recruited. These collateral vessels are likely derived via the enlargement of extant minute connections or anastomoses of arterial branches with distal vessels. For example, superficial femoral artery occlusions often produce minimal symptoms and may even be asymptomatic. This is due to the rich collaterals of the geniculate arteries which connect the profunda femoris with the popliteal artery. These channels usually provide adequate blood flow to meet the metabolic needs of the resting tissue and often are sufficient to meet moderate increases in skeletal muscle demands. This is not so with more distal popliteal and proximal tibial disease. Here there are often inadequate collateral vessels, and distal disease often causes more severe ischemia with rest pain and tissue loss.

A good exercise program can dramatically increase walking distance in the claudicant. It was long believed that this improvement was due to the development of new collaterals. Although this mechanism may contribute, studies of limb blood flow have demonstrated little, if any, increase in local blood flow capacity despite significantly improved symptoms with exercise training. Evidence now indicates that exercise improves the efficiency of oxidative metabolism in skeletal muscle and that this adaptation at the cellular level accounts for the improvement.[13] The cellular changes induced by exercise are characterized by an increased activity of oxidative enzymes and mitochondrial volume. The higher activity of mitochondrial enzymes allows more complete extraction and utilization of oxygen from the limited amount of blood perfusing the ischemic leg. Similar enzymatic adaptation of the muscle also has been observed in endurance training. Although an increase in myoglobin content, capillary density, or capacity for anaerobic metabolism also can enhance local oxygen transport, these adaptive changes have not been found uniformly in the ischemic limb muscle.

MICROCIRCULATORY DISTURBANCES IN ISCHEMIA

Vessels of the microcirculation are the conduits that are responsible for the local delivery and transfer of cell substrates and metabolites. Normally, blood flow in the microcirculation is maintained by the endothelium, by metabolic and myogenic autoregulation, as well as by neurohormonal activation.[14] Under the conditions of hypoperfusion and tissue hypoxia, there is initial compensatory vasodilation, largely mediated by local skeletal muscle metabolites such as adenosine. With sustained ischemia, a number of pathophysiologic alterations occur that tend to reverse this vasodilation. Increased permeability of the endothelial cells and vascular smooth muscle occurs, and this cellular edema can further impair oxygen and nutrient transfer. Local activation of clotting factors and complement occurs. This abnormality, together with the reduced shear stress, promotes platelet aggregation and neutrophil adherence to the vessel wall. Release of oxygen-derived free radicals from the activated neutrophils causes further cellular injury. Red cell deformability is of particular importance for the flow properties of blood in the microcirculation. An impairment of red cell membrane flexibility, mediated by reduced intracellular ATP availability, will increase blood flow viscosity in the microcirculation and leads to pathologic aggregation. These alterations initiate a vicious positive feedback cycle of flow retardation, enhanced aggregation, increased viscosity, and further reduction in flow until permanent stasis emerges, resulting in microcirculatory occlusive disease.

CLINICAL EVALUATION

History

Chronic PAD is clinically manifested by intermittent claudication and, when severe, can cause rest pain, ischemic ulceration, or gangrene. It is important to emphasize that many patients with PAD experience no symptoms whatsoever. In patients with symptomatic disease, about 70 percent complain of intermittent claudication only, whereas the remainder present with ischemic rest pain, cutaneous ulceration, or frank gangrene. In its mildest form, intermittent claudication is commonly described as cramping or fatigue of the leg with walking. Occasionally, this pain is limited to cramping in the foot (as with isolated infrapopliteal arterial disease). Most often, however, symptoms involve the calf (with stenosis of the superficial femoral artery) and may even involve the thigh and buttocks (as with iliofemoral arterial disease). Severe claudication of the buttock and thigh from aortoiliac disease is frequently associated with erectile impotence in men (Leriche syndrome). In any patient, the pain is reproducible after walking a certain distance; symptoms are exacerbated by walking uphill, by carrying additional weight, or by increasing the pace. The pain abates when the patient simply stands still. This is in contrast to the leg pain induced by lumbar spinal stenosis, also known as *pseudoclaudication*. The aching discomfort of pseudoclaudication mimics that of intermittent claudication, but relief can be obtained only by sitting down or leaning against a support. These patients often have low back pain or a history of back trauma and may have some manifestations of neurologic damage (parasthesias or broad-based gait).

Venous claudication may be mistaken for true arterial claudication. The pain is characterized by a sensation of bursting, tightening, or heaviness and is caused by occlusion of proximal (iliofemoral) venous channels. At rest, collateral venous networks permit venous outflow to match arterial inflow without development of high venous pressure. However, the substantial increase in arterial flow during exercise outstrips venous outflow. This can lead to striking increases in venous and tissue pressure, thereby limiting microvascular nutrient flow. These patients can be differentiated from patients with arterial insufficiency because they often have a history of deep-vein thrombosis, and examination reveals stigmata of deep-vein insufficiency.

As PAD progresses, the patient becomes increasingly limited. It is important to gauge the effects of the disease on lifestyle, because this will affect the choice of therapeutic options. A 60-year-old mail carrier may feel significantly limited by three-block claudication, whereas an 80-year-old retiree may feel unencumbered by claudication occurring at 100 yards. One would be more inclined to pursue angiography and intervention in the former patient than in the latter. The indication for more aggressive intervention becomes clear when the patient presents with rest pain or tissue loss. Generally, these patients undergo angiography and revascularization if possible. Rest pain may be described as a severe ache (similar in quality to toothache) or numbness, which may be associated with intermittent episodes of lancinating pain and is often worse at night. The pain diffusely involves the foot, often distal to the metatarsal level. These patients obtain partial relief by placing the legs in a dependent position. Elevation and reduced ambient temperature increase the severity of rest pain. Severe nocturnal foot pain is often accompanied by ischemic ulceration. Common sites for the ulcer are in the heel, toes, fingers, or feet and less likely in the pretibial area. Skin ulceration often occurs as a result of minor trauma. Lesions fail to heal because the increased metabolic demand of healing tissue cannot be met by the reduced blood supply.

It is important to determine whether there are symptoms reflecting arterial disease in other circulations (i.e., coronary or carotid), and a careful review of systems often elicits symptoms of myocardial or cerebrovascular ischemia. One also should search for risk factors predisposing to PAD, such as tobacco use, hyperlipidemia, hypertension, diabetes mellitus, and family history. Approximately 75 percent of these patients use tobacco; those who do not generally have disorders of lipid or carbohydrate metabolism. In patients without obvious risk factors for atherosclerosis, less common causes of chronic arterial occlusive disease should be considered: vasculitides, disorders of coagulation, homocystinemia, popliteal entrapment, and less well characterized lipid disorders such as elevated levels of Lp(a) liproprotein.

Physical Examination

The physical examination includes an evaluation for disease in other arterial circulations as well as associated conditions predisposing to atherosclerosis. Blood pressure should be taken in both arms to detect evidence of subclavian stenosis; a pressure difference of more than 20 mmHg confirms the diagnosis. In cases of occlusion of the origin of the subclavian artery, the pulse of the ipsilateral radial artery may be delayed compared with that of the contralateral vessel. When asked, a minority of these patients describe claudication of the upper extremity with use. Most patients are asymptomatic, but subclavian stenosis is a worrisome finding because of its frequent association with significant carotid artery disease.

"Cigarette-paper facies" (fine diffuse wrinkling of the facial skin) and staining of the teeth and fingers are common stigmata in this patient population. Xanthelasmas and xanthomas are specific but not sensitive indicators of hypercholesterolemia. Examination of the fundi may reveal "copper wiring" and arteriovenous nicking characteristic of patients with hypertension and diffuse atherosclerosis or may reveal the retinopathy of diabetes. The carotid arteries are always auscultated before palpation to avoid compromising a high-grade stenosis. A clue to the latter condition is a bruit extending into diastole; this finding indicates a hemodynamically significant lesion (75 percent or greater luminal obstruction).

An increased anteroposterior diameter of the chest and reduced breath sounds denote chronic obstructive pulmonary disease (COPD), which is not uncommon in this group and may warrant further evaluation with spirometry for patients in whom vascular surgery is considered. Another common auscultatory finding in these patients is a fourth heart sound, reflecting diastolic dysfunction, usually due to long-standing hypertension. A third heart sound denotes more significant ventricular dysfunction, as with ischemic cardiomyopathy. The abdomen is always auscultated for the presence of bruits that may signify aortoiliac, mesenteric, or renal artery occlusive disease. The astute examiner will carefully palpate the abdomen for the presence of an aortic aneurysm. Most often these are palpated in retrospect after their incidental detection on a radiologic study for another condition, but careful examination should reveal these earlier. Occasionally, patients' obesity may preclude palpation of the aortic aneurysm, and in such patients, computed tomography (CT) or ultrasound examination of the abdomen should be performed, especially if the patients are at increased risk for aneurysm (if they are hypertensive or hyperlipidemic or have a family history of aneurysms).

Careful palpation of the pulses may disclose much information. An irregular pulse may provide a clue to the origin of a peripheral arterial embolism; most of these cases occur in elderly patients with atrial fibrillation. The attenuation or absence of a peripheral pulse often establishes the level of significant disease. Although repeatability and interobserver agreement are low, sensitivity and positive predictive value are moderate for detecting lower extremity arterial disease. A reduced femoral pulse (often with a bruit) denotes aortoiliac occlusive disease. A popliteal pulse cannot be obtained in patients with superficial femoral arterial occlusion. One should carefully palpate the popliteal region so as not to miss the opportunity of detecting a popliteal aneurysm; these aneurysms have a tendency to thrombose, often with drastic sequelae. Furthermore, 50 percent of these patients also have an abdominal aortic aneurysm. Absence of the dorsalis pedis pulse, when bilateral, may be an anatomic variant in up to 12 percent of normal individuals. By contrast, absence of the posterior tibial pulses is always an indication of peripheral arterial occlusive process. An occasional patient has no pulses in the lower extremities but admits to only mild claudication. These patients almost always have an aortic occlusion and have developed a rich supply of collaterals circumventing the obstruction. Conversely, an occasional patient may complain of intermittent claudication but have a normal arterial examination at rest. These patients should be asked to walk to the point of claudication (e.g., walk up and down stairs) and then are reexamined. Many will now demonstrate a reduction in ankle pulses (or pressure); they have an isolated iliac artery stenosis and are often good candidates for balloon angioplasty.

The hand-held Doppler probe is a very useful tool in the office. The probe is placed over the artery to be examined, and the quality of the signal is evaluated. In normal young individuals, the signal will be strong and clearly biphasic (and in some cases triphasic); with progression of atherosclerosis, the signal becomes less biphasic and eventually monophasic. With severe arterial occlusive disease, the signal is faint and monophasic or absent entirely. To further quantitate the severity of arterial occlusive disease, one may obtain an ankle-brachial pressure index (ABI) test. This is done by obtaining simultaneous ankle and brachial systolic blood pressures and expressing these as a ratio. To obtain the ankle pressure, one simply places the blood pressure cuff above the malleoli, positions the Doppler probe over the dorsalis pedis or posterior tibial artery, and inflates the cuff to suprasystolic pressures. Upon deflation of the cuff, the pressure at which the signal returns is the ankle pressure. The ABI is useful in quantitating the severity of the obstruction, as well as in following patients in the long term (Table 3-1). However, in a subset of patients the ABI is not helpful owing to arterial calcification. Elderly patients and those

Table 3-1. Ankle-Brachial Index (ABI)

ABI*	Condition
1.0–1.2	Normal
≤ 0.85	Mild
≤ 0.70	Moderate
≤ 0.50	Severe

*Pressures obtained with the patient at rest. In the elderly and diabetic patient, pressures at the ankle may be artifactually elevated due to arterial calcification.

with diabetes often have substantial calcification of the infrapopliteal vessels. These vessels are resistant to compression by the blood pressure cuff, and the systolic pressures obtained are artifactually elevated. If the ankle systolic pressure is 75 mmHg or more higher than the arm systolic pressure and/or the ABI is greater than 1.3, arterial wall calcification is virtually certain.[15] In these patients there is a discordance between ankle pressures and other clinical clues regarding tissue perfusion (i.e., elevation pallor, dependent rubor, and nutritive changes secondary to ischemia). Pulse volume recordings will be markedly reduced.

Elevation pallor is detected by raising the extremity to an angle of 45 degrees and observing the digits. Pallor occuring within 60 seconds denotes mild ischemia; within 30 seconds, moderate ischemia; and within 15 seconds, severe ischemia. If pallor is noted at rest, the extremity is in jeopardy. Subsequently, the lower extremities are placed in a dependent position, the venous filling time is determined, and the patient is observed for dependent rubor. Normally, the superficial veins of the foot fill within 10 to 15 seconds with dependency. A filling time of 20 to 30 seconds denotes mild ischemia; 30 to 45 seconds, moderate ischemia; and over 45 seconds, severe ischemia. Dependent rubor is also noted in patients with significant disease. Additional evidence of reduced tissue perfusion may be obtained by observing the capillary refill time. A digit is pinched lightly so that it blanches; in a normal individual, the color will return almost immediately upon release of the digit; conversely, with significant arterial occlusive disease (or vasospasm), the return of normal color (capillary refill) is sluggish.

Nutritive changes are also seen in patients with significant long-standing ischemia. The subcutaneous tissues atrophy, lending a shiny appearance to the skin. Hair loss is evident. With severe ischemia, cutaneous ulcers occur at sites of pressure (the heel, malleoli) and at sites of contact between the digits ("kissing" ulcers). The ischemic ulcer may be differentiated from others because of its location, because it is covered with a thick black eschar, and because the periphery of the ulceration is painful to touch. These ulcers are usually rounded and well circumscribed ("punched out"). If the eschar is removed, the base of the ulcer usually consists of poorly developed grayish granulation tissue and will bleed less than expected with manipulation. Neurotropic ulcers also cluster in the pressure points or calluses but are typically painless and bleed easily with probing. The ulcer crater is deep and surrounded by chronic inflammatory changes. The venous ulcers, which are caused by stasis and high venous pressure from chronic venous insufficiency, are typically located in the medial malleolar area and lower third of the leg and are surrounded by chronic pigmentary changes from hemosiderin deposits. The ulcers are shallow with irregular edges. When exudate is removed, pink well-perfused granulation tissue is seen at the base. Less commonly, systemic vasculitis can produce cutaneous ulcers of the leg, which are extremely painful and appear as multiple punched-out or serpigenous ulcerations, with surrounding erythema and occasionally livedo reticularis (a netlike pattern of cyanosis or hemosiderin deposition). From a therapeutic standpoint, an understanding of the etiology of the ulceration is essential for appropriate management.

One also may detect evidence of a recent atheroembolic event that has precipitated or exacerbated the patient's symptoms. A cyanotic toe or livedo reticularis of the foot, calf, thigh, or buttocks is a clue to significant proximal occlusive or aneurysmal disease (the source of atheroembolism). If these findings are bilateral, the patient has an aortic aneurysm or a severely atherosclerotic, ulcerated ("shaggy") aorta, which is the source of the atheroembolism. If the findings are unilateral, the patient most likely has ruptured plaque of the ipsilateral iliac artery or a popliteal aneurysm which is responsible for the thromboembolic event. Evidence of atheroembolism is an indication for further evaluation and possibly intervention, since these patients may be at risk for recurrent embolic events leading to renal failure, mesenteric insufficiency, or peripheral arterial occlusion. Moreover, they may be at risk for rupture of an aortic aneurysm or thrombosis of a popliteal aneurysm.

LABORATORY STUDIES

The seasoned clinician recognizes arterial occlusive disease of the extremities, and laboratory studies are not necessary for a diagnosis of intermittent claudication, rest pain, or ischemic ucleration. However, noninvasive vascular laboratory studies are helpful in quantitating the severity and progression of the disorder. These tests are also useful in patients in whom spinal stenosis is responsible for a component of their symptoms. In such patients, computed tomography or magnetic resonance imaging of the spine and electromyography help determine the extent to which spinal stenosis is contributing to their disability.

The most commonly utilized noninvasive studies are segmental pressure measurements, pulse volume recordings, and ABIs at rest and after exercise. Segmental pressure measurements are performed by placing blood pressure cuffs at the thigh, above the knee, below the knee, and above the ankle; these allow for detection of systolic pressure gradients at the iliofemoral, superficial femoral, popliteal, and infrapopliteal levels, respectively. A pressure decrement of 15 percent from one level to the next denotes a hemodynamically significant lesion between those levels. These measurements at rest are supplemented by measurements of ankle systolic pressure before and after exercise. Treadmill exercise should include continuous 12-lead electrocardiographic (ECG) recordings to detect evidence of exercise-induced myocardial ischemia. Exercise is discontinued at the point of significant claudication, and supine ankle and brachial systolic blood pressures are taken for calculation of a postexercise ABI. Blood pressure measurements and ECG records are taken every 3 minutes until these values return to baseline. In a normal individual, the ABI is 1.0 to 1.2 at rest and does not change with exercise. In the claudicant, the resting ABI is usually less than 0.85 and drops still further with exercise. In the patient with an isolated iliofemoral lesion, the ABI may be normal at rest but will drop below 0.85 with exercise. Severe claudication is characterized by a marked drop in the ABI, occurring at a low level of exertion and persisting well into the rest period.

As mentioned, systolic pressure measurements and ABI readings may be artifactually elevated owing to arterial calcification in the elderly and in diabetics. Finding of incompressible arteries (i.e., suprasystolic blood pressure > 1.3 times brachial pressure) at the ankle level makes the ABI an inaccurate index of arterial disease. Instead, determination of the toe systolic blood pressure and/or index (TSP/TSPI) permits a more accurate assessment of vascular status in the presence of proximal vessel calcification. Radiographic studies in diabetics have demonstrated that most of the arterial wall calcification occurs proximal to the toe vessels. Two cutoff values of toe systolic pressure measurements are of clinical utility. For screening purposes, a TSPI (toe systolic pressure/brachial pressure index) of greater than 0.60 is normal. In a patient with ischemic ulcer, an absolute toe pressure of less than 30 mmHg indicates that the ulcer is unlikely to heal without some form of revascularization.[15]

Pulse volume recordings (PVRs) are obtained simultaneously with the segmental pressure measurements. With significant arterial occlusive disease, the amplitude of the pulse volume is reduced and its contour altered from a biphasic waveform, with a clearly evident dicrotic notch, to a monophasic waveform. In patients with vascular calcification, PVRs are usually markedly abnormal, and a pulse waveform may not be detectable. This is a valuable, but qualitative, observation. Some laboratories use other diagnostic tools, such as transcutaneous oximetry or laser Doppler spectroscopy, to further quantitate tissue perfusion. The latter is a semiquantitative technique in which a probe affixed to the skin delivers a low-energy infrared laser light to illuminate the underlying cutaneous microcirculation (with a hemispheric sampling volume of approximately 1 mm). The laser light is reflected back to the probe with a Doppler shift in its frequency, which is related to the average velocity of the red cells coursing through the microvasculature. The intensity of the reflected signal is inversely proportional to the volume of red cells in the microvasculature, because the laser light is absorbed by the heme moiety of the red cells. Therefore, an estimate of the red cell volume and velocity can be obtained, allowing for a semiquantitative estimation of microvascular flow. The advantage of this technique is that it exclusively reflects cutaneous blood flow, with a short time constant. A disadvantage is that the sampling volume is small and the measurements are only semiquantitative. The same weaknesses are characteristic of cutaneous oximetry.

Both techniques have been used to determine local cutaneous perfusion at the site of an ulcer, with the goal of predicting whether the ulcer will heal without surgical intervention. However, the predictive value of these tests has been challenged.

Color flow Doppler ultrasonography is used increasingly in the noninvasive vascular laboratory. This technique allows for direct visualization of the major conduit vessels and estimation of the flow through them. This technique is particularly useful in the postoperative assessment and long-term follow-up of saphenous vein bypass grafts in the lower extremity. This technique can be used to detect technical problems (retained valve leaflets, arteriovenous anastomoses, misplaced sutures, and thrombus) that may be repaired before the graft fails. Disadvantages of this technique include its dependence on the skill of the operator and the time required to perform a careful examination.

MANAGEMENT

Understanding of the pathophysiology, natural history, and prognosis of peripheral occlusive arterial disease, as well as judicious use of noninvasive vascular studies, greatly facilitates decision making regarding various treatment options. Importantly, the complete medical regimen should be designed to attain at least one of these four objectives: (1) to improve functional capacity (i.e., walking distance), (2) to prevent acute ischemia and limb loss, (3) to arrest progression or induce regression of atherosclerotic plaques, and (4) to reduce cardiovascular morbidity and mortality.[16] In this regard, the vascular internist is in an excellent position to coordinate the necessary care required to accomplish these objectives in a cost-effective manner with limited and rational use of technology. An increasing number of procedures is being performed for patients with PAD, too often with questionable therapeutic benefit and always with economic impact on health care cost, which should not be ignored. A recently published study conducted in Maryland confirms the sharp increase in procedures for PAD.[17] Between 1979 and 1989, the age-adjusted annual rate of balloon angioplasty for PAD has dramatically increased by 24-fold, and peripheral bypass surgery has doubled

in volume. Despite an increase in these interventions, the annual rate of lower extremity amputation remained unchanged. These data may indicate excessive use of interventional procedures, with a consequent increase in complications. It should be emphasized that interventional therapy for PAD will not improve the patient's life expectancy, which is shortened due to coronary and cerebrovascular disease. Only aggressive medical therapy will reduce the likelihood of future vascular events and mortality in these patients.

Referral for Arteriography and Revascularization

On the other hand, seasoned clinicians recognize when to refer a patient for arteriography and appropriate intervention. Critical ischemia presenting as rest pain, cutaneous ulcerations, or digital gangrene is a well-accepted indication for angiography with a view toward revascularization. If untreated, these patients will eventually sustain tissue loss or require amputation. Therefore, all patients in this category should receive early intervention for limb salvage. In a variable but small number of claudicants, the exercise-induced pain may become incapacitating and prevent them from performing tasks required for their livelihood or from engaging in desired recreational activity. In such cases, a more aggressive approach is also warranted. Absent femoral pulses in claudicants indicate aorto-iliac involvement, with lesions that are often readily amenable to angioplasty or stenting. Above the inguinal ligament, catheter interventions are usually successful in restoring pulsatile flow and have excellent long-term patency. Angioplasty or atherectomy below the inguinal ligament is associated with a high rate of restenosis in the range of 30 to 40 percent in the superficial femoral artery and 40 to 50 percent below the knee.[18] The presence of diabetes, poor runoff, unfavorable lesions (i.e., long-segment occlusions), and severe ischemia adversely affects the outcome of interventions.

Premature PAD

Intermittent claudication is a rare symptom in patients under the age of 40 years.[19] Young claudicants should undergo an aggressive investigation,

tion, since in half the cases a treatable pathology other than atherosclerosis is found. In addition, the long-term prognosis for these young patients may be improved if risk factors can be identified and treated. Premature atherosclerosis remains the most common cause in this age group and is frequently associated with multiple cardiovascular risk factors, especially heavy tobacco smoking. However, other cardiovascular risk factors such as homocystinemia and elevated Lp(a) should be considered. The heterozygote form of homocystinuria is not uncommon and is estimated to be present in 1 to 2 percent of the population.[20] Several reports have shown a strong association between elevated plasma homocystine concentration and peripheral occlusive arterial disease.[21] Homocysteine is generally thought to initiate premature atherosclerosis by damaging endothelial cells. Since elevated levels of homocystinemia can be reduced by folic acid supplementation in the heterozygote condition, young patients with premature atherosclerosis should be screened for this abnormality. Many younger claudicants with premature atherosclerosis have significant lesions in the aortoiliac segments, which are readily treatable by balloon angioplasty. In some surgical series, almost half of patients with this localized lesion are women with a characteristic clinical picture that is often termed *hypoplastic aorta syndrome*.[22]

Buerger's disease (thromboangiitis obliterans) is an occlusive arterial disease that is distinct clinically and pathologically from atherosclerosis. Affected individuals are heavy smokers and usually young males, although the prevalence of the disease in young women is increasing in association with their increased use of tobacco. Most often these patients present with symptoms of digital ischemia, but in more advanced cases they also may have foot claudication. They often have a history of migratory superficial thrombophlebitis. Examination discloses normal pulses in the proximal vessels but evidence of severe digital artery disease. With increasing severity, involvement occurs of the infrapopliteal vessels as well as the radial and ulnar arteries.

More proximal vessels are rarely involved. Arteriography reveals pristine proximal vessels with severe distal disease. Characteristic "corkscrew collaterals" (Martorell's sign) can be seen following the course of occluded infrapopliteal vessels. These vessels represent the dilated and tortuous vasa vasorum of the major named conduits that have enlarged in an attempt to increase tissue perfusion. Histologic examination of an involved artery reveals a nonnecrotizing vasculitis with diffuse round cell infiltrate involving the intima, media, adventitia, and even adjacent nerves. A highly cellular thrombus within the lumen, often containing giant cells, is pathognomonic.

Arterial thromboemboli are frequently potential sources for acute ischemia. However, emboli from cardiac sources or abdominal aorta lesions also may cause chronic ischemia. A less common cause of claudication is in situ thrombosis as a result of the hypercoagulable state seen in antiphospholipid antibody syndrome and protein C and S and antithrombin III deficiencies. Usually these syndromes are manifested by venous thrombosis; when arterial involvement occurs, it is usually distal vessels that are affected. This is also true of the hypercoagulable state that is associated with some neoplasms (usually adenocarcinomas).

Extravascular compression is an unusual cause of claudication, more commonly seen in young individuals. Patients with popliteal artery entrapment sydrome are usually between the ages of 20 and 30. The underlying lesion is an abnormal origin of the gastrocnemius, usually the medial head, which compresses the artery and causes intermittent claudication. Clinical clues to this disease are normal resting ankle pulse, low postexercise ankle pressures, and flattened PVR and reduced pulses with gastrocnemius contraction. If left untreated, the compressed artery may become occluded with thrombus or develop a poststenotic aneurysm. Bilateral arteriography with and without active plantar flexing should disclose the abnormality. Cystic adventitial disease is an uncommon condition in which the lumen of the popliteal artery is compressed by a cyst developing in the media. Onset of claudication is often abrupt and due to cyst rupture and hemorrhage. Arteriography may demonstrate a "scimitar" sign due to compromise of the arterial lumen. Treatment is either surgery or needle aspiration. Other rare causes of claudication in the young are arteritis, fibromuscular dysplasia of the iliac artery, and coarctation of the aorta.

Assessment of Other Circulations

Peripheral occlusive arterial disease is a marker of a similar atherosclerotic process affecting other vascular beds, most importantly the carotid and coronary circulations. Early detection and appropriate treatment may prevent a catastrophic vascular event in these patients. In population-based studies, the prevalence of coronary artery disease and cerebrovascular disease in subjects with intermittent claudication is several-fold greater than that in the general population. Significant and correctable coronary artery disease (> 70 percent stenosis) is found in approximately 60 percent of patients evaluated for elective peripheral arterial surgery.[23] Less than 10 percent of this population have normal coronary arteries. The prevalence of cerebrovascular disease in patients with PAD is not well established. Depending on the criteria used, studies have yielded a wide range of prevalence (from 0.5 to 56 percent).

It is well recognized that coronary artery disease is the leading cause of early and late mortality associated with vascular surgery. However, the optimal strategy of preoperative cardiac assessment of these patients is still debated, and what to do with the information obtained has become increasingly controversial. The methods of risk stratification include clinical indices, exercise stress testing, dipyridamole-thallium scanning, gated blood pool ejection fraction measurement, continous electrocardiographic monitoring for silent ischemia, dobutamine echocardiography, and/or coronary angiography.

The presence of more than three clinical risk factors (age > 70 years, diabetes, angina, Q wave on electrocardiogram, or ventricular arrhythmias), or high scores on the indexes developed by Goldman or Detsky, is associated with higher perioperative cardiac complications. Conversely, patients with none of the clinical risk factors or low scores on these indices are not likely to have perioperative cardiac events. Unfortunately, the largest segment of the claudicant population falls into an intermediate risk profile. These patients can be further stratified by a number of functional tests, including Holter monitoring for silent ischemia or dipyridamole-thallium or dobutamine echocardiography.

Once this information is obtained, it is not clear how it should alter further management.

Many of these patients are referred for angiography and subsequently receive catheter or surgical revascularization before the vascular surgery. It has been argued that subjecting the patient to three procedures (coronary angiography, coronary revascularization, and vascular surgery) after an abnormal noninvasive study may not reduce overall risk compared with the risk of a single vascular procedure (with intensive medical management to reduce myocardial ischemia). Indeed, there is recent evidence that the latter approach reduces adverse perioperative cardiovascular events. Clinical trials are needed to compare the cost-efficacy of these different strategies.[24]

General Measures

Patient compliance can be a significant problem unless time is taken to emphasize the rationale, goals, and importance of the medical treatment. Ischemia limits wound healing and response to infection. Minor trauma that would normally heal may progress to ulceration in the ischemic foot; thus immediate attention to cuts and blisters is critical in proper management. These patients must therefore be advised to protect the ischemic extremity from trauma. Approximately 75 percent of amputations in this patient population result from a nonhealing wound due to preventable trauma (such as poorly fitting shoes, inadvertent injury during clipping of the nails, or a puncture wound incurred while ambulating). Ambling about with bare feet is a luxury these patients can ill afford. Emollients applied twice daily after a bath or shower maintain the skin in a supple and hydrated condition to prevent drying and fissuring, which can create a portal of entry for bacteria. For the same reason, fungal infections should be treated aggressively. In addition, lamb's wool placed between adjacent toes prevents pressure necrosis and "kissing" ulcers.

Reducing the load that the exercising leg muscles must bear can increase walking distance. The symptoms of claudication can be improved markedly in obese patients by weight loss. Modifications in the workplace may allow patients to adjust to their limitations; for example, the heavy tool belt of a maintenance worker may be replaced by a push cart.

Certain medications, such as ergot preparation for migraine, should be avoided in patients with occlusive arterial disease because they may further reduce blood supply by virtue of their vasoconstrictor properties. On the other hand, many well-designed studies have shown clearly that beta blockers do *not* affect walking distance in patients with intermittent claudication.[25] However, Raynaud's phenomenon can be exacerbated by beta blockers, and may necessitate withdrawal of beta-blocker therapy.

Risk-Factor Modification

The use of tobacco is the most prevalent risk factor, with 80 to 90 percent of claudicants acknowledging a history of smoking. In the Framingham Study, heavy smokers had a twofold higher risk of developing claudication compared with nonsmokers with similar risk-factor profiles. The relative risk for female smokers was greater than for males.[3] A conservative medical management strategy can be successful in symptomatic improvement of 85 percent of patients who have ceased smoking, compared with only 20 percent of patients who continue to smoke.[2] The persistent use of tobacco is also a predictor of a poor long-term outcome. In a study from the Mayo Clinic, claudicants who abstained from tobacco did not incur any tissue loss over a 5-year period.[6] Of those who continued to smoke, approximately 10 percent underwent amputation for ischemic gangrene over the same period. Saphenous vein bypass grafts (in the coronary or peripheral circulations) are more likely to fail if the patient continues to smoke. When claudication is due to Buerger's disease, approximately 50 percent of patients who continue to smoke will suffer tissue loss, whereas only 5 percent of those who desist will incur this complication. A simple admonition from the physician will be sufficient stimuli for a minority of patients. A written contract between the physician and the patient, stating that the patient will discontinue the use of tobacco before the next office visit, has been shown to significantly increase the number of patients who abstain. These simple counseling techniques, combined with the use of nicotine patches or gums, produces long-term abstention in 30 percent of patients. This figure can be further increased up to 60 percent with the addition of biofeedback, group therapy sessions, and frequent follow-up by nurse-practitioners.

There is increasing evidence that aggressive reduction of serum cholesterol level can reduce progression, and even induce regression, of atherosclerotic plaque. In an angiographic study, Blankenhorn and Hodis[26] demonstrated that this approach was successful in inducing regression of atherosclerotic disease in the superficial femoral artery. A number of studies have confirmed this work and extended it to the coronary circulation. In patients with diabetes, triglyceride concentration appears to have greater predictive power for both cardiac and peripheral vascular disease than in the general population.[15] Improving glycemic control helps normalize elevated triglyceride concentration in diabetics. Data from the Diabetic Control and Complications Trial (DCCT) suggest that intensive insulin treatment (≥ 3 injections per day or insulin pump therapy) dramatically reduces microvascular complications (retinopathy and nephropathy) by 35 to 45 percent. In addition, when macrovascular (cardiovascular, cerebrovascular, or peripheral vascular) events were examined, there was a trend in the reduction of risk in the intensive insulin treatment group.[27] Because the number of total macrovascular events is small, further studies are necessary to confirm these findings. Hypertension is also a risk factor for atherosclerotic arterial occlusive disease. Treatment of severe hypertension limits its vascular complications (stroke, myocardial infarction). Clinicians have long observed that hypertensive patients are more likely to suffer the ravages of atherosclerosis. It has been postulated that hypertension causes "barotrauma," with resultant endothelial injury or dysfunction. Indeed, reduced endothelium-dependent relaxation has been observed in patients with essential hypertension. Whether this abnormality is secondary to the elevated blood pressure or is the primary cause of hypertension in some individuals is under investigation. In the Framingham Study, hypertension was present in about one-third of claudicants, and as a risk factor, elevated arterial pressure increased the incidence of claudication by 2.5- to 4-fold.[3] No studies have yet been performed to determine whether treatment of hypertension reduces the progression of PAD. Furthermore, hypertension in the patient with claudication should alert the physician to the possibility of renovascular disease. Therefore, if such a patient requires angiographic evaluation of the peripheral vessels, consideration should be given to aortography and possibly selective renal arteriography during the same procedure.

Exercise Rehabilitation

The most potent medical measure in the treatment of claudication is an exercise program.[1,6,16,28,29] Most patients can double their walking distance within 3 months with a daily exercise routine. If they understand that surgery and angioplasty are not curative and are only meant to extend the walking distance, they may choose a more conservative approach, knowing that a significant improvement in walking distance can be expected. More important, regular exercise is associated with lower incidence of overall cardiovascular events and, in the elderly population, better neuromuscular function and joint mobility. In the few controlled clinical trials, the improvement in pain-free walking distance varies from 88 to 190 percent.[28] It has been suggested, among other factors, that duration and intensity of the exercise training may explain the variation. The mechanism for the improved walking distance with exercise training is under investigation. Proposed mechanisms include improved oxidative metabolism in the skeletal muscle of the limb, growth of collateral vessels, and refined walking technique.[6,28] Although an increase in macrovascular blood flow is probably not a dominant factor, regular exercise may enhance hemorrheologic properties, thereby increasing microcirculatory flow, which is influenced by changes in viscosity.

From the available data, an organized, supervised program is generally more effective than a purely home-based program. The usual prescription for walking program is a goal of 30 to 60 minutes, 4 to 5 days weekly, at a pace of 2 mi/h or more. Patients should take breaks for moderately severe pain during the walk. If an indoor machine is used instead, a treadmill is preferable to the nonbearing stationary bicycle or rowing machine for optimal results. Positive results of the exercise program frequently reinforce the patient's compliance for modification of other risk factors. Nevertheless, the majority of controlled studies on exercise training are short term, and the few long-term studies yield conflicting data on the effect of exercise on arterial disease progression. Not surprisingly, compliance with any long-term physical activity regimen can diminish significantly with time; therefore, regular feedback between patient and physician becomes an essential prerequisite for durable success.

Pharmacologic Treatment
ANTIPLATELET TREATMENT

Antiplatelet therapy reduces the thrombotic complications associated with many vascular disorders. It reduces acute closure of saphenous vein bypass grafts and substantially decreases the incidence of acute thrombosis after coronary angioplasty. It also reduces coronary thrombosis and, in the setting of an acute coronary occlusion, can reduce myocardial damage by reducing the time required to restore patency with thrombolytics and by reducing reocclusion. Antiplatelet treatment also appears to reduce progression of PAD, probably by inhibiting the accretion of thrombus. Moreover, the same process that induces unstable angina or an acute myocardial infarction (plaque rupture followed by luminal thrombosis) can exacerbate claudication, precipitate rest pain, or produce an acute occlusion jeopardizing viability of the limb. In addition, platelet aggregation may release vasoactive substances such as serotonin and stimulate local vasospasm. These processes are inhibited by antiplatelet therapy.

Aspirin is the prototypical cyclooxygenase inhibitor that diminishes both prostacyclin production by the endothelium and thromboxane production by platelets. Its latter effect, irreversible for the lifespan of the platelets, is responsible for its antiaggregatory properties. There have been two randomized, placebo-controlled studies of high-dose aspirin (>900 mg/day), with and without dipyridamole, and both suggest a delay in angiographic progression of occlusive arterial disease.[30,31] Neither study, however, was large enough to assess any benefit in reducing the risk of subsequent major vascular ischemic events. In the recent U.S. Physician Heath Study, chronic administration of low-dose aspirin (325 mg on alternate days) to apparently healthy men was shown to reduce the need for peripheral arterial surgery.[32] The minimal dose of aspirin required to have a significant beneficial effect on these processes is not known, but one baby aspirin (81 mg) is probably sufficient. Aspirin alone appears to be as effective as a combination of aspirin and dipyridamole therapy in inhibiting platelet aggregation. Another recently introduced antiplatelet agent, ticlopidine, inhibits platelet aggregation by antagonizing ADP-dependent activation of glycoprotein II_b/III_a receptors. A large Swedish trial in patients with intermittent claudication showed that ticlopidine reduced the risk of stroke, myocardial infarction, or vascular death by about 20 percent. Ticlopidine also was found to improve claudication in a small placebo-controlled study.[33] Nevertheless, ticlopidine is expensive, requires initial monitoring for neutropenia, and has yet no proven superiority over aspirin in reduction of overall ischemic complications. The drug is an excellent alternative for those who cannot tolerate aspirin. Indobufen and suloctidil are antiplatelet agents that also have been shown in small trials to provide an increase in pain-free walking distance, but further clinical studies are required to confirm the benefit.

Eicosapentanoic acid (EPA) and docasahexanoic acid (DHA) are omega3 unsaturated fatty acids and important constituents of marine lipids. The omega3 unsaturated fatty acids compete with arachidonic acid as a substrate for cyclooxygenase. In contrast to arachidonic acid, EPA and DHA are metabolized to an inactive form of thromboxane (TxA_3). However, like arachidonic acid, these substances may be converted to an active form of prostacyclin (PGI_3). Therefore, EPA and DHA shift the balance of cyclooxygenase metabolism from a vasoconstrictor/proaggregatory prostanoid to one with vasodilator/antiaggregatory properties. This may explain the observation that populations consuming large amounts of marine lipids (e.g., Greenland Eskimos) manifest reduced platelet reactivity (i.e., increased bleeding time) and incur less cardiovascular mortality. Experimentally, fish oil reduces the progression of atherosclerosis in animal models and improves endo-

thelial function. These observations have led to the use of fish oils and/or their omega3 fatty acid constituents in the treatment of various vascular diseases. However, the beneficial effects of fish oil appear to be only modest in humans. In addition, large amounts of omega3 fatty acids (approximately 10 g) are required to equal the effect of one aspirin; these large doses are often associated with gastrointestinal side effects. Nevertheless, on the basis of the experimental and epidemiologic data, it seems rational to advise patients to increase the amount of fish in their diet.

HEMORRHEOLOGIC THERAPY

Increased blood viscosity can exacerbate the microcirculatory disturbance that occurs with chronic ischemia. Alterations in membrane fluidity of the red cells and platelets, as well as increased plasma concentration of fibrinogen, are known to increase blood viscosity and resistance to blood flow. Red cell deformability is of particular significance for the flow properties of blood in the microcirculation. The erythrocyte has to change its shape continuously in response to the microvessel geometry in order to travel freely in the capillary bed. An impairment of the deformability will increase viscosity, which can be further aggravated by pathologic aggregation. In PAD, tissue ischemia and hypoxia adversely affect the membrane fluidity of circulating bood cells. Thus the rationale for using a hemorrheologic agent in severe PAD is to restore blood fluidity in the microcirculation and hence improve oxygen delivery to the ischemic tissue.

Pentoxifylline is the only oral hemorrheologic agent approved by U.S. Food and Drug Administration for treatment of intermittent claudication.[34] The drug was discovered in Germany in the 1950s while investigators were searching for vasodilator derivatives of theobromine. However, it became apparent that the drug had no vasodilating property, since it did not change heart rate, arterial blood pressure, or systemic vascular resistance. Pentoxifylline has since been studied extensively, and its rheologic properties have been reported widely. Besides reducing red cell rigidity and aggregation, it lowers fibrinogen concentration and thereby causes a decrease in whole blood viscosity. Some studies also have suggested that the drug stimulates the endothelium to elaborate prostacyclin. Finally, it appears to inhibit leukocyte adherence to the vessel wall.

Pentoxifylline is of modest clinical utility in the treatment of intermittent claudication. In the double-blind, placebo-controlled study conducted by Porter and colleagues,[35] the drug increased the duration of treadmill exercise time by 45 percent, compared with a 23 percent improvement in placebo-treated controls at 24-week follow-up. Much of the improvement (as demonstrated in the placebo group) may have been a training effect as the patients adapted to walking on a treadmill.

In our experience, only a minority of patients gain significant relief with pentoxifylline. If a patient has not noted a significant improvement after 3 months of treatment, we discontinue the drug. In only a few cases have we observed worsening of symptoms after discontinuing treatment. Because of its probable salutory effects on the microcirculation, this drug may have greater utility in patients with ischemic or venous stasis ulcers, in whom there is a disorder of microcirculation characterized by platelet aggregation, leukocyte adherence, and increased viscosity. The recommended dose of pentoxifylline is 400 mg orally three times a day; it is preferably taken with meals to minimize its gastrointestinal side effects.

Ketanserin, a selective antagonist of serotonin receptors (5-hydroxytryptamine-2), has been assessed as therapy for intermittent claudication. In addition to its inhibitory action on serotonin-induced platelet aggregation and vasoconstriction, ketanserin improves hemorrheologic properties, particularly red cell deformability. However, no consistent benefit in claudication has been observed with this drug.

VASODILATOR THERAPY

The use of vasodilators in intermittent claudication has been disappointing. Many clinical trials have been carried out using a variety of vasodilators without any beneficial effect. This lack of effect extends to all classes of vasodilators, including alpha-adrenergic antagonists, beta-adrenergic agonists, calcium channel antagonists, angiotensin converting enzyme inhibitors, and so-called direct-acting vasodilators such as hydralazine. Although numerous other vasodilators such as tolazolin, nicotinyl, alcohol, and cyclandelate have been prescribed for intermittent claudication for many years, there is no evidence that these agents are of any benefit. In fact, deterioration of symptoms due to steal phenomenon has been reported in patients treated with vasodilators. From a pathophysiologic viewpoint, vasodilator therapy is unlikely to improve blood flow further or change the workload on skeletal muscle during exercise because the distal vessels in the resting muscle are already maximally dilated.

ANTIOXIDANT THERAPY

As mentioned, oxidation of low density lipoprotein (LDL) cholesterol is an important factor in the pathogenesis of atherosclerosis. It is believed that the native tissue antioxidant system that protects against naturally occurring free radicals consists of enzymatic (i.e., glutathione reductase) and nonenzymatic systems (i.e., vitamins E, C, and beta-carotene).[36] These enzymes and endogenous antioxidants form a synergistic, multilevel defense system against free radical injury to the vessel wall. Accumulating data from animal experiments, epidemiologic studies, several large prospective cohort studies, and ongoing clinical trials suggest that antioxidant vitamins E, C, and beta-carotene, consumed either in foods or in supplements, inhibit the progression of atherosclerosis and reduce the risk of cardiovascular disease. Currently, a large-scale study of combination antioxidant theraphy in patients with PAD is under way. In this study, the effect of an antioxidant cocktail consisting of vitamin E (400 IU bid), vitamin C (500 mg bid), and beta-carotene (30 mg/day) is being studied. The *French paradox* refers to the observation that despite their consumption of a cholesterol-rich diet, the French have a lower rate of cardiovascular events than other Europeans. This paradox has been attributed to the Gallic love of red wine, which has been reported to have salutory effects on the vascular system. Indeed, red wine contains a number of tannins that have antioxidant properties. Of note is the fact that the tannins are contained in the grape skin and not the pulp. For this reason, most white wine lacks these antioxidant substances.

Antioxidants not only inhibit the oxidation of LDL cholesterol but also protect the activity of endothelium-derived nitric oxide. Nitric oxide is inactivated by oxidized LDL and other oxygen-derived free radicals. Because nitric oxide is a potent vasodilator and inhibitor of atherogenesis, its preservation by antioxidents may be an important mechanism by which these agents exert their beneficial effects.

MEDICAL TREATMENT OF CRITICAL ISCHEMIA

Limb-threatening ischemia manifested as rest pain or an ischemic ulceration occurs when resting blood flow is insufficient to satisfy basal metabolic requirements for nonexercising tissue and is an absolute indication for arteriography.[37] Several parameters obtained by noninvasive tests may aid the decision for early interventions, including amputation. In general, an ABI $\leq$ 0.40 in association with the symptoms described above will require intervention for limb salvage. In the presence of noncompressible vessels, especially in diabetics, the toe systolic blood pressure (TSBP) may provide additional predictive information of wound healing. A TSBP < 20 mmHg is associated with a 30 percent healing rate, compared with a healing rate of 92 percent for a TSBP of $\geq$ 30 mmHg.[15] Similarily, a tissue P_{O_2} < 10 mmHg is generally not compatible with healing. Occasionally, the angiogram reveals that the disease is not correctable surgically or with catheter techniques. Thrombolytic therapy is often used in such cases, but long-term patency is low in patients with compromised runoff. These patients are more likely to be elderly and diabetic. Patients with vasculitis, or with thromboangiitis obliterans, often have noncorrectable distal disease. Most often these patients require an amputation, but about 30 percent of ischemic ulcers will heal with vigorous medical therapy. In acute ischemia caused by thromboembolism or in situ thrombosis, rest pain will usually improve with bed rest, systemic heparinization, and pain control as collateral circulation develops and/or the occlusion recanalizes. Ambulation should be limited, since this reduces perfusion to an area of severe arterial insufficiency. If the ulcer is infected, oral antibiotics are insufficient, and intravenous administration must be used to achieve therapeutic levels locally. Wet-to-dry soaks are used to debride the thick black eschar from these ischemic ulcerations. The foot should be kept protected in a bulky, warm dressing or in a thermal boot (a Rooke boot). Patients should be cautioned not to apply a warming pad to the extremity; because of the markedly reduced blood flow, local thermoregulation is grossly impaired, and the skin is vulnerable to a burn if a heating pad is applied. Surgical sympathectomy should be considered; this often allows healing of a cutaneous ulcer. Ischemic pain must be well controlled with narcotics; pain control also reduces vasoconstriction induced by sympathetic activation.

Effective pharmacologic therapy in the treatment of critical ischemia is still lacking. Vasodilators are ineffective because the metabolites of ischemic tissue have already induced maximal vasodilation. Use of hemorrheologic agents such as pentoxifylline have not yielded consistent benefits. In fact, the rheologic agent ancrod, which decreases fibrinogen concentration and blood viscosity, has not been shown to improve ischemic rest pain. Topical epidermal growth factors appear to have some benefit for venous stasis ulcers, but it is unlikely that they will be applied successfully to ischemic ulceration.

Prostaglandin derivatives have stimulated considerable interest in their use in treatment of critical ischemia.[37,38] These agents have antiaggregatory and cytoprotective effects that may improve the microcirculatory disturbance in these patients. Uncontrolled studies as early as 1973 reported beneficial effects of intraarterial infusion of prostaglandin (PG) E_1 on healing of ischemic ulcers. However, these early prostanoids, PGE_1 and prostacyclin (PGI_2), are difficult to use, since they are unstable and require special preparation and intraarterial administration. In fact, it is possible that the inconsistent effects of these prostanoids in treating rest pain and ischemic ulcer are the result of poor stability of these agents. An analysis of the studies evaluating prostanoids in the treatment of critical ischemia was recently reported in the European Consensus Document on Critical Leg Ischemia. There is substantial experience with stable analogues of prostacyclin which can be infused intravenously. When administered as an intermittent intravenous infusion at 2 ng/kg/minute or less for 2 to 4 weeks, the collective data demonstrated that iloprost reduced rest pain and improved ulcer healing in 40 to 60 percent of patients with critical leg ischemia, including diabetic patients, and delayed amputation in the majority of responding individuals during 6 to 12 months of follow-up.[38] Similar efficacy also has been demonstrated in patients with ulcers due to thromboangiitis obliterans and Raynaud's phenomenon. Objective measurements of blood flow in the affected limb were not substantially affected by iloprost. More trials are needed in the United States to further improve the criteria for patient selection and to determine optimal regimens. Oral and topical forms of these prostanoids are being developed and may overcome the difficulty of lengthy intravenous therapy.

Future Therapeutic Strategies

Pharmacotherapy for vascular disease is expanding, with new agents based on a better understanding of thrombosis, thrombolysis, restenosis, and atherogenesis. Many approaches are being explored to prevent or induce regression of established lesions and hence preserve vascular function. Human trials with antioxidants in PAD are underway. Antiplatelet agents similar to ticlopidine but with fewer side effects may prove to be useful alternatives to aspirin in reducing vascular morbidity and mortality. Results showing that calcium channel blockers (CCBs) preserve endothelial function and retard atherosclerosis in animal models have led to clinical trials to assess the effect of these agents on the progression of atherosclerosis in humans.[39] The INTACT trial and Montreal Heart Institute studies revealed that CCBs of the dihydropyridine class inhibit the formation of new lesions but do not affect the progression of established lesions. Unfortunately, the results of the MIDAS trial, which assessed the antiatherogenic effect of Isradipine on carotid lesions in hypertensive patients, were negative.

The antiatherogenic and platelet antiaggregatory properties of endogenous nitric oxide (NO) are now well appreciated. NO donors such as molsidomine are under investigation for their efficacy in inhibiting vascular lesion formation; a preliminary report indicates that molsidomine reduces angiographically demonstrable restenosis after coronary angioplasty.[40]

For symptoms of claudication, there are several new drugs in clinical development, some of these with novel mechanisms of action. These include agents which enhance skeletal muscle oxidative metabolism, improve collateral flow, or reverse microcirculatory derangements in patients with PAD. For patients with critical ischemia, oral prostanoid analogues are under development. Finally, the novel concept of therapeutic angiogenesis is being explored. Vascular endothelial growth factor (VEGF) is a potent angiogenic factor. In an animal model of limb ischemia, intra-arterial injection of VEGF augmented the development of significant collateral vessels, as demonstrated by angiography and histology, in association with significant hemodynamic improvement.[41]

The era of gene therapy has arrived and, with it, potential new approaches to vascular disease. Gene supplementation has been attempted to improve the lipid profile in patients with familial hypercholesterolemia. These patients lack functioning LDL receptors. Wilson and colleagues[42] genetically engineered hepatocytes derived from liver biopsies of the affected individuals, transfecting these cells with a plasmid construct containing a normal LDL receptor. These engineered cells were injected intravenously into the subjects, where they appear to take up residence in the liver. In these few subjects, cholesterol levels have fallen. It remains to be seen what the long-term efficacy and safety of this approach will be. Other molecular strategies are being investigated at Stanford and other centers using local delivery of antisense or "decoy" oligonucleotides or even plasmid constructs encoding for antiproliferative genes (i.e., NO synthase) to prevent restenosis and atherogenesis. To summarize, there has been significant progress in the past decade in diagnosis and therapeutic modalities for management of peripheral arterial disease. However, the rate of this progress will be exceeded in the next 10 years as the insights gleaned from vascular biology are translated into clinical practice.

REFERENCES

1. Vogt M, Wolfson S, Kuller L: Lower extremity arterial disease and the aging process: A review. J Clin Epidemiol 1992;45:529.
2. Pentecost M, Criqui M, Spies J: Guidelines for peripheral percutaneous transluminal angioplasty of the abdominal aorta and lower extremity vessels. Circulation 1994;89:511.
3. Kannel W, McGee D: Update on some epidemiologic features of intermittent claudication: The Framingham Study. J Am Geriatr Soc 1985; 33:13.
4. Criqui MH, Fronek A, Gabriel S: The sensitivity, specificity, and predictive value of traditional clinical evaluation of peripheral arterial disease: Results from noninvasive testing in a defined population. Circulation 1985;71:516.
5. Fowkes F, Housley E, Prescott R: Edinburgh Artery Study: Prevalence of asymptomatic and symptomatic peripheral arterial disease in the general population. Int J Epidemiol 1991;20:384.
6. Cooke J: Medical management of chronic arterial disease. *In* Cooke J, Frohlich E (eds): Current Management of Hypertensive and Vascular Diseases. St Louis, Mosby–Year Book, 1992, pp 203–208.
7. Coffman J: Intermittent claudication—Be conservative. N Engl J Med 1991;325:577.
8. Hertzer N: The natural history of peripheral vascular disease. Circulation 1991;81(suppl I):I-12.
9. McDaniel M, Cronenwett J: Basic data related to the natural history of intermittent claudication. Ann Vasc Surg 1989;3:273.
10. Criqui M, Langer R, Fronek A, et al: Mortality over a period of 10 years in patients with peripheral arterial disease. N Engl J Med 1992;326:381.
11. Ross R: The pathogenesis of atherosclerosis. N Engl J Med 1986;314:488.
12. Cooke J: Endothelial function and peripheral vascular disease. *In* Spittell J (ed): Contemporary Issues in Peripheral Vascular Disease. Philadelphia, FA Davis, 1992, pp 1–17.
13. Jansson E, Johanson J, Sylvén E, Kaijser L: Calf muscle adaptation in intermittent claudication: Side-differences in muscle metabolic characteristics in patients with unilateral arterial disease. Clin Physiol 1988;8:17.
14. Schönharting M, Musikié P, Müller R: The hemorrheological and antithrombotic potential of pentoxifylline (Trental): A review. Pharmatherapeutica 1988;5:159.
15. Orchard T, Strandness D, et al: Assessment of peripheral vascular disease in diabetes: Report and recommendations of an international workshop. Circulation 1993;88:819.
16. Duprez D, Clement D: Medical treatment of peripheral vascular disease: Good or bad. Eur Heart J 1992;13:149.
17. Tunis S, Bass E, Steinberg E: The use of angioplasty, bypass surgery, and amputation in the management of peripheral vascular disease. N Engl J Med 1991;325:556.
18. Isner JM, Rosenfield K: Redefining the treatment of peripheral artery disease: Role of percutaneous revascularization. Circulation 1993;88:1534.
19. Hallett J Jr, Greenwood L, Robison J: Lower extremity arterial disease in young adults: A systematic approach to early diagnosis. Ann Surg 1985; 202:647.
20. Clarke R, Daly L, Graham I, et al: Hyperhomocysteinemia: An independent risk factor for vascular disease. N Engl J Med 1991;324:1149.
21. Malinow NR, Karg SS, Taylor LM, et al: Prevalence of hyperhomocysteinemia in patients with peripheral arterial occlusive disease. Circulation 1989;79:1180.
22. Brewster D: Clinical and anatomical considerations for surgery in aortoiliac disease and results of surgical treatment. Circulation 1991;83(suppl I):I-42.
23. Wong T, Detsky A: Preoperative cardiac risk assessment for patients having peripheral vascular surgery. Ann Intern Med 1992;116:743.
24. Mason J, Owens D, Hlatky M: The role of coronary angiography and coronary revascularization prior to non-cardiac vascular surgery. In preparation.
25. Thadini U, Whitsett TL: β-adrenergic blockers and intermittent claudication: Time for reappraisal. Arch Intern Med 1991;151:1705.
26. Blankenhorn D, Hodis H: Arterial imaging and atherosclerosis reversal. Arterioscler Thromb 1994; 14:177.
27. The Diabetes Control and Complications Trial Research Group: The effect of intensive treatment of diabetes on the development and progression of long-term complications in insulin-dependent diabetes mellitus. N Engl J Med 1993;329:977.
28. Ernst E, Flalka V: A review of the clinical effectiveness of exercise therapy for intermittent claudication. Arch Intern Med 1993;153:2357.
29. Radack K, Wyderski R: Conservative management of intermittent claudication. Ann Intern Med 1990;113:135.
30. Hess H, Mietaschk A, Deichsel G: Drug-induced inhibition of platelet function delays progression of peripheral occlusive arterial disease. Lancet 1985;1:415.
31. Libretti A, Catalano M: Treatment of claudication with dipyridamole and aspirin. Int J Clin Pharmacol Res 1986;6:59.
32. Goldhaber S, Manson J, Hennekens C, et al: Low-dose aspirin and subsequent peripheral arterial surgery in the Physician's Health Study. Lancet 1922;340:143.

33. Janson L, Bergqvist D, Boberg D, et al: Prevention of myocardial infarction and stroke in patients with intermittent claudication: Effects of ticlopidine. Results from STIMS, the Swedish Ticlopidine Multicentre Study. N Engl J Med 1990;301:962.

34. Cameron H, Walker P, Ramsay L: Drug treatment of intermittent claudication: A critical analysis of the methods and findings of published clinical trials, 1965–1985. Br J Clin Pharmacol 1988;26:569.

35. Porter JM, Cutler BS, Lee BY, et al: Pentoxifylline efficacy in the treatment of intermittent claudication: Multicenter controlled double-blind trial with objective assessment of chronic occlusive arterial disease patients. Am Heart J 1982;104:66.

36. Manson J, Gaziano J, Hennekens C, et al: Antioxidants and cardiovascular disease: A review. J Am Coll Nutr 1993;12:426.

37. European Working Group on Critical Leg Ischemia: Second European consensus document on chronic critical leg ischemia. Circulation 1991; 84(suppl IV):IV-1.

38. Grant S, Goa K: Iloprost: A review. Drugs 1992;43:890.

39. Henry P: Calcium channel blockers and progression of coronary artery disease. Circulation 1990; 82:2251.

40. The ACCORD Study Investigators: Nitric oxide donors reduce restenosis after coronary angioplasty: The ACCORD Study (abstract). J Am Coll Cardiol 1994;23:59A.

41. Takeshita S, Zheng L, Isner J: Therapeutic angiogenesis: A single intra-arterial bolus of vascular endothelial growth factor augments revascularization in a rabbit ischemic hind limb model. J Clin Invest 1994;93:662.

42. Wilson JM, Grossman M: Therapeutic strategies for familial hypercholesterolemia based on somatic gene transfer. Am J Cardiol 1993;72:590.

4

The Hypercoagulable Syndromes

MAGRUDER C. DONALDSON
ANTHONY D. WHITTEMORE

It is convenient to conceptualize hypercoagulability as either (1) primary, with a specific, usually familial abnormality, or (2) secondary, with a more complex, acquired abnormality[1] (Tables 4-1 and 4-2). Secondary hypercoagulability occurs as a physiologic accompaniment of stress and trauma and also plays a prominent role in the pathophysiology of various disease processes. Both venous and arterial thrombotic complications related to hypercoagulability usually occur only in the presence of one or more other predisposing risk factors. Thus, even though patients may have harbored a primary hypercoagulable state since birth, clinical manifestations may not arise for several decades, when other circumstances such as pregnancy, surgery, or vascular disease become operative.

CONGENITAL HYPERCOAGULABLE STATES

Most primary congenital hypercoagulable states result from abnormalities in the proteins that help regulate the thrombotic and fibrinolytic cascades (see Table 4-1). Quantitative deficiency of these proteins is most common, but mutant molecules that are dysfunctional also have been discovered.

Antithrombin III (AT III) is a circulating anticoagulant synthesized in the liver that acts as a cofactor with heparin to bind and deactivate thrombin.[1,2] AT III deficiency is inherited in an autosomal dominant heterozygous pattern and has a prevalence of 1 per 2000 to 5000 in the general population. Homozygous inheritance is apparently incompatible with life. Patients with AT III levels below 60 percent of normal may exhibit resistance to heparin and are at increased risk of significant venous and arterial thromboembolism.[3]

Protein C is a vitamin K–dependent glycoprotein synthesized in the liver.[1,2,4] It is activated by thrombin, with greatly accelerated activation at the vascular intimal surface by the cofactor thrombomodulin. Activated protein C inhibits clot formation by inactivating activated factors V and VIII and may enhance fibrinolysis by inhibiting tissue plasminogen activator inhibitor. It has been found recently that many patients with venous thromboembolism exhibit resistance to activated protein C.[5] Protein S is another vitamin K–dependent protein that functions as a cofactor for the anticoagulant activities of protein C.[6] Patients with autosomal dominant homozygous inheritance of protein C deficiency develop venous thrombotic complications very early in life. Heterozygotes without thrombosis and 25 to 50 percent of normal protein C levels may occur in as many as 1 per 200 to 300 unselected blood donors,[7] with thromboembolism if additional risk factors develop. There are few reported cases of primary arterial thromboembolism related solely to familial protein C or protein S deficiency.[3]

Congenital dysfibrinogenemia has been recognized in which an abnormal fibrinogen molecule forms a fibrin gel that is resistant to normal

Table 4-1. Primary Hypercoagulable States

Antithrombin III deficiency

Protein C, protein S deficiency

Fibrinolytic disorders
  Hypoplasminogenemia
  Abnormal plasminogen
  Plasminogen activator deficiency

Dysfibrinogenemia

Factor XII deficiency

Abnormal platelet reactivity

---

removal by the fibrinolytic system. This abnormality may be detected by a prolonged thrombin time, and 10 percent of affected families suffer thrombotic complications.[8] Plasminogen deficiency or quantitatively normal but dysfunctional plasminogen detectable by immunoelectrophoresis occurs in association with both venous and arterial thromboembolism.[9,10] There is also a rare familial defect in the release of plasminogen activator from vessel walls.[11]

ACQUIRED HYPERCOAGULABILITY

As part of the normal homeostatic response to stress and injury, a stereotypic response follows major surgery, including vascular surgery,[12] with elevated levels of *acute-phase reactants,* which include platelets and leukocytes, as well as various plasma proteins such as fibrinogen, factor VIII, alpha$_1$-antitrypsin, plasminogen activator inhibitor, and antiplasmin. The transient reduction in fibrinolytic capabilities during the acute-phase reaction has been described as "fibrinolytic shutdown."[13] Platelets may become hyperreactive, and AT III, protein C, and protein S deficiencies also frequently follow major surgery or trauma, further shifting the balance toward coagulation.[12]

Enhanced coagulability accompanies a host of pathologic conditions[1,2] (see Table 4-2). Acquired AT III, protein C, and protein S deficiencies may occur because of decreased synthesis associated with severe liver disease and malnutrition and increased loss with the nephrotic syndrome, massive thrombosis, and disseminated intravascular coagulation. Malignancy produces hypercoagulability in association with acute-phase reactants, tissue thromboplastin, fibrinolytic dysfunction, and lu-

pus anticoagulant, as well as by activation of platelets by tumor cells and production of procoagulant proteins by mononuclear and tumor cells. Chemotherapy can enhance coagulation by depression of regulatory protein levels, as, for example, in AT III deficiency caused by L-asparaginase. Hematologic malignancies and myeloproliferative disorders such as polycythemia vera increase viscosity and capillary sludging. Hyperlipidemia and diabetes have been associated with increased sensitivity of platelets to in vitro aggregation reagents. In addition, there is evidence of increased platelet thromboxane, decreased vessel wall prostacyclin, and increased platelet turnover in diabetics.[14]

Immune-mediated secondary acquired hypercoagulability has been recognized more frequently in recent years. Most prominent is the antiphospholipid syndrome (APS), in which a heterogeneous group of autoantibodies interferes with phospholipid-dependent biochemical reactions.[1,2,15–17] Among these reactions are the in vitro coagulation cascades measured by the partial thromboplastin time (PTT) and Russell's viper venom time (RVVT). Prolongation of these assays among a minority of patients with lupus erythematosus led to the term *lupus*

Table 4-2. Secondary Hypercoagulable States

Abnormalities of coagulation and fibrinolysis
  Malnutrition
  Malignancy/chemotherapy
  Nephrotic syndrome
  Consumptive coagulopathy
  Antiphospholipid syndrome
  Pregnancy, use of oral contraceptives
  Trauma/surgery

Abnormalities of platelets
  Myeloproliferative disorders
  Paroxysmal nocturnal hemoglobinuria
  Hyperlipidemia
  Diabetes mellitus
  Heparin-induced platelet activation

Abnormalities of blood vessels and rheology
  Stasis of blood flow
  Hyperviscosity (polycythemia, leukemia, sickle cell disease, cryo/macroglobulinemia)
  Thrombotic thrombocytopenic purpura
  Vasculitis, collagen-vascular diseases
  Homocystinuria
  Chronic peripheral vascular disease
  Vascular trauma
  Artificial surfaces

anticoagulant, broadened more recently to *lupus-like anticoagulant* upon discovery of the larger group of patients with normal PTT and RVVT but with specific anticardiolipin antibodies, present in 40 to 60 percent of patients with lupus. APS is associated with both arterial and venous thrombosis and not with bleeding unless there is a coincident platelet or protein coagulopathy. The mechanism by which APS causes thrombosis is not clear. Though APS may occur with no overt signs of associated illness, it is present in many patients with lupus and other autoimmune or "collagen-vascular" disorders, cancer, and infectious diseases, and antibody levels may parallel waxing and waning of the underlying illness.

Heparin-induced platelet activation (HIPA) is an acquired hypercoagulable state present in about 6 percent of patients exposed to heparin.[18,19] All types of heparin have been implicated. HIPA may be detected after intravenous or subcutaneous exposure and even after infusion of fluids through heparin-coated catheters.[20] Sensitized patients produce antibodies to platelet membrane antigens resulting in enhanced platelet aggregation. Because rapid consumption of platelets results, a relative thrombocytopenia usually, but not always, occurs. Thrombocytopenia occurs as early as 4 days after initiation of daily heparin but may develop on the first day if the patient has had previous heparin exposure. In addition to a falling platelet count, relative resistance to heparin may signal the presence of the antibody. HIPA may become undetectable in as little as 8 days, although it can persist for up to 28 months.[18] This phenomenon is distinct from the more common idiosyncratic thrombocytopenia that occurs in about 15 percent of patients within a few days of exposure and usually resolves without sequelae during continuation of heparin.

HYPERCOAGULABILITY AND VASCULAR SURGERY

Superimposition of hypercoagulability is likely to have a deleterious impact on the success of efforts to revascularize patients with arterial disease. Endovascular injury, hemodynamic fluctuation, and systemic acute-phase responses are part and parcel of percutaneous and surgical therapy. In the immediate postoperative period, anatomic lesions such as intimal scrapes, plaque fractures, flaps, and retained valve leaflets present reactive foci on the lumenal surface. Injudicious choice of inferior, small veins or extremely compromised outflow tracts during bypass introduces unfavorable hemodynamics. In the later postoperative period, intimal hyperplasia and disease progression eventually add to the imbalance toward terminal thrombosis.[21]

Hypercoagulable syndromes have been identified among many young patients with precocious vascular disease. In a study of 20 patients under age 51 with severe leg ischemia, regulatory protein deficiencies or APS were found in 45 percent and platelet hyperaggregability was found in 47 percent of those tested.[22] A study of 51 patients under age 40 identified findings suggesting hypercoagulability in 6 of 8 patients with recurrent unexplained arterial thromboembolism.[23] Defects in the fibrinolytic system have been found in patients with unexplained postoperative graft or spontaneous arterial thrombosis.[24,25]

Congenital or acquired antithrombin III deficiency has been documented in association with unexplained spontaneous or postoperative arterial thrombosis.[26–28] Serial assays have shown a clear correlation between AT III, transferrin, and albumin, varying with the state of nutrition and postoperative protein catabolism. Low AT III levels were found in 48 percent of patients with serum albumin levels less than 3.0 g/dl prior to vascular reconstruction. Early femorodistal bypass failure occurred in 33 percent of patients with low AT III levels and in only 13.4 percent of patients with normal levels.[29]

APS is associated with an increased incidence of spontaneous arterial thromboembolic complications, occurring in patients who are more frequently young, female, and nonsmoking than in the general atherosclerotic population, with a high incidence of early thrombosis after bypass surgery.[16,17,30,31] In a series of 18 vascular and 33 nonvascular surgical procedures in 23 patients with APS, 11 thromboembolic complications occurred in 4 patients. Nine of the

18 vascular procedures were complicated by thrombosis, and only 2 of the 33 nonvascular procedures were complicated. Steroids, aspirin, and anticoagulants appeared to confer protection against thrombosis after vascular procedures in this series.[32]

In a series of 455 in situ saphenous vein grafts, thrombosis within 30 days of surgery occurred in 28 grafts (6.2 percent) due to 37 contributing causes, 8 (22 percent) of which were linked to evidence of hypercoagulability.[21] One failure occurred in a patient with proven HIPA, one with APS, and one with AT III deficiency. The additional 5 patients included 2 with associated systemic malignancy or collagen-vascular disease and 3 with clinical evidence of enhanced platelet reactivity producing the "white-platelet thrombus" phenomenon.

In a preoperative screening program designed to identify hypercoagulable states (Table 4-3), 272 vascular surgical patients underwent preoperative assay for AT III, proteins C and S, plasminogen, APS, and HIPA.[33] Thirty-seven (14 percent) of the 272 patients harbored abnormalities (Table 4-4). Thrombotic complications occurred within 30 days of surgery in 11 (8 percent) of 137 of these patients who subsequently underwent surgical revascularization, consisting of 5 infrainguinal graft thromboses, 2 myocar-

Table 4-4. Hypercoagulable States in 272 General Vascular Patients

Antithrombin III deficiency	3
Protein C deficiency	11
Protein S deficiency	4
Plasminogen abnormality	1
Antiphospholipid syndrome	18
Heparin-induced platelet activation	5

Note: 42 abnormalities in 37 patients (13.6%).

dial infarctions, 3 cerebrovascular events and 1 deep venous thrombosis. Within the group of 137 patients, 3 of 14 patients (27 percent) with documented hypercoagulable conditions sustained graft thrombosis, while only 2 failures (2 percent) occurred among the 123 patients with normal coagulation tests. Among the 3 infrainguinal graft occlusions associated with hypercoagulability, HIPA was present in 2 and APS in the other.

In a larger subsequent study of 185 infrainguinal grafts, preoperative assays were positive for HIPA in 1.7 percent and for APS in 12.4 percent. Graft occlusion occurred within 30 days in 7.0 percent and during late follow-up in 10.3 percent. Preoperative HIPA or APS assays were positive in 23.1 percent of grafts that suffered early occlusion and in only 8.1 percent of patent grafts and were positive among 31.6 percent of grafts that occluded during the entire follow-up period compared with 6.6 percent of patent grafts.

MANAGEMENT OF HYPERCOAGULABILITY

Given the potentially deleterious impact of hypercoagulability on patients with vascular disease, it is worthwhile to attempt to prospectively identify patients who may be at increased risk (Table 4-6). Evaluation should include a careful history and assessment of concurrent illness, focusing on past clotting disorders or the presence of one or more of the conditions listed in Tables 4-1 and 4-2. Patients younger than age 45 should receive particular attention. Routine laboratory evaluation should include prothrombin time, partial thromboplastin time, thrombin time, hematocrit, platelet count, and erythrocyte sedimentation rate, with

Table 4-3. Hypercoagulability Screening Panel

Laboratory Test	Normal Value
Regulatory proteins*	
Antithrombin III	75–120%
Protein C	60–125%
Protein S	60–140%
Plasminogen	80–120%
Antiphospholipid syndrome	
Russell's viper venom time	< 30 s
Anticardiolipin antibody	< 22 IU
Heparin-induced platelet activation	Absent
Prothrombin time	
Activated partial thromboplastin time	
Thrombin time	
Hematocrit, white cell count	
Platelet count	
Erythrocyte sedimentation rate	

*Functional assays with results expressed as percentage of activity in control pooled plasma.

Table 4-5. Therapy of Hypercoagulable States

Fresh-frozen plasma
Regulatory protein deficiencies (AT III, proteins C and S)
Antiplatelet agents
Aspirin—most patients with HIPA; APS with no clinically active other illness
Iloprost—intraoperative infusion with heparin in HIPA
Anticoagulants
Heparin—all conditions except HIPA
Dextran 40—perioperative substitute for heparin in HIPA; adjunct in high-risk circumstances
Ancrod—perioperative substitute for heparin in HIPA
Coumadin—perioperative substitute for heparin in HIPA; long-term therapy for APS with active associated disease; long-term therapy for chronic regulatory protein deficiencies, fibrinolytic abnormalities

Table 4-6. Preoperative Management Strategy

If:
History of—hypercoagulable state (Table 4-1)
          Predisposing illness or condition (Table 4-2)
          Previous unexplained thrombosis
Age less than 45 years
High-risk reconstruction planned
Elevated routine PTT, PT, Hct, WBC, platelets
Diagnosis:
Hypercoagulability panel (Table 4-3)
Therapy:
? Alternatives to interventional therapy
Preoperative aspirin
Agents specific to condition (Table 4-5)

further assays as appropriate to confirm one of the known hypercoagulable syndromes (see Table 4-3).

Evidence supports a policy of routine preoperative screening of all patients with infrainguinal disease for APS and HIPA. APS usually can be detected by a combination of Russell's viper venom time and anticardiolipin antibody. The most common assay for HIPA involves mixing the patient's platelet-poor plasma with pooled platelet-rich plasma in a standard aggregometer and observing aggregation upon addition of heparin. Should HIPA be detected, assay can be repeated testing against patient or donor platelet-rich plasma after acetylation with aspirin to assess drug efficacy in vitro.[34] Since antiplatelet drugs may ablate HIPA, patients with negative HIPA while on antiplatelet agents should continue to be treated until the risk of heparin exposure is over. Some investigators have suggested HIPA testing only if

daily serial platelet counts fall while the patient is under heparin therapy.[19]

Should unexplained thrombosis occur during or soon after vascular intervention, full investigation for the more frequent causes of hypercoagulability is warranted (Table 4-7). Assessments of protein C and protein S are currently recommended despite their apparent infrequent association with arterial thrombosis. Protein C, protein S, and AT III may all be transiently reduced during active thrombosis and in the perioperative period, so assessment should be repeated after recovery before concluding that a chronic deficiency exists. In addition, heparin reduces circulating levels of AT III,[35] and coumadin therapy will reduce proteins C and S because they are vitamin K–dependent. Tests for fibrinolytic inhibitors and platelet hyperreactivity and immunoelectrophoresis to identify patients with abnormal plasminogen subspecies should be reserved for problematic patients in whom the other more common entities are found to be absent.

Optimal therapy of hypercoagulability includes general preventive measures designed to reduce the impact of stress, surgery, and intercurrent illness during the perioperative period. There is some evidence, for example, that epidural anesthesia and postoperative analgesia may reduce coagulability.[36–38] In addition, the importance of gentle, precise surgical technique aimed at protecting intimal surfaces cannot be overemphasized.

Routine preoperative therapy with antiplatelet or anticoagulant drugs is a reasonable strategy, with an acceptably low level of hemorrhagic morbidity as long as other unusual risk factors for

Table 4-7. Postoperative Management Strategy

If no preoperative data and:
Unexpected early thrombosis
Diagnosis:
Exclude technical, hemodynamic cause
Platelet count, HIPA assay
Therapeutic adjuncts to revision:
Aspirin
HIPA likely—alternatives to heparin (Table 4-5)
HIPA unlikely—heparin, dextran
   consider postoperative Coumadin
Confirm hypercoagulable state with postoperative panel (Table 4-3)

bleeding are not present. Many experienced vascular surgeons rely on liberal use of these measures without attempting to vigorously screen patients preoperatively for hypercoagulable states, arguing that screening is imprecise, of low yield, costly, and usually results in institution of the same preventive measures that would have been used in the first place. Our experience would support limited screening, since some patients suffer disastrous thrombotic complications despite broad antithrombotic measures, most particularly in the case of HIPA, in which heparin is contraindicated.

Currently, we recommend routine preventive therapy with 325 mg aspirin daily starting prior to surgery or percutaneous intervention and continued through the indefinite postoperative period. Patients at increased risk for thrombosis because of the need for small-vessel reconstruction in the presence of other risk factors such as malignancy, malnutrition, hyperlipidemia, diabetes, or low-flow vascular prostheses probably also should be treated with intraoperative and postoperative low-molecular-weight dextran (20 ml/h) or heparin (500 to 750 units/h) for a few days, though clear data on efficacy are not yet available.

Should specific hypercoagulable states be suspected or proven preoperatively, consideration should first be given to use of noninterventional strategies to manage the vascular problem. When postponement is not feasible, or when unexpected thrombosis has led to the diagnosis postoperatively, specific therapy to correct the hypercoagulable state must be used (see Table 4-5). Deficiencies in AT III and proteins C and S can be treated easily with replenishment using fresh-frozen plasma at the time of intervention and during early recovery.[28] Abnormalities in fibrinolysis are adequately treated by heparin followed by chronic coumadin anticoagulation.[24] Patients who have active collagen-vascular or other diseases associated with APS may benefit from treatment of the primary illness using steroids, antimetabolites, or other appropriate medications in addition to anticoagulation with heparin followed by long-term coumadin.[32] The presence of APS without an associated active clinical illness probably can be managed adequately with aspirin alone unless extra precautions seem warranted because of the presence of other risk factors for thrombosis.

When HIPA is suspected, heparin should be avoided or promptly stopped while confirmatory testing is performed. If intervention can be postponed, most patients with HIPA will revert to normal within a few months provided they are not reexposed to heparin in any form during the interim.[18] The ill effects of HIPA may be blunted by perioperative aspirin in the majority of patients such that a single dose of heparin during vascular clamping may be possible under aspirin coverage despite the presence of HIPA.[39,40] Alternatively, or if it is possible to demonstrate preoperatively that aspirin will not ablate in vitro platelet aggregation in the presence of heparin, a combination of coumadin started 1 to 3 days preoperatively and intraoperative low-molecular-weight dextran (500 ml) is the most practical alternative to heparin when short clamp times are anticipated.[41] Among other options is the heparinoid ORG 10172, which does not cause platelet aggregation in the presence of antibody.[42] The defibrinating agent ancrod also has been employed successfully as a surgical anticoagulant.[43] Another strategy consists of the use of the prostaglandin analogue iloprost infused intravenously at the time of heparin administration.[34,40,41]

A number of studies have examined the impact of antiplatelet drugs on intermediate and late graft failure without regard to the presence of identifiable hypercoagulable states. No efficacy has been demonstrated for vein graft patency,[44] but there appears to be a small benefit for prosthetic grafts as long as the agents are started preoperatively.[45,46] Most surgeons currently recommend indefinite postoperative aspirin because of the associated reduction in late myocardial events.[44,47] Anticoagulation with coumadin also appears to have a beneficial effect on late patency of both vein grafts and prosthetics, though at the expense of a small but finite number of hemorrhagic complications. For example, a randomized, controlled trial demonstrated a significant improvement in 30-month cumulative graft patency among patients treated with coumadin after vein bypass for critical ischemia.[48] In an uncontrolled series of prosthetic grafts placed in infrageniculate positions, coumadin was associated with 4-year cumulative primary patency of 37 percent, comparing favorably with reports of similar grafts without anticoagulation.[49]

REFERENCES

1. Schafer AI: The hypercoagulable states. Ann Intern Med 1985;102:814.
2. Hart RG, Kanter MC: Hematologic disorders and ischemic stroke: A selective review. Stroke 1990;21:1111.
3. Coller BS, Owen J, Jasty J, et al: Deficiency of plasma protein S, protein C, or antithrombin III and arterial thrombosis. Atherosclerosis 1987;7:456.
4. Clouse LH, Comp PC: The regulation of hemostasis: The protein C system. N Engl J Med 1986;314:1298.
5. Svensson PJ, Dahlback B: Resistance to activated protein C as a basis for venous thrombosis. N Engl J Med 1994;330:517.
6. Engesser L, Broekmans AW, Briet E, et al: Hereditary protein S deficiency: Clinical manifestations. Ann Intern Med 1987;106:677.
7. Miletich J, Sherman L, Broze G: Absence of thrombosis in subjects with heterozygous protein C deficiency. N Engl J Med 1987;317:991.
8. Mammen EF: Congenital coagulation disorders: Dysfibrinogenemia. Semin Thromb Hemost 1983;9:4.
9. Aoki N, Moroi M, Sakata Y, et al: Abnormal plasminogen. A hereditary molecular abnormality found in a patient with recurrent thrombosis. J Clin Invest 1978;61:1186.
10. Soria J, Soria C, Bertrand O, et al: Plasminogen Paris I: Congenital abnormal plasminogen and its incidence in thrombosis. Thromb Res 1983;32:229.
11. Stead NW, Bauer KA, Kinney TR, et al: Venous thrombosis in a family with defective release of vascular plasminogen activator and elevated plasma factor VIII/von Willebrand's factor. Am J Med 1983;74:33.
12. McDaniel MD, Pearce WH, Yao JST, et al: Sequential changes in coagulation and platelet function following femorotibila bypass. J Vasc Surg 1984;1:261.
13. Kluft C, Verheijen JH, Jie AFH, et al: The postoperative fibrinolytic shutdown: A rapidly reverting acute phase pattern for the fast-acting inhibitor of tissue-type plasminogen activator after trauma. Scand J Clin Lab Invest 1985;45:605.
14. Davi G, Catalano I, Averna M, et al: Thromboxane biosynthesis and platelet function in type II diabetes mellitus. N Engl J Med 1990;322:1769.
15. Greenfield LJ: Lupus-like anticoagulants and thrombosis. J Vasc Surg 1988;7:818.
16. Bacharach JM, Lie JT, Homburger HA: The prevalence of vascular occlusive disease associated with antiphospholipid syndromes. Int Angiol 1992;11:51.
17. Asherson RA, Khamashta MA, Gil A, et al: Cerebrovascular disease and antiphospholipid antibodies in systemic lupus erythematosus, lupus-like disease, and the primary antiphospholipid syndrome. Am J Med 1989;86:391.
18. Laster J, Cikrit D, Walker N, et al: The heparin-induced thrombocytopenia syndrome: An update. Surgery 1987;102:763.
19. Kakkasseril JS, Cranley JJ, Panke T, et al: Heparin-induced thrombocytopenia: A prospective study of 142 patients. J Vasc Surg 1985;2:382.
20. Laster J, Silver D: Heparin-coated catheters and heparin-induced thrombocytopenia. J Vasc Surg 1988;7:667.
21. Donaldson MC, Mannick JA, Whittemore AD: Causes of primary graft failure after in situ saphenous vein bypass grafting. J Vasc Surg 1992;15:113.
22. Eldrup-Jorgensen J, Flanigan DP, Brace L, et al: Hypercoagulable states and lower limb ischemia in young adults. J Vasc Surg 1989;9:334.
23. Hallet JW, Greenwood LH, Robison JG: Lower extremity arterial disease in young adults: A systematic approach to early diagnosis. Ann Surg 1985;202:647.
24. Towne JB, Bandyk DF, Hussey CV, et al: Abnormal plasminogen: A genetically determined cause of hypercoagulability. J Vasc Surg 1984;1:896.
25. Towne JB, Hussey CV, Bandyk DF: Abnormalities of the fibrinolytic system as a cause of upper extremity ischemia: A preliminary report. J Vasc Surg 1988;7:661.
26. Shapiro ME, Rodvien R, Bauer KA, et al: Acute aortic thrombosis in antithrombin III deficiency. JAMA 1981;245:1759.
27. Karl R, Garlick I, Zarins C, et al: Surgical implications of antithrombin III deficiency. Surgery 1981;89:429.
28. Towne JB, Bernhard VM, Hussey C, et al: Antithrombin deficiency—A cause of unexplained thrombosis in vascular surgery. Surgery 1981;89:735.
29. Flinn WR, McDaniel MD, Yao JST, et al: Antithrombin III deficiency as a reflection of dynamic protein metabolism in patients undergoing vascular reconstruction. J Vasc Surg 1984;1:888.
30. Baker WH, Potthoff WP, Biller J, et al: Carotid artery thrombosis associated with lupus anticoagulant. Surgery 1985;98:612.
31. Shortell CK, Ouriel K, Green RM, et al: Vascular disease in the antiphospholipid syndrome: A comparison with the patient population with atherosclerosis. J Vasc Surg 1992;15:158.
32. Ahn SS, Kalunian K, Rosove M, et al: Postoperative thombotic complications in patients with the lupus anticoagulant: Increased risk after vascular procedures. J Vasc Surg 1988;7:749.
33. Donaldson MC, Weinberg DS, Belkin M, et al: Screening for hypercoagulable states in vascular surgical practice: A preliminary study. J Vasc Surg 1990;11:825.

34. Kappa JR, Fisher CA, Berkowitz HD, et al: Heparin-induced platlet activation in sixteen surgical patients: Diagnosis and management. J Vasc Surg 1987;5:101.

35. Marciniak E, Gockerman JP: Heparin-induced decrease in circulating antithrombin III. Lancet 1977;2:581.

36. Tuman KJ, McCarthy RJ, March RJ, et al: Effects of epidural anesthesia and analgesia on coagulation and outcome after major vascular surgery. Anesth Analg 1991;73:696.

37. Christopherson R, Besttie C, Frank SM, et al: Perioperative morbidity in patients randomized to epidural or general anesthesia for lower extremity vascular surgery. Anesthesiology 1993; 79:422.

38. Rosenfeld BA, Beattie C, Christopherson R, et al: The effects of different anesthetic regimens on fibrinolysis and the development of postoperative arterial thrombosis. Anesthesiology 1993;79:435.

39. Laster J, Elfrink R, Silver D: Re-exposure to heparin of patients with heparin-associated antibodies. J Vasc Surg 1989;9:677.

40. Kappa JR, Cottrell ED, Berkowitz HD, et al: Carotid endarterectomy in patients with heparin-induced platelet activation: Comparative efficacy of aspirin and iloprost (ZK36374). J Vasc Surg 1987;5:693.

41. Sobel M, Adelman B, Szentpetery S, et al: Surgical management of heparin-associated thrombocytopenia: Strategies in the treatment of venous and arterial thromboembolism. J Vasc Surg 1988;8:395.

42. Makhoul RG, Greenberg CS, McCann RL: Heparin-associated thrombocytopenia and thrombosis: A serious clinical problem and potential solution. J Vasc Surg 1986;4:522.

43. Cole CW, Bormanis J: Ancrod: A practical alternative to heparin. J Vasc Surg 1988;8:59.

44. McCollum C, Alexander C, Kenchington G, et al: Antiplatelet drugs in femoropopliteal vein bypasses: A multicenter trial. J Vasc Surg 1991; 13:150.

45. Green RM, Roedersheimer LR, DeWeese JA: Effects of aspirin and dipyridamole on expanded polytetrafluoroethylene graft patency. Surgery 1982; 92:1016.

46. Clyne CAC, Archer TJ, Atuhaire LK, et al: Random control trial of a short course of aspirin and dipyridamole (Persantine) for femorodistal grafts. Br J Surg 1987;74:246.

47. Steering Committee of the Physicians' Health Study Research Group: Final report on the aspirin component of the ongoing physicians' health study. N Engl J Med 1989;321:129.

48. Kretschmer G, Wenzl E, Piza F, et al: The influence of anticoagulant treatment on the probability of function in femoropopliteal vein bypass surgery: Analysis of a clinical series (1970 to 1985) and interim evaluation of a controlled clinical trial. Surgery 1987;102:453.

49. Flinn WR, Rohrer MJ, Yao JST, et al: Improved long-term patency of infragenicular polytetrafluoroethylene grafts. J Vasc Surg 1988;7:685.

5

Prosthetic Vascular Grafts: Materials and Their Properties

LUKE S. ERDOES
VICTOR M. BERNHARD

Vascular surgery would be quite simple if we could repair any diseased vessel with a replacement graft off the shelf. Unfortunately, the perfect vascular prosthesis does not exist, and we are still plagued by intimal hyperplasia and the need for autogenous conduits. A revolution in vascular surgery began in 1952 when Voorhees and associates[1] demonstrated that fabric grafts could function as an arterial substitute in dogs. Since that time, a huge volume of research and clinical experience has accrued in search of the ideal vascular graft. In this chapter we will attempt to outline the development and evolution of vascular prostheses, discuss the properties of the existing materials, and look to the future to outline modifications of existing materials and touch on new polymers and graft configurations.

An ad hoc committee of the Joint Councils of the Society for Vascular Surgery and the International Society for Cardiovascular Surgery reported on the evaluation and performance standards for arterial prostheses in April of 1993.[2] The ideal prosthesis should have a satisfactory feel and appearance, be clean and sterile, be low in cost, have no need for preclotting, handle well during implantation, be resistant to thrombosis and infection, match the viscoelastic properties of the system in which it is implanted, and prove durable without dilation or breakdown over the life of the recipient.

Nylon, Ivalon, and Orlon were rejected early on due to their loss of tensile strength after implantation. Both Dacron (polyethylene terephthalate) and PTFE (polytetrafluoroethylene, or Teflon) were found to maintain tensile strength in the host, and these polymers have become the standard materials for prostheses employed in contemporary vascular surgery.[3] The properties and configurations of these two materials will be presented, and then the two will be compared.

DACRON PROSTHESES

Dacron yarn contains many small continuous filaments and can be configured in three ways: weaving, knitting, or braiding.[4] Braided Dacron was discarded as a vascular prosthesis due to its bulk and ungainly handling characteristics. Knitted and woven prostheses are available commercially at present. Woven fabric yarn is interlaced in an over-and-under pattern (Fig. 5-1). This results in minimal stretch in any direction and, depending on the tightness of the weave, minimal to virtually no porosity. However, woven fabric has a tendency to fray and unravel and thus may require heat sealing to avoid this problem. By contrast, knitted fabric is made up of threads looped to form a a continuous chain (Fig. 5-2). Knitting imparts a moderate stretch in both length and width (the warp and woof) but mainly diagonally (the bias). Knitted

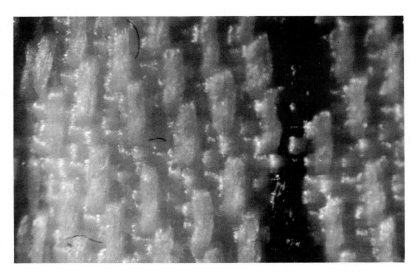

Figure 5-1. Woven Dacron graft showing the over-and-under pattern of the yarn. The black thread is part of the line used for orientation of the graft at the time of implantation (× 25).

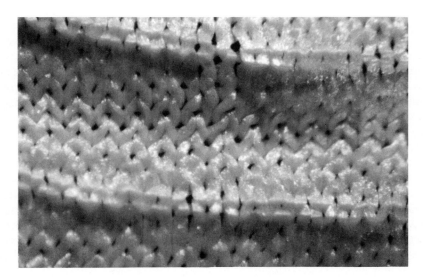

Figure 5-2. Knitted crimped Dacron graft with looped threads forming a pattern of continuous chains (× 20).

material has a much higher porosity than woven material and is also prone to more immediate and long-term dilation.

Some degree of porosity is desirable to allow tissue ingrowth and graft incorporation. The porosity of a vascular prosthesis is defined as the volume of water in milliliters per minute that will pass through a square centimeter of fabric. It has been stated that the ideal porosity of a graft for healing purposes is 10,000 ml/cm^2 per minute.[5] Unfortunately, this results in excessive bleeding, even if the graft is preclotted. Commercially available knitted Dacron grafts have porosities in the range of 1200 to 1900 ml/cm^2 per minute prior to preclotting. In order to reduce porosity without tightening the weave, Dacron grafts have been impregnated with various biodegradable substances in an attempt to create an initially nonporous implant which with degradation of the sealant behaves like the porous implant, allowing tissue ingrowth.[6-9] Considerable success has been obtained in these endeavors, and these grafts will be discussed subsequently.

A modification of the manufacturing process in both knitted and woven prostheses is to have some of the yarn project upward from the surface, creating a plush, velvety surface. This "velour" surface can be placed inside, outside, or on both sides of the prosthesis.[10] The velour surface is felt to promote more effective and stable tissue incorporation by creating a mechanical scaffold for cell growth, and indeed, excellent cellular ingrowth has been shown in several investigations.[11] Some reports have shown a benefit with velour prostheses; however, whether velour actually imparts a significant advantage in terms of graft healing, resistance to infection, lack of late prosthetic degeneration, or long-term patency has not been clearly demonstrated. Incorporation occurs with nonvelour Dacron prostheses, although adhesion to surrounding tissue is much less intense. Most commercially available Dacron prostheses are marketed with velour because it may be beneficial and certainly does not appear harmful.

Early work by Wesolowski et al.[12] showed better incorporation in the more porous Dacron grafts. This was not supported by a more recent graft healing study that disclosed no difference in the pseudointima seen with woven and knitted prostheses with water porosities between 200 and 1200 ml/cm^2 per minute.[13] No configuration or porosity of Dacron will support spontaneous ingrowth of a confluent endothelial lining in humans.[14] For these reasons, the choice of a specific Dacron prosthesis is mainly based on the ease of intraoperative placement and surgeon preference.

As stated, knitted Dacron fabric has significantly more elasticity than the woven fabric. Further elasticity can be imparted by crimping either configuration. Most currently available grafts are produced with a crimp, particularly in aortic sizes. In high-flow, large-diameter systems such as the aorta, the crimping has no effect on long-term patency; however, in the lower-flow, smaller-diameter prostheses, crimped grafts show a decreased patency over their uncrimped counterparts as well as more fibrin accumulation in the convexities of the crimps.[15] Some workers have noted improved healing of noncrimped prostheses and decreased thrombogenicity.[16] The advantages of crimping are both increased elasticity, particularly in woven grafts, and also a greater ability to conform to the recipient vessel. Despite these apparent advantages of crimping noted at the time of insertion, the elasticity is progressively reduced as incorporation occurs, and the prosthesis reverts to the status of a nonelastic tube.[17,18]

Woven Dacron grafts are preferred for reconstructions involving the thoracic aorta, where a relatively less porous graft is desirable to limit blood loss. Woven prostheses are also usually chosen for repair of ruptured aortic aneurysms for the same reason. Most surgeons use a knitted Dacron graft for elective abdominal aortic procedures because of the ease of handling and excellent conformability. Regardless of the type of prosthesis, Dacron in the aortic position has a patency at 5 years of about 85 percent and 75 percent at 10 or more years.[19]

Dacron also has performed well as an extraanatomic conduit, particularly in the axillofemoral position. Both 3- and 5-year patencies are in the range of 60 to 78 percent.[20,21] Long subcutaneous grafts, especially in the axillofemoral position, are often externally supported with polypropylene rings. However, whether this reduces the likelihood of external compression–induced thrombosis has not been clearly defined.[22,23] Dacron also has fared quite well in the above-knee femoral-to-popliteal position, with reported patencies at 5 years of 60 percent.[24] One recent report comparing femoral-to-popliteal grafts of Dacron with PTFE actually found a better long-term patency with Dacron,[25] and another recent large experience with Dacron both above and below the knee reports very favorable patencies.[26] For below-knee grafts, or more distal grafts, the available Dacron prostheses do not function as well, with very limited long-term patencies, especially when extended to the tibial level.[27]

Although Dacron has performed well for the past 35 years, it has been plagued by several shortcomings. Despite perioperative antibiotics and careful aseptic techniques, 1 to 2 percent of Dacron grafts become infected, usually requiring removal of the graft.[19] Often extraanatomic revascularization is also needed, and these combined complex procedures are associated with a high morbidity and mortality.

Thromboses of aortic Dacron grafts occur primarily with bifurcation prostheses and usually involve only one graft limb, with the remainder of the prosthesis remaining patent.[28] These occlusions are normally the result of outflow obstruction, usually due to intimal hyperplasia or progression of vascular disease. In most cases, the occluded aortofemoral graft limb can be reopened by thrombectomy and outflow revision, most commonly utilizing profundaplasty. Similar good results can be obtained from occluded extraanatomic grafts, however, occluded infrainguinal grafts are more difficult to reopen with either thrombolysis or thrombectomy.[27]

Dacron grafts in general and knitted Dacron grafts in particular tend to show significant dilation both immediately after implantation and over the long term.[29] Up to a 15 percent dilation occurs immediately with restoration of flow due to the force of intraarterial pressures and is probably acceptable.[30] However, a greater frequency and extent of dilation have been observed recently with increased length of time after implantation.[31] Our group recently analyzed the degree of graft dilation, based on caliper measurements from computed tomographic scans, compared with the manufacturer's measured diameter. Knitted grafts were found to dilate 63.6 ± 45.5 percent, and when serial data were available, it appeared that this dilation continued and was not limited to initial prosthetic enlargement due to arterial pressure.[29] Such graft dilation may be the harbinger of graft failure, and indeed, there are several reports of massively dilated grafts that have become aneurysmal or have ruptured.[31] In our personal experience, we have seen four late ruptures of Dacron grafts, three of which were fatal. Our most recent graft rupture occurred in an 18-mm graft that expanded to 68 mm prior to posterior longitudinal rupture of the fabric. There was no associated pseudoaneurysm. Dilated grafts also may contain laminated thrombus, which has the potential for embolization. With dilation, the hemodynamics and flow patterns in the graft are markedly altered, which may potentiate graft thrombosis.

Pseudoaneurysms occur in 3 to 6 percent of Dacron grafts followed over the long term. When pseudoaneurysms occur, they are bilateral in 70 percent of patients, and 15 percent of these will have a concomitant aortic anastomotic pseudoaneurysm.[32,33] Since pseudoaneurysms can promote anastomotic occlusion, embolization, or rupture, repair of anastomotic pseudoaneurysms is almost always indicated.

The implantation of any vascular prosthesis creates a systemic response with an increase in fibrinolysis, platelet, white cell, and complement activation.[34–36] This response may have long-term effects with regard to intimal hyperplasia and patency. Several studies have shown a higher degree of platelet and complement activation with Dacron as opposed to PTFE.[37,38] Shoenfeld et al.[34] described a baboon model with an ex vivo perfusion circuit in which Dacron and PTFE grafts were placed in series and platelet uptake measured by gamma counting indium 111–labeled platelets.[39] In all experiments, platelet uptake on PTFE was increased when there had been previous exposure in the circuit to Dacron. The clinical implications of these findings are unknown. There has been one carefully documented report of anaphylaxis resulting from exposure to Dacron fibers in several patients.[40] Although this is exceedingly rare, if it is observed, one should remove the prosthesis and convert to autogenous tissue or another synthetic material if this is possible. Anaphylaxis has not been reported with PTFE.

As mentioned earlier, Dacron grafts have been impregnated with several materials in an attempt to decrease the need for preclotting yet maintain the advantages of Dacron. The impregnating substances currently used are mammalian gelatin, bovine collagen, or albumin.[6–9] Regardless of the impregnating substance employed, it is removed completely in weeks to months, and long-term healing of the prosthesis does not appear to be altered. One animal study did show delayed dissolution of sealant in the albumin-impregnated grafts and possibly delayed and inferior healing.[41] However, this does not appear to be a problem in reported human experiences. The albumin-impregnated grafts are not currently marketed in the United States but are available in Europe. There also has been a question of the antigenicity to bovine collagen. However, two carefully done studies have documented only a weak immunologic response to bovine collagen in human recipients, and this response had no clinical significance.[42,43]

It is somewhat surprising that one randomized study did not demonstrate a significant difference with regard to blood loss with impregnated Dacron compared with conventional Dacron.[44] By contrast, another nonrandomized study did show a marked decrease in blood loss using impregnated prostheses. Regardless, the impregnated grafts tend to handle well and definitely save time, since preclotting manuevers are unnecessary. One investigator found an increased patency rate but also an increased rate of pseudoaneurysm formation in impregnated Dacron grafts.[45] Most other series report patencies comparable with conventional Dacron series and have not identified an increased rate of aneurysm formation. Long-term follow-up data are just now becoming available on the impregnated prostheses, and it appears that the their long term behavior will be similar to that of nonimpregnated counterparts, with overall exemplary results.[46]

Impregnated Dacron grafts have been found to be an excellent medium for the binding of various biologically active compounds.[47–51] Most commonly employed antibiotics have been bonded, but growth factors, inhibitors of intimal hyperplasia, or anticoagulants are other possibilities being investigated. Animal reports and one clinical series have shown excellent results with rifampicin-bonded impregnated Dacron grafts.[52] This initial experience suggests that in situ placement of antibiotic-bonded grafts may be possible in infected fields in selected patients.

Dacron grafts are quite pliable and to date have proven to be the most useful prostheses for endovascular grafting. The Dacron graft is stented at both ends and compressed to fit in a catheter-based system.[53,54] For repair of abdominal aortic aneurysms, the device is introduced via a femoral artery cutdown, and once the correct position is confirmed using imaging techniques, the stents and graft are deployed and expanded for fixation to the arterial wall using balloon catheters. This procedure excludes the aneurysm. Early reports have been very encouraging, although much longer follow-up will be required. Broadening clinical applications for prosthetic insertion by endovascular techniques are being reported, including the treatment of arteriovenous fistulas and even occlusive disease after balloon angioplasty or closed atherectomy/endarterectomy.[55,56] PTFE is being used for some of these applications, but current systems mainly employ Dacron prostheses.

POLYTETRAFLUOROETHYLENE PROSTHESES

Polytetrafluoroethylene (PTFE, or Teflon) is a highly electronegative and hydrophobic polymer of carbon and fluorine. Teflon was initially made into fibers and woven to form a graft. Experience with these grafts was limited due to the very tight weave, which gave the graft very poor handling characteristics. Tissue incorporation also was poor due to the low porosity, and the graft was plagued with early thromboses and late disruptions. For these reasons, the woven Teflon graft was abandoned.[57] Since the initial development of PTFE as an electrical insulator, it has found many nonmedical uses, including nonstick cooking surfaces and "breathable" but waterproof clothing. Ben Eiseman, Glenn Kelly, and W. L. Gore considered the possibility of using this material as a vascular prosthesis after Mr. Gore showed off his white Teflon tie after a day of skiing in the Colorado Rockies.[58] This proved to be an idea that spawned another revolution in clinical vascular surgery.

The subsequent evolution of Teflon as a vascular prosthesis was based on extrusion of the polymer producing a configuration of microfibrils attached to nodes (Fig. 5-3). This characteristic appearance is created by a heating and mechanical stretching process that results in a prosthesis called *expanded PTFE*.[59] For the remainder of this discussion, the abbreviation PTFE will refer to expanded PTFE.

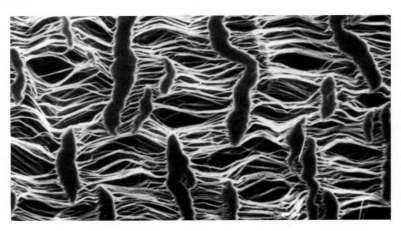

Figure 5-3. Expanded PTFE graft showing the characteristic pattern of nodes with interconnecting microfibrils (SEM; × 1000). (*Courtesy of W. L. Gore and Associates, Flagstaff, Arizona.*)

The first reported clinical use of PTFE was by Norton and Eiseman in 1971 to replace a segment of portal vein in a patient with pancreatic carcinoma.[60] The first arterial bypasses were reported by Campbell et al.[61] in 1976. Initial animal trials defined the optimal internodal distance to minimize bleeding but still allow for tissue ingrowth.[62] When the internodal distance is varied, the porosity of the graft is altered. Commercially available PTFE has an internodal distance of 30 μm; however, research continues on PTFE with varying internodal distances. PTFE with a 30-μm internodal distance allows endothelial ingrowth only 2 to 3 cm from the anastomosis, and complete coverage of the graft by endothelium does not occur.[63,64] Using a 60-μm internodal distance prosthesis in a baboon model, increased endothelialization was noted, with complete coverage of these grafts. Endothelial cell movement is seen as a sheet of cells and is based on both proliferation and migration. Despite the endothelial coverage, there is an increased cellular turnover, possibly indicative of chronic cellular damage, but the endothelial coverage is durable. Similar experiments using 90-μm internodal grafts have shown complete endothelialization; however, there was some late endothelial loss, with patches of bare graft seen at late explantation.[65] Capillary ingrowth between the nodes has been demonstrated histologically and may result in the formation of

endothelial islands. The formation of endothelium based on pleuripotent stem cells is still an unproven mechanism of endothelialization. A possible exception to the lack of spontaneous endothelialization of the 30-μm internodal distance PTFE was recently reported by Marin and colleagues.[56] An endovascular PTFE graft was placed for ileofemoral occlusive disease which required revision to a more distal anastomotic site. At revision, a segment of the graft was excised and was noted to be covered 4 cm from the anastomosis with endothelial cells. The endothelial nature of these cells was confirmed by immunohistochemical methods.

Early PTFE grafts suffered from aneurysm formation and thus were altered either with the placement of a thin external wrap of PTFE or by making the graft thicker with or without external reinforcing rings.[66] Despite fears of decreased healing with these modifications, tissue incorporation and prosthesis healing have not been affected. One laboratory investigation found a higher strength of soft tissue bonding to PTFE at anastomoses as opposed to Dacron.[67] This is felt by many to be one reason why there appear to be fewer pseudoaneurysms with PTFE versus Dacron.

PTFE was initially researched as a graft for medium sized arteries and is still used most widely for these indications. Numerous studies have been performed with PTFE grafts used for femoral-to-popliteal bypass. If the distal anastomosis is to the above-knee segment of the popliteal artery, 5-year primary patency rates of 40 to 65 percent have been reported.[24,68,69] If the distal anastomosis is below the knee, patency rates drop to the 50 percent level.[70] When used as a femoral-to-tibial graft, 3-year patency rates have been in the range of 12 to 35 percent.[70,71] These data prompted the recommendation that PTFE was an acceptable conduit for femoral-to-popliteal bypass but was only to be used for tibial reconstructions if autogenous vein was not available. These recommendations have been challenged recently as a result of a report of a modified distal anastomosis by Taylor et al.[72] Using the so-called Taylor patch, 5-year patency rates for femoral-to-tibial reconstructions were reported at 54 percent. Despite the encouraging results by Taylor et al. when distal anastomoses are below the knee, there is no question that autogenous vein still yields superior results and remains the "gold standard." Clinical trials are in progress to see if other groups can duplicate the encouraging results of Taylor et al. Some surgeons have made the recommendation that PTFE is the conduit of choice for femoral-to-popliteal bypass in order to save the ipsilateral saphenous vein for future reconstructions to a more distal level.[68]

Ring-reinforced PTFE has become the conduit of choice for most extraanatomic reconstructions. Harris et al.[73] have reported an 85 percent primary patency rate with a mean follow-up of 2 years and 4 months for ring-reinforced PTFE axillobifemoral grafts. Others' results have not been as good but are at least equal to those obtained with Dacron prostheses.

Most surgeons feel that there is an increased resistance to infection with PTFE as opposed to Dacron, which has prompted the suggestion that PTFE is preferable in the face of existing infection.[74,75] We will comment further on this later.

When autogenous arteriovenous fistulas cannot be constructed for hemodialysis access, PTFE has become the graft of choice for the construction of these dialysis shunts. Studies comparing PTFE with bovine carotid artery grafts have generally shown superior results with PTFE, with a lower incidence of thrombosis and aneurysm formation.[76–79] When thrombosis occurs, thrombectomy and revision are performed more easily with PTFE than with the bovine conduits. Of all available vascular prostheses, PTFE is the easiest to thrombectomize by mechanical means or by use of thrombolytic agents due to its smooth inner surface. PTFE as a patch material also has functioned very well, particularly in high flow systems such as the carotid artery and aorta.[80] PTFE is also a preferred graft for carotid-subclavian bypass and other short, high-flow bypasses in the neck.[81]

PTFE has functioned better than other prostheses when placed in the venous circulation. As noted, the first clinical use of PTFE was to replace the pancreatic segment of the portal vein in patients undergoing Whipple resection for pancreatic carcinoma. In this initial report, two of three patients maintained long-term patency.[60] Replacement of the vena cava, iliac veins, internal jugular, and other large veins has been reported with PTFE.[82] Usually, a large, externally supported conduit is used, often with an adjunctive arteriovenous fistula. There are also several applications for PTFE grafts in the treatment of portal hypertension, such as the mesocaval H graft and the mesoatrial bypass for the Budd Chiari syndrome.[83]

PTFE aortic grafts have been available for over 10 years. Results have been excellent and at least comparable with Dacron in this area.[84–86] Despite these good results, the use of PTFE in the aortic position has lagged well behind that of Dacron. The reasons for this bring us to the downside of PTFE. Particularly in the larger grafts, PTFE is relatively stiff and difficult to conform to body contours and anastomoses. Kinking of the graft, particularly at the bifurcation as the graft dips posteriorly over the sacrum into the pelvis and at the heel of an end-to-side anastomosis, has been problematic. PTFE grafts also have virtually no longitudinal stretch, and thus length measurements must be very precise. Bleeding from needle holes also can be very troublesome.

In an attempt to overcome these problems, one of the major graft manufacturers has altered the manufacturing process such that the internodal fibrils are microcrimped, which results in a more supple, stretchable graft (Fig. 5-4). When the graft is stretched to the appropriate length, there is no microscopic difference in appearance between the

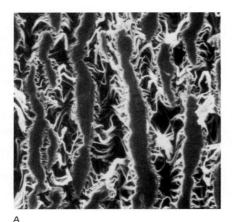

A

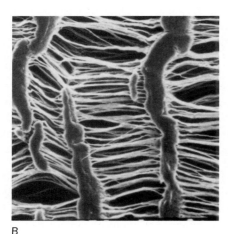

B

Figure 5-4. A. Relaxed configuration of a stretch expanded PTFE graft with crimped microfibrils. **B,** Tensioned appearance of a stretch expanded PTFE graft. Note the similarity in appearance to a conventional expanded PTFE graft shown in Fig. 5-3. (SEM; × 1000). *(Courtesy of W. L. Gore and Associates, Flagstaff Arizona.)*

immunosuppressed patient. During follow-up by clinical examination and computed tomography we have identified no evidence of significant graft dilation or elongation and no pseudoaneurysm formation. Subjectively, the stretch PTFE graft handles well, and needle hole bleeding has been markedly reduced, although precise needle hole volume loss and time to spontaneous cessation of needle hole bleeding have not been studied prospectively. Thus it appears that the stretch PTFE graft has overcome many of the shortcomings of its predecessors. Stretch PTFE is now available in multiple sizes and configurations. Patency rates appear comparable with conventional PTFE grafts in similar positions.

Several investigators have found an increased resistance to infection in PTFE grafts as opposed to Dacron.[74,75] Although the absolute rates of infection with any prosthesis are low, the consequences are so devastating that any increased resistance to infection is advantageous. Despite this purported advantage of PTFE, there is at least one study clinically comparing Dacron with PTFE that showed a decreased rate of graft infection with Dacron.[85] Most vascular surgeons prefer PTFE grafts when insertion is required in potentially infected fields. Excellent results have been reported with in situ replacement of grafts involved with low-grade infection, generally *Staphylococcus epidermidis,* after adequate debridement.[89]

Similar to impregnated Dacron grafts, many substances have been bonded successfully to the surface of PTFE grafts, including penicillin, cefoxitin, and ciprofloxin, with maintenance of antibiotic activity for days to weeks.[90,91] Carbon coating of PTFE was done in an attempt to decrease the surface electronegativity and to decrease the thrombogenicity. Unfortunately, this technology did not result in improved patency rates in a canine study.[92] Photodynamic treatment of the PTFE surface is developing and may provide a method for bonding almost any biologic molecule to this material. These bonded polymer surfaces are currently being investigated in our laboratories and others.

Investigators in Atlanta have designed a system for local drug delivery in and locally around PTFE grafts. Utilizing a slow infusion through the

stretch and conventional material. This new prosthetic configuration became available for clinical use early in 1991. One early clinical experience was favorable, with 100 percent patency with a mean follow-up of 10 months.[87] We recently prospectively analyzed our initial experience with 106 stretch PTFE grafts in the aortic position.[88] At a mean follow-up of 14 months we have 98 percent primary patency and 100 percent secondary patency. There has been 1 graft infection, manifest at 11 months postoperatively in a high-risk wall of the graft, local concentrations of active drugs can be delivered.[93] By infusing hirudin (a reversible antithrombin) around a PTFE graft, a significant decrease in intimal hyperplasia was observed at the site of an arterial injury distal to the graft in a baboon model. Similar systems obviously could be designed for a variety of substances and could prove to be useful clinically.

COMPARISON OF DACRON AND PTFE

There have been three relatively large studies reported (two randomized and one retrospective) comparing Dacron and PTFE aortic grafts.[84–86] All three found comparable and excellent patency rates and very low rates of complications. The retrospective study compared 312 patients over a 9-year period and found the 4-year cumulative patency rate of Dacron to be 90 percent and PTFE to be 97 percent.[86] Significant complications were seen in 13 percent of patients in the Dacron group and 4 percent in the PTFE group. All six graft infections and all double-limb graft thromboses were observed with Dacron. Intraoperative blood requirements were substantially less with PTFE than with Dacron.

This favorable report for PTFE was tempered somewhat by the randomized study of Lord et al.,[84] who found no significant differences in the complication rate or transfusion rate in 80 patients followed through the perioperative period. Although this was a randomized study, the comparison Dacron group consisted of whichever type of Dacron the surgeon chose to use. Polterauer et al.[85] found no difference in patency during a 3-year follow-up in 165 randomized patients (95 percent for both Dacron and PTFE). However, all graft infections (1.8 percent) and early graft failures (3.6 percent), occurred in patients with PTFE grafts. This study reported a high incidence of kinking of the back wall of the distal femoral anastomoses felt to be due to the stiffness of the PTFE graft. This may have been a factor contributing to the higher rate of graft failure with PTFE in this study.

All three of these studies were with conventional PTFE grafts. As stated earlier, our results with 106 stretch PTFE grafts have been quite gratifying.[88] It remains to be seen if stretch PTFE will prove a better conduit than conventional PTFE for aortic reconstruction and how it will compare with conventional and impregnated Dacron. A multicenter prospective study is currently being implemented to shed some light on these questions. Regardless, it appears safe to conclude that both Dacron and PTFE are excellent prosthetic substitutes for aortoiliac reconstructions.

The other areas of significant overlap of indications for Dacron and PTFE are in extra-anatomic grafts, femoral-to-popliteal grafts, and patch angioplasty, particularly in the carotid artery. As mentioned earlier, the best reported results for axillobifemoral grafts were presented by Harris et al.[73] Good results using Dacron have been reported by others.[20] Specifically designed prostheses for axillobifemoral reconstruction fabricated from stretch PTFE and impregnated Dacron are now available. However, long-term comparative results have not been documented with these grafts.

Both PTFE and Dacron are acceptable prostheses for above-knee femoral-to-popliteal reconstruction. As noted, one recent retrospective series actually showed better results with Dacron.[25] However, others have shown exemplary results with PTFE.[70] There is currently a prospective, randomized study underway comparing Dacron with PTFE in the femoral-to-popliteal position. Neither prosthesis yields results comparable with autogenous vein, particularly in below-knee popliteal, tibial, or pedal locations.

Many investigators have reported favorable results with carotid patching using either Dacron, PTFE, or vein.[94–96] None has disclosed significant differences between the patch material. Rosenthal et al.[80] looked at 400 carotid endarterectomies, with groups of 100 being performed by primary closure, vein patch, Dacron patch, and PTFE patch angioplasties. No significant differences could be found between any of the groups with regard to stroke, acute thrombosis, or late restenosis. It is still controversial whether patch angioplasty is beneficial in carotid surgery; however, it appears that both Dacron and PTFE can function as suitable patches with good clinical results and probably no significant difference in performance.

SEEDING AND SODDING OF VASCULAR PROSTHETIC GRAFTS

In an attempt to decrease the thrombogenicity of the prosthetic surface and hopefully to modulate the intimal hyperplastic response, several laboratories have been attempting to line the lumenal surface of prosthetic grafts with a confluent layer of endothelial cells.[97] Surprisingly little is known of the behavior of endothelial cells on various polymer surfaces, and it is not known why human endothelial cells will not migrate or bud out from ingrowing capillaries and line available prosthetic grafts. It has been found that endothelial cells can be grown on protein-treated Dacron or PTFE and that these monolayers remain adherent under conditions of high shear stress.[98]

The more common approach has been to harvest large-vessel autologous endothelial cells, grow them in culture, and then seed them onto a treated graft prior to implantation. This process typically takes 1 to 3 weeks.[99,100] Animal models have shown decreased platelet and fibrin deposition and increased patency in seeded grafts. Others have shown persistence of the endothelial cell monolayer on long-term follow-up.[83,101] There also develops a subendothelial neointima comprised mainly of smooth muscle cells and matrix proteins. One recent clinical trial that randomized patients with infrainguinal vascular disease to receive a seeded or bare graft disclosed not only a persistent endothelial lining on the seeded grafts but also an improved patency.[100]

In our laboratories, Williams et al.[102,103] have developed a method of covering the lumenal surface of the graft with confluent endothelial cells in a short period of time with an operating room compatible method. Subcutaneous fat is removed by liposuction, followed by collagenase digestion and centrifugation to isolate a pellet of cells separate from the adipocytes. These cells have been characterized extensively and found to be almost exclusively microvascular endothelial cells. After filling the graft interstices with pressurized cellular growth media and autologous serum (a process called *denucleation*), the endothelial cells are pressure "sodded" onto the prosthetic, which results in a monolayer of endothelial cells that are resistant to high shear stress. Study of a sodded mesoatrial shunt revised 9 months after placement confirmed a confluent layer of endothelial cells.[83] Likewise, we have explanted several sodded hemodialysis grafts, after thrombosis or patient demise, etc., and again have documented a confluent endothelial layer without evidence of inflammatory cells or platelet deposition (Fig. 5-5). The endothelial nature of the cells has been confirmed with immunohistochemical staining. Unfortunately, the sodded grafts have not consistently prevented neointimal hyperplasia; however, it does appear to modulate the process. Canine experiments with 4-mm PTFE grafts interposed in the carotid circulation show a patency advantage with sodded grafts as compared with the bare grafts.[104] Other experiments have shown decreased platelet and fibrin deposition on sodded grafts as opposed to unsodded grafts. Initial clinical results with sodded tibial PTFE grafts are promising. Relatively little clinical work has been done with seeding or sodding Dacron grafts; however, it is known that Dacron can be a suitable medium to seed endothelial cells.[98] It also may be possible to alter the endothelial cells to express or make different proteins to affect any number of biologic processes. The field of endothelial cell biology is rapidly expanding, and it will undoubtedly yield valuable advancements in the relatively near future.

As mentioned earlier, the field of endovascular grafting is rapidly developing. Marin and colleagues[56] have early experience with endovascular grafting for occlusive aortoiliac and femoropopliteal disease, and as stated earlier, they reported an interesting case of a portion of a patent graft explanted as part of a distal revision. An endothelial monolayer was seen on the lumenal surface of this PTFE endovascular graft a full 4 cm from the nearest anastomosis.[56] Thus it appears as though endovascular grafts may endothelialize spontaneously. Possibly, some autocrine or paracrine response to the host vessel allows this to occur. Obviously, much more research needs to be done in this exciting area.

OTHER VASCULAR GRAFTS

There is ongoing work with a graft consisting of an inner lining of spun Corethane (a modified

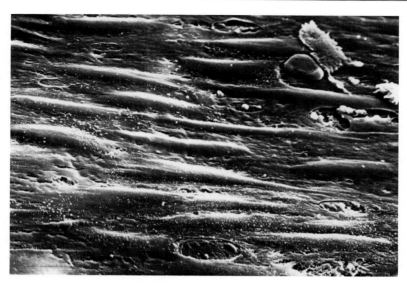

Figure 5-5. Lumenal surface of the midgraft portion of a patent "sodded" PTFE dialysis access graft explanted postmortem from a patient who died of causes unrelated to the graft. A confluent layer of cells is seen, and their endothelial origin was confirmed using immunohistochemical staining (SEM; × 850).

polyurethane) and a knit Dacron outer surface with the entire graft impregnated with a heparin-gelatin complex. In a canine model, patency of 4-mm grafts was superior with the Corethane-Dacron than with PTFE.[105] The process of glow-discharge polymerization has been used to bond an ultrathin layer of tetrafluoroethylene to a thin woven Dacron graft externally supported with an adherent polypropylene helix. This graft has been evaluated for hemodialysis angioaccess yet was inferior to PTFE controls and exhibited exuberant intimal hyperplasia; it also was very difficult to open with thrombectomy once thrombosis occurred.[106]

Some vascular grafts are a composite of synthetic and biologic materials. Some of these composites have already been discussed in the form of Dacron or PTFE impregnated or bonded with various proteins. Another of this genre is the human umbilical vein graft. Fresh human umbilical veins are cleaned and the collagen cross-linked with glutaraldehyde. The resulting tube is extracted multiple times with ethanol to remove soluble proteins. The graft is then covered with a Dacron mesh to impart more strength. Despite the Dacron mesh, um-

bilical vein grafts have been plagued by late aneurysmal degeneration, and they are quite difficult to thrombectomize or revise.

Dardik et al.[107] have reported 5-year patency rates of 53 percent for human umbilical vein femoral-to-popliteal grafts and 27 percent for tibial grafts in a large group of patients with ischemic tissue loss or rest pain. A contemporary series by Jarrett and Mahood[108] showed overall patency at 1 year of 70 percent, 44.5 percent at 5 years, and 29 percent at 10 years in 211 grafts placed mainly for limb salvage indications. Thus, although human umbilical vein is an acceptable conduit for infrainguinal reconstruction, it does not compare with autogenous saphenous vein and still eludes the standards for the ideal vascular graft.

Bioresobable arterial prostheses have been studied in several animal models. It has been demonstrated that the material can be a scaffolding for the native tissue, and once the scaffold is absorbed, there remains an autologous endothelial-lined tube. The most studied of this genre are the lactide-glycolide copolymeric bioresorbable prostheses.[109,110] Grossly and histologically, polyglycolic acid is resorbed between 4 weeks and 3 months following implantation. Animal studies are ongoing and encouraging. Biodegradable polymers also have been designed as a possible temporary stent for endovascular interventional procedures. Work continues in this area in our laboratories and others. Significant problems remain, particularly in previously diseased arterial segments and in the presence of hyperlipidemia. Regardless, this will probably be an area of fruitful experimentation in the future.

Other groups have utilized cell-free arterial allografts in an animal model with encouraging results.[111] Yet another approach has been to design an intestinal submucosal autograft that is used as an arterial substitute in dogs.[112] The interesting twist to this model is that the intestinal submucosal grafts seem to have a remarkable resistance to infection.

SUMMARY

The ideal vascular graft, prosthetic or otherwise, does not yet exist. Dacron and PTFE have excellent results in high-flow, large-diameter vascular systems. Both Dacron and PTFE are acceptable conduits for extraanatomic reconstructions. For medium-sized arteries, PTFE seems to have a mild patency advantage over Dacron, particularly with the distal anastomosis below the knee. Both prosthetics have inferior patencies as compared with autogenous vein in any infrainguinal reconstructions. Impregnated Dacron grafts and stretch PTFE grafts are both advances in technology that make the grafts easier to use; however, it is not clear as to whether they will result in any improvement in long-term results.

Lining of prosthetic grafts with autologous endothelial cells has been attempted with varying success for the last decade. Recent advances in seeding and sodding techniques have finally brought some of these grafts to limited clinical trials. There is no question that one can create a viable, durable endothelial layer that is resistant to fibrin and platelet deposition, but it is not known whether this will inhibit long-term intimal hyperplasia or result in improved patency.

Novel synthetic, biologic, and combined technology grafts are currently being researched. Although none are yet in clinical trials, much basic research and many animal trials have yielded promising results. The expanding field of endovascular surgery also may give an opportunity to study a new prosthetic blood interface that may be different than any known to date.

REFERENCES

1. Voorhees AB Jr, Jaretzki A III, Blakemore AH: The use of tubes constructed from Vinyon "N" cloth in bridging arterial defects. Ann Surg 1952;135:332.
2. Abbott WM, Callow AD, Moore W, et al: Evaluation and performance standards for arterial prostheses. J Vasc Surg 1993;17:746.
3. Creech O Jr, Deterling RA Jr, Edwards WS, et al: Vascular prostheses. Report of Committee for study of vascular prostheses for the Society for Vascular Surgery. Surgery 1957;41:62.
4. Stanley JC, Lindenauer SM, Graham LM, et al: Biologic and synthetic vascular grafts. *In* Moore WS (ed): Vascular Surgery: A Comprehensive Review, 4th ed. Philadelphia, W. B. Saunders Company, 1993, p 370.
5. Wesolowski SA, Dennis C. Fundamentals of Vascular Grafting. New York, McGraw-Hill, 1963.
6. Freischlag JA, Moore WS: Clinical experience with a collagen-impregnated knitted Dacron vascular graft. Ann Vasc Surg 1990;4:449.
7. Drury JK, Ashton TR, Cunningham JD, et al: Experimental and clinical experience with a gelatin impregnated Dacron prosthesis. Ann Vasc Surg 1987;1:542.
8. Quindon R, Snyder R, Martin L, et al: Albumin coating of a knitted polyester arterial prosthesis: An alternative to preclotting. Ann Thorac Surg 1984; 37:457.
9. Patel M, Kaplan A, Sauvage LR, et al: Comparative evaluation of the elasticity and flexibility of bioimpregnated knitted grafts. Ann Vasc Surg 1992; 6:127.
10. Lindenauer SM, Weber TR, Miller TA, et al: Velour vascular prosthesis. Trans Am Soc Artif Intern Organs 1974;20:314.
11. Sauvage LR, Berger K, Wood SJ, et al: An external velour surface for porous arterial prostheses. Surgery 1971;70:940.
12. Wesolowski SA, Fries CC, Karlson KE, et al: Porosity: Primary determinant of ultimate fate of synthetic vascular grafts. Surgery 1961;50:91.

13. Sottiurai VS, Lim Sue S, Hsu MK, et al: Pseudo-intima formation in woven and knitted Dacron grafts. J Cardiovasc Surg 1989;30:808.

14. Greisler HP: New Biologic and Synthetic Vascular Prostheses. Austin, R. G. Landes Company, 1991, p 5.

15. Takebayashi J, Kamatani M, Katagami Y, et al: A comparative study on the patency of crimped and-noncrimped vascular prostheses with emphasis on the earliest morphological changes. J Surg Res 1975;19:209.

16. Lucer C, Noszczyk W: Comparative studies on healing of crimped and flat arterial prostheses. Pol Med J 1972;11:168.

17. Gozna ER, Mason WF, Marble AE, et al: Necessity for elastic properties in synthetic arterial grafts. Can J Surg 1974;17:176.

18. Hokanson DE, Strandness DE: Stress strain characteristics of various arterial grafts. Surg Gynecol Obstet 1968;127:57.

19. Szilagyi DE, Elliott JP, Smith RF, et al: A thirty-year survey of the reconstructive surgical treatment of aortoiliac occlusive disease. J Vasc Surg 1986;3:421.

20. El-Massry S, Saad E, Sauvage LR, et al: Axillofemoral bypass with externally supported, knitted Dacron grafts: A follow-up through twelve years. J Vasc Surg 1993;17:107.

21. Ray LI, O'Connor JB, Davis CC, et al: Axillofemoral bypass: A critical reappraisal of its role in the management of aortoiliac occlusive disease. Am J Surg 1979;138:117.

22. Cavallaro A, Sciacca V, DiMarzo L, et al: The effect of body weight compression on axillo-femoral by-pass patency. J Cardiovasc Surg 1988;29:476.

23. Jarowenko MV, Buchbinder D, Shah DM: Effect of external pressure on axillofemoral bypass grafts. Ann Surg 1981;193:274.

24. Rosenthal D, Evans RD, McKinsey J, et al: Prosthetic above-knee femoropopliteal bypass for intermittent claudication. J Cardiovasc Surg 1990;31:462.

25. Pevec WC, Darling RC, L'Italien GJ, Abbott WM: Femoropopliteal reconstruction with knitted, non-velour Dacron versus expanded polytetrafluoroethylene. J Vasc Surg 1992;16:60.

26. El-Massry S, Saad E, Sauvage LR, et al: Femoropopliteal bypass with externally supported knitted Dacron grafts: A follow-up of 200 grafts for one to twelve years. J Vasc Surg 1994;19:487.

27. Mosley JG, Marston A: A 5-year follow-up of Dacron femoropopliteal bypass grafts. Br J Surg 1986;73:24.

28. Bernhard VM, Ray LI, Towne JB: The reoperation of choice for aortofemoral graft occlusion. Surgery 1977;82:867.

29. Hunter GC, Berman SS, Smyth SH, et al: Computed tomographic surveillance of aortic grafts: Is it warranted? (abstract). J Vasc Surg 1993;17:1120.

30. Nunn DB, Freeman MH, Hudgins PC: Postoperative alterations in size of Dacron aortic grafts. Ann Surg 1989;189:741.

31. Greenlaugh RM: Dilation and stretching of knitted Dacron grafts associated with failure. In Bergan JJ, Yao JT (eds): Surgery of the Aorta and Its Body Branches. New York, Grune & Stratton, 1979.

32. Treiman GS, Weaver FA, Cossman DV, et al: Anastomotic false aneurysms of the abdominal aorta and iliac arteries. J Vasc Surg 1988;8:268.

33. Schellack J, Salam A, Abouzeid MA, et al: Femoral anastomotic aneurysms: A continuing challenge. J Vasc Surg 1987;6:308.

34. Vohra R, Drury JK, Shapiro D, et al: Sealed versus unsealed knitted Dacron prostheses: A comparison of the acute phase protein response. Ann Vasc Surg 1987;1:548.

35. De Mol van Otterloo JCA, Van Bockel JH, Ponfoort ED, et al: The effects of aortic reconstruction and collagen impregnation of Dacron prostheses on the complement system. J Vasc Surg 1992;16:774.

36. Brothers TE, Graham LM, Till GO: Systemic effects of prosthetic vascular graft implantation. Surgery 1988;104:375.

37. De Mol van Otterloo JCA, Van Brockel JH, Ponfoort ED, et al: Systemic effects of collagen-impregnated aortoiliac Dacron vascular prostheses on platelet activation and fibrin formation. J Vasc Surg 1991;14:59.

38. Shepard AD, Gelfand JA, Callow AD, O'Donnell TF Jr: Complement activation by synthetic vascular prostheses. J Vasc Surg 1984;1:829.

39. Shoenfeld NA, Connolly R, Ramberg K, et al: The systemic activation of platelets by Dacron grafts. Surg Gynecol Obstet 1988;166:454.

40. Roizen MF, Rogers GM, Valone FH, et al: Anaphylactoid reactions to vascular graft material presenting with vasodilation and subsequent disseminated intravascular coagulation. Anesthesiology 1989;71:331.

41. Hake U, Gabbert H, Iversen S, et al: Healing parameters of a new albumin-coated knitted Dacron graft. Thorac Cardiovasc Surg 1991; 39:208.

42. Norgren L, Holtas S, Persson G, et al: Immune response to collagen impregnated Dacron double velour grafts for aortic and aorto-femoral reconstructions. Eur J Vasc Surg 1990;4:379.

43. The Canadian Multicenter Hemashield Study Group. Immunologic response to collagen-impregnated vascular grafts: A randomized prospective study. J Vasc Surg 1990;12:741.

44. De Mol van Otterloo JCA, Van Bockel JH, Ponfoort ED, et al: Randomized study on the effect of

collagen impregnation on knitted Dacron velour prostheses on blood loss during aortic reconstruction. Br J Surg 1991;78:288.

45. Hirt SW, Dosis D, Siclari F, et al: Collagen-presealed or uncoated aortic bifurcation Dacron prostheses: A 5-year clinical follow-up study. Thorac Cardiovasc Surg 1991;39:365.

46. Reid DB, Pollock JG: A prospective study of 100 gelatin-sealed aortic grafts. Ann Vasc Surg 1991; 5:320.

47. Avramovic JR, Fletcher JP: Rifampicin impregnation of a protein-sealed Dacron graft: An infection-resistant prosthetic vascular graft. Aust NZ J Surg 1991;61:436.

48. Avramovic J, Fletcher JP: Prevention of prosthetic vascular graft infection by rifampicin impregnation of a protein-sealed Dacron graft in combination with parenteral cephalosporin. J Cardiovasc Surg 1992;33:70.

49. Goeau-Brissonniere O, Leport C, Bacourt F, et al: Prevention of vascular graft infection by rifampin bonding to a gelatin-sealed Dacron graft. Ann Vasc Surg 1991;5:408.

50. Colburn MD, Moore WS, Chvapil M, et al: Use of an antibiotic-bonded graft for in situ reconstruction ofter prosthetic graft infections. J Vasc Surg 1992; 16:651.

51. Lundell A, Bergquist D, Lindblad B, Leide S: The acute thrombogenicity of an infection-resistant rifampicin-soaked Dacron graft: An experimental study in sheep. Eur J Vasc Surg 1992;6:403.

52. Torsello G, Sandmann W, Gehrt A, Jungblut RM: In situ replacement of infected vascular prostheses with rifampin-soaked vascular grafts: Early results. J Vasc Surg 1993;17:768.

53. Chuter TAM, Green RM, Ouriel K, et al: Trans-femoral endovascular aortic graft placement. J Vasc Surg 1993;18:185.

54. Parodi JC, Palmaz JC, Clem MF, et al: Transfemoral intraluminal graft implantation for abdominal aortic aneurysms. Ann Vasc Surg 1991; 5:491.

55. May J, White G, Waugh R, et al: Transluminal placement of a prosthetic graft-stent device for treatment of subclavian artery aneurysm. J Vasc Surg 1993;18:1056.

56. Marin ML, Veith FJ, Panetta TF, et al: Minimally invasive aorto-iliac reconstruction: The use of stented grafts for limb salvage in patients with co-morbid medical illnesses. Unpublished data presented at the 22nd Annual Meeting of the Society for Clinical Vascular Surgery, Tucson, Arizona, 1994.

57. Boyd DP, Midell AI: Woven Teflon aortic grafts: An unsatisfactory prosthesis. Vasc Surg 1971;5:148.

58. Kelly GL, Eiseman B: Development of a new vascular prosthetic. Arch Surg 1982;117:1367.

59. Gupta SK, Veith FJ, Ascer E, Wengerter KR: Expanded polytetrafluoroethylene vascular grafts. In

Rutherford RB (ed): Vascular Surgery, 3rd ed. Philadelphia, W. B. Saunders Company, 1989, p 460.

60. Norton L, Eiseman B: Replacement of portal vein during pancreatectomy for carcinoma. Surgery 1975;77:280.

61. Campbell CD, Brooks DH, Webster MW, et al: The use of expanded microporous polytetrafluoroethylene for limb salvage: A preliminary report. Surgery 1976;79:485.

62. Campbell CD, Goldfarb D, Roe R: A small arterial substitute: Expanded microporous polytetrafluoroethylene. Patency versus porosity. Ann Surg 1975; 182:138.

63. Clowes AW, Kirkman TR, Reidy MA: Mechanisms of arterial graft healing. Am J Pathol 1986; 123:220.

64. Clowes AW, Kirkman TR, Clowes MM: Mechanisms of arterial graft failure. II. Chronic endothelial and smooth muscle cell proliferation in healing polytetrafluoroethylene prostheses. J Vasc Surg 1986;3:877.

65. Golden MA, Hanson SR, Kirkman TR, et al: Healing of polytetrafluoroethylene arterial grafts is influenced by graft porosity. J Vasc Surg 1990; 11:838.

66. Campbell CD, Brooks DH, Webster MW, et al: Aneurysm formation in expanded polytetrafluoroethylene prostheses. Surgery 1976;79:491.

67. Quinones-Baldrich WJ, Ziomek S, Henderson T, Moore WS: Primary anastomotic bonding in polytetrafluoroethylene grafts. J Vasc Surg 1987; 5:311.

68. Prendiville EJ, Yeager A, O'Donnell TF, et al: Long-term results with the above-knee popliteal expanded polytetrafluoroethylene graft. J Vasc Surg 1990;31:731.

69. Kram HB, Gupta SK, Veith FJ, et al: Late results of two hundred seventeen femoropopliteal bypasses to isolated popliteal artery segments. J Vasc Surg 1991; 14:386.

70. Veith FJ, Gupta SK, Ascer E, et al: Six-year prospective multicenter randomized comparison of autologous saphenous vein and expanded polytetrafluoroethylene grafts in infrainguinal arterial reconstructions. J Vasc Surg 1986;3:104.

71. Cranley JJ, Hafner CD: Revascularization of the femoropopliteal arteries using saphenous vein, polytetrafluoroethylene, and umbilical vein grafts. Arch Surg 1982;117:1543.

72. Taylor RS, Loh A, McFarland RJ, et al: Improved technique for polytetrafluoroethylene bypass grafting: Long-term results using anastomotic vein patches. Br J Surg 1992;79:348.

73. Harris Jr JE, Taylor LM, McConnell DB, et al: Clinical results of axillobefemoral bypass suing externally supported polytetrafluoroethylene. J Vasc Surg 1990;12:416.

74. Bergamini TM, Bandyk DF, Govostis D, et al: Infection of vascular prostheses caused by bacterial biofilms. J Vasc Surg 1988;7:21.

75. Schmitt DD, Bandyk DF, Pequet AJ, Towne JB: Bacterial adherence to vascular prostheses: A determinant of graft infectivity. J Vasc Surg 1986; 3:732.

76. Anderson CB, Sicard GA, Etheredge EE: Bovine carotid artery and expanded polytetrafluoroethylene grafts for hemodialysis vascular access. J Surg Res 1980;29:184.

77. Bone GE, Pomajzl MJ: Prospective comparison of polytetrafluoroethylene and bovine grafts for dialysis. J Surg Res 1980;29:223.

78. Butler HG III, Baker LD Jr, Johnson JM.: Vascular access for chronic hemodialysis: Polytetrafluoroethylene (PTFE) versus bovine heterograft. Am J Surg 1977;134:791.

79. Tellis VA, Kohlberg WI, Bhat DJ, et al: Expanded polytetrafluoroethylene graft fistula for chronic hemodialysis. Ann Surg 1979;189:101.

80. Rosenthal D, Archie JP, Garcia-Rinaldi R, et al: Carotid patch angioplasty: Immediate and long-term results. J Vasc Surg 1990;12:326.

81. Ziomek S, Quinones-Baldrich WJ, Busuttil RW, et al: The superiority of synthetic arterial grafts over autologous veins in carotid-subclavian bypass. J Vasc Surg 1986;3:140.

82. Gloviczki P, Pairolero PC, Cherry KJ, et al: Reconstruction of the vena cava and of its primary tributaries: A preliminary report. J Vasc Surg 1990; 11:373.

83. Park PK, Jarrell BE, Williams SK, et al: Thrombus-free, humanendothelial surface in the midregion of a Dacron vascular graft in the splanchnic venous circuit: Observations after nine months of implantation. J Vasc Surg 1990; 11:468.

84. Lord RSA, Nash PA, Raj BT, et al: Prospective randomized trial of polytetrafluoroethylene and Dacron aortic prosthesis: I. Perioperative results. Ann Vasc Surg 1988;2:248.

85. Polterauer P, Prager M, Holzenbein TH, et al: Dacron versus polytetrafluoroethylene for Y-aortic-bifurcation grafts: A six-year prospective randomized trial. Surgery 1992;111:626.

86. Cintora J, Pearce DE, Cannon JA: A clinical survey of aorto-bifemoral bypass using two inherently different graft types. Ann Surg 1988; 208:625.

87. DeMasi RJ, Wheeler JR, Gregory RT, et al: Clinical evaluation of the Gore-Tex stretch vascular graft in the aortic position. Unpublished data presented at the 4th Winter Meeting of the Peripheral Vascular Surgery Society, Breckenridge, Colorado, 1994.

88. Erdoes LS, Bernhard VM, Berman SS, et al: Initial experience with a stretch PTFE graft for aortic reconstruction. Ann Vasc Surg (submitted).

89. Bandyk DF, Kinney EV, Riefsnyder TI, et al: Treatment of bacteria-biofilm graft infection by in situ replacement in normal and immune-deficient states. J Vasc Surg 1993;18:398.

90. Greco RS, Harvey RA: The biochemical bonding of cefoxitin to a microporous polytetrafluoroethylene surface. J Surg Res 1984;36:237.

91. Kinney EV, Bandyk DF, Seabrook GA, et al: Antibiotic-bonded PTFE vascular grafts: The effect of silver antibiotic on bioactivity following implantation. J Surg Res 1991;50:430.

92. Akers, DL, Du YH, Kempczinski RF: The effect of carbon coating and porosity on early patency of expanded polytetrafluoroethylene grafts: An experimental study. J Vasc Surg 1993;18:10.

93. Lumsden AB, Salam T, Allen RC, Hanson SR: Local drug delivery for prevention of restenosis. Unpublished data presented at the 4th Winter Meeting of the Peripheral Vascular Surgery Society, Breckenridge, Colorado, 1994.

94. Katz D, Snyder SO, Gandhi RH, et al: Long-term follow-up for recurrent stenosis: A prospective, randomized study of ePTFE patch angioplasty versus primary closure after carotid endarterectomy. J Vasc Surg 1994;19:198.

95. Ten Holter JBM, Ackerstaff RGA, Thoe Schwartzenberg GWS, et al: The impact of vein patch angioplasty on long-term surgical outcome after carotid endarterectomy: A prospective follow-up study with serial duplex scanning. J Cardiovasc Surg 1990;31:58.

96. Hertzer NR, Beven EG, O'Hara PJ, Krajewski LP: A prospective study of vein patch angioplasty during carotid endarterectomy: Three-year results for 801 patients and 917 operations. Ann Surg 1987;206:628.

97. Greisler HP: Endothelial cell transplantation onto synthetic vascular grafts: Panacea, poison or placebo. In New Biologic and Synthetic Vascular Prostheses. Austin, R. G. (ed.) Landes Company, 1991, p 47.

98. Vohra R, Thompson GJ, Carr HM, et al: The response of rapidly formed adult endothelial-cell monolayers to shear stress of flow: A comparison of fibronectin-coated Teflon and gelatin impregnated Dacron grafts. Surgery 1992;111: 210.

99. Schneider PA, Hanson SR, Price TM, Harker LA: Durability of confluent endothelial cell monolayers on small caliber vascular prostheses in vitro. Surgery 1988;103:456.

100. Zilla P, Deutsch M, Meinhart J, et al: Clinical in vitro endothelialization of femoropopliteal bypass grafts: An actuarial follow-up over three years. J Vasc Surg 1994;19:540.

101. Muller-Glauser W, Zilla P, Lachat M, et al: Immediate shear stress resistance of endothelial cell monolayers lined in vitro on fibrin glue-coated ePTFE prostheses. Eur J Vasc Surg 1993; 7:324.

102. Williams SK, Jarrell BE, Rose DG, et al: Human microvessel endothelial cell isolation and vascular graft sodding in the operating room. Ann Vasc Surg 1989;2:146.

103. Williams SK, Schneider T, Kapelan B, Jarrell BE: Formation of a functional endothelium on vascular grafts. J Electron Microsc Tech 1991; 19:439.

104. Williams SK, Rose DG, Jarrell BE: Microvascular endothelial cell sodding of ePTFE vascular grafts: Improved patency and stability of the cellular lining. J Biomed Mater Res 1994.

105. Wilson GJ, MacGregor DC, Klement P, et al: A compliant Corethane/Dacron composite vascular prosthesis: Comparison with 4-mm ePTFE grafts in a canine model. ASAIO J 1993;39:M526.

106. Farmer DL, Goldstone J, Lim RC, Reilly LM: Failure of glow-discharge polymerization onto woven Dacron to improve performance of hemodialysis grafts. J Vasc Surg 1993;18:570.

107. Dardik H, Miller N, Dardik A, et al: A decade of experience with the glutaraldehyde-tanned human umbilical cord vein graft for revascularization of the lower limb. J Vasc Surg 1988;7:336.

108. Jarrett F, Mahood BA: Femoropopliteal bypass with stabilized human umbilical vein: Long-term results. Unpublished data presented at the 22nd Annual Meeting of the Society for Clinical Vascular Surgery, Tucson, Arizona, 1994.

109. Greisler HP, Ellinger J, Schwarcz TH, et al: Arterial regeneration over polydioxanone prostheses in the rabbit. Arch Surg 1987;122:715.

110. Greisler HP, Kim DU, Dennis JW, et al: Compound polyglactin 910/polypropylene small vessel prostheses. J Vasc Surg 1987;5:572.

111. Allaire E, Guettier C, Bruneval P, et al: Cell-free arterial grafts: Morphologic characteristics of aortic isografts, allografts, and xenografts in rats. J Vasc Surg 1994;19:446.

112. Badylak SF, Coffey AC, Lantz GC, et al: Comparison of the resistance to infection of intestinal submucosa arterial autografts versus polytetrafluoroethylene arterial prostheses in a dog model. J Vasc Surg 1994;19:465.

Aneurysmal Disease

6

Infrarenal Aortic Aneurysms

MICHAEL B. SILVA, JR.
ROBERT W. HOBSON, II

HISTORY

Aneurysms of the abdominal aorta have been recognized as dangerous and potentially lethal for literally thousands of years. Antyllus performed the first recorded successful operation for aneurysm, which was ligation and evacuation, in the second century.[1] Over the years, a number of techniques for treating aneurysms have been developed by surgeons including ligation, intraluminal wiring, periaortic injection of sclerosing agents, and wrapping of the aneurysm with cellophane or skin grafts. These methods, aimed at promoting thrombosis or controlling expansion, proved to be largely unsuccessful, but without a suitable alternative, they were being used even through the first half of this century.

The modern era for treatment of aneurysms of the abdominal aorta began in 1951, when C. Dubost and colleagues[2] described the successful surgical management of an infrarenal aortic aneurysm by resection and replacement using an interpositional homograft harvested from a cadaveric thoracic aorta. This was followed by the introduction of synthetic grafts by Voorhees and colleagues,[3] also in the early 1950s. Modifications by others, notably the method of endoaneurysmorrhaphy introduced by Oscar Creech,[4] along with contemporary improvements in surgical and anesthetic techniques have led to the routine and safe surgical treatment of aneurysms today.

DEFINITIONS

The Ad Hoc Committee on Reporting Standards of the Society for Vascular Surgery (SVS) and the International Society for Cardiovascular Surgery (ISCVBS) define an *aneurysm* as "a permanent and localized dilatation of an artery to at least 1.5 times the expected normal diameter for that particular artery."[5] The normal diameters of arteries depend on many factors, most notably sex, age, and blood pressure. The inclusion of the descriptive term *localized* allows one to differentiate an aneurysm from diffusely enlarged arteries. Diffuse dilatation of the arterial tree is a condition known by a variety of terms including *ectasia, arteriectasis, arteriomegaly, dolichomegaarteries,* or *arteria magna syndrome.*[6]

Of note, the term *dissecting aneurysm* is a misnomer occasionally used to represent a process that is more aptly described as *aneurysmal dilatation from aortic dissection.* An aortic dissection results from degeneration of the media of the aorta and the creation of a false lumen within the wall of the aorta itself. This leads to an overall increase in aortic diameter typical of an aneurysm. This is a pathogenesis distinct from that responsible for the usual aneurysmal degeneration, of which dissection is not a common sequella. Most simply stated, aortic dissections generally become aneurysmal, but aortic aneurysms do not generally dissect.

INCIDENCE

According to data from the National Center for Health Statics in 1987, approximately 1.2 percent of all men and 0.6 percent of women in the United States die of aortic aneurysms. Aortic aneurysms have been implicated as the thirteenth most common cause of death in the United States,[7] and recent estimates indicate that in the population above age 60, at least 5 percent will have abdominal aortic aneurysms.[8] It is clear that detection of aneurysms has improved as a result of enhanced diagnostic methodology, particularly the widespread use of computed tomography and ultrasound in the workup of a variety of abdominal complaints. It is also clear that the actual incidence of aneurysmal disease is also increasing significantly. A well-known epidemiologic study documented a significant increase in the incidence of abdominal aortic aneurysms over a 30-year period; between the years 1950 and 1960, there were 8.7 new aneurysms diagnosed per 100,000 person-years, while there was a greater that threefold increase to 36.5 new aneurysms discovered per 100,000 person-years from 1971 to 1980.[9] Additionally, as the average life span of our population increases, we can expect an increase in the number of aneurysms identified and amenable to treatment.

Other Statistical Associations

There are a number of associated aneurysms and conditions that accompany infrarenal aortic aneurysms. The male-to-female ratio of aneurysm formation is 4:1.[10] Cigarette smokers have an 8 times greater ratio of aneurysm occurrence than nonsmokers. Hypertension is a common finding, occurring in 40 percent of patients with aneurysms.

There is a known strong familial occurrence of abdominal aneurysms; reportedly as many as 11 to 15 percent of patients with infrarenal aneurysms present with a family history of aneurysmal disease.[7] As many as 20 percent of patients with infrarenal aneurysms will have a first-degree relative with the same disorder. This association is particularly important for male siblings.[11]

Common or internal iliac aneurysms are found in association with abdominal aortic aneurysms in up to 41 percent of patients and femo-ropopliteal aneurysms in about 15 percent of patients. If a patient has a unilateral popliteal aneurysm, his or her incidence of aortic aneurysm is approximately 8 percent, and if bilateral popliteal aneurysms are present, this association may be as high as 35 percent.[10] Stenosis of the carotid arteries or tortuous internal carotid arteries also may exhibit a high degree of correlation with aortic aneurysms (10 and 40 percent, respectively).[12,13]

PATHOGENESIS

Pathogenesis of abdominal aortic aneurysm remains ill-defined. Traditionally, atherosclerotic changes resulting in degeneration of the supporting structures have been implicated. More recently, an inherited disorder manifested as an imbalance in the enzymatic regulation of deposition and absorption of collagen and elastin in the media of the aorta has been presented as an etiologic factor. Additionally, aneurysmal dilatation can be explained as a function of aortic design, with the physical principles of mechanical stress and flow dynamics as described by Bernoulli and Laplace coming to bear on cylinders subjected to 60 or 70 years of forceful pulsations.

Currently, it is probably most accurate to consider the etiology of aneurysms to be multifactorial, with a variety of pathogenic mechanisms contributing to their occurrence, growth, and eventual rupture.

Degenerative Aortic Aneurysm Disease

Aneurysmal degeneration of the aortic wall traditionally has been thought to represent a sequela of atherosclerotic changes occurring within the aorta. This has not been a completely satisfying explanation, however, since other areas within the arterial tree which are frequently afflicted by obliterative atherosclerotic changes (the infrapopliteal circulation or carotid bifurcation, for instance) are unusual sites of aneurysmal degeneration. Also, it has been observed that many patients with aortic aneurysmal disease do not have concomitant occlusive vascular disease of the iliac or femoral segments, and estimations suggest that no more than

25 percent of aortic aneurysms are associated with significant occlusive disease.[14]

More recent study has focussed on the biochemical aspects of elastin and collagen metabolism. Elastin is a component of virtually every tissue in the body and plays a critical role in maintaining the integrity of the aorta. Alterations in the metabolism of aortic elastin are being investigated as primary components in the pathogenesis of aneurysm formation. The major catabolic enzyme for the breakdown of mature elastin is the proteolytic enzyme elastase. Elastase, in turn, has its activity modulated by the major serum proteinase inhibitor alpha$_1$-antitrypsin. Thus the ratio between elastase and alpha$_1$-antitrypsin is a critical determinant in the degradation of tissue elastin.

Cohen[15] measured elastase and alpha$_1$-antitrypsin in patients with different aortic diseases.[15] The various groups included patients with occlusive disease, patients with abdominal aortic aneurysms, patients with multiple aneurysms, and patients with ruptured aortic aneurysms. Cohen reported a significant increase in the ratio of elastase to alpha$_1$-antitrypsin in abdominal aortic aneurysms, multiple aneurysms, and ruptured abdominal aortic aneurysms as compared with aortic segments with occlusive disease only. This suggests that an imbalance between synthesis and degradation of arterial connective tissue may be responsible for the development of atherosclerotic aneurysms. Rizzo et al.[16] observed differences in the concentration of both collagen and elastin in infrarenal aortas for nonaneurysmal age-matched control subjects and in abdominal aortic aneurysms.[16] Further evidence implicating the possible imbalance of circulating elastase and elastase inhibitors would be the association of aortic aneurysm rupture and chronic obstructive pulmonary disease.[16] Patients with chronic obstructive pulmonary disease (COPD) have reduced alpha$_1$-antitrypsin levels and increased levels of elastase both in their alveoli and circulating in their serum.[17]

Experimental evidence for the genetic transference of specific defects in collagen and elastin metabolism has been obtained through study of the blotchy mouse. In this model, the mice, which routinely develop aneurysms early in life, exhibit a defect in cross-linking of elastin and collagen due to an aberration in the functioning of the enzyme lysyl oxidase. This enzyme requires copper as a cofactor for proper linkage of collagen and elastin.[18] Further, skin biopsies from patients in families with an apparent genetic predisposition to the formation of aneurysms demonstrated deficiencies in copper, and these patients exhibited decreased hepatic copper reserves as well.[19,20]

Inflammatory, Infectious, and Congenital Etiologies

Less commonly, inflammation or infection may result in arterial aneurysms. In the past, syphilis was the most common cause of aortic aneurysms, with a predilection for the ascending aorta. Other infections may result in mycotic arterial aneurysms, including a variety of gram-positive and gram-negative bacteria. *Staphylococcus* species have surpassed the more classic *Salmonella* species as the most common infectious pathogen.[21] Noninfectious arteritis such as giant cell arteritis or polyarteritis nodosa also may result in arterial aneurysms. However, these most commonly affect medium-sized arteries.

Congenital aneurysms occur in Ehlers-Danlos syndrome and Marfan's syndrome as a result of alterations in collagen metabolism.

Mechanical Considerations

Regardless of the etiology of aneurysmal development, increased lateral pressure and tension and resultant enlargement and rupture are predicted by Bernoulli's theorem and the law of Laplace. Bernoulli's theorem predicts that acceleration of flow past a point of narrowing creates slower flow lateral to the jet stream beyond the stenosis and increased lateral pressure. The law of Laplace states that tension in the wall of a hollow structure or tangential stress T, is directly proportional to the product of radius R and transmural pressure P: $T = PR$. Therefore, once dilatation of the aorta has begun (an increase in R), for any given transmural blood pressure P, there will be an increase in transmural tension T. This law explains several clinical findings: Aneurysms get larger, hypertension increases the risk of rupture, and the larger the aneurysm, the greater is the risk of rupture.

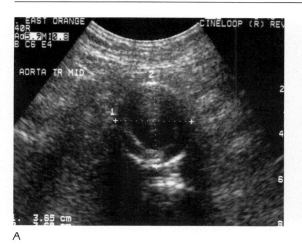
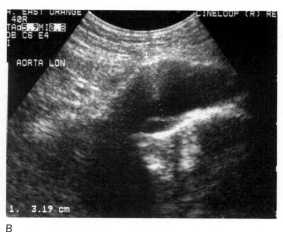

A   B

Figure 6-1. A, B-mode ultrasonogram of a small abdominal aortic aneurysm viewed in the transverse plane. Numbers 1 and 2 represent diameter measurements of the aneurysm taken in the transverse and anteroposterior planes. **B,** Same aneurysm viewed in the longitudinal plane. The patient's head is to the viewer's left. The measurement numbered 1 is 3.19 cm and is an anterior-to-posterior diameter.

DIAGNOSIS

Diagnosis of abdominal aortic aneurysms may be achieved by a thorough physical examination in most patients (up to 90 percent) by abdominal palpation.[22] The patient's body habitus is a significant consideration, since obesity substantially limits the ease of detection by physical examination alone. The presence of a pulsatile abdominal mass, detected during examination, should prompt further investigation to determine the presence and size of the abdominal aortic aneurysm. Associated abdominal pain radiating to the flank, groin, or back may suggest the presence of an expanding aortic aneurysm and warrants immediate attention.

The majority of abdominal aortic aneurysms are asymptomatic and are found serendipitously during the workup for other frequently nonrelated medical conditions. For instance, many unsuspected aortic aneurysms are first noted on abdominal radiographs, lumbar spine films, or intravenous pyelograms, where a fine rim of calcium representing the aortic wall is seen. This is not always reliable, however, since there may not be enough calcium present in the aneurysmal wall to determine maximal aortic size, and plain radiographs generally are not considered as accurate screening tests.

B-mode ultrasonography (Fig. 6-1) is used frequently as an initial screening test for direct evaluation of the size of the abdominal aorta and is sometimes used to follow aneurysms to determine rate of enlargement. Color duplex ultrasonography may be preferred to standard B-mode ultrasonography because of the more sophisticated appearance of images produced (Fig. 6-2), but the information the two studies provide is roughly equivalent.

Alternatively, computed tomography (CT) can be used as a screening method and may be preferred, since considerations such as abdominal distension from gas, which limit ultrasound examinations, do not impair the diagnostic accuracy of CT (Fig. 6-3). Additional information regarding unexpected intraabdominal pathology such as gallstones or tumors of the colon, kidney, or liver or the presence of anatomic variations that might affect the approach to repair of the aneurysm such as the presence of a retroaortic left renal vein or a horseshoe kidney also can be obtained from a CT scan more readily than from ultrasonography. This and the dependably readable nature of the hard copy of the CT scan have made it the preferred study of many vascular surgeons for the diagnosis and planning of repair of abdominal aortic aneurysms.

Magnetic resonance imaging (MRI) and magnetic resonance arteriography (MRA) may offer

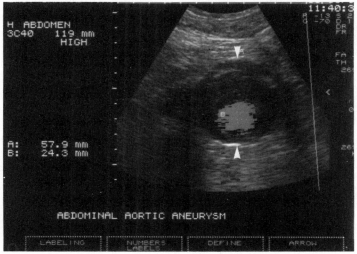

A

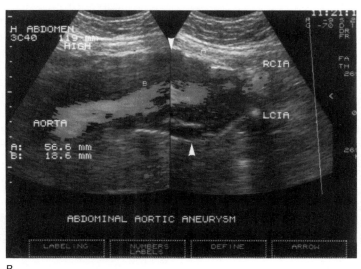

B

Figure 6-2. A, Larger aneurysm as viewed by color flow Duplex ultrasonography. The arrows and *A* represent the anterior-to-posterior diameter of the aneurysm wall, measuring 5.79 cm. The inner channel or aortic lumen is arbitrarily assigned the color red, and its diameter is designated by *B*, measuring 2.43 cm. The difference between *A* and *B* represents the extent of mural thrombus accumulation. **B**, Composite view in the longitudinal plane of the same aneurysm. Again, the patient's head is to the viewer's left. The right and left common iliac arteries are identified. The arrows and *A* represent anterior-to-posterior diameter.

additional information, such as the detection of associated atherosclerotic arterial disease present within the renal, mesenteric, and iliac arteries (Fig. 6-4). Further, MRA has the benefit of not requiring intravenous contrast administration, with its

attendant risks and complications. However, to date, cost and availability have prevented the widespread acceptance of MRI and MRA as screening tests.

Conventional contrast arteriography is not used for diagnosing and sizing aortic aneurysms,

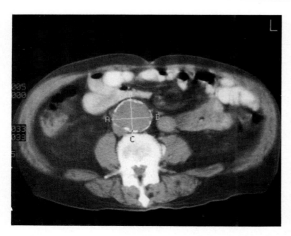

Figure 6-3. Conventional computed tomographic scan of an abdominal aortic aneurysm. Transverse and anterior to posterior diameters are measured. An eccentric ring of aortic calcification can be seen.

since the presence of mural thrombus typically leads to significant underestimation of the size of the aneurysm. However, arteriography does provide important information about concomitant renal and visceral atherosclerotic disease, the distal extent of aneurysmal involvement, and the presence or absence of disease within the runoff vessels (Fig. 6-5). The availability of nonionic contrast material and the refinement of arteriographic technique have significantly reduced the number of complications associated with performing arteriography in the patient with aortic aneurysmal disease. The contributions to planning of the surgical alternatives of repair obtained with arteriography and its relatively low risk have lead many authors to advocate its frequent, if not routine, preoperative use.

INDICATIONS FOR OPERATION, RISKS, NATURAL HISTORY, AND TREATMENT CONSIDERATIONS

Even though aneurysms can cause symptoms and serious consequences from thrombosis and distal embolization, rupture is the most dangerous risk, and recommendation for elective repair of an abdominal aortic aneurysm is driven by the fact that the chance for survival is poor once the aneurysm

has ruptured. Approximately 50 percent of people who experience a ruptured abdominal aortic aneurysm die before they reach the hospital.[10] Of the remaining 50 percent, 24 percent die before surgery is possible, and 42 percent develop fatal complications following emergent aneurysm repair, resulting in an overall mortality rate of between 60 and 80 percent.

It has been established that the size of an aneurysm is the most important factor that determines risk of rupture. The 5-year risk of rupture of a 4-cm aneurysm is less than 15 percent, while it is 95 percent for an aneurysm over 7.0 cm in diameter.[17,23] The risk of rupture rises sharply as the aneurysmal diameter exceeds 5 cm. Thus, 5 cm is the aneurysmal size identified as critical for a clinical decision regarding elective repair of the aneurysm by the SVS-ISCVS committee in their recently published guidelines for practice standards.[5] However, the authors note this value should not be used as a firm dividing line for recommending surgical correction, since smaller aneurysms do rupture.

Autopsy studies reported by Darling and associates[24] showed that 23.4 percent of aneurysms 4.1 to 5.0 cm rupture, and the same is true for up to 10 percent of aneurysms less than 4.0 cm

Figure 6-4. Magnetic resonance image of an abdominal aortic aneurysm reconstituted in the sagittal plane.

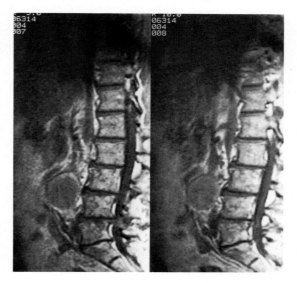

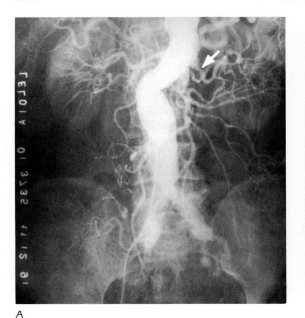
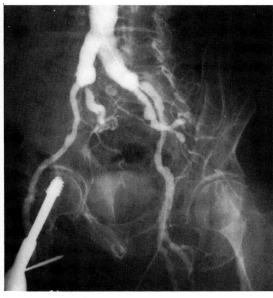

A   B

Figure 6-5. A, Contrast aortogram of a patient with a 6-cm infrarenal aortic aneurysm. Note that it is not possible to determine the outside diameter of the aneurysm. This patient has a stenosis of the left renal artery identified by the arrow. **B,** Contrast aortogram with runoff view shows proximal involvement of both iliac arteries. This patient underwent successful aortobifemoral bypass grafting with a saphenous vein graft placed from the body of the graft to the left renal artery.

in diameter. Cronenwett et al.[17] reported that "small" aneurysms 4.0 cm in diameter were associated with a rupture rate as high as 20 percent per year if hypertension and chronic obstructive pulmonary disease were present. Such data have led many surgeons to recommend repair of almost all aortic aneurysms in good-risk patients.

As we have seen, once dilatation of an arterial segment has begun, the tendency is toward continued enlargement, although this is not always the case. The average rate of growth of aortic aneurysms, as reported by Bernstein et al.,[25] is approximately 4 mm per year. Since this is an average figure, any particular aneurysm may grow more slowly, more rapidly, or not at all. While serial measurements, obtained usually by ultrasound, are helpful in following the change in size of an aneurysm that is not repaired surgically at the time of initial detection, it remains impossible to predict which aneurysm will rupture in which patient. However, in the elderly patient with major risk factors, such follow-up has been accurate. Cronenwett et al.[26] demonstrated that patients with small

aneurysms who have well-controlled blood pressure can be followed with ultrasonography at 6-month intervals and undergo elective repair when the diameter reaches 5 to 6 cm. Additional factors that may affect the decision to repair rather than follow a smaller aneurysm include poorly controlled hypertension, rapid growth rate documented by serial examinations, family history of ruptured aneurysm, and the presence of symptoms that cannot be distinguished from those caused by acute expansion.

Conversely, patients with larger aneurysms and altered mental status or prohibitive medical risks may be followed by serial examinations. The issue of what constitutes a prohibitive medical risk, however, is not always certain. When the diameter of an aneurysm exceeds 6 cm, the risk of death from rupture exceeds that of elective repair for almost all patients regardless of coexisting cardiac and pulmonary disease. With careful preoperative optimization and intraoperative management, many high-risk patients can undergo elective repair of their large abdominal aortic aneurysm.

In a modern medical center, overall operative mortality for elective aneurysm repair should be 5 percent or less.[27] If high-risk cases are eliminated, the mortality rate for uncomplicated infrarenal abdominal aortic aneurysm repair approximates 2 percent.[28]

While the size of an aneurysm is related to its risk of rupture, the correlation is not inviolate, and size should not be the absolute determinant of need for surgical repair; indeed, the presence of an aortic aneurysm may be more important than its diameter as an indication for surgical treatment.

PREOPERATIVE EVALUATION

Thorough preoperative evaluation of the patient with an aortic aneurysm is essential to limit postoperative morbidity and mortality. Typically, all aspects of the patient's vascular system should be evaluated prior to surgical treatment of the aneurysm. Cardiac, pulmonary, and renal systems should be optimized, and the cerebrovascular and peripheral vascular systems should be evaluated for concomitant disease.

Clinical factors predictive of increased risk for postoperative cardiac complications include advanced age, diabetes mellitus, a history of previous myocardial infarction, congestive failure, angina pectoris, and an abnormal preoperative electrocardiogram.[29] Noninvasive evaluation of the cardiac status may be performed by stress MUGA scanning or by dipyridamole-thallium myocardial stress testing on patients with any two or more of these risk factors. If reversible areas of myocardial ischemia are identified, cardiac catheterization is performed. Percutaneous transluminal coronary angioplasty (PTCA) or coronary artery bypass grafting prior to repair of the asymptomatic aneurysm may be indicated. In patients with myocardial dysfunction not requiring treatment with PTCA or surgery, preoperative Swan-Ganz catheterization and fluid adjustment can assist in optimizing perioperative cardiac and renal function.

In patients with a history of smoking or known pulmonary compromise, pulmonary function screening tests can be helpful in planning the surgical and anesthetic management. Preoperative bronchodilator therapy may be begun to minimize ventilatory effort and enhance gas exchange.

Renal function also should be assessed and optimized prior to angiography and operation. Evidence of either renal insufficiency or renovascular hypertension should prompt study of the renal arteries at the time of aortic angiography. Significant renal artery stenosis can be treated preoperatively by balloon angioplasty if indicated. Alternatively, renal artery reconstruction at the time of aneurysm repair can be anticipated.

Signs or symptoms of cerebrovascular insufficiency should be assessed routinely by noninvasive duplex scanning of the carotid arteries. Patients with either symptomatic carotid artery stenosis or bilateral high-grade asymptomatic carotid artery stenosis should undergo carotid endarterectomy prior to elective aneurysm surgery.

All prospective aneurysm repair candidates should have segmental Doppler studies and documentation of ankle-brachial indices as an objective baseline prior to angiography and operation. This is invaluable in identifying the patient who develops complications from embolization following cross-clamping of the aortoiliac segments. For the patient with evidence of peripheral arterial occlusive disease or of concomitant aortoiliac occlusive disease, aortography with lower extremity runoff should be obtained to assist in planning reconstructive options.

SURGICAL REPAIR AND MANAGEMENT OF ASSOCIATED PATHOLOGY

Surgical repair of the abdominal aortic aneurysm may be accomplished using either a midline abdominal incision, a transverse abdominal incision, or a retroperitoneal flank approach. The particular approach used is dictated by the surgeon's preference or by circumstances presented by each particular patient. The retroperitoneal approach may offer some benefit in the patient with severe chronic obstructive lung disease or the patient with previous multiple abdominal operations.

General anesthesia is typically used for aortic aneurysm repair; it is often combined with a continuous epidural anesthesia catheter to lessen the amount of inhalation agents used and to provide control of postoperative pain. Invasive cardiovascular monitoring with a radial artery catheter and a pulmonary artery catheter is standard practice in most circumstances. Foley catheterization and nasogastric tube insertion for decompression are performed once the patient is anesthetized. Prior to surgery, all patients receive prophylactic intravenous antibiotics and undergo a mechanical bowel preparation.

In our generally preferred midline abdominal approach, an incision is made from the xyphoid to the pubis. Care is taken to thoroughly explore the abdomen for evidence of associated pathology. Given the usual age of the population undergoing repair of an abdominal aneurysm, associated pathology is not uncommon. Malignancies of the colon, lung and prostate are most common and may occur in up to 4 percent of patients.[30]

For patients who have a colon carcinoma discovered at the time of laparotomy for aneurysm repair, treatment should be directed toward the symptomatic lesion first. If the colon carcinoma is near obstructing, it should be removed and the abdomen closed and the aneurysm repaired at a later time. There are reports of aneurysm rupture following laparotomy. However, if the retroperitoneal space is not violated, that risk appears to be low. If the colon lesion is small and the aneurysm represents the greatest risk to survival, then the aneurysm should be repaired and the colon lesion removed after a 4- to 6-week interval. Simultaneous removal of the colon lesion with repair of the aneurysm would expose the graft to an increased risk of infection and should be avoided.

Cholelithiasis is present in 5 to 20 percent of patients with abdominal aortic aneurysms. Because of the difficulty in diagnosing postoperative cholecystitis following a large intraabdominal procedure and the resultant increase in morbidity, some authors recommend concomitant chelecystectomy for asymptomatic gallstones with aneurysm repair.[31] This is performed after the aortic graft has been placed and the retroperitoneum closed. For patients with symptomatic cholelithiasis and a stable aneurysm, preoperative laparoscopic cholecystectomy could be performed in anticipation of aneurysm repair. Other inflammatory intraabdominal processes such as diverticulitis should addressed prior to aneurysm repair, if possible, to limit the chance of graft infection.

Renal carcinomas are occasionally diagnosed preoperatively by CT scan or angiography. It is acceptable and probably preferable to remove the affected kidney at the time of aneurysm repair. Again, the graft is placed, the retroperitoneum closed, and the kidney removed.

There is an association of aortic aneurysms with inguinal hernias, possibly secondary to altered collagen and elastin metabolism. Herniorraphy can be performed safely and effectively by an abdominal approach following aneurysm repair.

After assessing the abdomen for associated pathology, the nasogastric tube is positioned manually in the fundus of the stomach, and a self retaining retractor is placed to provide for exposure of the peritoneum covering the aneurysm and its surrounding structures. The ligament of Treitz is divided as necessary to facilitate lateral displacement of the duodenum and small bowel. The retroperitoneal tissue above the neck of the aneurysm is then sequentially ligated and divided. Care is taken to ligate all major lymphatics, reducing the risk of postoperative chylous acites. The dissection is typically carried cephalad to the level of the left renal vein as it crosses anteriorly over the neck of the aneurysm. Additional exposure may be obtained by thorough mobilization of the left renal vein with cephalad retraction. Occasionally, it may be necessary to divide the left renal vein in order to obtain a suitable segment of nonaneurysmal aorta for placement of the proximal anastomosis. This is usually well tolerated if the left adrenal and gonadal veins are spared. Following completion of the aortic repair, reanastomosis of the divided renal vein may or may not be performed.

Several anatomic anomalies arise that can complicate the dissection of the infrarenal aorta. Vena caval anomalies encountered include either a left sided inferior vena cava (0.2 to 0.5 percent of cases) or duplication of the vena cava with one segment on each side of the aorta (up to 3 percent of cases).[32] In both instances, major venous channels can course either anterior or posterior to the aortic aneurysm. A retroaortic left renal vein, either alone or in addition to a normally occurring anteriorly placed renal vein can be present (1.8 to 2.4 percent of cases) and, if not identified prior to dissection, represents a particularly dangerous obstacle to those who routinely obtain circumferential control of the neck of the aneurysm prior to clamping.[33] Venous collars are circumferential venous channels that wrap the aorta and occur even more frequently (8.7 percent of cases). If injured, any of these posteriorly located venous channels may require division of the aorta to facilitate control of hemorrhage.

Horseshoe kidneys, while rare, represent a particular hindrance to infrarenal aortic aneurysm repair. The isthmus typically passes anterior to the aneurysm, but extensive mobilization usually allows for posterior passage of the graft without the need for division. More challenging may be the presence of multiple renal arteries arising from either the aneurysm or the iliac arteries. The collecting system and ureters also may be aberrantly placed and complicate dissection and repair of the aneurysm.

Once sufficient exposure of the neck of the aneurysm is obtained to allow for aortic control and creation of the proximal anastomosis, attention is turned toward identifying the distal extent of the aneurysm. Care is taken to avoid division of the tissue crossing the left common iliac artery because it is possible to damage autonomic nerve fibers that affect sexual function in men.[34] Resultant retrograde ejaculation, as well as its consequences regarding sterility, is a troublesome complication, particularly in a younger man. If the proximal iliac arteries are spared from involvement, then they can be clamped and a tube graft placed. If they too are aneurysmal, then they are individually dissected beyond their area of involvement to facilitate clamping and placement of a bifurcated prosthesis. Circumferential control of the aorta and iliac arteries is generally unnecessary and may lead to injury of adjacent structures. Similarly, care must be taken to identify and preserve both ureters, which normally course anterior to the bifurcation of the common iliac arteries. If possible, antegrade flow to at least one of the internal iliac arteries should be preserved in order to minimize the risk of postoperative left colon ischemia.

The patient is systemically anticoagulated at this juncture with intravenous heparin to prevent thrombosis during aortic and iliac occlusion. Placement of distal clamps first may reduce the occurrence of distal embolization from aortic cross-clamping. The proximal clamp is placed, and the aneurysm is entered sharply and divided longitudinally along its anterior surface. The intraluminal thrombus is removed, and any bleeding lumbar arteries are oversewn with figure-of-eight silk sutures. The origin of the inferior mesenteric artery (IMA) is examined for patency and volume of back-bleeding. Either occlusion or vigorous back-bleeding would suggest that replantation of the artery may not be necessary, especially if hypogastric circulation is to be maintained. If the origin of the inferior mesenteric artery is occluded by the presence of the aneurysm and its intraluminal thrombus, then the left colon is receiving blood via its collateral circulation. Similarly, vigorous back-bleeding suggests the adequacy of collateral circulation within the left colon mesentery. If the back-bleeding is minimal and the collateral circulation therefore is in question, evaluation by continuous-wave Doppler,[35] or photoplethysmography[36] or measurement of inferior mesenteric backpressure[37] is recommended. Noninvasive assessment is easily performed prior to aortic cross-clamping during temporary occlusion of the IMA. Either absence of a Doppler signal or loss of pulsatility as determined by photoplethysmography within the left colonic mesentery suggests inadequate collateral arterial flow and indicates that replantation of the IMA is necessary. Alternatively, an IMA backpressure less than 40 mmHg also would suggest the need for replantation.

Once intraaneurysmal back-bleeding is controlled, the proximal and distal arterial cuffs are fashioned by extending the anterior arteriotomy into the normal nonaneurysmal segment and then dividing the wall laterally. The aortic cuff is sized, and either a tube or bifurcated synthetic prosthesis of appropriate size is selected. The proximal anastomosis is created using a running monofilament vascular suture. The proximal occluding clamp is moved below the anastomotic line, and the anastomosis is inspected for hemostasis. Prior to completion of the distal anastomosis, adequate intravascular volume resuscitation should be accomplished in anticipation of restoration of prograde flow to the lower extremities. This should limit declamping hypotension from alterations in hemodynamics and flushing of myocardial depressants built up during the periods of lower extremity ischemia and reperfusion.

As is well known, the abdominal aortic aneurysm is no longer resected at the time of repair. Rather, the walls of the aneurysm are left behind, and the aneurysmal aortic segment is replaced with the prosthetic graft. This endoaneurysmorrhaphy allows for repair of the aneurysm without the need for actual resection, which formerly led to much higher intraoperative blood losses. Requirements for perioperative transfusion can be reduced even further by the use of intraoperative autotransfusion devices and by preoperative donation of blood by the patient for autologous blood transfusion.

Once hemostasis is ensured, the left colon inspected for adequacy of perfusion, and the distal circulation examined for any evidence of embolization, the graft should be covered and excluded from the peritoneal cavity. This usually can be accomplished by reapproximating the walls of the aneurysm anteriorly over the graft. Occasionally, insufficient tissue remains to allow for this manner of graft exclusion. In these instances, a well-vascularized pedicle of omentum can be isolated and used to separate the graft and anastomotic suture lines from the overlying duodenum.

Ruptured Aneurysm

Preoperative and operative considerations for a ruptured aneurysm are different from those employed for an elective repair. Patients presenting with a pulsatile mass, hypotension, and abdominal, back, or flank pain should be taken directly to the operating room for repair of a presumed ruptured abdominal aneurysm. There should be no hesitation for diagnostic workup once the diagnosis is suspected. Frequently, the initial rupture has been contained at the time of presentation by a combination of the patient's hypotensive state and the partial impediment to expansion provided by the retroperitoneal space. Vigorous fluid resuscitation with elevation of blood pressure should therefore be delayed until the patient is in the operating room and control of the aorta above the site of rupture has been accomplished.[38] Similarly, the patient should be prepared and draped prior to being anesthetized, and the operating surgeon must be ready to make the incision at the time of induction. Severe hypotension often ensues as a result of the vasodilating effects of anesthesia combined with the relaxation of the abdominal wall musculature and elimination of its tamponading effect.

If the rupture is contained, division of the crura of the diaphragm through the lesser omentum will facilitate placement of a supraceliac aortic clamp. Once the infrarenal neck of the aneurysm is identified, the clamp can be moved caudally and flow restored to the abdominal viscera. Blood volume replacement should proceed and hemodynamic stability achieved prior to restoration of flow to the lower extremities. Other methods of controlling hemorrhage may be necessary in cases of free intraperitoneal rupture. Manual compression of the aorta at the level of the diaphragm without prior dissection can be followed by subsequent placement of an intraluminal occluding balloon catheter introduced proximally through the opened infrarenal portion of the aorta.

Heparin is usually not given for repair of a ruptured aortic aneurysm because bleeding and coagulopathy are common sequelae of the massive blood loss and subsequent replacement. Adequate administration of blood, fresh-frozen plasma, and platelets will contribute to achieving patient survival.

Inflammatory Aneurysm

Inflammatory aneurysms of the abdominal aorta may occur in 2.5 to 5.0 percent of patients.[39] These aneurysms can be identified preoperatively by their appearance on CT scan, which shows a thickened anterior wall, substantial periaortic reaction, and obliteration of tissue planes.[40] Additionally, they exhibit a characteristic halo effect of enhancement following intravenous contrast injection. The inflammatory aneurysm tends to be larger and may be tender to palpation.[41] These patients frequently have an elevated sedimentation rate and may describe weight loss. At laparotomy, there is an intense retroperitoneal desmoplastic reaction with dense fibrous tissue connecting the aortic wall with the surrounding structures, including the duodenum, left renal vein, inferior vena cava, and ureters. While rupture is less common in inflammatory aneurysms, it occurs, and endoaneurysmorrhaphy should be performed. At surgery, dissection is limited, with care taken to avoid the duodenum and ureters, and suprarenal clamping may be required. Histopathologic evaluation of the aortic wall shows distinct differences from other aortic aneurysms, with a thickened media and prominent infiltration of T lymphocytes. Once the aneurysm is repaired, the surrounding inflammatory response typically subsides.

COMPLICATIONS

Early Complications

Intraoperative and perioperative complications account for the majority of morbidity and mortality associated with aneurysm repair. Myocardial events are probably the most common serious complication. Myocardial ischemia is the most common cause of death following aneurysm surgery, and nonfatal myocardial infarction is reported to occur in from 3.1 to 16 percent of patients depending on the criteria used to define infarction.[10]

Hemorrhage, either during surgery or in the immediate postoperative period, occurs and can be life-threatening. Areas of more common injury are often venous and include the lumbar venous branches around the aneurysm neck and the branches of the left renal vein, gonadal or adrenal veins, and the left common iliac vein, which passes beneath the right common iliac artery. Postoperative tachycardia, hypotension, and falling hematocrit should prompt early reexploration of the abdominal cavity.

Technical injury to the bowel or ureters can occur, usually in the case of bowel injury secondary to adhesions from previous surgery and for the ureters as a result of displacement by the aneurysm. If the bowel is entered prior to placement of the aortic prosthesis for elective aneurysm repair, conventional treatment is to close the enterotomy, close the abdomen, and repair the aneurysm at a later date in order to avoid possible graft contamination. With a complete bowel preparation (4 liters of oral electrolyte solution preoperatively and systemic antibiotics) and no soiling from a limited enterotomy, one may consider proceeding with repair. Ureteral injuries should be stented and repaired at the time of identification.

Renal failure is an infrequent but particularly morbid complication. The mortality associated with renal failure in patients undergoing elective repair of an infrarenal aneurysm is as high as 70 percent despite the use of hemodyalisis.[42] Renal parenchymal injury may occur even without hypotension or suprarenal clamping. A number of causes have been proposed, including atheromatous embolization from manipulation of the perirenal aorta, delayed tubular necrosis from contrast material used for preoperative arteriography, and reflexive renal vasoconstriction causing a resultant decrease in renal blood flow following aortic cross-clamping. Renal failure following ruptured aortic aneurysm is more common than for elective repair, occurring in up to one-fifth of survivors.

Paraplegia is a devastating but fortunately infrequent complication of infrarenal aneurysm repair. The mechanism may involve interruption of blood flow to the anterior segment of the spinal cord via obliteration of an inferiorly originating artery of Adamkiewicz (artery magna radicularis). There is a 50 percent mortality associated with this complication, which occurs more frequently after ruptured aneurysms (hypotension probably plays a significant role here).[43] Unfortunately, there is no way to predict which patients will develop this complication, and it is effectively not preventable.

Impotence following aneurysm repair is a recognized complication and may be either vasculogenic or neurogenic in origin. Retrograde ejaculation is also known to occur as a result of division of autonomic nerves along the aorta and iliac arteries.[34] Careful preoperative and postoperative interrogation is necessary to identify this complication and should always be performed.

Ileus following infrarenal aortic aneurysm repair is not uncommon and is effectively treated with nasogastric decompression. There is a reduction in postoperative ileus in patients who undergo retroperitoneal rather than abdominal repair. A high duodenal obstruction, however, can occur with either approach as a result of edema from periduodenal dissection or hematoma formation. This too will usually resolve with nasogastric decompression. Postoperative pancreatitis is occasionally seen and probably results from retraction injury to the pancreas.

Ischemia of the left colon or rectum can occur and, as described previously, is a result of disturbances to the inferior mesenteric circulation and the hypogastric circulation. Severity of colon ischemia ranges from a transient ischemic colitis involving only the mucosa, to muscularis involvement that may result in stricture formation, to full-thickness infarction requiring resection and colostomy formation.[44] Bloody diarrhea during the first 24 to 48 hours postoperatively should prompt colonoscopy. Evidence of transmural involvement necessitates resection. Mortality from postoperative colon ischemia following aortic aneurysm surgery manifested by full-thickness necrosis and peritonitis approaches 90 percent.

Distal embolization or thrombosis following interruption of blood flow to the lower extremities may occur with cross-clamping of the aorta or iliac arteries. It is imperative that preoperative evaluation of lower extremity perfusion be performed in order to assist in identifying the occurrence of this complication, whose findings may range from subtle to profound. Before closing the abdomen, distal perfusion must be reassessed and corrective measures such as balloon catheter embolectomy performed as indicated.

Late Complications

There are a number of complications that may occur remote to the repair of the abdominal aortic aneurysm and which result from the implantation of the prosthetic conduit. Prosthetic aortic graft infection is rare, probably occurring in about 1 percent of patients and most commonly occurring within the first 2 years following graft placement but reported as late as 7 years following the surgical procedure.[45] Patients with graft infections present with a wide clinical spectrum of symptoms from an indolent chronic malaise to massive upper gastrointestinal hemorrhage resulting from an aortoduodenal fistula. The mortality rate from this complication is as high as 75 percent.

Anastomotic aneurysms are a late complication of aortic aneurysm repair. They occur most commonly at the site of femoral anastomoses (3 percent) and less commonly at iliac anastomoses (1.2 percent), and they are least likely to form at the proximal aortic anastomoses (0.2 percent).[46] While a number of factors may be involved (indolent infection, disruption of the suture line from suture failure, compliance mismatch between graft and artery), progressive degeneration of the native artery is thought to represent the most common abnormality. Treatment once the diagnosis is made is surgical repair with prosthetic replacement.

ENDOLUMINAL REPAIR

Currently, one of the most active areas of interest and research in vascular surgery is the development and deployment of endoluminal stent graft devices for the treatment of aortic aneurysms. These devices are made of an expandable wire-mesh stent with an attached tube of prosthetic material and are inserted over a guidewire placed through the femoral artery by a cutdown performed in the operating room. The proximal stent is deployed at the level of the neck of the aneurysm, and blood flow is diverted centrally through the lumen of the prosthetic graft. The distal aspect of the tube is then secured to the aorta above the bifurcation with a second stent. This second stent is necessary to prevent retrograde flow around the sides of the stent graft. Alternatively, a bifurcated stent graft can be placed with plication of the distal limbs within the iliac arteries or at the femoral arteries with additional stent deployment. Early reports of this alternative to transabdominal or retroperitoneal aneurysm repair are encouraging, with apparently satisfactory results in high-risk patients.[47] With technical refinements in the stent grafts and delivery systems and expansion of patient selection criteria, it is feasible that this shall become a preferred method of treatment for abdominal aortic aneurysms in the not distant future.

REFERENCES

1. Rutherford RB: Arterial aneurysms: Etiologic considerations. *In* Rutherford RB (ed): Vascular Surgery, 3rd ed. Philadelphia, W. B. Saunders Company, 1989, pp 238–245.

2. Dubost C, Allary M, Deconomos M: Resection of an aneurysm of the abdominal aorta: Reestablishment of the continuity by a preserved human arterial graft with results after five months. Arch Surg 1952;64:405.

3. Voorhees AB, Jaretski A, Blakemore AH: The use of tubes constructed from Vinyon N cloth in bridging arterial defects. Ann Surg 1952;135:332.

4. Creech O Jr: Endo-aneurysmorrhaphy and treatment of aortic aneurysms. Ann Surg 1966; 164:935.

5. Johnston KW, Rutherford RB, Tilson MD, et al: Suggested standards for reporting on arterial aneurysms. J Vasc Surg 1991;13:452.

6. Hollier LH, Stanson AW, Glovicski P, et al: Arteriomegaly: Classifications and morbid implications of diffuse aneurysmal disease. Surgery 1983; 93:700.

7. Majumber PP, St Jean PL, Ferrell RE, et al: On the inheritance of abdominal aortic aneurysm. Am J Hum Genet 1991;48:164.

8. Svensson LG, Crawford ES: Aortic dissection and aortic aneurysm surgery: Clinical observations, experimental investigations, and statistical analyses, part 3. Curr Probl Surg 1993;30(1):1.

9. Bickerstaff LK, Hollier LH, Van Peenen HJ, et al: Abdominal aortic aneurysms: The changing natural history. J Vasc Surg 1984;1:6.

10. Taylor LM, Porter JM: Basic data related to clinical decision making in abdominal aortic aneurysms. Ann Vasc Surg 1980;1:502.

11. Cole CW, Barber GG, Bouchard AG, et al: Abdominal aortic aneurysm: Consequences of a positive family history. Can J Surg 1989;32:117.

12. Bengtsson H, Ekberg O, Aspelin P, et al: Abdominal aortic dilatation in patients operated on for carotid artery stenosis. Acta Chir Scand 1988; 154:441.

13. Mukherjee D, Mayberry JC, Inahara T, Greig JD: The relationship of the abdominal aortic aneurysm to the tortuous internal carotid artery: Is there one? Arch Surg 1989;124:955.

14. Zarins CK, Glagov S: Aneurysms and obstructive plaques: Differing local responses to atherosclerosis. *In* Bergan JJ, Yao JST (eds): Aneurysms: Diagnosis and Treatment. New York, Grune & Stratton, 1982, pp 61–82.

15. Cohen J: Pathogenesis of aortic aneurysms. Perspect Vasc Surg 1990;3:103.

16. Rizzo R, McCarthy WJ, Dixit SN, et al: Collagen types and matrix protein content in human abdominal aortic aneurysms. J Vasc Surg 1989;10:365.

17. Cronenwett JL, Murphy TF, Zelenock GB, et al: Actuarial analysis of variables associated with rupture of small aortic aneurysms. Surgery 1985;98:472.

18. Rowe DW, McGoodwin EB, Martin GR, Grahn D: Decreased lysyl oxidase activity in the aneurysm-prone, mottled mouse. J Biol Chem 1977;252:939.

19. Tilson MD, Davis G: Deficiencies of copper and a compound with ion-exchange characteristics of pyridinoline in skin from patients with abdominal aortic aneurysms. Surgery 1983;94:134.

20. Tilson MD: Decreased hepatic copper levels: A possible chemical marker for the pathogenesis of aortic aneurysms in man. Arch Surg 1982;117:1212.

21. Parson R, Gregory J, Palmer DL: *Salmonella* infections of the abdominal aorta. Rev Infect Dis 1983;5:227.

22. Rob CG, Williams JP: The diagnosis of aneurysms of the abdominal aorta. J Cardiovasc Surg 1961;2:55.

23. Bernstein EF, Chan EL: Abdominal aortic aneurysm in high risk patients: Outcome of selective management based on size and expansion rate. Ann Surg 1984;200:255.

24. Darling RC, Messina CR, Brewster DC, Ottinger LW: Autopsy study of unoperated aortic aneurysms. Circulation 1977;56(suppl 2):161.

25. Bernstein EF, Dilley RB, Goldberher LE, et al: Growth rates of small abdominal aortic anerrysms. Surgery 1976;80:765.

26. Cronenwett JL, Sargent SK, Wall MH, et al. Variables that affect the expxansion rate and outcome of small abdominal aortic aneurysms. J Vasc Surg 1990;11:260.

27. Thompson JE, Hollier LH, Patman RD, et al: Surgical management of abdominal aortic aneurysms. Ann Surg 1975;181(5):654.

28. Brown OW, Hollier LH, Pairolero PC, et al: Abdominal aortic aneurysms and coronary artery disease. Arch Surg 1981;116:1484.

29. Eagle KA, Coley CM, Newell JB, et al: Combining clinical and thallium data optimizes preoperative assement of cardiac risk before major vascular surgery. Ann Intern Med 1989;110:859.

30. Szilagyi DE, Elliott JP, Berguer R: Coincidental malignancy and abdominal aortic aneurysm. Arch Surg 1967;95:402.

31. Ouriel K, Ricotta JJ, Adams JT, DeWeese JA: Management of cholelithiasis in patients with abdominal aortic aneurysm. Ann Surg 1983; 198:717.

32. Seib GA: The azygos system in American whites and American Negroes, including observations on the inferior vena cava. Am J Phys Anthropol 1934;19:39.

33. Brener BJ, Darling CR, Frederick PL, et al: Major venous anomalies complicating abdominal aortic surgery. Arch Surg 1974;108:159.

34. DePalma RG: Impotence in vascular disease: Relationship to vascular surgery. Br J Surg 1982;69:514.

35. Hobson RW II, Wright DB, Rich NM, et al: Assessment of colonic ischemia during aortic surgery by Doppler ultrasound. J Surg Res 1976; 20:231.

36. Ouriel K, Fiore WM, Geary JE: Detection of occult colonic ischemia during aortic procedures: Use of

an intraoperative photoplethysmographic technique. J Vasc Surg 1988;7:5.

37. Ernst CB: Prevention of intestinal ischemia following abdominal aortic reconstruction. Surgery 1983; 93:102.

38. Crawford ES: Ruptured abdominal aortic aneurysm: An editorial. J Vasc Surg 1991;13:348.

39. Goldstone J, Malone JM, Moore WS: Inflammatory aneurysms of the abdominal aorta. Surgery 1978;83:425.

40. Ramirez AA, Riles TS, Imparato AM, et al: CAT scans of inflammatory aneurysms: A new technique for preoperative diagnosis. Surgery 1982; 91:390.

41. Pennell RC, Hollier LH, Lie JT, et al: Inflammatory abdominal aortic aneurysms: A 30-year review. J Vasc Surg 1985;2:859.

42. Castronuovo JJ Jr, Flanigan DP: Renal failure complicating vascular surgery. In Bernhard VM, Towne JB (eds): Complications in Vascular Surgery, 2nd ed. Orlando, Fla, Grune & Stratton, 1985, pp 259–273.

43. Ferguson LRJ, Bergan JJ, Conn J Jr, et al: Spinal ischemia following abdominal aortic surgery. Ann Surg 1975;181:267.

44. Boley SJ, Brandt LF, Veith FJ: Ischemic disorders of the intestines. Curr Probl Surg 1978;15:1.

45. Goldstone J, Moore WE: Infection in vascular prostheses: Clinical manifestations and surgical management. Am J Surg 1974;128:225.

46. Szilagyi DE, Smith RF, Elliott JP, et al: Anastomotic aneurysms after vascular reconstruction: Problems of incidence, etiology, and treatment. Surgery 1975;78:800.

47. Parodi JC, Palmaz JC, Barone HD: Transfemoral intraluminal graft implantation for abdominal aortic aneurysms. Ann Vasc Surg 1991;5:491.

CHAPTER

7

Juxtarenal, Pararenal, and Paraanastomotic Aneurysms of the Abdominal Aorta

GIAN LUCA FAGGIOLI
JOHN J. RICOTTA

DEFINITION

From the Greek *para* (= "at the site of, along-side") and the Latin *renal* (= "of the kidney"), the definition of *pararenal aneurysm* indicates an aneurysm that involves the origin of the renal arteries[1] (Fig. 7-1). Several authors classify such aneurysms as *suprarenal*,[2,3] while others restrict suprarenal aneurysms to involvement of the superior mesenteric artery and the celiac trunk.[4] This may lead to an overlap with type IV thoracoabdominal aneurysms of Crawford's classification and may further confuse the issue.[5] *Juxtarenal aneurysms* (from the Latin *juxta* = "near, beside") are defined as aneurysms that originate immediately below the renal arteries, leaving no space for infrarenal aortic clamping and suture[2-4] (Fig. 7-2). These two kinds of aneurysms (pararenal and juxtarenal) will be discussed together in this chapter, since they present similar technical problems of surgical exposure, clamping site, and protection from both renal and spinal cord ischemia.

Paraanastomotic aneurysms occur in the same area of the aorta but are complicated by the presence of a prior aortic graft. These may represent true aneurysm of the aortic remnant or false aneurysm of the proximal aortic suture line[6,7] (Fig. 7–3). These cases combine issues of exposure and visceral perfusion with those of reoperation and are some of the more difficult problems encountered in abdominal aortic surgery.

INCIDENCE

Juxtarenal and Pararenal

The true incidence of juxtarenal and pararenal aortic aneurysms is difficult to determine. There are differences in terminology in reported series. Some authors limit the definition of *pararenal* to those aneurysms with proximal extension below the superior mesenteric artery; others include suprarenal aneurysms with involvement of the other visceral vessels (Crawford's type IV thoracoabdominal aneurysms).[5] There is in addition an effect of referral patterns on reported incidence; i.e., the centers reporting the largest series are generally major referral centers. It is reasonable to conclude that the reported figures are often an overestimation of the real incidence.[1]

In 1991, 1719 of 29,656 (5.8 percent) procedures performed in the United States for any kind of aortic disease (i.e., aneurysmal or occlusive) involved either the juxtarenal or the pararenal aortic segment.[4] In the 1984 experience of aortic procedures from Stoney et al.,[8] this incidence was as high as 16 percent (90 of 560). Considering only the aneurysmal disease, Qvarfordt et al.[2] reported an incidence of juxtarenal and pararenal aneurysms of 20 percent (77 of 375), with 54 (14.4 percent) juxtarenal aneurysms and 23 (6.1 percent) pararenal ones. Lower incidences were reported by both Green et al.[9] (30 of 431, 6.9 percent) and by Breckwoldt et al.[10] (23 of

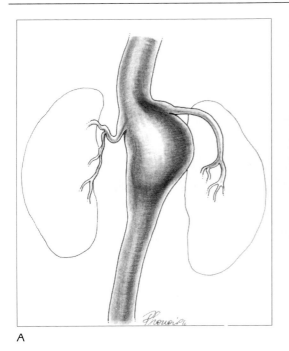

A

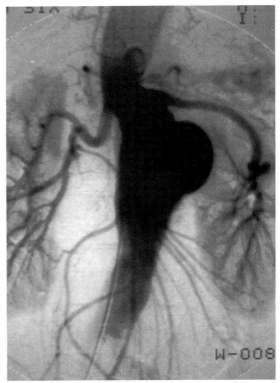

B

Figure 7-1. Artist's interpretation (**A**) and angiography (**B**) of a typical juxtarenal aneurysm. The aneurysm originates just below the renal arteries, and there is no space for infrarenal aortic clamping.

205, 11 percent). These latter figures are similar to those of two European prospective studies in which aneurysmal involvement of the renal arteries occurred in 8 percent of nonruptured aneurysms and in 13.6 percent of ruptured ones.[11,12] The surgical series usually report the highest incidence of juxtarenal and pararenal aneurysms, since some remain unrecognized until surgery.[9,13,14] Some nonsurgical series report an incidence of from 2 to 4 percent.[15,16] Juxtarenal aneurysms seem to be twice as common as pararenal ones.[1]

Crawford et al.[13] identified these lesions as group V in a series of 82 thoracoabdominal and abdominal aneurysms involving the visceral vessels. The incidence of these type V lesions was 14.6 percent (12 of 82) in their series.

ASSOCIATED LESIONS

Crawford et al.[5,13,17] report 16 of 71 cases of atherosclerotic involvement of visceral arteries (22 percent) in patients with either pararenal or tho-

racoabdominal aneurysms and 20 of 101 renal artery involvement in juxtarenal aortic aneurysms. Allen et al.[4] performed 7 of 31 (22.5 percent) renal artery reconstructions during juxtarenal aneurysms resection. In Qvarfordt's series,[2] 11 of 77 patients demonstrated unilateral renal disease, 32 of 77 had bilateral disease, and only 34 of 77 (44 percent) patients had no renal stenosis. Poulias et al.[14] reconstructed one or both renal arteries in 6 of 38 patients (15.8 percent) with juxtarenal aneurysms. The reason for this high incidence of renal lesions in this series is not clear, but it is reasonable to assume that the more proximal localization of the aneurysmal atherosclerotic disease causes atherosclerotic involvement of the adjacent arterial vessels. The functional or even hemodynamic significance of all these lesions is uncertain, however, since moderate lesions may have been subjected to prophylactic surgery during aneurysm resection. There have been reports[2] of an increased incidence of multiple renal arteries (22 percent),

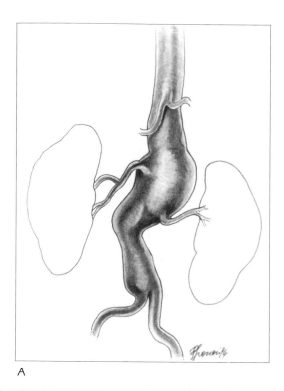

A

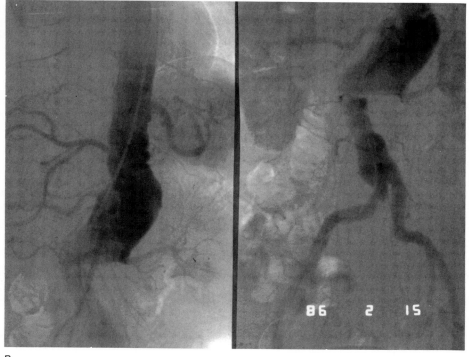

B

Figure 7-2. Artist's interpretation (**A**) and angiography (**B**) of pararenal aneurysm. The aneurysm involves the origin of both renal arteries. The aorta is tortuous, and the left renal artery appears to be ectopic.

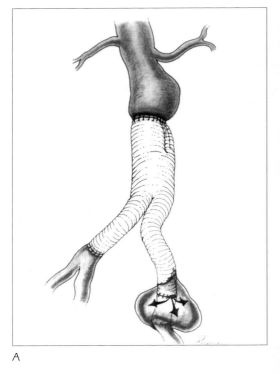

A

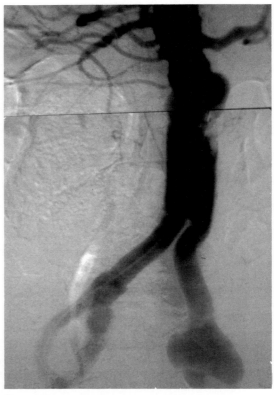

B

Figure 7-3. Artist's interpretation (**A**) and angiography (**B**) of a paraanastomotic aneurysm that developed 2 years after the operation performed in a suburban hospital. Bilateral iliac anastomotic aneurysms are evident. CT scan subsequently showed that the paraanastomotic aneurysm was a true aneurysm and the iliac aneurysms were false. The proximal aneurysmal dilatation was probably caused by incomplete resection of the aortic aneurysm during the primary operation.

but this is an inconsistent finding. Aneurysmal degeneration of renal arteries is rare and is reported in the 1 percent range.[2]

Iliac artery occlusive disease was reported in 13 of 101 patients by Crawford et al., while Allen et al.[4] found 17 of 65 (26.2 percent) patients with iliac disease that was either aneurysmal or occlusive. Symptomatic aortoiliac obstruction also was present in approximately 30 percent of patients in two other series.[2,14]

Paraanastomotic

The overall incidence of paraanastomotic aneurysms is also difficult to assess. Few reports give an estimate of the frequency of this late complication

after aortic graft replacement. Early, retrospective series reported an overall incidence of paraanastomotic aneurysms of less than 1 percent.[18–20] These papers reported only false anastomotic aneurysms. However, when a routine surveillance program was employed for detection of late graft complications, the incidence of paraanastomotic aneurysms increased dramatically. In the study by Edwards et al.,[21] there was a 5 percent incidence of either true or false paraanastomotic aneurysm at 8 years. At 15 years, the authors estimated, by life-table analysis, that almost one-third of the patients would develop an aortic paraanastomotic aneurysm.[21] Paraanastomotic false aneurysms occurred in 4.8 percent of 437 patients in the series of Van den Akker et al.[22] By life-table analysis, the incidence in their series was 7.7 percent and 28.4 percent at 15 and 20 years, respectively. It is important to note that para-anastomotic aneurysms may develop at any time postoperatively; therefore, their incidence continues to increase with the length of postoperative interval. Differences in length and completeness of follow-up make accurate assessment of the incidence of this condition difficult.[22]

Crawford et al.[13] described 5 true paraanastomotic aneurysms in a series of 101 juxtarenal aneurysms. True paraanastomotic aneurysms occurred in 8 percent of patients operated on primarily for an abdominal aortic aneurysms in the series from Edwards et al.,[21] where a routine screening follow-up examination was performed within a 12-month interval. False aneurysms are approximately two or three times more common than true aneurysms. Pseudoaneurysms had an incidence of 20 percent and true aneurysms 9 percent at 15 years in the series of Edwards et al.[21] Similarly, Fulenwider et al.[23] revised 11 paraanastomotic aneurysms (7 false and 4 true) found in 76 patients undergoing abdominal aortic reintervention. Curl et al.[6] found 12 false and 9 true aneurysms in 21 cases of paraanastomotic aneurysm.

ETIOLOGY

Juxtarenal and Pararenal

The etiology of juxtarenal and pararenal forms is similar to that of infrarenal abdominal aneurysms; they are generally classified as *nonspecific degenerative* in origin and are commonly called *atherosclerotic*.[24] Crawford et al.[13] found 92 percent of 101 juxtarenal aneurysms to be atherosclerotic; 7 percent were "inflammatory" and 1 percent secondary to Marfan's syndrome. It is not clear whether the term *inflammatory* used by Crawford et al. indicates the inflammatory variant of nonspecific aneurysms or rather a true inflammatory etiology.[24] Similarly, Qvarfordt et al.[2] found 91 percent "atherosclerotic" and 9 percent "inflammatory" forms. In the series of Poulias et al.,[14] there were 38 juxtarenal aneu-

rysms, of which 35 were atherosclerotic, 1 was inflammatory, and 1 was dysplastic. The etiology of one case was not reported.[14] Several series do not specify the etiology, thus implying that all the cases were nonspecific—"atherosclerotic." In general, the etiology of these forms is the same as that of the infrarenal ones,[1] and they can be considered as proximal extension of infrarenal aneurysms.

Paraanastomotic

The etiology of paraanastomotic aortic aneurysms involves degeneration of the aortic wall or prosthetic material and may be different for false and true aneurysms. False paraanastomotic aneurysms are caused by a discontinuity occurring at the anastomotic line. Systemic factors, such as hypertension, extension of atherosclerotic disease, and collagen defects[6,7,18,19,22,25,26] may be involved as well as dilatation, disruption from material fatigue, or anastomotic compliance mismatch.[18,19,22,26,27] Most authors, however, agree that disruption of the arterial wall rather than the prosthetic material occurs in the majority of false aneurysms.[6,7,18,19,22] Mechanical factors may play a major role, since end-to-side anastomoses have a significantly greater incidence of false aneurysms when compared with end-to-end anastomoses.

True paraanastomotic aneurysms usually occur as a late complication of operations performed for aneurysmal rather than for aortic occlusive disease.[7] In several series, true paraanastomotic aneurysms were seen almost exclusively in patients whose original operation was aneurysm resection. They are generally considered a proximal extension of the original aneurysmal process. Some authors speculate that a subgroup of patients with defined enzymatic abnormalities is particularly exposed to the risk of aneurysm recurrence. Although most true anastomotic aneurysms involve the pararenal portion of the aorta and can occur proximally to a graft correctly placed just below the renal arteries, a significant number affect only the infrarenal aorta.[7] Inadequate resection at the primary aneurysm resection may contribute to the occurrence of some cases in this latter group (see Fig. 7-3).

DIAGNOSIS

Juxtarenal and Pararenal

It is interesting to note that in many series[9,13,14] the presence of the aneurysm was detected in an institution different from the one in which it was eventually treated. Patients are often referred to tertiary care institutions either because of the large size of the aneurysm or because of the known involvement of renal vessels. Owing to the importance of technical considerations in the treatment of pararenal, juxtarenal, and paraanastomotic aneurysms, it is important to define as much morphologic information as possible preoperatively.

Ultrasonography, although helpful in the initial detection of an abdominal aneurysm with renal artery involvement, does not permit adequate assessment of the proximal extent of the lesion or visceral artery involvement in most instances.[12,28–30] Computed tomographic (CT) scan is presently the diagnostic tool of choice for defining proximal and distal aneurysm extent, visceral artery involvement, and accurate aneurysm size[15] (Figs. 7-4, 7-5, and 7-6). Presence of an inflammatory variant of an aneurysm, venous anomalies, and other extravascular pathologies also can be detected by this technique.[31–33]

Angiography, which is not performed routinely in infrarenal aortic aneurysms by many authors,[15,34] is essential in these patients. It is important to detail possible visceral artery occlusive disease, the relationship between renal and mesenteric vessels and the aneurysm, and the presence of multiple renal vessels. If a tortuous aorta is present, angiography may be necessary to interpret CT scan results, which can be imprecise in identifying renal artery involvement.[12,13,15,16] Although some authors believe that a single anteroposterior angiographic projection may be sufficient when the digital subtraction technique is used,[12] an additional lateral view is important in detailing proximal aortic dilatation and/or tortuosity[9,13] (Fig. 7-7).

Magnetic resonance imaging (MRI) might eventually substitute for both CT and angiography. It is reliable in detecting proximal and distal extent of the aneurysm and demonstrative visceral artery involvement, including visceral artery flow, and it can provide different projections.[28–30] However, its use is still limited by its expense, the need to exclude patients with pacemakers or other metallic devices (i.e., clips, stents), and the relative lack of experience available when compared with other diagnostic modalities.[28–30] Other diagnostic techniques, particularly spiral CT scan, are promising

Figure 7-4. CT scan of a small juxtarenal aneurysm with contained posterolateral rupture (*asterisk*). Rupture also can occur in these small aneurysms.

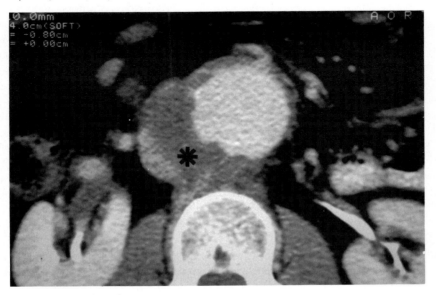

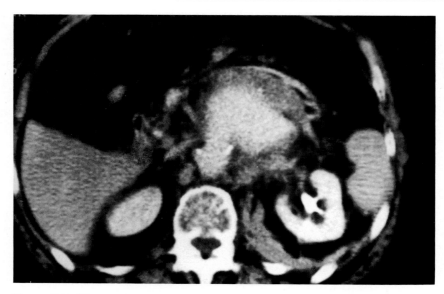

Figure 7-5. CT scan of a large pararenal aneurysm with contained rupture in a symptomatic patient.

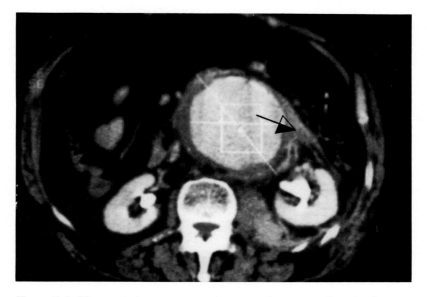

Figure 7-6. CT scan of a large symptomatic pararenal aneurysm. Contained rupture is shown (*arrow*).

and allow a complete three-dimensional view of the aorta and its branches.[34,35] Experience and availability of this diagnostic tool are presently limited.

Paraanastomotic

The diagnostic evaluation of paraanastomotic aneurysms is similar to that of pararenal and juxtarenal aneurysms, but several specific points should be emphasized. Patients with a paraanastomotic false aneurysm have a high incidence of concomitant distal pseudoaneurysms. While false aneurysms in the groin are easily appreciated by simple clinical observation, their presence at the iliac level has to be investigated carefully by CT scan.[36] Rupture is not

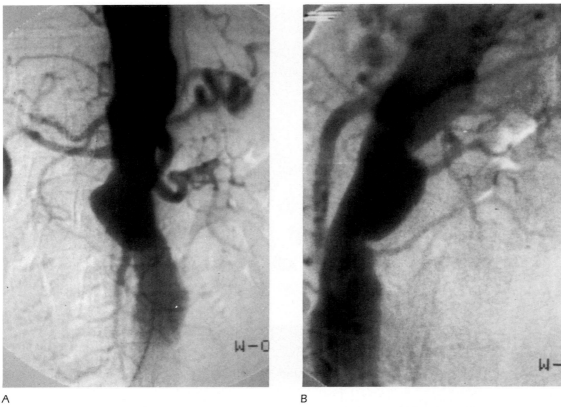

A   B

Figure 7-7. Biplane angiography of a pararenal aneurysm. The lateral view (**B**) demonstrates the proximal extension of the dilatation, which was difficult to assess by conventional anteroposterior view (**A**).

uncommon in paraanastomotic aneurysms, ranging from 15 to 55 percent,[6,13,37,38] particularly when a screening program is not performed routinely (Figure 7-1).[21,39] In emergency cases, there is usually no time available for complete preoperative assessment, and as soon as a diagnosis of rupture is suspected, operation must performed.

Infection may be the cause of the paraanastomotic false aneurysm.[22,40] It should be considered and, whenever possible, excluded in all cases of paraanastomotic false aneurysm, since the surgical approach is completely different in these patients.[40] If an infection is suspected at CT scan by the presence of unidentified fluid collection around the graft and/or the pseudoaneurysm, a more sensitive evaluation, such as leukocyte-labeled scintigraphy, should be performed.[41] Treatment

of an infected aortic prosthesis generally requires graft excision and extraanatomic bypass.

TREATMENT

The treatment of all proximal abdominal aortic aneurysms depends more on the proximal extent of the lesion than on its etiology. Therefore, the treatment of paraanastomotic forms is similar to that of pararenal or juxtarenal true aneurysms and is well described in the literature.[1,3,5–7,42–51] Choices include the transabdominal approach (with or without medial visceral rotation), the extended retroperitoneal approach, and thoracoabdominal incisions. A standard transabdominal approach can provide adequate exposure for most cases of juxtarenal aneurysms and

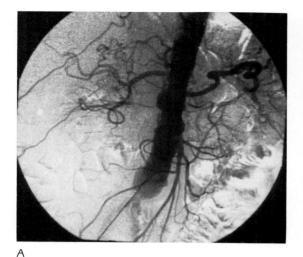

A

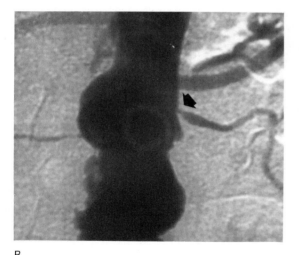

B

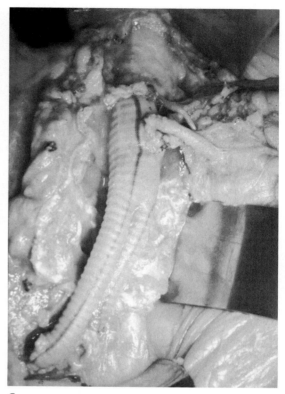

C

Figure 7-8. Angiography of a pararenal anuerysm with a left renal artery stenosis. **A**, The right renal artery is absent. **B**, A detail of the left renal artery stenosis (*arrow*). **C**, The intraoperative image of the anuerysm repair shows the reimplantation of the left renal artery which was previously endarterectomized.

for some paraanastomotic aneurysms, if infrarenal clamping can be anticipated (see Fig. 7-3B) and is most familiar to vascular surgeons. This approach, when combined with medial visceral rotation, allows a good exposure of the entire abdominal aorta and probably is the approach of choice when a concomitant lesion of the right iliac artery is associated with a small juxtarenal aneurysm. It allows also inspection of the abdominal contents. Suprarenal control is best obtained above the celiac axis by division of the gastrohepatic ligament and enlargement of the aortic hiatus.[9] This allows

placement of an infrarenal suture line in juxtarenal aneurysms. When visceral rotation is performed, care must be taken to avoid injury to spleen, pancreas, and adrenal gland during their dissection, mobilization, and retraction. Bleeding from the adrenal gland, rupture of the spleen, and postoperative pancreatitis are potential complications of this approach.[42] In reoperative cases, useful adjunctive maneuvers to facilitate exposure and avoid injuries to surrounding structures are the placement of a ureteral stent and division of the left renal vein.[44] Alternatively, the left kidney also can be displaced anteromedially, allowing access to the posterolateral aorta. However this approach has several disadvantages compared with a retroperitoneal exposure.

The transabdominal exposure can be difficult in case of reoperation; therefore, it is a second-choice option in the treatment of paraanastomotic aneurysms, even when their extension is limited to the infrarenal aorta.[7,45] A left retroperitoneal approach allows exposure of the proximal and distal abdominal aorta through an oblique left flank incision with the patient placed in lateral position. When this approach is performed with the incision beginning at the end of the twelfth rib, the infrarenal aorta is accessible; however, for the treatment of juxtarenal and pararenal aneurysms, the extended approach, as described by Williams et al.,[47-49] is necessary. The incision needs to be carried up to the eleventh or the tenth rib depending on the extent of proximal exposure required. In approximately 10 percent of patients, there is potential to injure the intercostal nerve; this can be minimized by its identification and dissection away from the rib.[45] The retroperitoneal dissection can be performed either anteriorly or posteriorly to the left kidney. The first option, i.e., with the kidney in situ, is chosen usually when exposure of the middle third of the superior mesenteric artery is needed for visceral reconstruction or when a retroaortic left renal vein is encountered.[3,47,48] In most instances, however, a retrorenal exposure is preferable; with this approach, the left kidney renal vein and ureter are reflected anteriorly and are excluded from the surgical field. When this approach is chosen for the treatment of a paraanastomotic aneurysm, attention has to be paid to possible adherence of the ureter to the graft, particularly if a bifurcated graft was implanted in the primary operation.

Once the proximal aorta is exposed, the major structure that can be injured is the left renal artery. It is identified by finding and dividing the posterior lumbar vein, which drains into the left renal vein. The artery is then identified and traced to the kidney. Dissection proceeds posterior to this vessel. In some instances, when the aneurysm is very large or extends proximally, the retroperitoneal access can be extended into a thoracoretroperitoneal approach. This is achieved by dividing the

diaphragm circumferentially.[45,50] However, if significant disease involves the right iliac or the distal right renal artery, a true thoracoabdominal approach is required.

It is useful to avoid manipulation of the aneurysm in order to prevent embolization from endoluminal thrombus. Aortic control is most safely obtained proximally above both the superior mesenteric artery and the celiac trunk after division of the left crus of the diaphragm. Occasionally, in aneurysms restricted to the juxtarenal aortic segment, a clamp may be applied between the renal and visceral vessels, although this should be done with great care and only when the aortic segment to be clamped is normal. In most instances, this approach gives sufficient aortic exposure, and only occasionally is an extended thoracoabdominal exposure needed. Suprarenal aortic clamping has been associated with increased risk of atherosclerotic plaque and thrombotic trashing, and thus with increased mortality.[9,52] However, this is usually due to improper placement of the aortic clamp in a diseased segment of artery. Some authors suggest preclamping of the renal vessels,[46] but we have found this unnecessary when clamps are placed carefully and appropriately. Application of clamps between the renal and superior mesenteric vessels can cause vessel damage and limits exposure,[9] and most authors prefer to clamp at the supraceliac position.[2,4] In case of paraanastomotic aneurysm, supraceliac aortic clamping also allows an easier aortic exposure through an unexposed field without dealing with the previously dissected tissue in the renal artery area.

When dealing with a juxtarenal aneurysm, the suture line is usually directly below the ostium of the renal arteries and may include the inferior margin of the renal orifice. Occasionally, the graft can be beveled to avoid reimplantation of one or both renal arteries.[47] When necessary, the right renal artery can be reimplanted using the inclusion technique described by Crawford.[13] The left renal artery can be either reimplanted directly in the graft or bypassed with a small prosthetic segment originating from the aortic graft. If a right renal artery stenosis is present, the best way to correct it through this approach is by endarterectomy; bypass is possible but can be technically difficult.

Table 7-1. Reported Incidence of Patients Presenting with Rupture

Author	Year	Juxta/ Pararenal	Paraanastomotic
Plate et al.[37]	1985	—	54.5%
Crawford et al.[13]	1986	7%	—
Qvarfordt et al.[2]	1986	4%	—
Treiman et al.[38]	1988	—	33.3%
Curl et al.[6]	1992	—	14.3%
Edwards et al.[21]	1992	—	0%*

*By ultrasonography

Perfusion of the kidneys may be a useful adjunct in complex cases. Different techniques and types of fluid have been described.[4,9,54–56] Presently, renal perfusion to protect from ischemia is used selectively and is recommended particularly for patients at higher risk of renal failure (i.e., renal dysfunction, long clamping time). Most authors use cold solutions of dextrose or Ringer's lactate and/or external cooling of the kidney with iced slush when renal ischemia greater than 30 minutes is anticipated or when preoperative renal insufficiency is present.[3,4,55–57]

RESULTS

Juxtarenal and Pararenal

As seen earlier in this chapter, juxtarenal and pararenal aneurysms are similar in their presentation, diagnosis, and surgical treatment. The results obtained with their treatment are also similar (Table 7-2). Two recent large series have shown very favorable results in terms of mortality, comparable with those obtained with infrarenal aortic aneurysms.[2,4] Morbidity, however, remains high. In both series, mortality was around 1.5 percent and major morbidity around 30 percent. Similar results were obtained also by Shepard et al.,[3] who found no significantly different mortality and morbidity in complex aortic aneurysms—juxtarenal and pararenal, large infrarenal, obese patients—compared with simple, straightforward aneurysms approached either retroperitoneally or transperitoneally. In their series of 35 juxtarenal and pararenal aneurysms,

mortality for elective repair was 0 percent.[3] Amundsen et al.[11] found that extension of an aortic aneurysm above the renal arteries was not a predictor of perioperative mortality in a series of 444 aneurysms prospectively evaluated.

RENAL DYSFUNCTION AND PROTECTION

The problem of renal ischemia is significantly increased in pararenal aneurysms. The incidence of temporary renal insufficiency after suprarenal clamping ranges from 12 to 31 percent in the literature, and the combined incidence of temporary and permanent dialysis averages 5.5 percent.[4] When local renal hypothermia was used in the series of Allen et al.,[4] postoperative dialysis was not required in any patient. However, this observation has not been made by others.[2] Renal failure was the most common cause of early death in the series of Crawford et al.,[13] and was responsible for 62 percent of all fatalities. Clamp time correlated significantly with renal insufficiency in this series. Other series have shown that renal failure is one of the most common causes of early death.[8] From the literature, it appears that the selective use of cold renal perfusion may contribute to reducing the incidence of perioperative renal complications.

O'Hara et al.,[58] in a series of abdominal aortic aneurysms involving the renal arteries feeding horseshoe kidneys, found that the need for postoperative dialysis significantly correlated with preoperative abnormal renal function. They used cold Ringer's lactate perfusion to protect the renal parenchyma. Svensson et al.,[56] in reviewing Crawford's experience with thoracoabdominal aortic aneurysm repair, showed that intraoperative perfusion of the kidneys correlated with a lower incidence of postoperative renal failure. They found that the kidney tolerates a short period of ischemia well (<45 minutes) but should be protected with cold perfusion when prolonged clamping is needed or when renal dysfunction is present preoperatively.

SPINAL CORD ISCHEMIA

The greater medullary artery (Adamkiewicz) originates from the segment of the aorta between T9 and T12 in 75 percent of cases.[59–61] Portions of this segment of aorta will be at risk

Table 7-2. Results Obtained in Juxtarenal and Pararenal Aneurysm Management in the Literature

Author	Year	N	Mortality	Renal Failure (Permanent)	Cord Ischemia
Stoney et al.[8]	1984	30*	3.3%	NS	NS
Crawford et al.[13]	1986	101[†]	7%	7%	NS
Qvarfordt et al.[2]	1986	77	1.3%	2.5%	0%
Shepard et al.[3]	1991	35	0%	0%	0%
Poulias et al.[14]	1992	38*	5.2%	10.4%	0%
Breckwoldt et al.[10]	1992	23	NS[‡]	0%	0%
Allen et al.[4]	1993	65	1.5%	0%	1.5%

*Only juxtarenal aneurysms.
[†]Includes 5 paranastomotic aneurysms.
[‡]Mortality in this series was 1 of 39 (2.6%) for all aortic cases with suprarenal clamping.
NS-not specified

with supraceliac clamping. One would therefore expect an increased risk of spinal cord ischemia when a pararenal aneurysm is resected. However, this complication is reported at 0.1 to 0.3 percent incidence,[59–61] similar to the risk reported for infrarenal aortic surgery. The fact that an infrarenal anastomosis often can be performed even with supraceliac clamping may be important in avoiding permanent exclusion of lumbar vessels. In addition, the short clamp time for the proximal anastomosis, the reduced blood loss, and the frequent ability to avoid visceral implantation probably also play a role. Type IV thoracoabdominal aneurysms, which involve the suprarenal aorta more extensively, require visceral implantation, lumbar exclusion, and increased clamp time and blood loss and have a higher incidence of spinal cord ischemia—4 percent in Crawford's experience.[55,62] Maintenance of adequate collateral spinal cord circulation (e.g., through the hypogastric arteries) is also important in the prevention of paraparesis/paraplegia in abdominal aortic surgery.[59]

CONCOMITANT VISCERAL LESIONS

The management of concomitant renal lesions during infrarenal aortic reconstructions remains controversial. This continues to be a very important issue in the treatment of juxtarenal, pararenal, and perhaps paraanastomotic aneurysms due to the increased incidence of renal artery disease in these situations and the role of renal dysfunction in mortality. In aneurysms that require replacement of part of the visceral aorta, all diseased renal and visceral vessels should be revascularized.[2,9,63] However, the treatment of asymptomatic renal artery stenosis when infrarenal graft placement is possible remains controversial. Specific prospective data are not available on the combined repair of either juxtarenal or paraanastomotic aneurysms and renal artery stenosis. Many authors agree that asymptomatic lesions should be treated if greater than 75 to 80 percent diameter reduction, if greater than 50 percent diameter reduction in a solitary kidney, or if bilateral lesions are present. Moreover, a single lesion should be treated if present in a symptomatic patient (hypertension, renal dysfunction).[64–67] Preliminary data on the natural history of renal artery stenosis suggest progressive renal parenchymal loss develops in untreated patients.[68] Consideration should be given to repair of an asymptomatic severe stenosis if the surgeon is experienced in renal reconstruction and can anticipate good results. If technical difficulties in the treatment of a lesion are anticipated, asymptomatic solitary lesions are not treated at present.

Paraanastomotic Aneurysms

Results in the treatment of paraanastomotic aneurysms are less favorable than those which are juxtarenal or pararenal. Mortality can be as high as 17 percent in elective cases (Table 7-3). While some large series report a lower mortality (8 percent),[38] it seems that treatment of paraanastomotic aneurysms carries a higher surgical risk when compared with primary operations (see Tables 7-2 and 7-3). Several factors probably account for this increase. The patients are generally older

Table 7-3. Results Obtained in Paraanastomotic Aneurysm Elective Management in the Literature

Author	Year	Cases in the Series	Cases Treated	Mortality	Major Morbidity
Szilagyi et al.[18]	1975	4	3	0%	NS
Clagett et al.[72]	1983	2	2	0%	0%
Fulenwider et al.[23]	1983	11	11	36.3%	18%
Treiman et al.[38]	1988	12*	12	8.3%	33.3%
Griffiths et al.[71]	1990	2†	2	0%	50%
Edwards et al.[21]	1992	11	3	0%	NS
Curl et al.[6]	1992	18	18	17%	11.1%

*Two cases were at the iliac anastomosis.
†These cases were treated urgently but did not show frank rupture at surgery.
NS-not specified

Table 7-4. Results in Ruptured Paraanastomotic Aneurysms

Author	Year	Cases in the Series	Cases with Rupture	Mortality	Major Morbidity
Olsen et al.[69]	1966	4	4	100%	—
Szilagyi et al.[18]	1975	4	1	100%	—
Plate et al.[37]	1985	11	6	100%	—
Treiman et al.[38]	1988	18*	6	66.6%	—
Curl et al.[6]	1992	21	3	66.6%	—

*One case was at the iliac anastomosis

since the time for paraanastomotic aneurysm development averages 5.2 to 12 years from primary procedures.[6,21,23,38] Rupture of paraanastomotic, particularly false, aneurysms is also relatively frequent and occurs in 14.3 up to 55 percent of cases,[6,18,19,37,38] while rupture in juxtarenal and pararenal aneurysms is reported to be around 4 to 7 percent[2,13] (see Table 7-1). Experience with ruptured cases has been reported by other authors.[69] In these cases, mortality is usually very high[6,7,18,19,37,38,69] (Table 7-4). One must remember that these operations are reinterventions, and operative times, blood loss, and technical complications can be expected to be higher. These factors may all contribute to increased operative and perioperative mortality.[23,70] Expeditious aortic control is more difficult in paraanastomotic aneurysms due to the scar tissue present.

Mortality is related to the extent of proximal aortic involvement. Results are best when an infrarenal or pararenal anastomosis can be performed. Replacement of the visceral aorta with visceral revascularization is associated with the highest mortality, often related to perioperative blood loss. Use of the existing graft for distal anastomosis facilitates the operation and reduces postoperative complications.

The good results with elective paraanastomotic aneurysms, contrasted with difficulties encountered when emergent operation is required, suggest that some follow-up program of patients with aortic grafts is indicated. While the exact nature of the program has not been established, assumptions can be made from existing data. True aneurysms occur in patients with a history of aneurysmal disease and usually present 5 to 10 years after the initial procedure. False aneurysms are less predictable but also usually occur late after aortic grafts. False aneurysms are more common in occlusive disease when an end-to-side proximal anastomosis is performed or when some type of aortic endarterectomy is performed. Finally, the fact that an infrarenal anastomosis is possible in a significant number of these reoperative cases suggests that poor aortic wall was incorporated in the proximal suture line.

Yearly physical examination of all patients with aortic prostheses is indicated. Any suggestion of an abnormality on physical examination should prompt an imaging study. At 5 years, patients should be considered for a routine CT scan to evaluate their visceral aorta and proximal suture line. Subsequent follow-up at 3- to 5-year intervals, or more often, should allow early detection.

All false aneurysms should be electively repaired when detected. Aneurysmal change in the visceral aorta should be treated in the standard fashion, with intervention for rapid growth or size greater than 5 cm in diameter. Finally, placement of the proximal anastomosis near the renal orifices at the original surgery will reduce the incidence of later paraanastomotic problems.

REFERENCES

1. Stoney RJ, Rabahie GN: Management of juxtarenal and pararenal aortic atherosclerosis. *In* Bergan JJ, Yao JST (eds): Aortic Surgery. Philadelphia, W. B. Saunders Company, 1989, pp 161–173.
2. Qvarfordt PG, Stoney RJ, Reilly LM, et al: Management of pararenal aneurysms of the abdominal aorta. J Vasc Surg 1986;3:84.
3. Shepard AD, Tollefson DFJ, Reddy DJ, et al: Left flank retroperitoneal exposure: A technical aid to complex aortic reconstruction J Vasc Surg 1991;4:283.
4. Allen BT, Anderson CB, Rubin BG, et al: Preservation of reanl function in juxtarenal and suprareanl abdominal aortic aneurysm repair. J Vasc Surg 1993;17:948.
5. Crawford ES, Snyder DM, Cho GC, Rohem JOF: Progress in treatment of thoracoabdominal and abdominal aortic aneurysms involving celiac, superior mesenteric and renal arteris. Ann Surg 1978;188:404.
6. Curl GR, Faggioli GL, Stella A, et al: Aneurysmal change at or above the proximal anastomosis after infrarenal aortic grafting. J Vasc Surg 1992;16:855
7. Curl GR, Faggioli GL, Ricotta JJ: Proximal paraanastomotic aortic aneurysms. *In* Veith FJ (ed): Current Critical Problems in Vascular Surgery. St Louis, Quality Medical Publishers, 1993, pp 240–246.
8. Stoney RJ, Skioldebrand CG, Qvarfordt PG, et al: Juxtarenal aortic atherosclerosis: Surgical experience and functional results. Ann Surg 1984; 200:345.
9. Green RM, Ricotta JJ, Ouriel K, DeWeese JA: Results of supraceliac aortic clamping in the difficult resection of infrarenal abdominal aortic aneurysm. J Vasc Surg 1989;9:125.
10. Breckwoldt WL, Mackey WC, Belkin M, O'Donnell TF: The effect of suprarenal cross-clampingon abdominal aortic aneurysm repair. Arch Surg 1992; 127:520.
11. Amundsen S, Skjaerven R, Trippestad A, et al:Abdominal aortic aneurysms: A study of factors influencing postoperative mortality. Eur J Vasc Surg 1989;3:405.
12. Vowden P, Wilkinson D, Ausobsky JR, Kester RC: A comparison of three imaging techniques in the assessment of an abdominal aortic aneurysm. J Cardiovasc Surg 1989;30:891.
13. Crawford ES, Beckett WC, Greer MS: Juxtarenal infrarenal abdominal aortic aneurysms: Special diagnostic and therapeutic considerations. Ann Surg 1986;203:661.
14. Poulias GE, Doundoulakis N, Skoutas B, et al: Juxtarenal abdominal aneurysmectomy. J Cardiovasc Surg 1992;33:324.
15. Todd GJ, Nowyrgrod R, Benvenisty A, et al: The accuracy of CT scanning in the diagnosis of abdominal and thoracoabdominal aortic aneurysms. J Vasc Surg 1991;13:302.
16. Papanicolau N, Wittemberg J, Ferrucci JT, et al: Preoperative evaluation of abdominal aortic aneurysms by computed tomography. AJR 1986;146: 711.
17. Crawford ES: Thoracoabdominal and abdominal aortic aneurysms involving renal, superior mesenteric and celiac arteries. Ann Surg 1974;179: 763.
18. Szilagyi DE, Smith RF, Elliott JP, et al: Anastomotic aneurysms after vascular reconstruction: Problem of incidence, etiology and treatement. Surgery 1975;78:800.
19. Szilagyi DE, Elliott JP, Smith RF, et al: A thirty-year survey of the reconstructive surgical treatment of aortoiliac occlusive disease. J Vasc Surg 1986; 3:421.
20. Millili JJ, Lanes JS, Nemir P: A study of anastomotic aneurysms following aortofemoral prosthetic bypass. Ann Surg 1980;192:69.
21. Edwards JM, Teefey SA, Zierler RE, Kohler TR: Intraabdominal paraanastomotic aneurysms after aortic bypass grafting. J Vasc Surg 1992;15: 344.
22. Van den Akker PJ, Brand R, van Schilfgaard R, et al: False aneurysms after prosthetic reconstruction-sfor aortoiliac obstructive disease. Ann Surg 1989; 210:658.
23. Fulenwider JT, Smith RB, Johnson RW, et al: Reoperative abdominal arterial surgery—A ten-year experience. Surgery 1983;93:20.
24. Ad Hoc Committee on Reporting Standards, Society for Vascular Surgery, North American Chapter, International Society for Cardiovascular Surgery: Suggested standards for reporting on arterial aneurysms. J Vasc Surg 1991;13:452.
25. Sterpetti AV, Feldhaus RJ, Schultz RD, Blair EA: Identification of abdominal aortic aneurysm patients with different clinical features and clinical outcomes. Am J Surg 1988;154:466.

26. Dennis JW, Littooy FN, Greisler HP, Baker WH: Anastomotic pseudoaneurysms: A continuinig late complication of vascular reconstructive procedures. Arch Surg 1986;121:314.

27. Drury JK, Leiberman DP, Gilmour DG, Pollock JG: Operation for late complications of aortic grafts. Surg Gynecol Obstet 1986;103:251.

28. Amparo EG, Hoddick WK, Hricak H, et al: Comparison of magnetic resonance imaging and ultrasonography in the evaluation of abdominal aortic aneurysms. Radiology 1985;154:451.

29. Flak B, Li DKB, Ho BYB, et al: Magnetic resonance imaging of aneurysms of the abdominal aorta. AJR 1985;144:991.

30. Lee JK, Ling D, Heiken JP, et al: Magnetic resonance imaging of abdominal aortic aneurysms. AJR 1984;143:1197.

31. Ricotta JJ: Venous anomalies encountered during aortic reconstruction. In Ernst CB, Stanley JC (eds): Current Therapy in Vascular Surgery, 2nd ed. Philadelphia, B. C. Decker, 1991, pp 289–292.

32. Rapp JH, Pan XM: Magnetic resonance immaging, ultrasonography and computed tomography in assessment of abdominal aortic aneurysm. In Ernst CB, Stanley JC (eds): Current Therapy in Vascular Surgery, 2nd ed. Philadephia, B. C. Decker, 1991, pp 255–260.

33. Stella A, Gargiulo M, Faggioli GL, et al: Postoperative course of inflammatory abdominal aortic aneurysms. Ann Vasc Surg 1993;

34. Zeman RK, Fox SH, Silverman XX, et al: Helical (spiral) CT scan of the abdomen. AJR 1993; 160:719.

35. Costello P, Ecker CP, Tello R, Hartnell GG: Assessment of the thoracic aorta by spiral CT. AJR 1992;158:1127.

36. Mark A, Moss AA, Lusby R, Kaiser JA: CT evaluation of complications of abdominal aortic surgery. Radiology 1982;145:409.

37. Plate G, Hollier LA, O'Brien P, et al: Recurrent aneurysms and late vascular complications following repair of abdominal aortic aneurysms. Arch Surg 1985;120:590.

38. Treiman GS, Weaver FA, Cossman DV, et al: Anastomotic false aneurysms of the abdominal aorta and the iliac arteries. J Vasc Surg 1988;8:268.

39. Nevelsteen A, Suy R: Anastomotic false aneurysms of the abdominal aorta and the iliac arteries (letter). J Vasc Surg 1989;10:595.

40. Faggioli GL, Ricotta JJ: Aortic graft infection. In Veith FJ (ed): Current Critical Problems in Vascular Surgery, vol 4. St Louis, Quality Medical Publishers, 1992, pp 371–380.

41. Lawrence PF, Dries DJ, Alazraki N, Albo D: Indium 111–labeled leukocyte scanning for detection of prosthetic vascular graft infection. J Vasc Surg 1985;2:165.

42. Sauer L, Stoney RJ: Management of juxtarenal

aortic occlusive disease by transabdominal exposure of the pararenal and suprarenal aorta by medial visceral rotation. In Ernst CB, Stanley JC (eds): Current Therpay in Vascular Surgery, 2nd ed. Philadelphia, B. C. Decker, 1991, pp 406–409.

43. DeBakey ME, McCollum CH: Surgical treatment of nonruptured infrarenal and juxtarenal aortic aneurysms. In Ernst CB, Stanley JC (eds): Current Therpay in Vascular Surgery, 2nd ed. Philadelphia, B. C. Decker, 1991, pp 261–264.

44. Yao JST, Flinn WR, Rizzo RJ, et al: Recurrent aortic and anastomotic aneurysms. In Bergan JJ, Yao JST (eds): Aortic Surgery. Philadelphia, W. B. Saunders Company, 1989, pp 305–316.

45. Rutherford RB: Suprarenal aortic surgery: Exposures and techniques. In Veith FJ (ed): Current Critical Problems in Vascular Surgery, vol 5. St Louis, Quality Medical Publishers, 1993, pp 271–277.

46. Starret RW, Stoney RJ: Juxtarenal aortic occlusion. Surgery 1974;76:890.

47. Williams GM, Ricotta JJ, Zinner M, Burdick JF: The extended retroperitoneal approach for treatment of extensive atherosclerosis of the aorta and renal vessels. Surgery 1980;88:846.

48. Ricotta JJ, Williams GM: Endarterectomy of the upper abdominal aorta and visceral arteries through an extraperitoneal approach. Arch Surg 1980;192:633.

49. O'Mara C, Williams GM: Extended retroperitoneal approach for abdominal aortic aneurysm repair. In Bergan JJ, Yao JST (eds): Aneurysms: Diagnosis and Treatment. New York, Grune & Stratton, 1982, pp 327–343.

50. Pokrowski AV: Nonspecific aortoarteritis. In Rutherford RB (ed): Vascular Surgery, 3rd ed. Philadelphia, W. B. Saunders Company, 1989, pp 217–237.

51. DeBakey ME, Crawford ES, Garrett HE, et al: Surgical considerations on the treatment of aneurysms of the thoracoabdominal aorta. Ann Surg 1965;162:650.

52. Cohen JR, Mannick JA, Couch NP, Whittemore AD: Abdominal aortic aneurysm repair in patients with preoperative reanl failure. J Vasc Surg 1986; 3:867.

53. Gomes MMR, Bernatz PE: Aortoiliac occlusive disease: Extension cephalad to origin of reanl arteries with surgical considerations and results. Arch Surg 1970;101:161.

54. Nunn DB, Dupree EL, Renard A: A new method for preserving the kidney during aortic grafting and reimplantation of renal arteries. Surg Gynecol Obstet 1974;139:923.

55. Svensson LG, Crawford ES: Aortic dissection and aortic aneurysm surgery: Clinical observations, experimental investigations and statistical analysis, part III. Curr Probl Surg 1993;3:163.

56. Svensson LG, Crawford ES, Hess KR, et al: Thoracoabdominal aortic aneurysms associated with celiac,

superior mesenteric and renal artery occlusive disease: Methods and analysis of results in 271 patients. J Vasc Surg 1992;16:378.

57. Hollier LH: Thoracoabdominal aortic aneurysms associated with celiac, superior mesenteric and renal artery occlusive disease: Methods and analysis of results in 271 patients (discussion). J Vasc Surg 1992;16:378.

58. O'Hara PJ, Hakain AG, Hertzer NR, et al: Surgical management of aortic aneurysms and coexistent horseshoe kidney: Review of a 31 year experience. J Vasc Surg 1993;17:940.

59. Picone AL, Green RM, Ricotta JJ, et al: Spinal cord ischemia following operations on the abdominal aorta. J Vasc Surg 1986;3:94.

60. Gloviczki P, Cross SA, Stanson AW, et al: Ischemic injury to the spinal cord or lumbosacral plexus after aortoiliac reconstruction. Am J Surg 1991; 161:131.

61. Connolly JE, Sise MJ, Bronwell DA: Paraplegia after elective infrarenal aortic surgery. In Veith FJ (ed): Current Critical Problems in Vascular Surgery, vol 4. St Louis, Quality Medical Publishers, 1992, pp 236–241.

62. Svensson LG, Crawford ES: Aortic dissection and aortic aneurysm surgery: Clinical observations, experimental investigations and statistical analysis, part I. Curr Probl Surg 1992;821.

63. Muller-Wiefel H, Langkau G, Fahrenkemper T: Indications and techniques for renal revascularization during abdominal aneurysm repair. In Veith FJ (ed): Current Critical Problems in Vascular Surgery, vol 5. St Louis, Quality Medical Publishers, 1993, pp 247–255.

64. Tarazi RY, Hertzer NR, Beven EG, et al: Simultaneous aortic reconstruction and renal revascularization: Risk factors and late results in eighty-nine patients. J Vasc Surg 1987;5:707.

65. Sterpetti AV, Schultz RD, Feldhaus RJ, Peetz DJ: Aortic and renal atherosclerotic disease. Surg Gynecol Obstet 1986;163:54.

66. Hollier LH: Special problems in aortic aneurysm surgery. In Bergan JJ, Yao JST (eds): Techniques in Arterial Surgery. Philadelphia, W. B. Saunders Company, 1990, pp 56–69.

67. Perry OM, Silane MF: Management of renovascular problems during aortic operations. Arch Surg 1984;119:681.

68. Zierler RE, Bergelin RO, Isaacson JA, Strandness DE: Natural history of atherosclerotic renal artery stenosis: A prospective study with duplex ultrasonography. J Vasc Surg 1994;19(2):250.

69. Olsen WR, DeWeese MS, Fry WJ: False aneurysm of abdominal aorta. A late complication of aortic aneurysmectomy. Arch Surg 1966;92:123.

70. Crawford ES, Manning LG, Kelly TF: "Redo" surgery after operations for aneurysm and occlusion of the abdominal aorta. Surgery 1977;81:41.

71. Griffiths D, Scott DJA, Horrocks M: Spontaneous rupture of suprarenal aneurysms: A late sequela to infrarenal aortic aneurysm repair. Eur J Vasc Surg 1990;4:431.

72. Clagett GP, Salander JM, Eddleman WL, et al: Dilatation of knitted Dacron prosthesis and anastomotic false aneurysms: Etiologic considerations. Surgery 1983;93:9.

Thoracoabdominal Aortic Aneurysm

HAZIM J. SAFI
STEFANO BARTOLI

A thoracoabdominal aortic aneurysm is a dilatation of the aorta that involves the thoracic aorta and the abdominal aorta to varying extents. This type of aneurysm presents a technical challenge for the vascular surgeon, and until recently, repair of these aneurysms carried high rates of morbidity and mortality. The remaining most vexing problem regarding thoracoabdominal aortic aneurysm repair is the development of neurologic deficit (paraplegia or paraparesis) following surgical repair. In the last 10 years, many methods have been tried to protect the spinal cord during surgical intervention.[1,2] These techniques include shunts, cardiopulmonary bypass, left atrial to left femoral bypass via a BioMedicus pump, cerebrospinal fluid drainage both intraoperatively and postoperatively, and systemic and intrathecal drugs. These different methods have met with varied degrees of success.

It is known that the cause of neurologic deficit is multifactorial. The extent and type of thoracoabdominal aortic aneurysm, aortic clamp time, age of the patient, previous proximal surgery, and renal failure may all play a role. In this chapter we will review both the past and current methods used to protect the spinal cord at our institution and their impact on the incidence of paraplegia and paraparesis, particularly in patients with high-risk thoracoabdominal aortic aneurysms. We will describe in detail the technical aspects of thoracoabdominal aortic aneurysm repair and some of the modifications that have made the operation a safer one.

CLASSIFICATION

In the analysis of thoracoabdominal aortic aneurysm repair by different authors, confusion arises from the lack of a universal classification as well as the lumping together of descending thoracic and thoracoabdominal aortic aneurysm results. The importance of a thoracoabdominal aortic aneurysm classification is that there is a strong correlation between the extent of an aneurysm and the incidence of neurologic deficit following surgical repair. The most recent classification used at our institution was named after Crawford. Type I is a thoracoabdominal aortic aneurysm that extends from just distal to the left subclavian artery to the level of the celiac axis and also may involve the aorta opposite the superior mesenteric artery above the renal arteries. Type II extends from just distal to the left subclavian artery and involves the infrarenal abdominal aorta to the level of the aortic bifurcation. Type III extends from the middle of the descending aorta as defined by the sixth intercostal space and tapers to just above the infrarenal abdominal aorta to the iliac bifurcation. Type IV extends from the level of the twelfth intercostal space and tapers to above the iliac bifurcation (Fig. 8-1).

The incidence of neurologic deficit as it occurs within the four thoracoabdominal aortic aneurysm types is as follows[3]: For type I, it is about 15 percent, but if the etiology is dissection, then the incidence rises to 24 percent; for type II, it is 31 percent, and with dissection, it is 33 percent; for

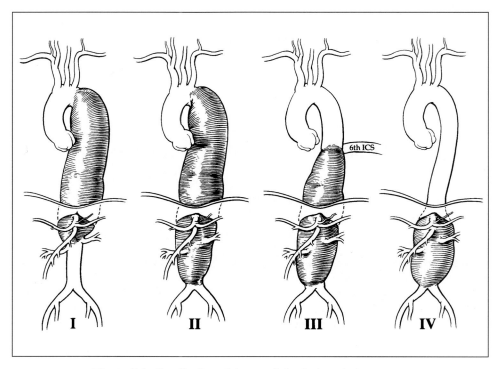

Figure 8-1. Classification of thoracoabdominal aortic aneurysms.

type III, the overall incidence is 7 percent; and for type IV, it is 4 percent. In certain cases, an aneurysm cannot be precisely classified. For example, an aneurysm that extends from the eighth intercostal space and tapers to just above the level of the celiac axis does not fall within any of the previously defined types. Such aneurysms have to be described according to anatomic landmarks in the chest and abdomen. A careful anatomic description of each thoracoabdominal aortic aneurysm will dispel confusion about the incidence of paraplegia following surgical repair.

NATURAL HISTORY

Prior to 1986 and a report by Crawford and DeNatale,[4] there was no study reflecting the natural history of thoracoabdominal aortic aneurysms. Crawford and DeNatale explored the nonsurgical management of patients with thoracoabdominal aortic aneurysm. Either these patients were at too high risk to be operated on due to associated disease or the patients actually refused operative repair of their aneurysms. There were 94 patients who were followed nonoperatively over a period of 25 years. The 2-year survival rate was 24 percent, with half the deaths due to rupture. Despite valid criticism of this study—that it was limited by reflecting only those thoracoabdominal aortic aneurysm patients who either refused the operation or were too sick to be operated on—the results revealed the same rate of rupture and death as patients with untreated aneurysms located in other segments of the aorta. A study of 607 patients who underwent thoracoabdominal aortic aneurysm repair revealed 70 percent survival at 2 years and 59 percent at 5 years.

ETIOLOGY

The most common etiology of thoracoabdominal aortic aneurysms is medial degeneration (Fig. 8-2). Microscopic examination generally shows a

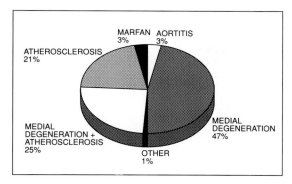

Figure 8-2. Etiology of thoracoabdominal aortic aneurysms. MD = Medial degeneration; ATH = Atherosclerosis.

loss and destruction of the elastic fibers and a increase in the mucopolysaccharide level. If the medial degenerative process is advanced, the smooth muscle is also affected, and the pathologic process is labeled as *medial necrosis*. Atherosclerosis, an intimal disease, can occur superimposed over the medial degenerative process. These changes can develop in patients with Marfan syndrome, in patients with aortic dissection, or in patients with other connective tissue disorders such as Ehlers-Danlos syndrome, as well as in older patients. Histologically, one cannot differentiate among aortic wall segments taken from a patient with Marfan syndrome, a patient with a medial degenerative process, or a patient with aortic dissection.

Marfan syndrome is a hereditary disease caused by a change in chromosome 15 that affects 50 percent of children born to parents with this disorder.[5] It is characterized by musculoskeletal changes, ocular deformity, and cardiovascular pathology in the form of aneurysm and/or dissection, aortic insufficiency, and/or mitral valve regurgitation.[6] Other connective tissue disorders such as Ehlers-Danlos syndrome are very rare. Aortitis is a combination of many inflammatory processes and involves diseases of the media and adventia such as Takayasu's syndrome, which has two forms, one occlusive and the other aneurysmal. Giant cell aortitis is another inflammatory process that affects the aorta.

Aortic dissection is the second most common cause of aneurysm in the thoracic and thoracoabdominal aorta and is due to the same medial de-

generative process described above (Fig. 8-3). It is associated with high blood pressure and most frequently develops in patients with Marfan syndrome but is sometimes due to trauma.[7] Survival studies show that death occurs within a few hours to 2 weeks in 74 percent of patients with thoracoabdominal aortic aneurysm dissection; hence the initial two weeks are known as the *acute phase* and the following period as the *chronic phase*.

SYMPTOMS AND SIGNS

Thoracoabdominal aortic aneurysms remain asymptomatic for extended periods of time.[8–9] The most common complaint is chest or abdomen pain. Pain in the chest occurs between the shoulder blades and usually as flank pain in the abdomen. Other symptoms are related to pressure on adjacent organs and are due to an extension of the aneurysm or rupture. Pressure on the trachea can cause stridor, wheezing, and cough. Pressure on the esophagus can cause dysphagia. Jaundice can be manifested as a result of pressure on the porta hepatis. Recurrent laryngeal nerve pressure causes hoarseness. An aneurysm can cause back pain due to pressure on the vertebral body and can cause erosion. The first clinical manifestation of a thoracoabdominal aortic aneurysm may be embolization to the lower extremities, especially to the foot (trash foot).

In an asymptomatic patient, the diagnosis of thoracoabdominal aortic aneurysm is usually suggested during a routine chest examination (Fig. 8-4), routine checkup, or investigation of heart or lung disease.

Figure 8-3. Dissection of thoracoabdominal aortic aneurysms.

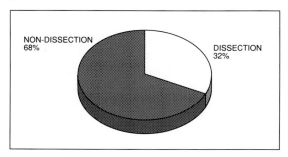

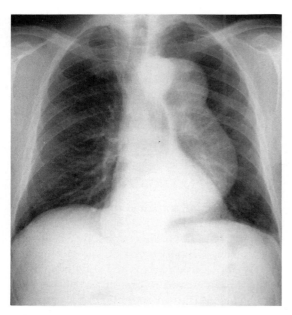

Figure 8-4. Chest x-ray of a thoracoabdominal aortic aneurysm.

When thoracoabdominal aortic aneurysm is suspected, the best noninvasive method for determining the diagnosis is computed tomography (CT). The CT scan of the chest and abdomen is essential in order to detect other associated aneurysms; 12.6 percent of aortic aneurysms are multiple.[10] CT scan provides an accurate measurement of the aortic diameter and characteristics of the aortic wall, the extent of the aneurysm, and the inside of the aortic lumen (thrombus), as well as assessment of surrounding organs in the chest and abdomen. The major disadvantages of CT are the cost and exposure to irradiation. In addition, any distinction between proximal thoracoabdominal aortic aneurysm and distal arch aneurysm is virtually impossible, and renal and visceral artery stenosis cannot be detected (Fig. 8-5).

Magnetic resonance imaging (MRI) is still evolving in its application for patients with aneurysmal disease. It has the same accuracy rate as the CT scan, and in addition, it can delineate major branch stenosis. The disadvantages are the high cost and the time required to perform the test, during which a patient has to remain stationary. MRI is contraindicated for patients with metallic clips or pacemakers and in patients who are claustrophobic (Fig, 8-6).

Aortography of the entire aorta supplies an important preoperative evaluation of the aorta, identifying stenosis or occlusion of branch vessels (Fig. 8-7). An aortogram provides a better anatomic delineation of the aorta than any other method. The drawbacks of routine aortography are that it is an invasive procedure with the potential complication of groin hematoma, injury to the femoral arteries, or possible dissection. Contrast media can have a deleterious effect on the kidneys, but this complication is less likely to occur if the patient is well hydrated (Table 8-1). Renal function is evaluated 24 hours after aortography, and if it is abnormal, surgery is postponed until renal function returns to normal.

Most patients with thoracoabdominal aortic aneurysm are affected by other associated diseases (Fig. 8-8). Five percent of our symptomatic patients have abnormal coagulation profiles. Cardiac evaluation includes transthoracic echocardiography, important in screening the patient for ejection fraction, and transesophageal echocardiography to best determine aortic size. In patients with a past history of ischemic heart disorders, a thallium stress test is important to detect coronary artery disease. If the test is positive or the patient is symptomatic for coronary artery disease, coronary angiography is performed. If the coronary artery disease requires surgical treatment, then coronary artery bypass grafting is done first. Six weeks later, the thoracoabdominal aortic aneurysm is repaired. For patients above age 60 or those who are symptomatic for carotid artery disease, a duplex scan

Table 8-1. Intravenous Hydration Before Aortography

Intravenously, the night before aortography:

25 g	Mannitol 25%
100 mEq	Sodium bicarbonate 8.4%
1000 cc	Dextrose 5% NS

Continue until 2 hours after examination

In patients with history of allergy
   Steroids
   Histamine blocker
   H_2 blocker
Orally 12 and 2 hours prior to examination

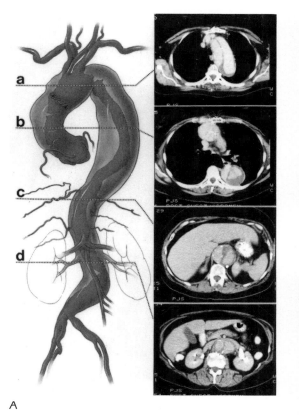

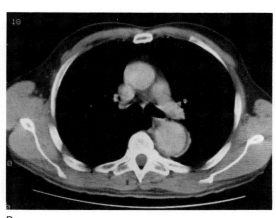

B

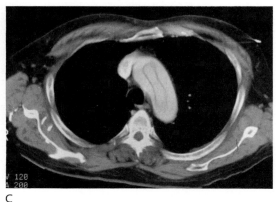

C

A

Figure 8-5. (**A**) CT scan and diagram of thoracoab-dominal aortic aneurysm with dissection. (**B**) CT scan of a thoracoabdominal aortic aneurysm. (**C**) CT scan of dissection involving the aortic arch.

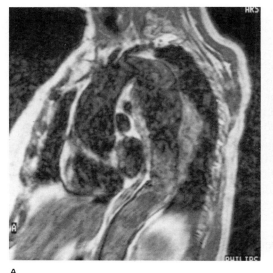

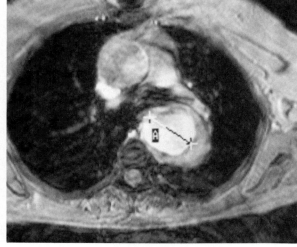

A   B

Figure 8-6. (**A**) MRI of thoracoabdominal aortic aneurysm, longitudinal view. (**B**) MRI of thoracoabdominal aortic aneurysm, transverse view.

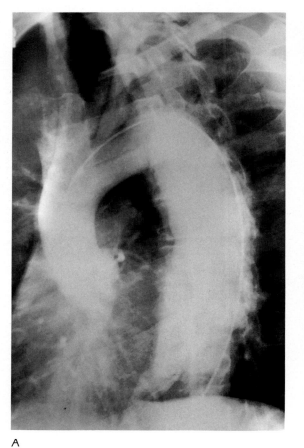

A

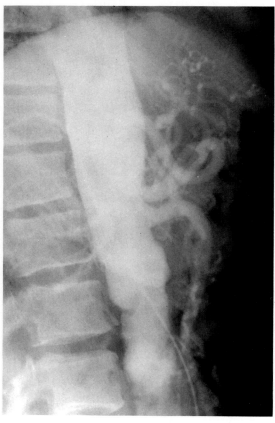

B

Figure 8-7. (A) Aortogram of thoracic portion of thoracoabdominal aorta. **(B)** Aortogram of lateral abdominal portion of thoracoabdominal aorta.

Figure 8-8. Associated diseases. COPD = Chronic obstructive pulmonary disease; ATH = Atherosclerosis; CD = Cerebrovascular disease; RI = Renal insufficiency.

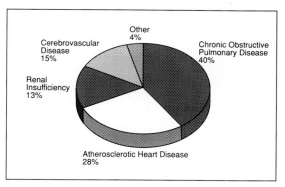

screening test of the carotid arteries is important. In patients in whom the duplex scan is positive or in those who are symptomatic, carotid arteriography is performed. If the carotid artery has over 90 percent stenosis, a carotid endarterectomy is done, and a few days later the thoracoabdominal aortic aneurysm is repaired. Magnetic resonance angiography (MRA) is being considered as an additional screening test for patients with carotid artery disease.

ANESTHESIA MONITORING

We routinely insert a double-lumen or double endotracheal tube for selective collapse of the left lung during repair of the thoracoabdominal aortic aneurysm and bilateral arterial lines for blood pressure monitoring. Blood pressure cannot be monitored from the left radial artery if the aortic clamp is applied proximal to the left subclavian artery. We insert a Swan-Ganz catheter for monitoring the volume status of the patient, upper extremity and jugular lines for intravenous fluid management, a Foley catheter to monitor urine output; nasopharyngeal and rectal temperature probes are important to monitor core temperature. A cell saver is needed in the operating room to collect blood and reprocess it for subsequent autotransfusion. Also, we are currently evaluating the use of transesophageal echocardiography (TEE) in the management of thoracoabdominal aortic aneurysms. In addition to hemodynamic measurement of the heart, TEE evaluates the junction between the transverse arch and the descending thoracic aorta. If that area contains a large amount of debris or is atherosclerotic, precluding the aortic clamp, cardiopulmonary bypass and profound hypothermia are employed in the repair of thoracoabdominal aortic aneurysms.

The patient is also given prophylactic antibiotics 12 hours prior to surgery. These are continued for 48 hours or until all catheters and chest tubes are removed. Sodium nitroprusside is administered when the proximal clamp is applied and is discontinued prior to release of the aortic clamp with restoration of the flow through the graft. Sodium bicarbonate solution is administered routinely by drip during the period of aortic cross-clamping to prevent acidosis. Currently, we insert the cerebrospinal fluid catheter in the lumbar space between L4 and L5 and drain the cerebrospinal fluid by gravity, keeping the spinal fluid pressure below 10 mmHg intraoperatively. Cerebrospinal fluid drainage is continued postoperatively for 3 days. Also, currently we are reevaluating the usefulness of somatosensory evoked potentials for monitoring spinal cord protection during thoracoabdominal aortic aneurysm repair.

PERIOPERATIVE BLOOD USE

Thoracoabdominal aortic aneurysm surgery is a procedure that must anticipate the need for large amounts of blood and blood components. Cooperation between blood bank personnel and the operating team is essential. Large aneurysms may contain up to 2000 ml of blood, emphasizing the indispensability of saved red blood cells via autotransfusion. Collection and transfusion of blood lost during surgery frequently makes it possible to save up to 45 units of packed washed red blood cells. Throughout the operation, hemoglobin and coagulation parameters are monitored carefully. Activated clotting time is used as a guide for the administration of protamine. Fresh-frozen plasma is administered throughout the operation. Additional fresh-frozen plasma and cryoprecipitate as well as platelets may be needed to correct deficiencies.

OPERATIVE TECHNIQUE

The patient is positioned in the right lateral decubitus position on an air-controlled "bean-bag" with the chest at 90 degrees and the left hip at 60 degrees to allow the easiest approach to the left groin. A left thoracoabdominal incision is made through the sixth intercostal space. Before 1986, the abdominal portion of the incision was a midline laparotomy extended to the xiphoid process and then connected with the thoracic portion of the incision. Blood supply in this area is dependent on the inferior epigastric artery, but the distal third of this artery is not sufficient for vascularization of this area of the chest and abdomen (Fig. 8-9A, B), making it vulnerable to an ischemic event. After 1986, the chest incision was made in between the vertebral border of the scapula and the spine, the incision curving around the angle of the scapula and crossing the thorax into the abdomen toward the umbilicus and, if needed, to the midline below the umbilicus. The sixth rib is always removed in patients with type I or type II thoracoabdominal aortic aneurysm to maximize exposure of the proximal aorta.

Following the skin incision, the latissimus dorsi is cut in half, the serratus anterior is cut flush with the rib attachment, and the rib is removed (Fig. 8-9C, D). The abdominal viscera are rotated medially and extraperitoneally, allowing exposure of the entire abdominal aorta. The diaphragm is split radially to the aortic hiatus. The Omni-Tract self-retaining retractor is put in place, and then the

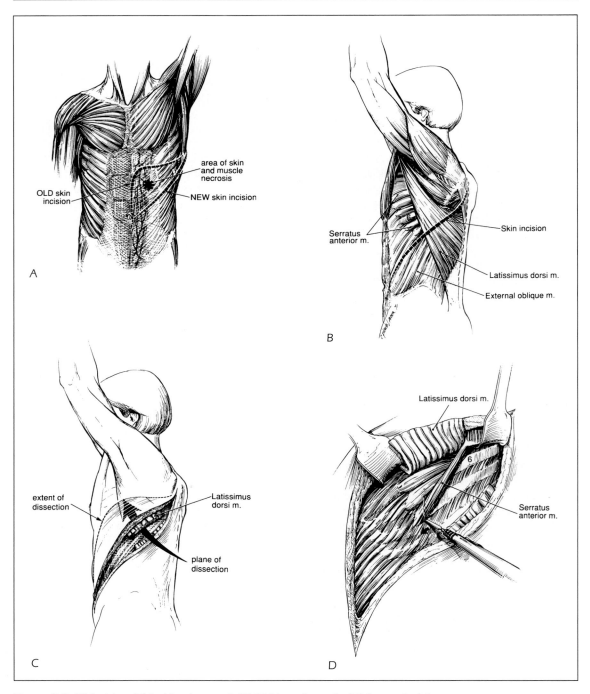

Figure 8-9. (**A**) Incision. (**B**) Incision (see text). (**C**) Division of muscle. (**D**) Removal of rib.

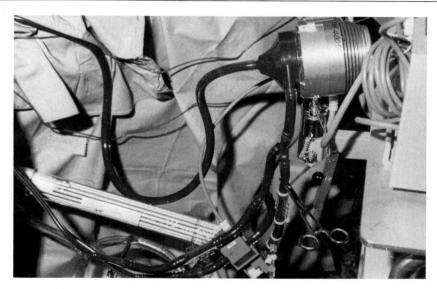

Figure 8-10. Photograph of head of BioMedicus pump, inflow/outflow, and background heat exchanger.

proximal descending thoracic aorta is dissected and separated from the esophagus. During this dissection, the left recurrent laryngeal nerve is protected. Following this, the proximal aorta distal to the left subclavian is transected completely in order to prevent graft esophageal fistula. A longitudinal incision is made in the left groin area in the majority of patients, but on rare occasions, this is done in the right groin. The common femoral artery is exposed and prepared for future cannulation. The pericardium is opened posterior to the left phrenic nerve, exposing the left atrial appendage. Using a pursestring suture and Rummel tourniquet, the venous portion of a 26F USCI aortic cannula is inserted into the left atrial appendage. The arterial end of a BioMedicus pump is inserted into the left or right common femoral artery and secured, and the pump is started (Fig. 8-10). If cannulation of the femoral artery is not possible, then the distal thoracic or abdominal aorta is used instead. At this time, the pump starts with a flow of over 500 ml/min (Fig. 8-11A, B).

An aortic clamp is placed either proximal or distal to the left subclavian artery depending on the anatomic configuration of the aortic aneurysm. Then a second clamp is placed on the descending thoracic aorta above the diaphragm at the level of the eighth intercostal space. The aneurysm is then opened longitudinally using an electrocautery and the walls of the aneurysm are retracted using no. 2 silk retraction sutures. In the event of chronic dissection, the partition between the false and true lumina has to be cut. A woven Dacron tube graft is used to replace the aneurysm. There are different kinds of woven Dacron tube grafts. Some come already albuminized or treated with collagen or gelatin. Any one of these is suitable for replacement. The proximal end of the graft is sutured to the proximal descending thoracic aorta just distal to the left subclavian artery using 3-0 Prolene suture in continuing fashion. Then the proximal anastomosis is checked for hemostasis.

The mid-descending thoracic aortic clamp is then moved down to the infrarenal abdominal aorta, and the remaining aorta is opened longitudinally. Back-bleeding from intercostal arteries T8 to L2 is controlled by no. 3 Fogarty catheters. The orifices of the celiac axis, superior mesenteric artery, and both renal arteries are perfused with oxygenated blood through a 9F Pruitt perfusion cannula using the BioMedicus pump (Figs. 8-11C and 8-12). A side

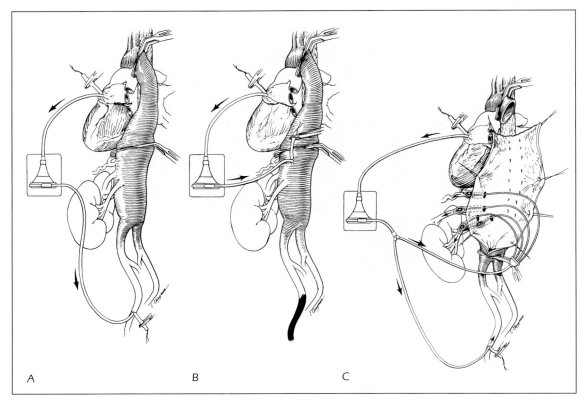

Figure 8-11. (A) Left atrial to left femoral artery bypass. **(B)** Left atrial to distal aorta bypass. **(C)** Visceral perfusion.

hole is cut into the graft, and the intercostal arteries from T8 to L2 are sutured to the graft using running 3-0 Prolene suture. Exceptions occur in the instance of acute dissection or calcified aorta, in which case we ligate the intercostal arteries. Reimplantation of the intercostal arteries of an acutely dissected or calcified aorta always leads to rupture either immediately or in the first 24-hour period postoperatively with catastrophic results.

After reimplantation of the intercostal arteries to the graft, attention is turned toward the visceral arteries. We do not advocate release of the proximal aortic clamp at this point because the flow in these arteries is low and leads to graft clotting. Another side hole is cut into the graft, to which the visceral arteries are reattached in a side-to-side fashion. The configuration of this anastomosis in the majority of cases is the celiac axis, superior mesenteric artery, and right renal artery in one patch. The left renal artery is reattached separately as a Carrel

patch. Five percent of our patients with thoracoabdominal aortic aneurysms have associated visceral artery stenosis or occlusion, and if this is the case, we perform endarterectomy of the visceral and/or renal arteries. However, if there is any question about the adequacy of the endarterectomy, then a bypass graft is done to the visceral artery orifices immediately.

Following this, the patient is placed in the head-down position, and the aortic graft and native aorta are flushed of air and debris. The proximal thoracic clamp is moved down and reapplied on the graft distal to the visceral vessel anastomosis, thus reestablishing flow to the reattached intercostal, visceral, and renal arteries. At the same time, visceral perfusion via the Bio Medicus pump is stopped. The aortic graft is then cut to the appropriate length and sutured end-to-end to the infrarenal abdominal aorta above the aortic bifurcation. Again, prior to

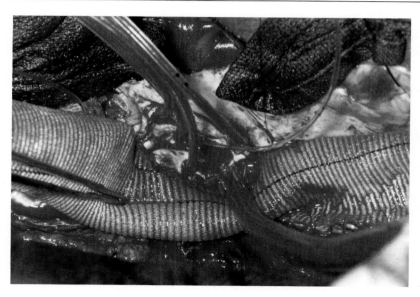

Figure 8-12. Visceral catheters in place.

completion of this distal aortic anastomosis, with the patient still in the head-down position, the graft and native aorta are flushed proximally and distally to remove all air and debris. Once there is adequate hemostasis, the Dacron graft is wrapped with the aneurysmal wall using running 2-0 Prolene suture. Femoral and atrial cannulas are removed. At each step of the sequential unclamping of the aorta, particularly when restoring flow to the visceral vessels and the lower extremities, the clamp should be opened slowly while the anesthesiologist provides a rapid infusion of blood and crystalloid. The anesthesiologist also has to frequently check cerebrospinal fluid pressure to maintain it below 10 mmHg (Fig. 8-13).

One of the significant factors in the development of neurologic deficits after thoracoabdominal aortic aneurysm repair is the total aortic clamp time. We also have learned that visceral ischemic time is a factor if it exceeds 45 minutes. Currently, we use visceral perfusion in all our patients. After reestablishing flow to the viscera and renal arteries, indigo carmine is injected intravenously to detect urine clearance time. We have found a urine clearance time of greater than 30 minutes to be a good prognostic indicator for renal failure.

Finally, the diaphragm is reapproximated with interrupted no. 2 Vicryl and running no. 1 Prolene sutures. Two large chest tubes are placed in the left side of the chest for drainage. The chest and abdomen are closed in layers in the standard fashion. Then the double-lumen endotracheal tube is changed to a straight endotracheal tube, and the patient is sent to the intensive care unit under close observation.

Elephant Trunk

The elephant trunk technique[11,12] for patients with extensive aneurysmal disease of the aorta can prevent the catastrophic complications that may occur during dissection of the proximal aorta, such as rupture of the aorta or tears of the pulmonary artery. Following replacement of the ascending and transverse arch, the aortic graft and the pulmonary artery are adherent to each other. If dissection were performed without this technique, the likelihood of a pulmonary artery tear leading to torrential bleeding would be high.

When the patient has already had repair of the ascending and arch aneurysm using the elephant trunk technique, the steps mentioned above for

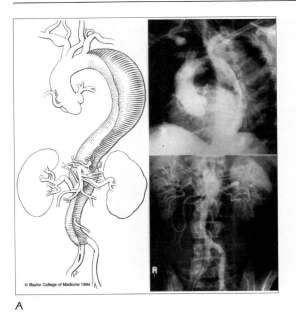

A

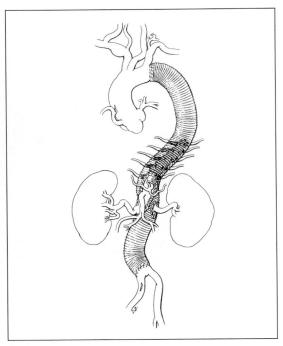

B

Figure 8-13. (A) Aortogram and diagram of thoracoabdominal aortic aneurysm due to chronic dissection type III. **(B)** Aortogram and diagram of postoperative repair.

general thoracoabdominal aortic aneurysm repair are followed except that proximal aortic dissection is not done. The proximal aorta is opened, and the graft in the descending thoracic aorta is clamped promptly, thus achieving proximal control of the graft. Because there is no longer any need to dissect between the pulmonary artery and the graft, the procedure is simplified tremendously (Fig. 8-14).

POSTOPERATIVE MONITORING

In the postoperative period the patient stays on the respirator for 1 to 2 days before extubation. Hemodynamic monitoring is essential for maintaining adequate filling pressure and a good urine output. Once the patient is awakened, he or she is evaluated neurologically. Blood pressure, arterial blood gases, cardiac indices, coagulation studies, and serum electrolytes are monitored frequently and kept within the preoperative normal ranges. Cerebrospinal fluid pressure is monitored for 3 days following surgery, and fluid is drained when

necessary to maintain a pressure of less than 10 mmHg. The patient is extubated when arterial blood gases can be sustained without support. Chest tubes are generally removed on the second or third postoperative day.

COMPLICATIONS

Pulmonary Complications

Pulmonary complications (see Table 8-2) include pulmonary insufficiency or respiratory failure and extended need for the ventilator for more

Table 8-2. Postoperative Complications

Factor	Incidence (%)
30-day survival rate	92
Pulmonary failure	33
Neurologic deficit	16
Cardiac complication	12
Renal failure (dialysis)	9
Bleeding	5

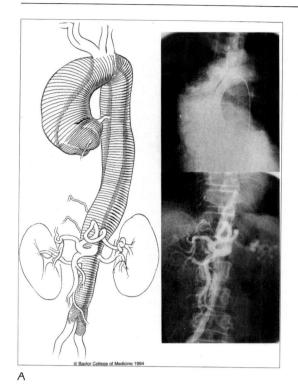

A

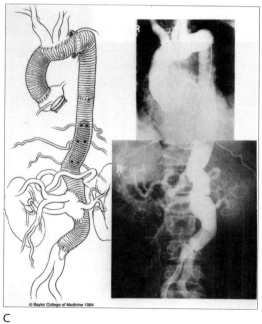

C

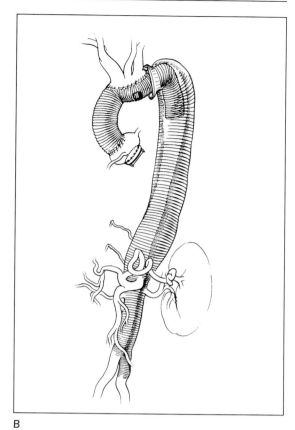

B

Figure 8-14. (**A**) Diagram and aortogram of extensive aortic aneurysm. (**B**) First-stage "elephant trunk" procedure. (**C**) Six-week postoperative aortogram and diagram thoracoabdominal aortic aneurysm repair.

than 3 days. Patients should be treated aggressively postoperatively. Early extubation from the ventilator is extremely beneficial. We place patients on a pulmonary ventilator regimen that consists of I and V regimen and subsequently CPAP extubation. We identify the independent predictors for pulmonary failure as previous pulmonary disease, smoking history, and cardiac and renal complications.[13] Preoperative preparation for patients includes cessation of smoking, bronchodilators, coughing and breathing exercises, and control of productive secretions with appropriate antibiotics.

Bleeding

Essentially all postoperative bleeding results from mechanical problems. Intraoperatively, good hemostasis is essential. Postoperatively, the patient should be monitored for excessive bleeding, and if in the first hour bleeding is above 400 ml through the chest tube, a trip to the operating room is in order to avoid hypotension and its harmful effects on spinal cord circulation and strong association with delayed paraplegia. Coagulopathy should be treated intraoperatively, or the PT/PTT and platelet function should be tested frequently and serially until normal. Subsequently, the patient is transferred to the intensive care unit in a stable hemodynamic condition. As alluded to previously, 5 percent of our patients will develop some kind of coagulopathy preoperatively, and the best treatment for such patients is to repair the thoracoabdominal aortic aneurysm.

Renal Failure

Several of our studies showed that renal failure is directly related to the preoperative renal status of the patient. If the patient has normal renal function as described by blood urea nitrogen (BUN) and creatinine levels preoperatively, the incidence of renal failure is around 4 percent, but if the creatinine level is abnormal, then the incidence of renal failure is about 25 percent, as defined by the 3 mg/dl of creatinine and/or hemodialysis. In the past we have tried a variety of methods to prevent renal failure.[14] One method was to use Ringer's

lactate solution perfused to the left renal artery under the assumption that if we can protect one kidney, this will function until the other kidney recovers from the ischemic insult. The disadvantages of Ringer's lactate perfusion are that it overloads the heart with 1 liter of Ringer's lactate solution and does lower the core body temperature markedly. We described a method in which the renal vein connection to the inferior vena cava is clamped and the renal vein is drained either by needle or by a side tributary to shed all the lactated Ringer's solution in the field without the deleterious effect on volume and the deleterious effect on the core temperature.[14] This method of protecting the kidney revealed a favorable trend but no statistical difference compared with use of the pump and simple clamping. We are currently evaluating perfusion of the kidney using oxygenated blood from the left atrium by means of a bifurcation cannula to see if the incidence of renal failure can be reduced.

Neurologic Deficit

Neurologic deficit remains the most daunting problem following thoracoabdominal aortic repair, especially in high-risk patients (types I and II). From our past experience, we have concluded that neurologic deficit is multifactorial in origin, with the major factors being aneurysm type and etiology, patient age, preoperative renal status, and previous proximal aortic repair.[3] However, most important, the longer the aortic clamp time and the deprivation of the blood supply to the spinal cord, the more likely is the chance of neurologic deficit. Moreover, we found the incidence of neurologic deficit to be higher in extended and dissected aneurysms.

A brief description of the anatomy of the spinal cord blood supply is warranted. The blood supply of the spinal cord, starting from the aorta, can be divided into three different levels. The primary level consists of vertebral, costocervical, intercostal, and lumbar arteries. The second is represented by the radicular arteries. These arteries, after embryonic development, where they are represented in every segment, remain sparse along the spine (one to two cervical, two to three thoracic, one to two lumbar). The largest and most developed radicular artery is the so-called artery of

Adamkiewicz,[15] or arteria radicularis magna. The site of origin of this artery is variable, from T9 to L3. In 75 percent of human subjects, it originates between T9 and T12, according to Djiian and Faure.[16] The terminal division is represented by the longitudinal pathways of blood flow, the anterior spinal artery that supplies over 75 percent of the blood to the spine, and the posterolateral spinal arteries. Some authors[17,18] tried a preoperative localization of the artery of Adamkiewicz with a selective spinal cord arteriography, but the procedure itself carries a risk of neurologic deficit. Experimental and clinical evidence favors reattachment of these critical intercostal arteries to reduce the incidence of neurologic deficit.

Many protective measures have been tried with the goal of prevention of neurologic deficit. Miyamoto et al.[19] in 1960 and Blaisdell and Cooley[20] in 1962 showed that cerebrospinal fluid drainage decreased paraplegia rates in dogs undergoing aortic cross-clamping. Oka and Miyamoto[21] in 1984 reconfirmed earlier experimental studies, and they strongly supported the hypothesis that spinal cord perfusion pressure is dependent not only on absolute arterial pressure below the cross-clamp but also on the relationship of distal aortic blood pressure minus cerebrospinal fluid pressure. Hollier et al.[22,23] first tried cerebrospinal fluid drainage intraoperatively and then later both intraoperatively and postoperatively. In their series, cerebrospinal fluid pressure was maintained at less than 10 mmHg, draining freely via gravity, and there was a significant reduction in the incidence of neurologic deficit. At our institution in a randomized study, high-risk thoracoabdominal aortic aneurysm type I and type II patients were treated with and without cerebrospinal fluid drainage with no appreciable difference between the groups for incidence of neurologic deficit.[24] The outstanding difference between Hollier's method of cerebrospinal fluid drainage and that used at our institution was the amount of fluid actually drained, with drainage here limited to 50 cc, whereas drainage for the Hollier studies was unlimited and continued into the postoperative period.

The use of left atrial-femoral bypass to improve blood flow to the distal aortic segment during clamping and thoracic aneurysm repair was proposed by Connolly et al.[25] in 1971. Using this method, they reported a 10 percent incidence of paraplegia in 10 patients with descending thoracic aortic aneurysms. The rationale for distal aortic perfusion is to increase distal aortic pressure to greater than 60 mmHg, increasing spinal arterial pressure and thus augmenting perfusion of the spinal cord during cross-clamp time. Somatosensory evoked potentials were attempted as intraoperative indicators of the critical intercostal arteries in the segmental thoracic and upper abdominal areas.[26] Crawford et al.[27] in 1988 presented a study to reevaluate distal aortic perfusion and somatosensory evoked potential monitoring in the prevention of paraplegia in aortic aneurysm repair. Unfortunately, the results showed no difference with or without distal aortic perfusion and somatosensory evoked potentials. In addition, false-positive results of somatosensory evoked potentials made it a totally unreliable indicator.

Medications used in an effort to lower the incidence of neurologic deficit include free radical scavengers, papaverine, steroids, and allopurinol. Unfortunately, studies investigating the success of these agents in limiting neurologic deficit have been limited in size and have encompassed too wide a range of aneurysm varieties, including thoracoabdominal aortic aneurysms of all types, as well as patients with descending thoracic aneurysms, making meta-analysis incomplete (Table 8-3).

Table 8-3. Prevention of Paraplegia in Thoracoabdominal Aortic Aneurysm Repair

Blood flow enhancement
  Shunts and bypasses
  Cerebrospinal fluid drainage
  Hypothermia
Drugs
  Intrathecal
  Systemic
Localization of the blood supply to the spinal cord
  Angiographic
  Hydrogen-induced current impulse
Monitoring spinal cord ischemia
  Evoked potentials
    Somatosensory
    Motor

Because of the variability of these results, in September of 1992, we decided to test the hypothesis that cerebrospinal fluid drainage and distal aortic perfusion enhances perfusion to the spinal cord. Proximal aortic clamping causes a marked drop in distal aortic pressure and a drop in spinal arterial pressure; cerebrospinal fluid pressure is increased, causing a decreased pressure to the spinal cord. There are two individual forces as a result of the combined use of distal aortic perfusion and cerebrospinal fluid drainage that will (1) augment the distal arterial pressure and have a beneficial effect on spinal arterial perfusion pressure and (2) decrease spinal fluid pressure and enhance perfusion on the spinal cord.[28,29] The result is ample time to perform thoracoabdominal aortic aneurysm repair which includes reattachment of intercostal arteries T8 to L2 and reattachment of visceral and renal arteries. This study was prospective but not randomized because of the established bias of the senior author toward simple cross clamping. The strength of the study was that all thoracoabdominal type I and type II aortic aneurysm patients were part of the study regardless of age, extent of aneurysm, previous surgery, or associated disease. We conducted a prospective study evaluating the possible prevention of postoperative neurologic deficit in high-risk patients with thoracoabdominal aortic aneurysms types I and II using perioperative cerebral spinal fluid drainage and distal aortic perfusion (Fig. 8-15).

Between September 18, 1992 and August 8, 1993, we evaluated 45 consecutive patients who

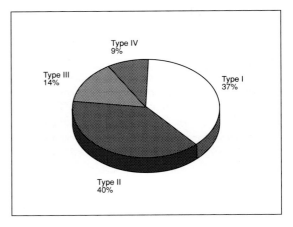

Figure 8-15. Classification of current series.

underwent thoracoabdominal aortic aneurysm repair (14 type I, 31 type II).[30] Thirty-six were male and nine were female. The median age was 63 years (range 28 to 88 years). There were 24 of 45 patients (53 percent) with dissection and 17 of 45 patients (38 percent) with prior proximal aortic replacement. All patients had perioperative cerebrospinal fluid drainage and distal aortic perfusion. Median aortic clamp time was 42 minutes. Thirty-five of 45 patients (78 percent) underwent intercostal artery reattachment.

The 30-day survival rate was 43 of 45 (96 percent). Early neurologic deficit occurred in 2 of 45 patients (4 percent), and late neurologic deficit also occurred in 2 of 45 (4 percent). We compared the neurologic deficit of our current group of 45

Table 8-4. Cerebrospinal Fluid Drainage and Distal Aortic Perfusion: Incidence of Neurologic Deficit According to Treatment Group

		Previous		Current		
Variable	Group	No. of Patients	No. of Deficits (%)	No. of Patients	No. of Deficits (%)	*p*-Value
—	All patients	112	35 (31%)	45	4 (9%)	0.0034
Extent	I	73	15 (21%)	14	0 (0%)	0.062
	II	39	20 (51%)	31	4 (13%)	0.0008
Dissection	Yes	32	9 (28%)	24	3 (12%)	0.16
	No	80	26 (32%)	21	1 (5%)	0.011
Clamp time	<45 min	68	14 (21%)	24	1 (4%)	0.061
	≥45 min	44	21 (48%)	21	3 (14%)	0.009

patients with the data of a previously unpublished study of 112 patients also from this center. Total neurologic deficit for the current group was 4 of 45 patients (9 percent) versus the previous group of 35 of 112 patients (31 percent) with a p value of 0.0034 (Pearson chi-square test) (Table 8-4). In cases of aortic dissection, the decline in the incidence of neurologic deficit also was significant, occurring in 28 percent of patients in the previous group and in 12 percent of the current group. The incidence of neurologic deficit in patients with an aortic clamp time of more than 45 minutes was 48 percent in the control group, while in our current study it was less than 14 percent.

We found that these combined methods had a profound influence on the reduction of neurologic deficits in patients with type I and type II thoracoabdominal aortic aneurysms despite age, clamp time, or etiology. Overall, neurologic deficits dropped from 31 percent in the control group to 9 percent in our current study and to 4 percent for early neurologic deficit (Table 8-4).

In conclusion, thoracoabdominal aortic aneurysm repair with spinal cord protection is still an evolving process requiring diligent attention to the analytical details of clinical trials as well as animal studies in order to reduce morbidity and mortality. We feel that cerebral spinal fluid drainage intraoperatively and for 3 days postoperatively combined with distal aortic perfusion via left atrial to left femoral artery or the distal aorta can effectively reduce neurologic deficits in patients with repair of type I and type II thoracoabdominal aortic aneurysms. We recommend this protocol in type I and type II aneurysm repair and suggest further study to explore the usefulness of these methods in types III and IV.

REFERENCES

1. Shenaq SA, Svensson LG: Paraplegia following aortic surgery. Cardiovasc Anesth 1993;7:81.
2. Kouchoukos NT, Rokkas CK: Descending thoracic and thoracoabdominal aortic surgery for aneurysm or dissection: How do we minimize the risk of spinal cord injury? Semin Thorac Cardiovasc Surg 1993;5(1):47.
3. Svensson LG, Crawford ES, Hess KR, et al: Experience with 1509 patients undergoing thoracoabdominal aortic operations. J Vasc Surg 1993; 17(2):357.
4. Crawford ES, DeNatale RW: Thoracoabdominal aortic aneurysm: Observations regarding the natural course of the disease. J Vasc Surg 1986; 3(4):578.
5. Kainulainen K, Pulkkinen L, Savolainen A, et al: Location on chromosome 15 of the gene defect causing Marfan syndrome. N Engl J Med 1990; 323:935.
6. Pyeritz RE: Editorial: Marfan Syndrome. N Engl J Med 1990;323:987.
7. Crawford ES: The diagnosis and management of aortic dissection. JAMA 1990;264:2537.
8. Svensson LG, Crawford ES: Aortic dissection and aortic aneurysm surgery: Clinical observations, experimental investigations, and statistical analyses. Curr Probl Surg 1992;29(11,12),819.
9. Svensson LG, Crawford ES: Aortic dissection and aortic aneurysm surgery: Clinical observations, experimental investigations, and statistical analyses. Curr Probl Surg 1993;30(1):1.
10. Crawford ES, Stowe CL, Crawford JL, et al: Aortic arch aneurysm: A sentinel of extensive aortic disease requiring subtotal and total aortic replacement. Ann Surg 1984;199:742.
11. Borst HG, Walterbusch G, Schaps D: Extensive aortic replacement using "elephant trunk" prosthesis. Thorac Cardiovasc Surg 1983;31:37.
12. Borst HG, Frank G, Scaps D: Treatment of extensive aortic aneurysms by a new multiple-stage approach. J Thorac Cardiovasc Surg 1988;95:95:11.
13. Svensson LG, Hess KR, Coselli JS, et al: A prospective study of respiratory failure after high-risk surgery on the thoracoabdominal aorta. J Vasc Surg 1991;14(3):271.
14. Svensson LG, Coselli JS, Safi HJ, et al: Appraisal of adjuncts to prevent acute renal failure after surgery on the thoracic or thoracoabdominal aorta. J Vasc Surg 1989;10(3):230.
15. Adamkiewicz A: Die Blutgefasse des menschlichen Rukenmarkesoberflache. Sitz dakadd wiss. Wien Math Natur Klass 1882;85:101.
16. Djindjian R, Faure C: Accidents medullariies de aortogram. J Belg Radiol 1967;50:207.
17. DiChiro G, Doppman J, Ommaya AK: Selective arteriography of arteriovenous aneurysms of spinal cord. Radiology 1967;88:1065.
18. Kieffer E, Richard T, Chiras J, et al: Preoperative spinal cord arteriography in aneurysmal disease of the descending thoracic and thoracoabdominal aorta: Preliminary results in 45 patients. Ann Vasc Surg 1989;3(1):34.
19. Miyamoto K, Ueno A, Wada T, et al: A new and simple method of preventing spinal cord damage following temporary occlusion of the thoracic aorta by draining the cerebrospinal fluid. J Cardiovasc Surg (Torino) 1960;16:188.

20. Blaisdell FW, Cooley DA: The mechanism of para-plegia after temporary thoracic aortic occlusion and its relationship to spinal fluid pressure. Surgery 1962; 51:351.
21. Oka Y, Miyamoto T: Prevention of spinal cord injury after cross-clamping of the thoracic aorta. Jpn J Surg 1984;14:159.
22. Hollier LH: Protecting the brain and spinal cord. J Vasc Surg 1987;5(3):524.
23. Hollier LH, Money SR, Naslund TC, et al: Risk of spinal cord dysfunction in patients undergoing tho-racoabdominal aortic replacement. Am J Surg 1992;164(3):210.
24. Crawford ES, Svensson LG, Hess KR, et al: A prospective randomized study of cerebrospinal fluid drainage to prevent paraplegia after high-risk sur-gery on the thoracoabdominal aorta. J Vasc Surg 1990;13(1):36.
25. Connolly JE, Wakabayashi A, German JC, et al: Clinical experience with pulsatile left heart bypass without anti-coagulation for thoracic aneurysms. J Thorac Cardiovasc Surg 1971;62:568.
26. Laschinger JD, Cunningham JN, Cooper MM, et al: Monitoring of somatosensory evoked poten-tials during surgical procedures on the thoraco-abdominal aorta I, II, III, IV. J Thorac Cardio-vasc Surg 1987;94(2):260.
27. Crawford ES, Mizrahi EM, Hess KR, et al: The impact of distal aortic perfusion and somatosensory evoked potential monitoring on prevention of para-plegia after aortic aneurysm operation. J Thorac Cardiovasc Surg 1988;95(3):357.
28. Shenaq SA, Svensson LG: Con: Cerebrospinal fluid drainage does not afford spinal cord protection during resection of thoracic aneurysms. J Cardiothorac Vasc Anesth 1992;6(3):369.
29. Nugent M: Pro: Cerebrospinal fluid drainage pre-vents paraplegia. J Cardiothorac Vasc Anesth 1992; 6(3):366.
30. Safi HJ, Bartoli S, Hess KR, et al: Neurological-deficit in high-risk patients with thoracoabdominal aortic aneurysms: the role of cerebral spinal fluid drainage and distal aortic perfusion. J Vasc Surg (in press).

9

Popliteal and Femoral Artery Aneurysms

JAMES A. DeWEESE

Popliteal and femoral artery aneurysms are the most common peripheral arterial aneurysms. During the period 1964 to 1979, 62 patients were admitted to Henry Ford Hospital with popliteal aneurysms, which represented only 1 of 5000 admissions per year.[1] During the years 1960 to 1971, 1488 patients with arteriosclerotic aneurysms of the abdominal aorta and its branches were admitted to The University of Michigan Hospital.[2] The diagnosis of popliteal and femoral aneurysms was made in only 36 (2.4 percent) and 37 (2.4 percent) of these patients, respectively. During the same period, 1470 abdominal aortic aneurysms were seen, suggesting that they were 41 times more common than popliteal aneurysms. Szilagyi and associates[1] found that operations for abdominal aortic aneurysms were 15 times more common than those for popliteal aneurysms. During the period 1958 to 1991, 1431 patients underwent operations for abdominal aortic aneurysms at the University of Rochester, and only 51 had operations for popliteal aneurysms.[3] Operations for aortic aneurysms were 26 times more common than those for popliteal artery aneurysms. These retrospective studies suggest that the incidence of popliteal and femoral aneurysm in patients with abdominal aortic aneu rysms is quite small, probably about 5 percent.

POPLITEAL ANEURYSMS

Although popliteal aneurysms are uncommon in patients with abdominal aneurysms, the presence of multiple aneurysms is common in patients with popliteal aneurysms. A collected series of 1179 patients with popliteal aneurysms indicates that if a patient has a popliteal aneurysm, there is a 48 percent chance that there is also a contralateral popliteal aneurysm[1,4–18] (Table 9-1).

Extrapopliteal aneurysms are also common[1,4–18] (Table 9-2). From a collected series of 964 patients with a popliteal aneurysm, there were 328 patients (34 percent) with aortic or aortoiliac aneurysms. There also were at least 175 patients (18 percent) with single or multiple iliac aneurysms. Thoracic aortic aneurysms were either not looked for or purposely not included in many references, since only 12 were reported. There were approximately 252 patients (26 percent) with femoral aneurysms.

Patients with bilateral popliteal artery aneurysms had an increased incidence of extrapopliteal aneurysms in the Whitehouse et al.[14] series. Extrapopliteal aneurysms were present in 78 percent of patients with bilateral popliteal aneurysms and 60 percent of those with single aneurysms. When bilateral popliteal aneurysms were present, aneurysms of the aorta, iliac artery, and femoral artery were seen in 70, 50, and 41 percent of patients, respectively. When single popliteal aneurysms were present, aortic, iliac artery, and femoral artery aneurysms were present in 56, 24, and 35 percent of patients, respectively. Only the differences in the case of iliac artery aneurysms proved significant.[14] Vermilion et al.[13] and Schellack et al.[16] found even more striking differences. The incidence of extrapopliteal aneurysm in their series of patients with

Table 9-1. Frequency of Bilateral Popliteal Artery Aneurysms

	Acquisition	Year of Report	Patients	Bilateral	Percent
Gifford[4]	1939–1951	1953	69	31	45
Crichlow[5]	1953–1965	1966	42	15	36
Baird[6]	1938–1964	1966	46	15	33
Wychulis[7]	1961–1968	1970	152	81	53
Bouhoutsos[8]	1958–1972	1974	71	32	45
Buda[9]	1951–1972	1974	64	22	34
Anton[10]	1952–1974	1986	56	17	30
Towne[11]	1954–1975	1976	80	39	49
Inahara[12]	1963–1977	1978	30	14	47
Szilagyi[1]	1964–1979	1981	62	25	40
Vermilion[13]	1960–1980	1981	87	60	69
Whitehouse[14]	1943–1982	1983	61	27	45
Reilly[15]	1958–1982	1983	159	85	53
Anton[10]	1975–1984	1986	54	33	61
Schellack[16]	1965–1985	1987	60	35	58
Farina[17]	1972–1988	1989	36	14	39
Dawson[18]	1958–1985	1991	50	21	42
			1179	566	48

bilateral popliteal aneurysms was 68 and 69 percent, as opposed to 21 and 32 percent for those with unilateral aneurysms, respectively.[13,16]

Pathogenesis

Popliteal aneurysms are the most common peripheral aneurysms. There have been some interesting theories as to why they occur. Matas[19] in 1912 stated, "The majority of these cases [popliteal aneurysms] occur in laboring men, very rarely in women, and . . . a history of syphilis, alcohol, and other causes of arterial degeneration is frequently present." Matas felt that the frequent occurrence in working men supported Delbet's theory that "the internal tunics [of the popliteal artery] are ruptured in violent lifting efforts in which the arterial tension is suddenly exaggerated while the leg is acutely flexed at the knee." Theis[20] did obtain a history of violent muscular strain while the knees were flexed in two of five patients with aneurysm. Wells and associates[21] also felt exertion could be a cause. More recently, however, the few reported cases of aneurysm secondary to trauma have been attributed to blunt or penetrating trauma and usually have been dissections or false aneurysms.[4,7,8] Matas' statement that popliteal aneurysms are

rarely seen in women remains true but unexplainable.[19] The collected series of Anton et al.[10] reported aneurysms in 35 women as compared with 664 men, an incidence of less than 0.5 percent. Matas[19] described syphilis as a frequent cause of popliteal aneurysms. Gifford et al.,[4] in a series from 1939 to 1951, included syphilis as a possible cause of six popliteal aneurysms, of which five had positive serology but only one had histologic proof. Wells and associates[21] pointed out that syphilitic aneurysms have been considered far more common in larger arteries such as the ascending thoracic aorta. They state, "However, in spite of an appalling lack of histologic proof, the frequency of 4+ Wassermann tests associated with popliteal aneurysms leaves little doubt as to the importance of this etiologic agent."[21]

The decline in syphilis and the increased appreciation of arteriosclerosis as the most commonly associated etiologic agent for aneurysms are best illustrated by the experience at Massachusetts General Hospital from 1908 to 1947.[22] Syphilis was listed as the cause of the popliteal aneurysm in 4 of 4 cases seen during 1908–1917, in 3 of 4 during 1918–1927, in 4 of 9 during 1928–1937, and in 0 of 25 during 1938–1947. Although arteriosclerosis is most commonly associated with

Table 9-2. Frequency of Extrapopliteal Aneurysms

					Iliac								
		Patients	Aortoiliac	Aorta	Iliac	Com.	Int.	Ext.	Thoracic	Femoral	COM	PF	SF
Gifford[4]	1953	69	8*						2				
Baird[6]	1966	46		8	7					5			
Crichlow[5]	1966	42		6							8		
Wychulis[7]	1970	152		53	28†	28	7	2	4		40		4
Bouhoutsos[8]	1974	71		23	5†	4		5			18		11
Buda[9]	1974	64		9			2	10	4		7		10
Towne[11]	1976	80	15*						1		14		
Inahara[12]	1978	30		11	3						5		
Szilagyi[1]	1981	62	25*							24			
Vermilion[13]	1981	87		35	22					30			
Whitehouse[14]	1983	61		38	22				1	23			
Anton[10]	1986	54	35*							13			
Schellack[16]	1987	60	32*										
Farina[17]	1989	36		12	13†	13	4				15	1	5
Dawson[18]	1991	50	18*								19	1	30
		964	133*	195	100	45	13	17	12	95	126	1	30
			14%	20%	10%	5%	1%	2%	1%	10%	13%	15%	3%

328 } 34%

75 } 8%

16%

*Number with iliac operations not given.
†Minimum possible number.

123

aneurysm, there are now those who question that it is responsible for the weakness of the wall that allows dilatation and aneurysm formation.[23]

That a localized disease process must be present, however, is not a new concept. Power[24] quotes Edvard Howe, the brother-in-law of John Hunter, as performing the following experiment: "Mr. Hunter laid bare the carotid artery for above an inch in length and afterwards dissected off the other coats layer by layer till what remained was so thin that the blood was plainly to be seen through it." Three weeks later, "the whole of the surrounding parts were consolidated . . . and the artery itself was neither increased nor diminished in size." He concluded that the artery that becomes aneurysmal must be diseased. It also led to his decision to treat aneurysms by ligation at a distance from the disease. Whatever the disease process, the reason for localized dilatations requires an explanation. Gedge et al.[25] proposed that popliteal artery aneurysms might well be examples of poststenotic dilatation. Halsted[26] in 1916 had experimentally produced dilatation of an artery distal to a partially occluding band. Halsted proposed this as an explanation of the occurrence of aneurysms secondary to constrictions of the subclavian artery as it passed through fibrous bands associated with cervical ribs.[26] Gedge et al.[25] suggested that the most common sites for popliteal artery aneurysms also were distal to constricting bands. Aneurysms are frequently found just distal to the tendinous hiatus of the adductor magnus muscle and are also seen just distal to the "sharp and prominent" arcuate popliteal ligament.[25] It should be noted that these two points of constriction are also the most frequent sites of stenotic "atherosclerotic" lesions, as described by Palma[27] and Boyd et al.[28] In addition, Cavallaro and associates,[29] in a collected series of 74 operative reports of popliteal entrapment, described "an aneurysmatic dilatation of the artery almost always downstream to stenosis or occlusion" on 31 occasions. Constriction by bands, tendinous structures, and atherosclerotic plaques, plus arteriosclerotic degeneration of the arterial wall, may explain the predilection of the popliteal artery for aneurysms.

Natural History

The threat to life and limb of popliteal aneurysms has been recognized for many centuries. Some of

Table 9-3. Complications in 49 Popliteal Aneurysms Seen at Admission to Mayo Clinic, 1939–1951

	Number	Percent
Thrombosis	20	41
Embolization	14	28
Gangrene	10	20
Venous compression	19	39
Nerve compression	10	20
Rupture	12	24

Adapted with permission from Gifford RW Jr, Hines EA Jr, Janes JM: An analysis and follow-up study of 100 popliteal aneurysms. Surgery 1953;33:284.

the earliest recorded operations were performed for the treatment of popliteal aneurysms.[19] The most dreaded of complications is death secondary to rupture. Percival Potts in 1779 is quoted by Friedman[30] as saying, "The artery is not only dilated and burst but it is also distempered someway above the dilatation." The loss of pulsation in a popliteal aneurysm was recognized as a cause of gangrene. The threat of rupture and thrombosis was aptly described by Guvendik and associates in the title of their article, "Popliteal Aneurysm: Sinister Harbinger of Sudden Catastrophe."[32] Gifford et al.[4] reported 100 popliteal aneurysms greater than 3 cm in diameter in 69 patients admitted to Mayo Clinic between 1913 and 1951 (Table 9-3). Forty-nine patients had aneurysms that were symptomatic from complications on admission to the hospital. Rupture had occurred in 12 patients (24 percent). There were 20 patients (41 percent) who presented with thrombosis. There were 14 patients (28 percent) who had thrombus in the aneurysm that had embolized to distal tibioperoneal or digital vessels. In other words, 34 patients (69 percent) presented with thromboembolic occlusive arterial symptoms. Ten patients (20 percent) had gangrene, of whom 7 required amputation. Venous compression was found in 19 (39 percent). Motor or sensory distal neurologic symptoms were seen in 10 (20 percent).

There were 45 popliteal aneurysms that were asymptomatic when first seen at Mayo Clinic and did not have operations performed.[4] During an average follow-up period of 44 months, complications occurred in 13 (29 percent) of the limbs. Gangrene and amputation occurred in 5 (11 percent). There were 14 aneurysms that were thrombosed on admission that were not treated, 2 (14 percent) developed gangrene, and 1 was amputated. There were 11 patients who had complications other than thrombosis on admission and had the worst outcome in the 59-month average follow-up. Five (45 percent) developed gangrene and required amputation. Overall, of the 70 aneurysms followed without operation, 12 (17 percent) developed gangrene and 11 (16 percent) required amputation. Vermilion et al.[13] followed 26 aneurysms in patients with medical contraindications to operations or who refused operation for a follow-up period that averaged 36 months. Eight (31 percent) of the 26 patients developed limb-threatening complications. In a collected series of 203 patients with uncomplicated aneurysms followed for less than 4 years average time, 31 percent became complicated.[4,7,13,14,18]

Diagnosis

The diagnosis of a popliteal artery aneurysm is usually suspected by the presence of a pulsatile mass in the popliteal space that is wider and more superficial than the usually difficult to feel popliteal artery. A thrombosed popliteal aneurysm also should be suspected if a hard, nonpulsatile mass is found in the popliteal space of a patient with symptoms of arterial insufficiency and diminished distal pulses. The diagnosis is not established nor discarded, however, until computed tomography (CT) or an ultrasound examination is performed. Chan and Thomas[33] performed ultrasonography on 122 extremities of patients with arteriomegaly. Of the 30 extremities suspected of having popliteal aneurysms, only 15 had positive scans. Of equal concern was that 41 aneurysms were found in 92 popliteal arteries not suspected of having aneurysms. Possible reasons for the falsely positive clinical examination are the presence of a Bakers cyst, or tumor, or overlying muscle. Ultrasound has been shown to be a reliable diagnostic test for popliteal aneurysms and also can visualize the presence of thrombus in the aneurysm sac[34-38] (Fig. 9-1A). Arteriography is most helpful in demonstrating thrombi, occlusive disease, and abnormal anatomy in the arteries proximal and distal to the aneurysm. Arteriography may assist in operative planning (Fig. 9-1B).

Anton and associates[10] found that during the years 1953–1974, only 30 percent (17 of 56) of contralateral aneurysms were recognized in patients with popliteal aneurysms at the Crile Clinic, whereas between 1975 to 1984, 61 percent (33 of 54) were recognized ($p = 0.002$). They felt that this trend might be attributed to the enhanced ability to recognize these aneurysms provided by ultrasonography. This also suggests that the incidence of bilateral aneurysms might be higher than the 48 percent reported in the collected series.

Indication for Operation

The complications of rupture, thromboembolic complications with disabling claudication, rest pain, gangrene, nerve compression, and vein compression are clear-cut indications for arterial reconstruction of popliteal aneurysms if possible because amputation may be the only alternative treatment available. The indications for operations on asymptomatic aneurysms are not as clear-cut. It has been shown that the development of complications is in general related to the size of the aneurysm. Whitehouse et al.[14] reported complications in 66 percent of 35 aneurysms greater than 2.0 cm in diameter but in only 9 percent of 11 aneurysms less than 2.0 cm in diameter. On the other hand, Inahara and Toledo[12] observed 9 limbs with acute ischemia secondary to thrombosis of popliteal aneurysms that were less than 2.5 cm in diameter. In addition, the mean size of thrombosed aneurysms observed by Inahara and Toledo[12] and Vermilion and associates[13] was 1.8 and 2.5 cm, suggesting that smaller aneurysms are indeed subject to thrombosis. It is reasonable to consider operation for a popliteal aneurysms greater than 2 cm in diameter in a patient without significant medical problems.

Surgical Treatment

Antyllus, a Greek surgeon in the second century A.D., according to Towne and associates,[11] and a Roman surgeon in the third century whose method most probably came from Greece, according to Henry,[39] are reported to have ligated the popliteal artery proximal and distal to an aneurysm, followed by an incision into and packing of

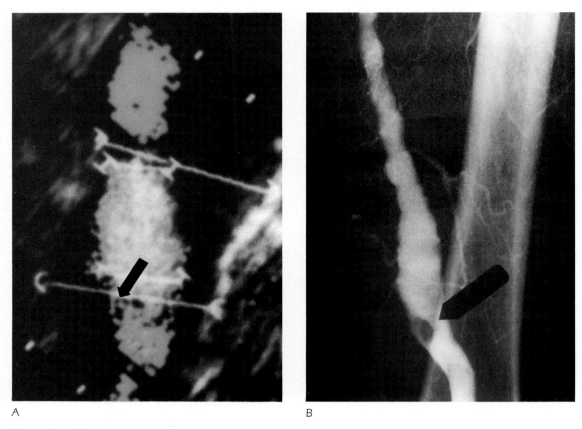

A   B

Figure 9-1. (A) Ultrasound of fusiform popiteal artery aneurysm containing a thrombus. **(B)** Arteriogram of the same popliteal artery aneurysm containing a thrombus.

the aneurysmal sac. Sporadically through the next several centuries, modifications of this method were reported. Some of these modifications involved various techniques for the use of ligatures alone. For example, in 1710, Anel, according to Matas,[19] ligated the artery immediately proximal to a brachial aneurysm. This technique was applied by others to popliteal aneurysms with variable results.[40] Some surgeons were very skeptical of arterial ligations, and the famous Potts, according to Power,[24] once said of a patient who had had a ligation, "I shall only remark that the patient died." A frequent cause of death was rupture of the diseased artery at the site of the ligature.

On December 12, 1785, John Hunter successfully ligated the femoral artery proximal to and at a distance from a popliteal artery aneurysm.

Friedman[30] quotes Homes' description of the operation, stating, "He began the operation by making an incision on the fore and inner part of the thigh rather than below its middle, which incision continued obliquely across the lower edge of the sartorius muscle. . . . the fascia which covers the artery was then laid bare for about three inches and the artery ligated." The patient died in 1787. At autopsy, which was witnessed by Hunter, it was determined that the patient's death was unrelated to the patient's popliteal aneurysm. The original specimen of the aneurysm and superficial femoral artery and profunda femoris artery are in the Hunterian Museum of the Royal College of Surgeons of England. It is frequently reported that Désault, on June 22, 1785, was the first to successfully ligate the femoral artery proximal to and at a distance from a popliteal artery aneurysm.[19] Matas' description of Désaults operation, however, identified the site of ligature as immediately below the opening of the adductor magnus muscle, which would have placed it on the proximal popliteal artery.[19]

Another variation of the use of ligation was ligation of the popliteal artery distal to an aneurysm, which, according to Matas,[19] was performed by Brasdor in 1798. Matas described this operation as being "so simple and comparatively safe that it is justifiable and is done with the view to favoring the deposition of the clot in the sac."[19] Matas indicated that it was best used for ligation distal to carotid aneurysms to avoid embolization from thrombus in the aneurysmal sac.

Another variation was ligation of the artery proximal and distal to the aneurysm without disturbing the aneurysm itself, which was performed by Pasquin in 1812 but did not become a popular procedure.[19] During the late 1800s and early 1900s, Hunter's ligation of the femoral artery at a distance from the aneurysm for the treatment of popliteal artery aneurysms remained popular. It was considered an easier operation than ligation immediately above the aneurysm because the dissection was through normal planes and the artery being ligated was more normal. The risk of bleeding was therefore decreased. Matas[19] considered the disadvantages of the Hunterian ligation to be the increased chance of gangrene secondary to the disturbance of an increased number of collaterals by the proximal ligature and the propagation or embolization of clot that would form in the aneurysm sac. Matas considered that ligation of the artery immediately proximal to the aneurysm would "shut off the circulation at once and allow drainage of its fluid contents, also allowing the old laminated clot to remain."[19] Matas concluded, "Therefore, it is evident that proximal ligation as near the sac as possible, as described by Anel, is the preferred method of ligation."[19] He further states, "However, the introduction of the proximal ligature (Hunter's) for the cure of aneurysm was an immense stride forward in the treatment of aneurysm."

Prior to the use of antiseptic technique in the operating room, early and late death secondary to sepsis was a frequent complication. Matas[19] quoted Delbet's statistics on the results of ligation by either Hunter's or Anel's technique for the treat-

ment of popliteal aneurysms, saying that the techniques resulted in a mortality rate of 19 percent in 1888, which was reduced to 8 percent in 1895. On the other hand, the rate of gangrene in 1888 was 7.6 percent and in 1895 was 8.3 percent. Matas[19] concludes that "Aseptic methods, while greatly reducing the mortality, have exercised very little if any influence upon the occurrence of gangrene."

Ligation was not the only technique being used for the treatment of popliteal aneurysms. Syme, according to Matas,[19] in 1857 revived and modified the technique of Antyllus. He made a small incision in the aneurysm and introduced his index finger, with which he identified minor or even major branches, which were then dissected and ligated from outside the sac. Matas' comment regarding the Syme operation was, "Few surgeons imitated his boldness as the penalty paid for such temerity by the profuse and almost uncontrollable hemorrhage from the distal end and the collaterals was too great to justify it." Mikulicz, according to Matas,[19] also performed a modification of the Antyllian operation. He would first apply a proximal ligature and allow the aneurysm to thrombose. At a later time he would either make a small incision or introduce a large trocar and evacuate the contents of the sac. Matas[19] felt that this carried a high risk of hemorrhage and gangrene and stated, "It has nothing to recommend it—except the prestige of the distinguished surgeon who first performed it."

Since early times, surgeons had performed "extirpation of aneurysms" (aneurysmectomy). Philagrius of Macedon in the fourth century is reported to have been the first to ligate above and below an aneurysm and excise it.[19] It also was performed by Paulus in the seventh century.[22] In 1680, Purmann reinvented the operation.[19] The operation was finally popularized by Trélat and Polosson in 1885.[19] Matas' description of the operation included the advice to excise all the sac, if possible, except when it was adherent to the vein, and then that portion should be left in place.[19] If the vein was entered, "the rent should be closed with the finest silk." Matas[19] also stated, "I believe that the preservation of the vein is a matter of decided importance to the vitality of the limb, and its sacrifice, when unavailable, must always be a source of anxiety and apprehension." Matas considered aneurys-mectomy and quoted Delbet's statistics. In 1888, the mortality rate for aneurysmectomy was 11 percent. This markedly improved with the advent of asepsis, and in 1895, 85 aneurys-mectomies were performed without a death. In 1888, gangrene occurred following 3 percent of aneurysmectomies. In 1895, the gangrene rate did not show significant improvement, with gangrene occurring following aneurysmectomy in 3 percent of operations. Matas[19] concluded that "it is evident therefore that not withstand-ing the enthusiasm of Delbet and his followers, the ideally safe operation has not been reached in extirpation."

Matas[19] therefore proposed a new technique he called "endoaneurismorrhaphy," an approach he had first applied on March 30, 1898 on a brachial artery aneurysm. It was soon applied to popliteal aneurysms. It was an operation performed by incis-ing the aneurysm and performing an intrasaccular repair. Three techniques were used, entitled *oblitera-tive, restorative,* and *reconstructive aneurismorrhaphies,* the last of which also was an *aneurismoplasty.*

Obliterative endoaneurismorrhaphy included the intrasaccular control of all branches of the artery by closing all visible orifices within the sac with fine chromic gut or suture.[19] The sac was then oblit-erated by approximating the wall with large buried catgut sutures. This type of procedure was best suited to popliteal artery aneurysms of the fusiform type. No attempt was made to restore the conti-nuity of the artery.

Restorative endoaneurismorrhaphy is possible only for the treatment of saccular aneurysms (pref-erably false aneurysms secondary to penetrating wounds). "After opening the aneurysmal sac, the opening between the more normal artery and the sac is identified and approximated with continuous sutures which penetrate all of the coats of the sac without narrowing the lumen of the parent artery."[19]

Reconstructive endoaneurismorrhaphy was per-formed by Matas on fusiform aneurysms that had well-defined openings between the proximal and distal main artery which were in close proximity but which had a surrounding firm and elastic wall of the sac.[19] The continuity of the artery was then "reconstructed" by making a new channel out of the sac walls.[19] A catheter was inserted between the two openings, and then the sac wall was brought together with continuous or interrupted sutures to re-form a new channel. The catheter was removed before tying the last suture. Matas[19] found that this operation was possible only in special cases where "the condition of the sac is especially favorable for rebuilding of the lost artery and cases in which there is good reason to fear the insufficiency of the collateral circulation." He con-sidered it frequently a temporary procedure to allow for the development of collateral circulation. In 1920, Matas recorded 154 endoaneurismor-rhaphies of the popliteal arteries, of which 103 were obliterative operations.[41] There was only 1 death. There were 8 cases of gangrene, of which 5 followed obliterative operations, 2 followed recon-structive operations, and 1 followed a restorative procedure. This operative mortality rate of 0.6 percent and amputation rate of 5.2 percent are, of course, superior to previous reports of the results of ligation for extirpation for the treatment of popliteal aneurysms.

Matas had developed a mechanical constrictor which he could place on the leg to occlude the femoral artery to evaluate the adequacy of the collateral blood supply prior to his operations.[42] In addition, he constricted the femoral artery just above the adductor hiatus with his device for 5 to 10 minutes every hour for several days prior to operation to improve the collateral circulation. This may have contributed to the low amputation rates following his operations.

Bird[42] in 1935 proposed that the collateral circulation also might be improved with a lum-bar sympathectomy in addition to the use of the Matas constrictor. He reported the successful use of these techniques in a patient on whom he performed an obliterative endoaneurysmorrha-phy of a popliteal artery aneurysm. Richards and Learmouth[43] in 1942 performed a lumbar sym-pathectomy 3 weeks prior to resecting a patent popliteal artery aneurysm. Within 24 hours of removal of the aneurysm, the toe skin tempera-ture had risen from room temperature to within 2°C of the opposite limb, and by 10 days after operation, the temperature was 4°C higher than the opposite limb. Lilly[44] in 1946 reported per-forming an obliterative endoaneurysmorrhaphy 3 days after performing an alcohol injection of the lumbar sympathetic trunk. He also performed ligation of a popliteal artery 2 days after a lumbar sympathectomy. Gage[45] also performed popliteal artery operations after lumbar sympathectomy.

Linton[22] in 1949 reported 14 patients with popliteal aneurysms who had lumbar sympathectomies performed in preparation for aneurysmectomy. One patient died following the sympathectomy. The remaining 13 patients had aneurysmectomies performed 7 to 11 days after the sympathectomy. After proximal and distal control with Bethune lung tourniquet clamps, the aneurysms were excised and the ends of the artery oversewn. No attempt was made to preserve the popliteal vein. Linton states, "this is contrary to Matas' advice—there seems little support to his [Matas'] view, since the popliteal vein was resected in 12 of them without serious effect to the extremities."[22] The operation was successful in the 13 survivors. No patient developed gangrene nor had an amputation. Linton preferred aneurysmectomy rather than Matas' operation "because of the difficulty encountered frequently in obliterating the aneurysm sac due to the rigidity of its walls from arteriosclerosis and calcification."[22] It is interesting that Linton reports[22] that the most common postoperative complication was edema, which developed in 5 (38 percent) of the patients, and of which 2 required continued elastic support. Janes and Ivins[46] in 1951 reported an additional 9 aneurysm resections preceded by lumbar sympathectomy. Three sympathectomies were performed immediately before the aneurysmectomy. All these patients returned to work. Austin and Thompson[47] also reported a successful use of this technique, although the patient did have postoperative claudication. Despite these isolated reports of successful results with this method of treatment, it was soon recognized that results were good only in carefully selected patients and that restoration of arterial continuity was most desirable.

Probably the earliest attempt to completely excise a popliteal aneurysm and restore arterial continuity by an end-to-end anastomosis was reported by Lexer in 1907, according to Matas.[19] Lexer "extirpated a sac about the size of the fist

connected with both the artery and vein." He then performed a "circular arteriorrhaphy and phleborrhaphy" with the assistance of Payr's magnesium rings. In addition, the knee was flexed to right angles for 6 weeks. The artery remained patent for at least 8 months. According to Matas,[19] Enderlen of Wurzburg in 1907 and Stich of Bonn in 1908 successfully performed resections of popliteal artery aneurysms and an anastomosis of the ends of the artery by "circular arteriorrhaphy" alone, as described by Carrel. This technique continued to be applied successfully when possible. Crawford et al.[48] in 1958 reported its use for the treatment of 10 popliteal aneurysms. Scattered reports of its application still appear.[5,11,14,49] However, the need for maintaining flexion of the knee and the development of satisfactory arterial substitutes seriously detract from its usefulness.

Carrel and Guthrie's demonstrations[50] that a short vein graft could be transposed between the cut ends of an excised vein provided new hope for the improved surgical treatment of popliteal aneurysms. Goyanes in 1906, according to Friedman,[31] successfully used the adjacent nonreversed popliteal vein to replace an excised syphlitic popliteal arterial aneurysm. Pringle[51] in 1913 replaced an excised popliteal aneurysm with "4 inches of the internal saphenous vein" which was reversed "in case there might be a valve in the portion of vein used." The graft remained patent for at least 3 months. Bernheim,[52] an associate of Halsted, reported in 1916 the use of a vein graft to successfully replace an excised syphlitic popliteal aneurysm in a 49-year-old man. It was not until the 1950s that interest was renewed in vein graft replacement of aneurysms using Carrel's techniques. Julian and associates[53] in 1955 reported the use of 5 autogenous saphenous reversed vein grafts to replace excised popliteal artery aneurysms through a posterior approach. Five grafts remained patent 3 days to 10 months following operation. One graft thrombosed immediately. One patient died of heart failure 3 days following operation. Lord[54] in 1957 reported the use of 4 vein grafts to replace resected aneurysms with "good" results.

Delbet in 1906, according to Matas,[19] had tried the "transplantation of a popliteal artery (obtained from a freshly amputated leg) in place of the artery excised in extirpating a femoropopliteal aneurism." It "failed because of extreme chalky degeneration of the arteries in the aneurismal patient." Julian and associates[53] in 1955 reported the use of three frozen homologous arterial grafts for replacement of excised popliteal arterial aneurysms. In one patient, the proximal artery was so large that the abdominal aortic portion of the homograft was sutured to the femoral artery at Hunter's canal, and one of the iliac limbs of the graft was anastomosed to the distal artery after oversewing the other limb. All grafts remained patent during a 3- to 10-month period of follow-up. During the 1950s, arterial homografts were used frequently in preference to veins. Satisfactory techniques for the preservation of the grafts (usually freezing or freeze drying) had been developed. The availability "off the shelf" and the easy suturing increased their popularity. In a collected series of 76 operations where homografts were used to replace or bypass popliteal aneurysms, short-term follow-up revealed very good patency rates. However, late follow-up, when available, revealed frequent thromboses, and 14 had developed graft aneurysms.[5,11,47–49,53,55–57] Few, if any, homografts were used as arterial grafts after 1958.

In the late 1950s and 1960s, a number of other graft materials became available for use "off the shelf." Edwards and Tapp[58] in 1956 reported the use of a nylon graft to replace a popliteal aneurysm that remained patent for 8 months. Crawford et al.[48] used four nylon grafts. A false aneurysm developed in one graft attributed to the fraying of the ends of the graft. Edmunds et al.[49] reported the thrombosis of three nylon grafts acutely postoperatively. Late aneurysmal dilatation of the grafts finally resulted in discontinuation of their production. Teflon grafts were available and were used by Friesen and associates[56] and Crichlow and Roberts[5] in 24 operations with patency or good results in 18 (75 percent) of the extremities. Crawford and associates[48] and Buda and associates[48] used 60 Dacron grafts, of which 43 (72 percent) were patent or "successful" in early follow-up. Autogenous vein and arterial grafts also were being used. Crichlow and Roberts[5] and Buda and associates[9] used vein grafts in 38 extremities, of which 37 (97 percent) were patent at 1 year or had good results. Edmunds et al.[49] in 1965 reported the use of 31 autogenous saphenous vein grafts. Twelve patients who were followed for

more than 3 years remained patent for up to 10 years following operation. Wylie[59] in 1964 described the use of the external iliac artery (which was replaced by a Dacron graft) to replace 6 popliteal aneurysms. All grafts were still patent 15 to 40 months after operation. The current graft material of choice would appear to be autogenous veins, although Dacron and polytetrafluoroethylene (PTFE) grafts continue to have their proponents.

Early operations were performed with the patient in a prone or semiprone position. Longitudinal or S-shaped incisions were made over the popliteal space. The aneurysms were resected. Grafts were inserted using end-to-end anastomoses (Fig. 9-2). Edmunds and associates[49] in 1965 reported resection of the aneurysm through a medial approach and replacement with a graft using end-to-end anastomoses. Crawford and associates[48] in 1958 reported 7 operations for patients with thrombosed or multiple aneurysms that were performed with the patient supine. A short groin incision and a medial incision over the distal popliteal artery were made for thrombosed aneurysms, and bypass grafts were inserted using proximal and distal end-to-side anastomoses. Friesen et al.[56] in 1962 described 10 patients in whom the aneurysms were "isolated" (presumably ligated) and femoropopliteal bypasses performed. It is not stated whether a medial or posterior incision was used. In 1965, through the medial approach, we successfully performed a femoropopliteal vein graft bypass of a popliteal aneurysm that was ligated proximally and distally (Fig. 9-3). Edwards[60] in 1969 reported 6 such operations without complications which popularized the exclusion approach. Towne and associates[11] and Wylie[61] did not ligate the artery proximal to the aneurysm when the superior geniculate vessels were patent in hopes of preserving these collateral vessels should graft thrombosis occur.

LATE RESULTS OF OPERATION

Patency Rates of Grafts

Results of life-table analysis of the long-term patency rates of grafting procedures have been reported (Table 9-4). At 5 years, cumulative patency rates for all grafts used for operative

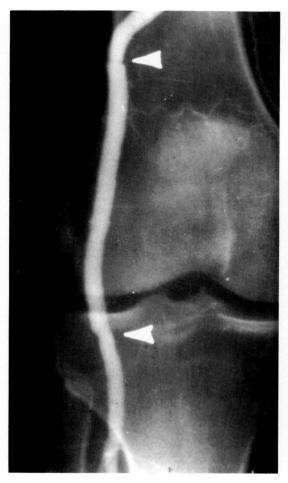

Figure 9-2. Arteriogram performed 11 years after resection of a 10-cm popliteal aneurysm followed by insertion of an autogenous saphenous vein graft through an S-shaped incision over the popliteal space.

repair of popliteal aneurysms have varied from 50 to 76 percent. At 10 years, the patency rates were 26 to 76 percent. At 15 years, patency rates of 16 and 64 percent were found in two series. Other series of long-term patency rates not reported by the life-table method are also available. Vermilion and associates[13] followed 99 reconstructions 1 to 14 years (average, 37 months) with patency rates of 68 percent.

The wide variation in reported results may in some instances be explained by the type of grafts used[10,15,16,18] (see Table 9-4). The patency rates of vein grafts at 5 years were 77 to 94 percent

and at 10 years 84 to 94 percent. These were individually significantly better than the reported prosthetic graft patency rates of 29 to 43 percent at 5 years and 27 to 41 percent at 10 years.

Figure 9-3. Arteriogram performed 70 months after ligation proximally and distal to a 4-cm-diameter popliteal aneurysm followed by insertion of an autogenous venous femoropopliteal bypass graft through a medial approach.

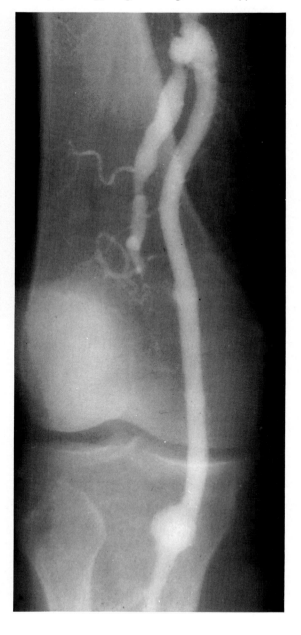

Table 9-4. Results of Operations for Popliteal Aneurysms

Result	Type	No.	Graft (%) Patency			Limb Salvage (%)		
			5 yrs	10 yrs	15 yrs	5 yrs	10 yrs	15 yrs
Overall								
Inahara[12]		40	76	76	—	—	—	—
Szilagyi[1]		50	50	26	16	—	—	—
Schellack[16]		62	61	—	—	—	—	—
Dawson[18]		42	75	64	64	95	95	95
Shortell[62]		51	67	47	—	94	94	
Type of graft								
Reilly[15]	Vein	114	77	—	—	—	—	—
	Dacron	40	30	—	—	—	—	—
Anton[10]	Vein	57	94	94	—	98	98	—
	Other	49	43	27	—	75	67	—
Dawson[18]	Vein	25	—	84	—	—	—	—
	Other	17	—	40	—	—	—	—
Shellack[16]	Vein	32	89	—	—	—	—	—
	Other	28	29	—	—	—	—	—
Complicated aneurysm								
Anton[10]	Uncomp.	55	82	82	—	93	93	—
	Comp.	68	54	48	—	82	79	—
Shellack[16]	Uncomp.	20	77	—	—	—	—	—
	Comp.	42	53	—	—	—	—	—
Shortell[62]	Uncomp.	32	92	—	—	100	—	—
	Comp.	19	39	—	—	84	—	—
Lilly[63]	Uncomp.	26	91	—	—	—	—	—
	Comp.	22	54	—	—	—	—	—
Runoff								
Shortell[62]	Good	30	89	64	—	93	—	—
	Poor	11	24	0	—	91	—	—
Lilly[63]	Good	22	84	—	—	—	—	—
	Poor	26	65	—	—	—	—	—

Variations in reported patency rate results also may be explained by the indication for operation[10,16,62] (see Table 9-4). There were differences in results between those who had uncomplicated aneurysms and those who were termed complicated or symptomatic or had limb-threatening complications usually secondary to thrombosis of the aneurysm or to distal emboli from the aneurysm. The 5-year patency rates for grafts used for uncomplicated aneurysms were 77 to 92 percent, compared with 39 to 54 percent for patients with complicated aneurysms.[10,16,62,63] Anton and associates[10] observed an 82 percent 5-year patency rate in asymptomatic limbs as compared with 48 percent in symptomatic limbs.

Whitehouse and associates[14] found no graft thromboses in operations performed on asymptomatic limbs.

Differences in patency rates also may be related to the preoperative status of the runoff vessels. Shortell et al.[62] observed 5- and 10-year patency rates of 89 and 65 percent, respectively, in patients with good two- to three-vessel runoff. This was compared with 24 and 0 percent patencies at 5 and 10 years, respectively, in limbs with no or one-vessel runoff due to distal embolization from the aneurysm or arteriosclerotic occlusion. Lilly et al.[63] observed a 5-year graft patency rate of 84 percent for limbs with two- to three-vessel runoff and a 65 percent patency when there was no or one-vessel runoff. Bouhoutsos and Martin[8] also have emphasized the importance of the patency of the runoff vessels for maintaining early and late graft patencies. Grafts were placed in 16 limbs with thrombosed popliteal aneurysms and patent runoff vessels, and only 1 (6 percent) required early or late amputation. On the other hand, 26 of 39 (67 percent) similar patients but with involvement of the runoff vessells required amputation.

Thrombolytic Therapy

For improved graft patency, it is apparent that it is important to restore patency of the runoff vessels whenever possible. This is most important in the patient with acute thromboembolic events. The use of balloon catheters has been disappointing for thrombectomy of the unstable lumen of the thrombosed aneurysm and fragile tibioperoneal arteries. Thrombolytic therapy provides an attractive alternative.

Schwarz et al.[64] in 1984 reported the successful treatment of an acutely thrombosed aneurysm with thrombolytic therapy. A 61-year-old man presented with a 4-day history of ischemic symptoms and an "egg-sized" mass in the popliteal space. An ultrasound confirmed the presence of a popliteal artery aneurysm, and the arteriogram confirmed that there was total occlusion of the popliteal artery with reconstitution of the tibioperoneal vessels, which contained thrombus. A catheter was introduced distally into the femoral artery and advanced to the popliteal artery. Streptokinase was infused at the rate of 5000 units per hour. Fourteen hours later, the runoff vessels were patent, but there was residual clot in the aneurysm. This clot was lysed within the next 4 hours. Intravenous heparin was administered continuously, and the next day the aneurysm was replaced with an interposed reversed vein graft. At discharge, the patient had a warm leg and a good dorsalis pedis pulse.

The recognition of a thrombosed popliteal aneurysm as the cause of an acutely ischemic limb has not always been easy. Bowyer and associates[65] suspected the presence of an aneurysm in 7 of 9 patients, but Ferguson and associates[66] suspected it in only 3 of 10. The diagnosis of the aneurysm was usually made on the basis of physical examination but was suspected in patients with contralateral popliteal or extrapopliteal aneurysm. Unsuspected thrombosed aneurysms have been identified in centers where thrombolytic therapy is being evaluated or is already standard therapy for the treatment of acutely ischemic limbs. Ferguson and associates[66] demonstrated popliteal aneurysms in 10 of 65 unselected patients. Lancashire et al.[67] treated 5 aneurysms in 40 selected patients. Ouriel et al.,[69] on the other hand, saw no popliteal aneurysms in 57 patients with acute limb ischemia randomized to thrombolytic therapy.

Thrombolytic drugs have been infused through catheters inserted antegradely into the ipsilateral femoral artery, as performed by Schwarz, but more commonly the catheters are introduced through the contralateral femoral artery and manipulated over the aortic bifurcation and into the femoral artery of the involved extremity. Currently, after passage of wires through the thrombus, catheters with single or multiple holes are positioned within the thrombus. During continuous infusion, arteriograms are repeated at 6- to 18-hour intervals for repositioning of the catheters. Streptokinase has been infused at rates of 5000 to 10,000 units per hour by some.[65,67] Others have given loading doses of 50,000 to 120,000 units per hour over a 4-hour period, followed by doses of 1000 to 8000 units per hour.[66] Urokinase has been administered at doses of 1000 to 4000 units per minute.[68,69]

Thrombolytic therapy for the preparation of patients for operative correction of popliteal aneurysms has shown promise (Table 9-5). Thirty-four popliteal aneurysms with acute thromboembolic complications have been treated and reported.[64–68,70] From this collected series there were 20 patients treated within 7 days of onset. Complete lysis of the thrombus in the aneurysm was achieved in 18 and partial lysis in 2. Complete lysis of thrombus in runoff vessels was achieved in 12 and partial lysis in 2. Seventeen patients had arterial reconstruction. Grafts were patent in all 17 extremities 3 days to 90 months later. Thrombolytic therapy was used in 4 patients greater than 10 days after onset. Aneurysm thrombus was lysed in all 4, but runoff vessels were improved in only 2 patients. Ferguson and associates[66] treated 10 limbs 0 to 28 days after the onset of their symptoms. Lytic

Table 9-5. Results of Thrombolysis for Popliteal Aneurysms (Collected Series)

Duration of Symptoms	Number	Aneurysm Lysis		Runoff Lysis		Recon-structed	Patency		Ampu-tation
		Complete	Partial	Complete	Partial		No. Patent	Time	
Acute, <7 days	20	18	2	12	2	17	17	3–9 mos.	0
Chronic, >10 days	4	2	0	2	0	2	2	4–? mos.	0
Unclassified, 0–28 days	10	?	?	?	?	5	5	6–24 mos.	3

therapy was successful in 7. The 5 patients who had arterial repair had patent grafts 6 to 24 months later. Lytic therapy was unsuccessful in 3 patients, and amputations were performed. Complications consisted of two groin hematomas, two retroperitoneal hematomas with one death, one late distal thrombosis, and three amputations. The short-term results of thrombolytic therapy are impressive and hopefully will be reflected in improved long-term graft patency rates.

Limb Salvage

Limb salvage rates following grafting procedures were reported to be 94 percent at 10 years by Shortell and associates[62] and 95 percent at 15 years by Dawson and associates[18] (see Table 9-4). The limb salvage rates were much better than the graft patency rates in the same patients, indicating that only 5 to 6 percent of the limbs required amputation despite a 36 to 53 percent graft thrombosis rate. Anton et al.[10] reported much better limb salvage rates with vein grafts compared with prosthetic grafts. Amputation rates 10 years following vein grafting were only 2 percent when 6 percent of the grafts were thrombosed. If prosthetic grafts were used, there was a 10-year amputation rate of 33 percent when 73 percent of the grafts were thrombosed. Shortell and associates[62] and Anton and associates[10] also found, as expected, that the limb salvage was better in uncomplicated aneurysms than in complicated aneurysms. The 5-year amputation rates were 0 and 7 percent when the thrombosis rate was 8 and 18

percent for operations on uncomplicated aneurysms.[10,62] These numbers increased to amputation rates of 16 and 18 percent with graft thrombosis rates of 61 and 46 percent for operations on complicated aneurysms.[10,62]

The discrepancy between amputation rate and graft thrombosis rate may be explained by the good collateral circulation through the geniculate arteries around the middle of the popliteal artery. Popliteal artery ligation for war related injuries in World War I and II resulted in a significant rate of limb loss.[71] In addition to popliteal artery injury, however, there also was associated soft tissue injury and damage to the collateral vessels. According to Matas,[19] Delbet reported the incidence of gangrene to be only 2.77 percent of 86 cases in which the popliteal aneurysm was "extirpated" without actual reconstruction. During the same period, ligation of popliteal aneurysms resulted in only a 7.65 percent incidence of gangrene.[19] The Antyllus method of incising the aneurysm and packing it resulted in only an 8.33 percent incidence of amputation.[19] Linton[22] reported that no amputations occurred after lumbar sympathectomy and aneurysm excision in 13 patients. Recent experience suggests that such good long-term results occur only in patients operated on before peripheral embolization or arteriosclerosis occurs. This concept is supported by observations that graft replacement is most successful in patients without outflow disease or in those in whom tibioperoneal occlusions are bypassed at the time of operation.[8,10,15] Improved collateral blood flow also may have occurred following gradual thrombosis of an aneurysm or of a graft.

New Aneurysms

Towne et al.[11] observed the development of new popliteal aneurysms proximal or distal to the original aneurysm in 6 of 69 popliteal operations. These were recognized between 5 months and 10 years after operation. Extrapopliteal aneurysms also may develop or become recognized during follow-up. Dawson and associates[18] reported 23 new aneurysms during a mean time of 5 years after operation. There were 6 thoracoabdominal, 11 femoral, and 6 contralateral popliteal aneurysms. One patient suffered a fatal rupture of an abdominal aortic aneurysm, and 2 developed acute thrombosis of a contralateral popliteal aneurysm and required amputation. These unusual complications point out the need for long-term careful follow-up of the patients.

Enlargement

Schellack and associates[16] described a patient who underwent proximal and distal ligation and bypass of a large popliteal aneurysm and continued to complain of discomfort. At reoperation, it was found that large geniculate collaterals were responsible for continued patency and enlargement of the aneurysm. Flynn and Nicholas[72] described two patients with similar findings. One patient had bypass of a ligated aneurysm 7 × 10 cm in size and returned 3½ years later with a painful 9 × 13 cm aneurysm. At operation, the aneurysm was evacuated of clot, and a geniculate artery "was seen to be feeding the aneurysm distally." The second patient had a similar exclusion operation for a 5 × 8 cm aneurysm. Thirteen months later he returned for increased swelling of the aneurysm, which was now 7 × 10 cm in size. "On opening the aneurysm, a large amount of clot and serum was removed. . . . A single geniculate artery was found back-bleeding into the aneurysm." Late enlargement or pain has been described in which no feeding collaterals were identified.[62] Roberts[73] described a thrombosed aneurysm which enlarged and from which he aspirated 700 ml of a "lymphatic type" fluid. This observation as well as that of Flynn, who found "serum" in the aneurysm, would suggest that in some patients the enlargement is a collection of serous fluid, akin to that frequently observed in resolving subcutaneous hematomas.

Patient Survival

The patient survival rates after popliteal artery reconstruction, as in all operations for complications of arteriosclerosis, are lower than those of the normal population of similar ages. Survival rates at 5 and 10 years are in the range of 60 and 40 percent, respectively.[10,13,18] Cardiac disease, usually of the coronary arteries, is responsible for 30 to 50 percent of the deaths. Stroke is responsible for 6 to 20 percent and ruptured aneurysms 3 to 6 percent of the deaths.

FEMORAL ARTERY ANEURYSMS

Femoral artery aneurysms, like popliteal artery aneurysms, are relatively rare. Dent and associates[2] found only 37 femoral artery aneurysms during a period when 1488 patients with aneurysms of the abdominal aorta and its branches were seen, an incidence of only 2.4 percent. When present, however, multiple aneurysms are frequently seen. From a collected series of patients with a femoral artery aneurysm, contralateral femoral artery aneurysms occur in 44 percent, abdominal aortic aneurysms are found in 38 percent, and popliteal artery aneurysms occur in 29 percent.[2,74,75]

Pathogenesis and Pathology

Femoral artery aneurysms may be associated with arteriosclerosis, blunt trauma, or needle puncture. False aneurysms secondary to catheterization and angiography are probably the most frequently seen femoral artery aneurysms and will not be discussed here. Anastomotic aneurysms and mycotic aneurysms secondary to the use of contaminated needles by intravenous drug abusers also will not be discussed. Whether blunt trauma is a cause is problematic, since arteriosclerosis is also usually present.[76] As with popliteal aneurysms, however, the possibility exists that proximal constriction of the artery between the inguinal ligament and the ilium is contributory to the aneurysm. Syphilis is rarely, if ever, incriminated.

The aneurysms most often involve the common femoral artery. A collected series of 157 femoral artery aneurysms were localized to the common femoral artery in 126, superficial femoral

Table 9-6. Complicated Femoral Aneurysms Admitted to Massachusetts General Hospital, 1952–1972

	Number	Percent
Expanding	9	20
Ruptured	9	20
Acute thrombosis	10	22
Chronic thrombosis	10	22
Distal thrombosis	7	16
	45	

artery in 30, and the profunda femoris artery only in 1 (see Table 9-2). From a practical standpoint, however, Cutler and Darling[75] found that common femoral artery aneurysms terminated enough proximal to the junction of the superficial and deep femoral arteries to allow preservation of the bifurcation in 24 of 45 (44 percent) cases. In the other 56 percent, the deep or superficial arteries were dilated proximally or the origins of the vessels were in continuity with dilatation of the common femoral artery.

Natural History

As with popliteal artery aneurysms, the threat to life and limb with femoral artery aneurysms has been recognized for centuries. The complications that prompted admission to Massachusetts General Hospital from 1952 to 1972 demonstrate the severity of these problems[75] (Table 9-6). Forty-five patients with 63 aneurysms were admitted with complications. Nine aneurysms (20 percent) were expanding and were producing localized pain, swelling, and tenderness, as well as femoral nerve irritation and distal venous engorgement in some. Nine aneurysms (20 percent) had already ruptured with preceding symptoms of expansion. Acute thrombsis had occurred in 10 (22 percent) of the aneurysms, of which 6 had gangrene or ischemic ulcerations. Chronic thrombosis producing claudication was present in 10 (22 percent) of the limbs. Seven limbs (16 percent) presented with distal occlusive disease due to embolization, thrombosis of popliteal aneurysms, or arteriosclerosis producing claudication. Tolstedt and associates[76] reported

thrombosis of 5 of 9 femoral artery aneurysms in less than 10 years of follow-up. Thrombosis led to amputation in all 5 patients. Thrombsis occurred in 16 percent (7 of 44) of femoral artery aneurysms in patients not considered fit for arterial reconstruction in less than 13 years in a series reported by Pappas and associates.[74]

Diagnosis

The diagnosis of a femoral artery aneurysm is easily made, except in unusual circumstances such as in very obese patients. It can be confirmed by ultrasound.[77] Because of the frequent association of abdominal aortic (38 percent) and popliteal artery aneurysms (29 percent), ultrasound also should be obtained of the abdomen and popliteal space. If operation is planned, arteriography is helpful to identify inflow or outflow disease.

Indication for Operation

Because of the threat of complications, ease of operation, low complication rate, and improved results when the operation is performed electively, operation for aneurysms greater than 2 cm in diameter should be considered in patients without medical contraindications.

Surgical Treatment

Although common femoral artery aneurysms are more easily recognized, they did not apparently attract the interest given to popliteal aneurysms by ancient physicians. The reason for this may be found in Matas' treatise,[19] where he discusses primarily femoral artery aneurysms distal to the bifurcation of the common femoral artery, "where circular elastic constriction is practical for hemostatic purposes." Matas considered common femoral artery aneurysms "surgically in the same light as iliofemoral or inguinal aneurisms." Barwell, according to Matas,[19] reported in 1883, prior to antisepsis, that the ligation of the common femoral artery below the origin of the epigastric and circumflex iliac branches in the presence of an aneurysm resulted in a 58 percent secondary hemorrhage rate and a 51 percent mortality rate.

However, in patients in whom the external iliac artery was ligated, there was secondary hemorrhage in only 22 percent. Delbet in 1895, according to Matas,[19] reported that with the advent of absorbable aseptic ligatures, the danger of secondary hemorrhage was practically eliminated, but gangrene still occurred following 19 percent of external iliac artery ligations for common femoral artery aneurysms. Matas[19] collected six cases of endaneurysmorrhaphy for the treatment of "high femoral aneurysms seated above the line of practicable circular elastic constriction." One patient died of rupture, another required amputation, and four cases were successful.

Matas did collect 43 cases of superficial femoral artery aneurysms managed by surgery.[19] There were 10 cases treated by ligation with "4 failures," and 2 developed gangrene. There were 9 cases treated by "extirpation" of the aneurysm without death or gangrene. There were 9 cases treated by the "Antyllian operation of double ligature, incision, and packing" without death or gangrene. There were 15 aneurysms treated with endoaneurysmorrhaphy, of which 8 aneurysms were obliterated with intrasaccular sutures. Of the other 7, 6 were "restorative" and 1 one was "reconstructive." There were no deaths nor gangrene.

Restorative endoaneurysmorrhaphy entails approximation of the more normal arterial wall found around the opening into a false or saccular aneurysm. *Reconstructive aneurysmorrhapy* consists of constructing a "tube" between the proximal and distal openings of a fusiform aneurysm by suturing the back wall of the aneurysm together. Blakemore[78] in 1947 described an innovation of this technique. He inserted a tube consisting of a segment of the superficial femoral vein tied over two vitallium tubes that were inserted into the proximal and distal openings of an incised common femoral aneurysmal sac. The vein graft remained patent "in excess of a year." Until the mid-1950s, ligation and endoaneurysmorrhaphy were still the treatment of choice for femoral artery aneurysms. For a period beginning in 1952, Cutler and Darling[75] still list the performance of 3 ligations and 5 aneurysmorrhaphies for the treatment of common femoral aneurysms. Pappas and associates,[74] for a period beginning in 1950, performed 3 endoanneurysmorrhaphies.

In the mid-1950s, resection of the aneurysm and replacement with a graft by performing end-to-end ansatomoses became the standard treatment for most aneurysms, including common and superficial femoral artery aneurysms. Arterial homografts were used in some cases by Crawford and associates,[48] in 7 cases by Cutler and Darling,[75] and in 10 cases by Pappas and associates.[74] Homografts were abandoned "because the deterioration of a homograft in this area was of such a degree that the overall results were not good."[74] Woven Teflon also was used but found unsatisfactory.[48,74,75] Wylie[59] described the use of autologous external iliac arteries that had been replaced by Dacron grafts for 10 common femoral artery aneurysms. Knitted Dacron and vein became the preferred grafts, although the saphenous vein was frequently not large enough. Polytetrafluoroethylene (PTFE) grafts are also commonly used.

Operative management for over half the common femoral artery aneurysms is straightforward. The usual aneurysm can be excised from distal to the inferior epigastric and circumflex arterial branches at the inguinal ligament to just proximal to the bifurcation. An interpositional graft can be inserted with end-to-end anastomoses. Instead of using a graft in two cases, Inahara and Toledo[2] were able to mobilize ectatic external iliac arteries and anastomose them end-to-end to the distal common femoral artery. If the superficial femoral artery is thrombosed, the distal anastomosis can be made end-to-end to the deep femoral artery. If removal of the aneurysm requires division of both the superficial femoral and deep femoral arteries, continuity of flow sometimes can be established to both vessels by using a small bifurcation graft. An alternative is to perform an end-to-end anastomosis to the superficial femoral artery and then anastomose the deep femoral artery end-to-side to the graft. Another alternative in the presence of quite normal vessels is to construct a new bifurcation. The deep and superficial arteries are placed side to side, and with scissors, a longitudinal incision is made through the open ends of the arteries down the coapted inner walls. The resulting cut edges of the two arteries are sutured together to reconstruct a bifurcation. The circumference of the end of this vessel will now equal the sum of the circumference of the two vessels and will approximate the size of the proximal common femoral artery, and a suitable graft can be anastomosed end-to-end to both vessels. Aneurysms of the superficial femoral arteries can be excised and replaced with short tube grafts. On occasion, these have been reconstructed with a direct end-to-end anastomosis.[48] Deep femoral artery aneurysms are extremely rare. An attempt to ligate one and bypass it with a Dacron graft by Cutler and Darling[75] was initially successful but occluded at 9 months. A vein graft should give hope for a longer-term success.

Long-Term Results

Cutler and Darling[75] reported a cumulative patency rate of 83 percent for autogenous vein and Dacron interpositional grafts at 5 years. There were 18 patients who had operations for uncomplicated aneurysms, and there was a 100 percent patency rate. There were 45 patients with complicated aneurysms. Nine patients underwent emergency operations for rupture, and all 4 patients who had reconstructions had patent grafts when last seen. Twenty patients were operated on for thrombosis of the aneurysm, and graft occlusion occurred in 5 patients, 8 remained symptomatic, and 2 required amputation. Nine patients had arterial reconstruction for prerupture symptoms with one graft occlusion. The increased patency rate and decreased incidence of amputations in patients operated on for asymptomatic aneurysms as compared with those operated on for complications support the aggressive resection of femoral artery aneurysms in those who are medically fit.

REFERENCES

1. Szilagyi DE, Schwartz RL, Reddy DJ: Popliteal arterial aneurysms. Arch Surg 1981;116:724.
2. Dent TL, Lindenauer SM, Ernst CB, et al: Multiple arteriosclerotic arterial aneurysms. Arch Surg 1972; 105:338.
3. DeWeese JA, Shortell C, Green R: Operative repair of popliteal aneurysms: Twenty-five years experience. In Yao JST, Pearce WH (eds): Long-Term Results in Vascular Surgery. Norwalk, Conn, Appleton & Lange, 1993, p 287.
4. Gifford RW Jr, Hines EA Jr, Janes JM: An analysis and follow-up study of one hundred popliteal aneurysms. Surgery 1953;33:284.
5. Crichlow RW, Roberts B: Treatment of popliteal aneurysms by restoration of continuity. Ann Surg 1966;163:417.
6. Baird RJ, Sivasankar R, Hayward R, et al. Popliteal aneurysms: A review and analysis of 61 cases. Surgery 1966;59:911.
7. Wychulis AR, Spittell JA Jr, Wallace RB: Popliteal aneurysms. Surgery 1970;68:942.
8. Bouhoutsos J, Martin P: Popliteal aneurysms: A review of 116 cases. Br J Surg 1974;61:469.
9. Buda JA, Weber CJ, McAllister FF, et al: The results of treatment of popliteal artery aneurysms. A follow-up study of 86 aneurysms. J Cardiovasc Surg 1974;15:615.
10. Anton GE, Hertzer NR, Beven EG, et al: Surgical management of popliteal aneurysms. Trends in presentation, treatment, and results from 1952 to 1984. J Vasc Surg 1986;3:125.
11. Towne JB, Thompson JE, Patman DD, et al: Progression of popliteal aneurysmal disease following popliteal aneurysm resection with graft: A twenty-year experience. Surgery 1976;80:426.
12. Inahara T, Toledo AC: Complications and treatment of popliteal aneurysms. Surgery 1978;84:775.
13. Vermilion BD, Kimmins SA, Pace WG, et al: A review of one-hundred forty-seven popliteal aneurysms with long-term follow-up. Surgery 1981; 90:1009.
14. Whitehouse WM Jr, Wakefield TW, Graham LM, et al: Limb-threatening potential of arteriosclerotic popliteal artery aneurysms. Surgery 1983; 93:694.
15. Reilly MK, Abbott WM, Darling RC: Aggressive surgical management of popliteal artery aneurysms. Am J Surg 1983;145:498.
16. Schellack J, Smith RB III, Perdue GD: Nonoperative management of selected popliteal aneurysms. Arch Surg 1987;122:372.
17. Farina C, Cavallaro A, Schultz RD, et al: Popliteal aneurysms. Surg Gynecol Obstet 1989;169:7.
18. Dawson I, van Bockel JH, Brand R, et al: Popliteal artery aneurysms. J Vasc Surg 1991;13:398.
19. Matas R: Aneurism. In Keen WW, DaCosta JC (eds):Keen's Surgery, vol 5. Philadelphia, W B Saunders Company, 1912, pp 255–290.
20. Theis FV: Popliteal aneurysms as a cause of peripheral circulatory disease: With special study of oscillographs as an aid to diagnosis. Surgery 1937;2:327.
21. Wells AH, Coburn CE, Walker MA: Popliteal aneurysm. JAMA 1936;106:1264.
22. Linton RR: The arteriosclerotic popliteal aneurysm. Surgery 1949;26:41.
23. Tilson MD: Atherosclerosis and aneurysm disease. J Vasc Surg 1990;12:371.
24. Power D: Hunter's operation for the cure of aneurysm. Br J Surg 1929;17:193.

25. Gedge SW, Spittel JA Jr, Ivins JC: Aneurysms of the distal popliteal artery and its relationships to the arcuate popliteal ligament. Circulation 1961;24:270.

26. Halsted WS: An experimental study of circumscribed dilation of an artery immediately distal to a partially occluding band, and its bearing on the dilation of the subclavian artery observed in certain cases of cervical rib. J Exp Med 1916;24:271.

27. Palma EC: Stenosed arteriopathy at Hunter canal and loop of adductor magnus. Am J Surg 1995; 83:723.

28. Boyd AM, Ratcliffe AH, Jepson RP, et al: Intermittent claudication: A clinical study. J Bone Joint Surg 1949;31B:325.

29. Cavallaro A, DiMarzo L, Gallo P, et al: Popliteal artery entrapment. Analysis of the literature and report of personal experience. Vasc Surg 1986;68:404.

30. Friedman SG (ed): Brothers Hunter. A history of vascular surgery. Mt. Kisco, NY, Futura, 1989, pp 33–44.

31. Friedman SG (ed): The arterial prosthesis: Arthur Voorhees. A history of vascular surgery. Mt. Kisco, NY, Futura, 1989, pp 131–139.

32. Guvendik L, Bloor K, Charlesworth D: Popliteal aneurysm: Sinister harbinger of sudden catastrophe. Br J Surg 1980;67:294.

33. Chan O, Thomas ML: Patients with arteriomegaly. Clin Radiol 1990;41:185.

34. Collins GJ Jr, Rich NM, Phillips J, et al: Ultrasound diagnosis of popliteal arterial aneurysms. Am Surg 1976;42:853.

35. Davis RP, Neiman HL, Yao JST, et al: Ultrasound scan in diagnosis of peripheral aneurysms. Arch Surg 1977;112:55.

36. Scott WW Jr, Scott PP, Sanders RC: B-scan ultrasound in the diagnosis of popliteal aneurysms. Surgery 1977;81:436.

37. Carpenter JR, Hattery RR, Hunder GG, et al: Ultrasound evaluation of the popliteal space. Comparison with arthrography and physical examination. Mayo Clin Proc 1976;51:498.

38. Neiman HL, Yao JST, Silver TM: Gray-scale ultrasound diagnosis of peripheral arterial aneurysms. Radiology 1979;130:413.

39. Henry AK: Some surgical aspects of aneurysm. Practitioner 943;150:136.

40. Chitwood WR: John and William Hunter on aneurysms. Arch Surg 1977;112:829.

41. Matas R: Endoaneurismorrhaphy. Surg Gynecol Obstet 1920;30:456.

42. Bird CE: Sympathectomy as a preliminary to the obliteration of popliteal aneurisms. Surg Gynecol Obstet 1935;60:926.

43. Richards RL, Learmonth JR: Lumbar sympathectomy in treatment of popliteal aneurysm. Lancet 1942;1:383.

44. Lilly GD: The management of aneurysms of the lower extremities. Ann Surg 1946;123:601.

45. Gage M: Editorial: The development of the collateral circulation in peripheral arterial aneurysms by sympathetic block. Surgery 1940;7:792.

46. Janes JM, Ivins JC: A method of dealing with arteriosclerotic popliteal aneurysms. Surgery 1951; 29:398.

47. Austin DJ, Thompson JE: Excision and arterial grafting in the surgical management of popliteal aneurysms. South Med J 1958;51:43.

48. Crawford ES, DeBakey ME, Cooley DA: Surgical considerations of peripheral arterial aneurysms. Arch Surg 1958;78:226.

49. Edmunds LH Jr, Darling RC, Linton RR: Surgical management of popliteal aneurysms. Circulation 1965;32:517.

50. Carrel A, Guthrie CC: Uniterminal and biterminal venous transplantation. Surg Gynecol Obstet 1906; 99:266.

51. Pringle JH: Two cases of vein-grafting for the maintenance of a direct arterial circulation. Lancet 1913;1:1795.

52. Bernheim BM: The ideal operation for aneurysm of the extremity. Report of a case. Bull Johns Hopkins Hosp 1916;27:93.

53. Julian OC, Dye WS, Javid H, et al: The use of vessel grafts in the treatment of popliteal aneurysms. Surgery 1955;38:970.

54. Lord JW Jr: Clinical behavior and operative management of popliteal aneurysms. JAMA 1957; 163:1102.

55. Taber RE, Lawrence MS: Resection and arterial replacement in the treatment of popliteal aneurysms. Surgery 1956;39:1003.

56. Friesen G, Ivins JC, Janes JM: Popliteal aneurysms. Surgery 1962;51:90.

57. Barner HB, DeWeese JA, Dale WA, et al: Aneurysmal degeneration of femoropopliteal arterial homografts. JAMA 1966;196:631.

58. Edwards WS, Tapp JS: Peripheral artery replacement with chemically treated nylon tubes. Surg Gynecol Obstet 1956;102:443.

59. Wylie EJ: Vascular replacement with arterial autografts. Surgery 1965;57:14.

60. Edwards WS: Exclusion and saphenous vein bypass of popliteal aneurysms. Surg Gynecol Obstet 1969; 128:829.

61. Wylie EJ: Popliteal Aneurysms (discussion). Surgery 1970;68:951.

62. Shortell CK, DeWeese JA, Ouriel K, et al: Popliteal artery aneurysms: 25-year surgical experience. J Vasc Surg 1991;14:771.

63. Lilly MP, Flinn WR, McCarthy WJ III, et al: The effect of distal arterial anatomy on the success of popliteal aneurysm repair. J Vasc Surg 1988;7:653.

64. Schwarz W, Berkowitz H, Taormina V, et al: The preoperative use of intra-arterial thrombolysis for a thrombosed popliteal artery aneurysm. J Cardiovasc Surg 1984;25:465.

65. Bowyer RC, Cawthorn SJ, Walker WJ, et al: Conservative management of asymptomatic popliteal aneurysm. Br J Surg 1990;77:1132.

66. Ferguson LJ, Faris I, Robertson A, et al: Intraarterial streptokinase therapy to relieve acute limb ischemia. J Vasc Surg 1986;4:205.

67. Lancashire MJR, Torrie EPH, Galland RB: Popliteal aneurysms identified by intra-arterial streptokinase: A changing pattern of presentation. Br J Surg 1990;77(12):1388.

68. Carpenter JP, Barker CF, Roberts B, et al: Popliteal artery aneurysms: Current management and outcome. J Vasc Surg 1994;19:65.

69. Ouriel K, Shortell CK, DeWeese JA, et al: A comparison of thrombolytic therapy with operative revascularization in the treatment of acute peripheral arterial ischemia. J Vasc Surg 1994;19:1021.

70. Garramone RR Jr, Gallagher JJ Jr, Drezner AD: Intra-arterial thrombolytic therapy in the initial management of thrombosed popliteal artery aneurysms: A report of three cases. Presented at the third annual meeting of the Peripheral Vascular Surgery Society, Breckenridge, Colorado, 1993.

71. DeBakey ME, Simeone FA: Vascular Surgery in World War II. Washington, DC: US Government Printing Office, 1955.

72. Flynn JB, Nicholas GG: An unusual complication of bypassed popliteal aneurysms. Arch Surg 1983;118:111.

73. Roberts B: Popliteal artery aneurysms: A 25-year surgical experience (discussion). J Vasc Surg 1991;14:771.

74. Pappas G, Janes JM, Bernatz PE, et al: Femoral aneurysms. JAMA 1964;190:489.

75. Cutler BS, Darling RC: Surgical management of arteriosclerotic femoral aneurysms. Surgery 1973;74:764.

76. Tolstedt GE, Radke HM, Bell JW: Late sequela of zarteriosclerotic femoral aneurysms. Angiology 1961;12:601.

77. Gooding GAW, Effeney DJ: Ultrasound of femoral artery aneurysms. AJR 1980;134:477.

78. Blakemore AH: Restorative endoaneurysmorrhaphy by vein graft inlay. Ann Surg 1947;126:841.

79. Inahara T: Aneurysms of the common femoral artery. Am J Surg 1966;111:759.

Endovascular Aneurysm Repair

TIMOTHY A. M. CHUTER

The advent of endovascular grafting as a means of aneurysm repair is part of a general trend in surgery toward "less invasive" treatment. With the help of new imaging techniques, surgeons have learned to operate through long, thin instruments that eliminate the need for direct surgical exposure. Considering endovascular graft technology in this wider perspective is instructive. For example, attention to some of the lessons of endoscopic and laparoscopic surgery can be applied to the dissemination and testing of endovascular grafting technology.

The main advantage of endovascular grafting is the avoidance of an abdominal operation. The graft is introduced through a remote artery, usually the common femoral artery. Effective aneurysm repair requires passage of the delivery system through the iliac arteries and secure, hemostatic implantation of the graft proximal and distal to the aneurysm. The ability of a given system of endovascular grafting to satisfy these requirements depends largely on its ability to accommodate variations in the anatomy of the arterial tree.

The most important step in the development of endovascular grafting was the use of the arterial stent as a means of graft attachment. All current systems rely on the structural functions of a stent, and the characteristics of the stent are primary determinants of system behavior.

Endovascular grafting requires sophisticated imaging. Access to the necessary but expensive imaging equipment is one factor that may determine who performs the procedure. Another factor is training; few vascular surgeons currently possess the necessary catheter skills to perform the procedure satisfactorily.

The arterial anatomy found in patients with aortic aneurysm is difficult to mimic in animal models. Therefore, clinical trials often provide the first opportunity to assess many aspects of system behavior. Moreover, the long-term fate of a graft inside an artery is entirely unknown. Early clinical trials should be designed to reflect these considerations.

ANEURYSM MORPHOLOGY AND DESIGN CONSIDERATIONS

Endovascular techniques are not as versatile or flexible as their conventional surgical counterparts. They are much more sensitive to variations in the anatomy of the arterial tree. Therefore, information on variant anatomy is an important consideration in system design. The goal is to produce a system that will be able to meet the challenges posed by the largest possible number of patients. The overall performance of a system often can be predicted by examining the function of its constituent elements in light of the common anatomic variants likely to be encountered in aneurysm repair. Anatomic information from preoperative imaging is also vital in patient selection.

Aneurysm Neck

Close apposition between the aorta and the proximal end of the graft is vital. Blood flowing onto a

Table 10-1. Length of the Proximal Neck and Distal Cuff in 22 Aortic Aneurysms by Three-Dimensional Reconstruction of CT Data

	≤ 10 mm	10.1–20 mm	> 20 mm
Neck	4	4	14
Cuff	18	3	1

poorly attached proximal graft orifice will inevitably produce leakage and graft displacement. Therefore, the feasibility of endovascular aneurysm repair with any of the current stent-attached grafts depends on the presence of a suitable site for stent implantation between the renal arteries and the aneurysm. The optimal site is long, straight, and cylindrical. A long neck confers several advantages:

1. A greater zone of apposition between the aorta and the graft, which may lessen the chance of leakage
2. More secure stent attachment
3. More leeway for variability in stent position

The length of neck that is considered necessary for aneurysm repair with any given system will therefore depend on the minimum requirements for each of these three functions of proximal graft attachment.

In a series of 22 patients studied by three-dimensional reconstruction of computed tomographic (CT) data,[1] 67 percent had a neck longer than 2 cm (Table 10-1). However, larger aneurysms tended to be associated with shorter necks. Only 38 percent of aneurysms larger than 6 cm had a neck longer than 2 cm.

Leakage will not occur if the graft is pressed tightly against the aorta by the struts of the stent. Generally, the better the stent conforms to irregularities in the aortic wall, and the greater the number of struts, the better will be the seal.

In the presence of a short neck, the security of stent implantation can be improved by implanting an uncovered portion of the stent at the level of the renal (or even mesenteric) arteries, the assumption being that the stent will neither occlude nor damage these aortic branches. Clearly, the validity of this assumption will depend on the characteristics of the particular stent. A still more radical version of this approach is to create holes in the graft, through which the visceral arteries can be perfused, while isolating the adjacent aneurysm from the circulation. Here the requirement is for very accurate imaging to localize the visceral branches.

Accurate placement depends on precise control of stent position during implantation and reliable information concerning the location of the relevant anatomic landmarks, specifically the renal artery orifices. It is rarely difficult to locate the renal arteries angiographically, but it is much more difficult to know their position at the time of implantation. Any movement in the imaging system, the patient, or the aorta may invalidate localization based on earlier angiograms. For example, most delivery systems will induce some straightening of a tortuous aorta. The resulting movement of the neck will not be detected unless the angiogram is repeated or there is a constant reference point, such as a guidewire in the renal artery. Minor degrees of aortic angulation in the region of the aneurysm neck are almost universal (mean 31.1 ± 19.3 degrees). Severe angulation (> 45 degrees) is unusual, occurring in approximately 18 percent of cases.

Distal Cuff

The creation of a hemostatic seal between the graft and nondilated artery is as important distally as it is proximally, even though the primary direction of blood flow at the distal end of the graft will tend to lessen the tendency for gross leakage at the distal implantation site. Indeed, a large gap between the aorta and the graft may not even produce sufficient retrograde perigraft flow for angiographic detection. However, such a gap will still transmit pressure to the aneurysm and may act as a route for leakage should rupture occur.

Secure hemostatic distal implantation of a straight, aortoaortic graft relies on the presence of a suitable segment of nondilated aorta between the aneurysm and the renal arteries (the distal cuff). The paucity of the distal cuff in the majority of aneurysms is a major limitation on endovascular repair of aortic aneurysms using straight grafts. In a series of 22 patients studied at the University of

Rochester, only 4 (18 percent) had a distal cuff longer than 1 cm, and only 1 (4.5 percent) had a cuff longer than 2 cm (see Table 10-1). All 4 were associated with small aneurysms (<5 cm).

Even when a suitable distal cuff is present, there is very little leeway for variation in the position of the distal stent, although a small degree of redundancy may be permissible with these large-diameter grafts. The resulting buckling and infolding is only apparent on evaluation with intravascular ultrasound. Even so, sufficiently accurate preoperative determinations of graft length are difficult. A more flexible option is the incorporation of some means of adjusting graft length intraoperatively. Alternatives include the use of a telescopic graft or a graft that is introduced in two or more pieces which can overlap to a variable degree to produce the desired length.

The limitations imposed by a short distal cuff can be avoided altogether by moving the distal implantation site into the common iliac arteries, thereby expanding the number of suitable patients and facilitating graft sizing. Exclusion of the aneurysm with a unilateral endovascular aortoiliac graft requires some form of contralateral common iliac artery occlusion and surgical bypass to the contralateral femoral artery. These limitations argue for the use of a bifurcated endovascular graft.

Iliac Tortuosity

The iliac arteries are often tortuous in patients with aortic aneurysms. Depending on the particular delivery system, iliac artery tortuosity may not be a significant impediment to graft insertion, but is an important potential cause of graft limb kinking and occlusion. One way to avoid kinking is to avoid traversing an iliac angulation with the graft. The use of thin-walled fabric also helps to prevent kinking. When kinks do occur, they can be eliminated by the insertion of additional stents, such as the Wallstent.

Iliac Artery Aneurysms

In the Rochester series, 11 iliac artery aneurysms were present in 7 patients. The presence of an iliac artery aneurysm is an absolute contraindication to straight graft repair, but iliac aneu-

rysms only prevent bifurcated graft repair if they leave no possible implantation site in the distal common iliac arteries.

Aneurysm Thrombus

Aortic aneurysms are almost always lined by some mural thrombus, which can make angiograms misleading as a basis for decisions regarding the anatomy of implantation sites. Mural thrombus is also important as a potential source of emboli, which is one of the most dreaded complications of endovascular aneurysm repair.[2] It is not yet possible, based on the small number of reported cases, to identify characteristic CT or magnetic resonance imaging (MRI) findings associated with this complication as a means of ruling out patients at risk. However, the irregular, nonhomogeneous thrombus and multiple lumens seen in patients whose presenting symptom is embolism may be prone to disruption and fragmentation.[3] These findings probably represent a relative contraindication to endovascular aneurysm repair.

It is also notable that the reported cases of embolism following endovascular repair were associated with "excessive instrumentation" of the aorta. An important goal of delivery system design and implantation technique should be to avoid the repeated endoluminal introduction of rigid instruments or instruments that have unprotected edges or points. An open technique with bifemoral clamping and flushing also may offer some protection against distal embolization.

HISTORY

Many alternative procedures have been developed over the years in an attempt to avoid the large abdominal operation required for conventional repair. Most of these procedures induced aneurysm thrombosis with varying degrees of success.[4,5] Unfortunately, aneurysm thrombosis alone has not been found to prevent rupture.[6] Indeed, nothing has been found to be as effective at preventing rupture as excluding the aneurysm from the circulation with a graft. Endovascular grafting aims to do just that while avoiding the need for abdominal operation by inserting the graft through the distal arterial tree, from the femoral artery in the groin.

Advances in arterial imaging, catheters, and guidewires all helped to make endovascular graft delivery feasible, but the principal element that led to the emergence of endovascular grafting as a viable clinical option was the development of a means of graft attachment in the form of the arterial stent. Even devices that were initially intended to be attached by staples or barbs[7] have come to rely largely on the expansile properties of a stent.[8] Moreover, "stentless" endovascular grafts[9,10] actually incorporate the structural properties of stents into the graft. The role of the stent is so central to endovascular grafting that many of the specific functional characteristics which differentiate the current systems from one another can be traced to the nature of the stent used in graft attachment. Stents and their associated systems of endovascular grafting, can be divided into two broad groups: the self-expanding and the balloon-expanded stents.

Self-Expanding Stents

The first coil-spring stents of Dotter were plagued by poor expansion rates and high rates of thrombosis.[11] Higher expansion ratios were observed with stents of Nitinol, which is pliant when cold but resumes its preformed shape as it warms.[12] Despite these improvements, simple spiral stents were never used clinically in the treatment of arterial occlusive disease. Nor have they assumed a role as a means of graft attachment. However, they deserve a mention in the history of endovascular grafting as the first stents to be used for experimental aneurysm repair in dogs. Another landmark in the development of endovascular grafting is to be found in a 1984 paper[13] describing several single- and double-helical stents in which Maas commented on Cragg's reported arterial repair and suggested that a stent might be used in conjunction with a graft for arterial repair, only to dismiss the idea on the grounds that a sufficiently impervious prosthesis would be prone to thrombosis.

Balko et al.[14] reported the first experimental use of covered stents for aneurysm repair. Their prosthesis was comprised of a polyethylene sleeve covering a frame of Nitinol stents. Three experi-

mental aortic aneurysms were repaired in sheep by endoluminal insertion at laparotomy.

The first transfemoral graft insertion using radiologic guidance was reported by Lawrence et al.[15] Their prosthesis was based on a framework of Gianturco Z-stents. A subsequent series of experimental canine aortic aneurysm repairs reported by Mirich et al.[16] employed a thin-walled nylon/Lycra fabric. In this remarkable series of experiments, the no. 12 French delivery system was inserted using percutaneous transfemoral technique. Despite such promising results, these experiments did not proceed to clinical application. However, several systems currently in clinical trials use the Gianturco Z-stent as a means of graft attachment. The closest relative of the system described by Mirich et al. is the one used by Semba et al.[17] to repair thoracic aneurysms. The only real difference was the method of joining stents; the Semba et al. system used sutures instead of little struts.

The grafts used by Chuter et al.[18] and by Ivanev et al.* both carried Gianturco Z-stents only at the graft orifices. As a result, these grafts lacked the column strength needed for graft extrusion using a simple pusher. Instead, these grafts relied, for extrusion from the delivery system, on their attachment to a central carrier. The main advantage of eliminating the stent endoskeleton was increased flexibility, which has permitted bifurcated graft insertion. Chuter et al.[18] reported the first animal insertions of a bifurcated endovascular graft in 1992. This was followed by the first clinical repair of aortic aneurysm with a bifurcated graft in 1993.[19]

Another Gianturco stent–based system seems to have been developed quite independently in Russia.[20] It has been used mainly as a means of expediting conventional surgical aneurysm repair. In addition, it appears that some grafts, in both bifurcated and straight configurations, have been inserted transluminally using a novel combined femoral and axillary approach.

The Wallstent is a form of spiral stent in which several wires are braided together to enhance structural stability and reduce shortening. Wallstents have been modified in a number of ways to reduce porosity and have been tested in experimental models of aortic aneurysm with variable results.

*Personal communication.

The system invented by Lazarus (Endovascular Technologies) is difficult to categorize, since it uses a balloon to enhance implantation of a self-expanding Gianturco Z-stent. The experimental work that led to the development of this device has not been published. The only guide to its history is to be found in the patent literature,[7,8] which suggests that the use of a balloon for stent implantation is a vestige of an earlier reliance on balloon-driven stapling. At the time of this writing, this is the only device to enter formal clinical trials in the United States under an Investigational Device Exemption (IDE) from the Food and Drug Administration (FDA). The design of this study is likely to set the pattern for other systems, which have to follow the same path to FDA approval.

Balloon-Expanded Stents

Parodi used a modified Palmaz stent in his pioneering experimental and clinical studies of endovascular aneurysm repair. Early canine experiments were presented by Palmaz et al.[21] in 1990. The technique of endovascular aneurysm repair and results of the first six clinical cases were described by Parodi et al.[22] in a landmark paper published in 1992. Interestingly, a similar system was described by Ersek[23] 20 years earlier. The solitary significant differentiating feature between the Ersek and Parodi systems was an angioplasty balloon to serve as the engine for stent expansion in the later device.

The Strecker stent has been manufactured in double-knit configuration and Dacron in an effort to reduce porosity so that it can be used for aneurysm repair. The co-knit version has been used clinically to repair aortic and iliac aneurysms with mixed results.[24] Multiple stents were used to achieve the desired length, an interesting solution to the problem of graft sizing plaguing all straight aortoaortic implantations for aneurysm repair.

CURRENT CLINICAL SYSTEMS

All systems of endovascular grafting must satisfy the same prerequisites of successful aneurysm repair, and in many cases the basic mechanisms are the same. However, certain differences, principally in the stents used for graft attachment, have important functional implications.

Parodi[2] has the largest experience with aortic aneurysm repair, now numbering 46 cases, with initial success in 80 percent. The system currently exists only in straight graft form, although a bifurcated version is under development. Graft attachment is accomplished by balloon expansion of Palmaz-type stents, which have been modified to increase expansion ratios. The first few cases were notable for perigraft leakage around the unstented distal end of the graft. Subsequently, Parodi has routinely employed stents both proximally and distally.

Stent implantation is accomplished by balloon inflation to approximately 110 percent of aortic diameter. The graft is squeezed between the stent and the aorta, resulting in a leakproof seal. The dimensions of these stents are remarkably stable, and the presence of the stent is likely to ensure secure, hemostatic graft attachment unless the aorta dilates. A recent case of stent dislocation suggests that this can occur.

The grafts in this system, like the stents, are manufactured in Argentina, and their only use is as part of this prosthesis. The thin-walled, weft-knit structure of the graft fabric confers some elasticity, which helps ensure an exact fit, even when the proximal and distal implantation sites are of different diameters. These grafts dilate up to 20 percent during their first year of implantation, and the potential for progressive graft dilatation is a concern. Thus far, however, dilatation has not been observed on follow-up studies.

The lack of a suitable distal aortic implantation site has led Parodi to adopt unilateral aortoiliac bypass in many cases of large aneurysm. Straight aortoaortic graft repair has been reserved for the smaller aneurysms.

The Parodi technique has been complicated by embolism on three occasions, two of them fatal.[2] In an attempt to limit the flow of particulate matter into the contralateral arterial system, Parodi has started to use temporary iliac artery balloon occlusion, via a sheath in the contralateral femoral artery.

These patients have been followed with serial CT and duplex scans. The only cases of aneurysm enlargement and rupture have been in association with perigraft leakage.

The system of endovascular aneurysm repair conceptualized by Lazarus and manufactured by Endovascular Technologies (EVT) is the only one currently undergoing formal clinical trials for approval by the FDA. It is also unique in its reliance on balloon augmentation of barb implantation. The volume occupied by the radially oriented barbs and the expansion balloon originally necessitated a relatively large delivery system with a steel introducer sheath. The substitution of more retractile barbs and small capsules around the stents has helped decrease the size and increase the flexibility of recent versions of the delivery system.

Two introducer sheaths are used, one within the other, because the loaded delivery system cannot traverse the iliac arteries by itself. It must be passed through a previously placed sheath. The hemostatic problems associated with the use of two introducer sheaths are not unique to this system but are magnified by its large size. To limit blood loss during the interval between removal of the dilator and insertion of the graft-bearing sheath, EVT has developed an ingenious two-valve mechanism.

The large size of the delivery system (no. 29 French, 9.5 mm) excludes many patients with small or tortuous iliac arteries. The other main limitation has been the relative scarcity of patients suitable for straight graft repair. A bifurcated version of this system is said to be undergoing animal trials. If it also works in patients, it will help to increase the number of suitable candidates.

Dake's system of thoracic aneurysm repair is built around an endoskeleton of Gianturco stents which are joined to one another by sutures. This gives the prosthesis the necessary column strength for it to be pushed the entire length of the introducer sheath from groin to aortic arch. The endoskeleton is clothed with a sleeve of woven polyester (Dacron). The relatively thick fabric of these (Cooley Verisoft) grafts contributes significantly to the overall volume of the prosthesis, necessitating a large (no. 24 French) introducer sheath. Dake's remarkable results are partly attributable to some very refined preoperative imaging, in the form of spiral CT scans and multiplane angiograms. At the time of this writing, 17 thoracic aneurysms have been repaired, with serious complications in only 2 patients. One died a month

after repair of largely unrelated causes, and the other suffered permanent paraplegia.

The group at the Royal Prince Alfred Hospital in Sydney (White and Yu) is in the unique position of having used all the devices currently available for infrarenal aortic aneurysms repair. These workers also have developed a system of their own. The concept is of a self-attaching graft, although in reality the "graft attachment devices" consist of multiple balloon-expanded Z-stents.

At the time of this writing, more than 30 patients have been treated. Initial success rates were dependent on the type of aortic anatomy encountered. In small aneurysms with clear distal implantation sites, 87 percent of insertions were successful, whereas the initial success rate was only 60 percent in larger aneurysms that lacked a distal cuff. Two attempted bifurcated graft insertions using their own system were unsuccessful.

The Gianturco stents responsible for attachment of the Chuter graft are found only at the proximal and distal orifices. Graft extrusion is accomplished through attachment to a central carrier, which is capable of applying the necessary traction to the upstream end of the graft. This carrier has an olive-shaped dilator near its tip. With the system closed and the olive in position at the tip of the sheath, the outer profile of the delivery system is smooth enough to permit insertion through the iliac arteries into the proximal aorta. No second sheath is needed. The ability to introduce the graft, its carrier, and its introducer sheath as a single preloaded system helps reduce the overall size and eliminates the hemostatic problems that occur with two-sheath systems.

One initial concern with this Gianturco Z-stent–based system was the potential for graft migration, especially with bifurcated grafts, which reflect and absorb a much higher proportion of the incident energy. Gianturco stents do not expand with the high forces that can be generated by a balloon, and they do not become as rapidly embedded within the aortic wall as Palmaz stents. The addition of barbs has at least in part alleviated this potential limitation. However, barb penetration probably plays very little part in stent attachment. Due to the flexibility of the barbs, the stents apply little force to the barb tips. The barbs are driven into the aorta neither by stent expansion nor by the expansion of a balloon. Only when the open stent displaces caudally do the barbs penetrate. Despite this, no stents have migrated spontaneously from their original site of implantation, either in animal experiments or in clinical experience with 34 patients for up to 14 months of follow-up.

The Chuter system is the only system to have entered clinical trials in bifurcated form. Figure 10-1 depicts the bifurcated graft and its delivery system. The proximal stent expands as soon as the sheath is removed, just as it would in a straight graft system. With the proximal stent deployed, the right limb of the graft resides in its final position in the right common iliac artery. However, the left limb of the graft and the associated stent have to be pulled out of the aorta into the left iliac artery. This is accomplished by applying traction to a catheter extending from the left femoral artery to the left limb stent (Figs. 10-2 and 10-3). This catheter is created by joining the catheter on the left limb of the graft with the cross-femoral catheter (Fig. 10-4). The distal stents are maintained in their compressed state by small, distinct sheaths until the left limb of the graft reaches its final position in the left common iliac artery. The left limb sheath can only be removed when the suture loop in its catheter is cut. The sheath around the left limb stent is attached to the carrier and comes off when the carrier is removed (Fig. 10-5).

It is clear, even from this rudimentary description, that bifurcated graft insertion includes many more maneuvers than straight aortoaortic graft insertion. Although bifurcated graft insertion is more complicated, the longer distal target zone (the common iliac arteries) makes the procedure much easier by allowing the operator to concentrate solely on the position of the aortic stent. The exact location of the distal stent is of little concern using a bifurcated graft, provided that the distal implantation sites are hemostatic and permit prograde flow into both iliac arteries.

Although the intraortic instrumentation necessary for bifurcated graft insertion theoretically carries a high risk of embolism, particulate matter has be found in blood flushed from the femoral arteries only once in 34 cases. Moreover, had any thrombus been dislodged from the inside of the aneurysm, bilateral common femoral artery clamping and flushing would have helped to ensure that

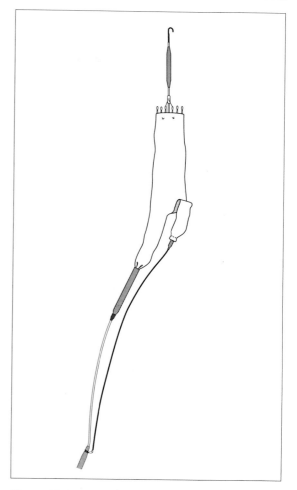

Figure 10-1. The bifurcated endovascular graft and its delivery system, with the sheath withdrawn.

none of it reached the distal circulation. None of the 34 patients showed any signs of embolism.

Careful assessment of the final result is arguably more important after bifurcated graft repair than after straight graft repair. The iliac limbs often traverse areas of acute angulation, which can cause kinking. In addition, even mild stenoses can constrict the small-diameter iliac limbs of a bifurcated graft to a significant degree. Placement of a Wallstent is a very effective remedy, as long as the problem is identified before the patient leaves the operating room. Figure 10-6 shows the widely patent graft limbs in which bilateral kinks were treated with Wallstents.

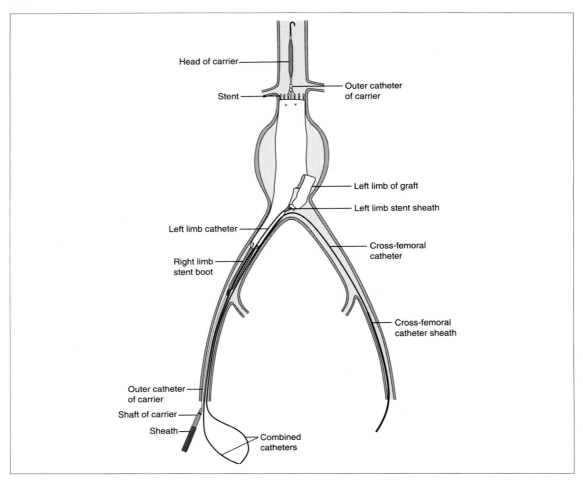

Figure 10-2. Bifurcated graft insertion showing the combined catheter looping from the left limb down through the right femoral arteriotomy, back up again, and down the other side to emerge from the left femoral arteriotomy.

The propensity of conventional graft materials for kinking highlights a previously neglected area in endovascular aneurysm repair: graft engineering. Graft manufacture can be modified to produce grafts with the specific properties needed for endovascular repair. The fabric developed for this system is an example of this point. It is thin-walled and kink-resistant. As a result of the preceding precautions, kinking and graft thrombosis have not occurred in any of the last 20 cases of bifurcated graft insertion.

PREOPERATIVE ASSESSMENT

The success of endovascular aneurysm repair depends largely on selecting the appropriate patients and the proper grafts based on preoperative imaging. The patient's arterial anatomy must lie within the functional limits of the system, as discussed above. Important parameters include the length and diameter of the aneurysm neck, the length and diameter of the cuff, the presence of iliac artery stenosis, angulation, or aneurysm, and the status of the mesenteric circulation.

Conventional CT scanning can be used to estimate diameters, although the measurements will be magnified if the plane of the scan is not perpendicular to the long axis of the vessel.[25] The length of the aneurysm and its neck can be estimated by identifying the scans that contain the renal artery orifices, the proximal and distal ends of the aneurysm, and the

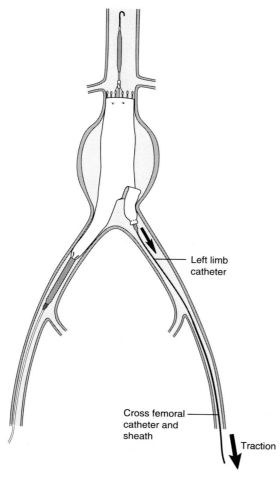

Left limb
catheter

Cross femoral
catheter and
sheath

Traction

Figure 10-3. Bifurcated graft insertion showing how traction on the combined catheter pulls the left limb of the graft into the left iliac artery.

aortic bifurcation. The narrower the interval between sections, the more accurate are the measurements. The same caveats regarding deviation of the vessel from the long axis of the scan apply.

MRI scans can be used in a similar way. The ability to generate longitudinal sections in coronal and sagittal planes facilitates measurements of length (Fig. 10-7). Three-dimensional reconstruction of MRI data in the form of an angiogram also can provide informative images of iliac and aortic angulation.

Angiography

Angiograms are invaluable in planning endovascular repair, but they suffer from two important limitations. First, the magnification factor is variable and sometimes difficult to measure, even using intraarterial calibrated guidewires or catheters. Second, the arteriogram displays only the lumen of the artery, not its wall. The appearance of the neck and cuff may be distorted by the presence of mural thrombus. This was illustrated in one of the early patients to receive bifurcated graft repair, in whom an overreliance on the angiographic appearance led to a small leak at a point in the neck where the proximal stent was seated only in thrombus. Interestingly, the leak was not apparent on completion angiography nor on follow-up intravenous digital subtraction angiograms but was revealed by duplex ultrasound and confirmed by CT scanning.

Accurate measurements of length may be made during angiography; either by using the bent wire pullback technique or by reference to the markings on a calibrated guidewire. Calculations based on the apparent length of a short segment of calibrating wire or catheter have proved to be inaccurate, possibly due to changes in the axis of the measured vessel.

Three-Dimensional Scanning

The images generated by three-dimensional reconstruction of conventional or spiral CT scans combines the spatial information of the scan with the anatomic detail of the angiogram. Specialized software is needed to make measurements of the distances through these three-dimensional constructs.

FOLLOW-UP

There are many unanswered questions concerning the long-term results of endovascular aneurysm repair which can only be addressed by follow-up examinations in clinical studies. One important question is whether the presence of the graft protects the patient from aneurysm growth and rupture. Follow-up imaging must be able to detect perigraft leakage and changes in the size of the aneurysm. Both CT scanning and duplex ultrasound accomplish this goal. These tests are also capable of

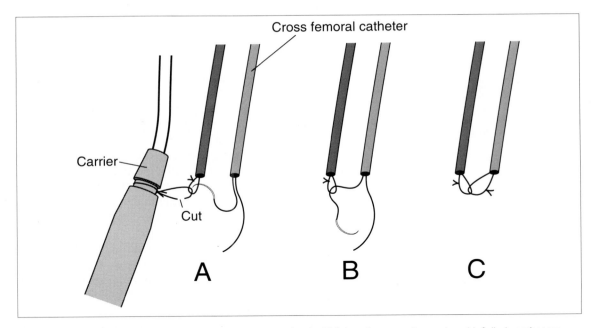

Figure 10-4. Bifurcated graft insertion showing the method of joining the cross-femoral and left-limb catheters.

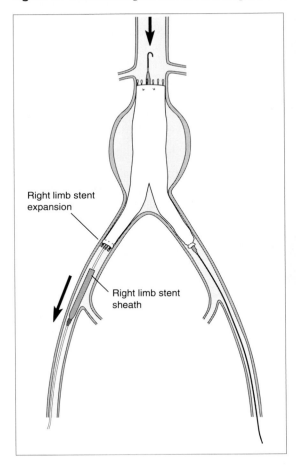

Right limb stent expansion

Right limb stent sheath

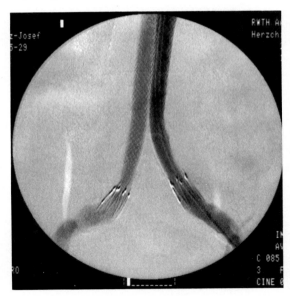

Figure 10-6. A completion angiogram showing bilaterally stented graft limbs.

Figure 10-5. Bifurcated graft insertion showing how removal of the delivery system deploys the right limb stent.

150

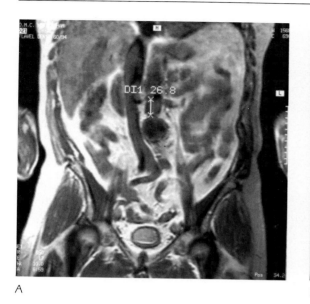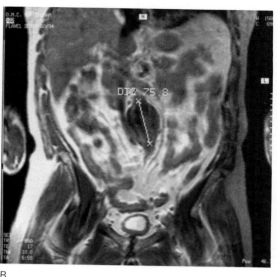

A   B

Figure 10-7. (A) Measurement of the length of the neck on an MRI scan. **(B)** Measurement of the length of the aneurysm on an MRI scan.

detecting luminal encroachment by kinks or thrombus. Although angiograms provide still better information on luminal anatomy, they give little information on the size of the aneurysm and may even fail to detect perigraft leakage.

FUTURE DIRECTIONS

Endovascular surgery is becoming a battleground for "turf wars" between surgeons, radiologists, cardiologists, and vascular medicine specialists. Rutherford's comments[26] on the politics of endovascular surgery are worth repeating:

> No one group can claim to have all the necessary skills and experience to provide comprehensive endovascular treatment of vascular disease. Surgeons generally lack the necessary catheter skills, and most radiologists lack a background in clinical patient care skills, while cardiologists and vascular internists fall somewhere in between. The ultimate solution is to fill the gaps in training, but the best short-term approach may be to combine the efforts of different groups to take advantages of their various skills.

Training

The economic incentives that fueled the explosive expansion of laparoscopic cholecystectomy are unlikely to have such a drastic effect on endovascular aneurysm repair because the FDA has tighter control over access to the necessary technology. Experience with endovascular aneurysm repair will be concentrated in the FDA study centers. Dissemination of these skills can then proceed in time with the schedule of the FDA approval process, allowing for better-organized training. The importance of adequate training and supervision is magnified in the case of endovascular aneurysm repair by the serious nature of potential complications. Slow ascent up a learning curve is unacceptable.

Clinical Study Design

The criteria for patient selection in early clinical trials of endovascular aneurysm repair vary widely among the different centers involved. Some take the view that only patients who are unsuitable for conventional treatment should be subjected to endovascular treatment. This policy is associated with a high-risk/

high-benefit policy because failed endovascular repair, under these circumstances, can be fatal, while success can be lifesaving. Others recommend that initial trials of the new procedure should occur only at the time of conventional operation, and subsequent trials should be confined to patients who would otherwise be candidates for conventional operative repair, a low-risk/low-benefit policy. Since the FDA takes a very dim view of poor outcomes, whatever the benefits in successful cases, I expect that industry will adopt the low-risk approach. Difficult cases will have to be performed outside formal studies on a compassionate-use basis.

Few systems are likely to emerge from animal testing in their final form, because animal models cannot mimic the arterial anatomy found in association with human aortic aneurysm. Therefore, early clinical trials must be designed to allow modifications in the criteria of patient selection, the operative technique, and the apparatus itself.

The role of prospective, randomized comparisons between endovascular repair and the conventional operation is a controversial subject. The FDA currently requires that such studies be performed early in clinical evaluation.

CONCLUSION

Anecdotal experience suggests that endovascular aneurysm repair holds promise as an exciting new therapeutic technique. The long-term fate of a graft within an artery, however, is entirely unknown. There are many other fundamental questions to be answered by clinical and experimental studies before endovascular grafting can be substituted for the traditional surgical technique, in the full range of patients. Despite these limitations, there is little doubt that endovascular grafting will play a significant role in the treatment of aortic aneurysmal disease.

REFERENCES

1. Chuter TAM, Green RM, Ouriel K, DeWeese JA: Infrarenal aortic aneurysm morphology: Implications for transfemoral repair. J Vasc Surg 1993; 17:1120.
2. Parodi JC: Abdominal aortic aneurysms. Presented at the SVS/ISCVS/NIH symposium on translumi-
nally placed endovascular prostheses, Bethesda, Maryland, March 26, 1994.
3. Pearce WH: Important vascular morphologic parameters. Presented at the SVS/ISCVS/NIH symposium on transluminally placed endovascular prostheses, Bethesda, Maryland, March 26, 1994.
4. Blakemore A: Progressive, constrictive occlusion of the abdominal aorta with wiring and electrothermic coagulation: One-stage operation for arteriosclerotic aneurysm of the abdominal aorta. Ann Surg 1951;133:447.
5. Karmody AM, Leather RP, Goldman M, et al: The current position of nonresective treatment for abdominal aortic aneurysm. Surgery 1983; 94:591.
6. Schanzer H, Papa MC, Miller CM: Rupture of surgically thrombosed abdominal aortic aneurysm. J Vasc Surg 1985;2:278.
7. Lazarus HM: Intraluminal graft device: System and method. US Patent Number 4,787,799, 1988.
8. Lazarus HM: Artificial graft and implantation method. US Patent Number 5,104,399, 1992.
9. de Vries. Instant tubular prosthesis. Presented at the workshop on transluminal treatment of aneurysms, Utrecht, Netherlands, January 28, 1994.
10. White GH, Yu W, May J, et al: A new nonstented balloon-expandable graft for either straight or bifurcated endoluminal bypass. Presented at the VIIth International Congress of Endovascular Interventions, Scottsdale, Arizona, February 14, 1994.
11. Dotter CT: Transluminally placed coilspring endarterial tube grafts: Long-term patency in canine popliteal artery. Invest Radiol 1969;4:329.
12. Cragg A, Lund G, Rysavy J, et al: Nonsurgical placement of arterial endoprostheses: A new technique using nitinol wire. Radiology 1983; 147:261.
13. Maas D, Zollikofer CL, Largiarder F, et al: Radiological follow-up of transluminally inserted vascular endoprosthesis: An experimental study using expanding spirals. Radiology 1984;152:659.
14. Balko A, Piasecki GJ, Shah DM, et al: Transfemoral placement of intraluminal polyurethane prosthesis for abdominal aortic aneurysm. J Surg Res 1986;40:305.
15. Lawrence DD Jr, Charnsangavej C, Wright KC, et al: Percutaneous endovascular graft: Experimental evaluation. Radiology 1987;163:357.
16. Mirich D, Wright KC, Wallace S, et al: Percutaneously placed endovascular grafts for aortic aneurysms: Feasibility study. Radiology 1989; 170:1033.
17. Semba CP, Dake MD, Mitchell RS, Miller DC: Endovascular grafting for the treatment of thoracic aortic aneurysms: Preliminary experience at Standord University Medical Center (abstract). Presented at the VIIth International Congress of Endovascular Interventions, Phoenix, Arizona, February 1994.
18. Chuter TAM, Green RM, Ouriel K, et al: Transfemoral endovascular aortic graft placement. J Vasc Surg 1993;18:185.

19. Scott RAP, Chuter TAM: Clinical endovascular placement of bifurcated graft in abdominal aortic aneurysm without laparotomy. Lancet 1994; 343:413.

20. Volodos NL, Karpovich IP, Troyan VI, et al: Clinical experience of the use of a self-fixing syn thetic prosthesis for remote endoprostheics of the thoracic and the abdominal aorta and iliac arteries through the remoral artery and as intraoperative endoprosthesis for aorta reconstruction. Vasa 1991; 33(S):93.

21. Palmaz JC, Parodi JC, Barone HD, et al: Transluminal bypass of experimental abdominal aortic aneurysm. Radiology 1990;177(S):202.

22. Parodi JC, Palmaz JC, Barone HD: Transfemoral intraluminal graft implantation for abdominal aortic aneurysms. Ann Vasc Surg 1991;5:491.

23. Ersek RA: Method for fixing prosthetic implants in a living body. US Patent Number 3,657,744, 1972.

24. Piquet P, Bartoli JM, Rolland PH, Mercier C: Tantalum Dacron co-knit stent for endovascular treatment of aortoiliac aneurysms: Experimental study and early clinical experience. Presented at the VIIth International Congress of Endovascular Interventions, Scottsdale, Arizona, February 17, 1994.

25. Ouriel K, Green RM, Donayre C, et al: An evaluation of new methods of expressing aortic aneurysm size: Relationship to rupture. J Vasc Surg 1992;15:12.

26. Rutherford RB: Political issues in endovascular surgery. Surg Clin North Am 1992;72:757.

Lower Extremity Arterial Occlusive Disease

Aortoiliac Reconstruction

BRUCE A. PERLER

PRESENTATION

Anatomy

Arteriosclerotic occlusive disease frequently involves the infrarenal abdominal aorta and iliac arteries, so-called inflow disease. In approximately one-third of patients with symptomatic inflow disease of sufficient severity to warrant revascularization, the hemodynamically significant occlusive process will be localized to the aorta and common iliac arteries, and in the remainder there also will be significant lesions in one or both external iliac arteries.[1] Furthermore, approximately two-thirds of patients who present with symptomatic aortoiliac occlusive disease suffer from multilevel disease, i.e., including significant occlusive lesions in the infrainguinal arterial tree.[1,2] Determining the relative hemodynamic significance of the aortoiliac and femoropopliteal components of the occlusive process is crucial in selecting the appropriate method of revascularization for the individual patient. When the relative contributions of aortoiliac and femoropopliteal disease are equivalent, or when the inflow component predominates, aortoiliac revascularization should be the initial therapeutic approach and will achieve significant symptomatic improvement in the majority of patients.[3]

While arteriosclerosis is the underlying pathologic entity responsible for aortoiliac occlusive disease in the overwhelming majority of patients, in a subset of this patient population the arteriosclerotic process involves a diffusely small infrarenal aorta and iliac arteries (Fig. 11-1). The so-called hypoplastic aortoiliac system is seen in 9 to 16 percent of patients who present with symptomatic aortoiliac occlusive disease.[4-6] This condition is seen predominately in women, although it has been described in men who present with aortoiliac occlusive disease. In one review of 408 peripheral arteriograms performed in males, 18 (4.4 percent) cases of hypoplasia of the abdominal aorta were identified.[7] In most patients one finds an unusually high aortic bifurcation, an acute angle at the aortic bifurcation, a relatively straight course of the iliac arteries without bowing, an infrarenal aortic diameter of 14 mm or less, and a common iliac artery diameter of 7 mm or less[5] (see Fig. 11-1). The etiology of the hypoplastic aortoiliac syndrome remains unclear, although trauma, congenital rubella, early exposure to therapeutic radiation, and oral contraceptive use, as well as other hormonal or inflammatory factors, have been proposed.[4,8] The frequent observation of single bifurcating lumbar arteries in many cases is consistent with the proposed etiology of congenital overfusion of the dorsal primitive aortas in the midline during the fourth week of embryonic development.[7,8] The average age at presentation of patients with the hypoplastic aortoiliac segment is approximately 10 to 15 years younger than those with more typical arteriosclerotic aortoiliac occlusive disease.[4,8] Furthermore, this syndrome poses special challenges to the surgeon undertaking aortoiliac revascularization.[9]

Demography

The patient population presenting primarily with symptomatic aortoiliac occlusive disease is

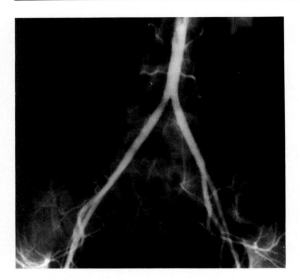

Figure 1. Aortogram in a 42-year-old woman with hypoplastic aortoiliac system.

approximately 10 years younger than those whose symptoms are related primarily to infrainguinal occlusive disease. Furthermore, the prevalence of hypertension and diabetes mellitus tends to be lower among the patient population with inflow disease, although the prevalence of hyperlipidemia may be somewhat greater when compared with those who present primarily with infrainguinal disease.[10] For these reasons and others, the survival of patients with aortoiliac occlusive disease is clearly superior to that of those who suffer predominantly from infrainguinal occlusive disease.[11] It should be noted, however, that patients with multilevel occlusive disease are older and more frequently have a history of hypertension and/or diabetes mellitus than patients with isolated aortoiliac disease.[12]

Whereas arteriosclerotic occlusive disease at other anatomic sites is characterized by an overwhelming male preponderance, females comprise roughly one-third of the patient population with aortoiliac occlusive disease,[1,13,14] and the prevalence of this disease in women appears to be increasing.[50] The development of aortoiliac occlusive disease in some women may be related to an underlying hypoplastic aortoiliac segment,[8] premature menopause, which eliminates the protec-

tive effect of estrogen,[16] cigarette smoking,[17] or a combination of these or other factors.[15]

WORKUP

History and Physical Examination

The classic presentation of aortoiliac disease, the Leriche syndrome, includes the clinical triad of absent femoral pulses, proximal leg claudication, and impotence in males. While the original description specifically denoted individuals with a complete aortic occlusion, this is seen in less than 10 percent of patients presenting with aortoiliac disease today.[1] Most patients with aortoiliac occlusive disease present with a history of progressive intermittent claudication affecting one or both legs. Symptoms typically involve the thigh, hip, or buttock regions. In many patients, however, pain may begin in the calf and move to the proximal muscle groups. In other patients, the pain will move from the proximal muscle groups to the calf with continued walking. In as many as 25 percent of patients with aortoiliac disease, however, claudication symptoms occur exclusively in the calf muscles.[18] Therefore, although proximal muscle claudication is indicative of inflow disease, symptoms only occurring in the calf do not rule out this diagnosis. Among male patients, difficulty achieving and maintaining an erection is further suggestive of aortoiliac occlusive disease. However, these symptoms are experienced by no more than 30 to 50 percent of men with aortoiliac occlusive disease.[12]

Limb-threatening ischemia, manifested by ischemic rest pain, nonhealing digital ulcerations, and frank gangrene, is extremely unusual in the patient with isolated aortoiliac occlusive disease. While these symptoms usually indicate multilevel occlusive disease, one important exception to this is the so-called blue toe syndrome, manifested by the acute onset of multiple small discrete areas of painful cyanotic discoloration on the feet and toes due to multiple microscopic atheroemboli.[19,20] The source is usually one or several ulcerative atheromatous lesions in the aorta. Since these patients usually have palpable pedal pulses indicative of patent proximal vessels, aortoiliac graft replacement is performed to eliminate the atherogenic focus rather than to improve distal arterial perfusion. Conversely, other patients have presented initially with peripheral thromboembolic occlusions of large vessels and have been found to have mural thrombus in the infrarenal abdominal aorta as the embolic source. This syndrome has been reported predominately in women and has been suggested by some to be a separate disease entity rather than typical aortoiliac atherosclerosis.[21] It has been proposed that cigarette smoking in association with hormonal drugs may result in a peculiar lesion characterized by intimal thickening and subsequent thrombus deposition in these patients.[21]

On physical examination, one will note the absence, or weakness, of the femoral pulses to palpation. There often will be abdominal or femoral bruits. However, in the patient who presents exclusively with intermittent claudication and who is asymptomatic at rest, a completely normal pulse examination at rest, including femoral pulses, is not inconsistent with a diagnosis of mild to moderate aortoiliac occlusive disease. It is in these patients that pre- and postexercise physical examination and noninvasive vascular laboratory testing can be quite helpful. Pedal arterial pulses that are palpable at rest may be become nonpalpable immediately after exercise. This "disappearing pulse syndrome" results from a drop in the distal perfusion pressure due to peripheral vasodilation and a pressure drop across proximal arterial stenotic lesions in association with increased cardiac output and flow across the lesion.

The differential diagnosis of intermittent claudication due to aortoiliac occlusive disease includes a number of musculoskeletal and vascular causes of leg pain (Table 11-1). Without question, one of the most important diagnostic considerations is *pseudoclaudication,* which is also known as *neurogenic claudication.*[22,23] In this condition, pain usually results from compression of the cauda equina due to a herniated disk, local cord pressure due to hypertrophic ridging in the intervertebral canal, or congenital narrowing of the spinal canal.[24–28] As the name implies, the symptoms experienced by the patient with neurogenic claudication in many respects mimic the complaints of the patient with vascular claudication, although careful attention to the history usually can elicit the correct diagnosis.

Table 11-1. Aortoiliac Disease: Differential Diagnosis

Pseudoclaudication
Arthritis
Osteoporosis
Lumbar disk disease
"Night cramps"
Arteritis

In neurogenic claudication, pain characteristically occurs in the hip or buttock and often is described as cramping in nature, although other patients describe the pain as sharp. While these complaints often are brought on by walking, the walking distance at which symptoms occur will vary greatly from day to day, from just a few steps on some days to several blocks at other times. In the patient with intermittent claudication, on the other hand, the walking distance is very consistent over protracted periods of time. Furthermore, in most patients with neurogenic claudication, symptoms can be brought on by standing or even prolonged sitting, whereas true claudication is invariably relieved by rest. In neurogenic claudication, the individual usually must change body position at rest to achieve symptomatic relief.

Vascular Noninvasive Laboratory Evaluation

While arteriography remains the "gold standard" diagnostic test, in most cases the clinical impression of arterial insufficiency due to aortoiliac occlusive disease can be confirmed by noninvasive vascular laboratory testing. The two most frequently employed conventional diagnostic technologies are Doppler ultrasound and the pulse volume recorder. Each of these technologies allows the rapid noninvasive assessment of segmental systolic blood pressure and arterial waveforms in both lower extremities. The preliminary noninvasive assessment provides quantitative data with respect to the severity of arterial insufficiency at rest, the anatomic location of the occlusive process (i.e., aortoiliac versus femoropopliteal/tibial), and is very useful in assessing the results of revascularization initially and during long-term follow-up. In the patient who presents with intermittent claudication, the examination should be performed at rest and immediately after treadmill exercise. It has been shown that the magnitude of the ankle blood pressure drop after exercise, as well as the time elapsed until return of pressure to baseline, is indicative of the severity of the proximal occlusive process.[29]

An important clinical issue in selecting therapy is an assessment of the hemodynamic significance of aortoiliac lesions among patients who present with multilevel arteriosclerotic occlusive disease. Essentially, the surgeon needs to predict the likelihood that inflow revascularization will provide sufficient clinical improvement to obviate the necessity for a synchronous or early metachronous infrainguinal bypass operation. Direct intraarterial pull-through pressure measurements, from the aorta to the femoral artery site of puncture, represent an objective method to document the hemodynamic severity of the inflow component.[30,31] A central aorta to femoral artery pressure gradient of 20 mmHg at rest or after intraarterial papaverine administration is indicative of significant inflow disease on that side, so aortoiliac revascularization should result in significant clinical improvement. In view of the invasiveness of this test, however, routine noninvasive vascular laboratory testing can be quite helpful in the preoperative evaluation. In one study, for example, three easily derived vascular laboratory criteria were found to be quite predictive of the need for infrainguinal bypass in the patient undergoing aortoiliac reconstruction.[3] For example, a thigh pressure index (thigh pressure divided by brachial pressure) greater than 0.6 was predictive of the need for an infrainguinal bypass. More sensitive indicators of the need for distal reconstruction were a thigh-ankle pressure gradient of 30 mmHg or greater or an index of runoff resistance (thigh-ankle pressure divided by brachial pressure) of 0.2 or greater.[3]

Most recently, conventional Doppler and pulse volume recorder testing has been supplemented, and in some centers replaced, by duplex and color flow duplex scanning. In addition to providing physiologic flow data, duplex technology can provide an image of the arterial tree. One can use changes in flow velocity data to localize the site of hemodynamically significant disease and to differentiate between stenoses and complete occlusions. To date, prospective trials have demonstrated duplex scanning to be highly accurate in identifying hemodynamically significant aortoiliac lesions, although accuracy declines in the setting of multilevel occlusive disease.[32,33] Duplex scanning can be quite useful in noninvasively identifying lesions that should be amenable to endovascular intervention and thus candidates for formal arteriography.[34,35] However, at the present time, duplex imaging has not sufficiently evolved to replace formal arteriography in the planning of major arterial surgical reconstructive procedures.[36]

Arteriography

Formal arteriography should be reserved for the patient in whom a decision to proceed with revascularization has been made based on the clinical and noninvasive assessments. Today, most studies are performed using the transfemoral Seldinger approach. In the patient with bilateral critical iliac artery stenoses/occlusions or an infrarenal aortic occlusion, the axillary or translumbar approach may be necessary. The complete study should include a biplane aortogram with visualization of the runoff to the pedal level. The celiac and superior mesenteric artery origins should be clearly delineated, especially if one identifies a meandering mesenteric artery suggestive of significant mesenteric occlusive disease. Likewise, the renal arteries and any accessory renal arteries should be visualized completely. An oblique pelvic run is essential to rule out significant profunda femoris orificial disease. Through digital subtraction technology, images have improved, and the contrast load required has been reduced. As noted earlier, pullback pressure measurements are an important physiologic adjunct to the overall study. Vigorous pre-angiography hydration is important to minimize the risk of contrast-induced renal dysfunction, especially in patients with preexisting renal functional compromise, diabetes mellitus, or other significant comorbidities.[37,38]

ANATOMIC RECONSTRUCTION

Aortofemoral Bypass

The first surgical bypass procedure for aortoiliac occlusive disease was performed by Oudot[39] in

1951 using an aortic homograft. The earliest synthetic grafts were constructed of nylon and were first used in aortic reconstruction by Blakemore and Voorhees[40] in 1954. Dacron prostheses were subsequently introduced in the late 1950s.[41] Over the last three decades, Dacron prostheses have proven to be extremely durable arterial substitutes. As a result, the number of aortofemoral bypass (AFB) procedures performed has dramatically increased, and this operation has emerged as the most frequently performed surgical procedure for aortoiliac occlusive disease, with approximately 30,000 procedures performed annually in U.S. today.[42] While Dacron prostheses continue to be used by most vascular surgeons, recently, improved polytetrafluoroethylene (PTFE) aortic prostheses are growing in popularity and providing comparable results[43] (see below).

TECHNICAL DETAILS

The operation is begun by exploring the femoral arteries through bilateral groin incisions. Most surgeons prefer longitudinal incisions. Although some have suggested that transverse incisions result in fewer local wound problems, there is little substantive evidence to confirm this viewpoint. Lymphatic tissue should be ligated carefully to minimize the risk of postoperative lymphorrhea or other wound complications. The common, superficial, and profunda femoris arteries are exposed individually and controlled with vessel tapes. The inguinal ligament on each side is incised slightly, and a tunnel into the retroperitoneal space is bluntly begun by finger dissection on each side in preparation for later tunneling of each graft limb.

The aorta is approached in most cases through either a midline transperitoneal incision or an extended left flank incision.[44] Each of these options has specific advantages or indications (Table 11-2). While the transperitoneal midline incision has been the conventional approach to the infrarenal abdominal aorta, experience over the past decade has clearly identified several clinical situations in which the retroperitoneal approach may convey advantage. For example, there is anecdotal evidence to support the retroperitoneal approach in the obese patient. Clearly, in the patient with a "hostile" abdomen due to multiple previous ab-

Table 11-2. Aortofemoral Bypass: Choice of Incision Transperitoneal (T) versus Retroperitoneal (R)

Issue	T	R
Obese patient		x
"Hostile" abdomen		x
Suprarenal aortic control		x
Bypass left renal artery		x
Bypass right renal artery	x	
Bypass celiac/SMA	x	
Endarterectomy visceral arteries		x
Exposure distal leg arteries	x	
Cardiac/pulmonary risk		x
End-to-side proximal anastomosis		x

dominal operations, the retroperitoneal approach allows more rapid exposure of the aorta while obviating the risk of inadvertent bowel injury. In terms of technical vascular considerations, suprarenal aortic exposure and control are generally more easily achieved via the left retroperitoneal approach. The left renal artery can be exposed along its entire course without difficulty if a synchronous bypass graft to that vessel is required as part of the AFB procedure. Since the right renal artery is not exposed from the left flank approach, however, concomitant right renal artery bypass mandates exploration through the conventional midline incision in most cases. On the other hand, since the origin of the celiac and superior mesenteric arteries, as well as the left renal artery, can be exposed via the left retroperitoneal incision, AFB bypass and concomitant visceral artery endarterectomy are indications for the retroperitoneal approach. Finally, there is some evidence that the patient experiences less physiologic insult in association with the retroperitoneal approach, so this incision may be indicated for the patient with limited cardiopulmonary reserve, although this remains controversial[45–48] (see below). One significant disadvantage of the left retroperitoneal approach is that due to the positioning of the patient on the operating table, operative exposure distal to the groins, especially on the right side, is limited. Since most patients undergoing AFB suffer from multilevel disease, and since extensive exposure of the profunda and at times other vessels distally is required, in the absence of specific indications, I still prefer to perform AFB via the conventional transperitoneal approach.

The abdomen is entered through a midline incision extending from the xiphoid to pubis, and the transverse colon is eviscerated and packed in moist towels on the abdominal wall. The ligament of Trietz is sharply incised, allowing lateral mobilization of the duodenum, and the small bowel is then placed in moist towels on the abdominal wall. The lymphatic tissue over the aorta is ligated and divided from the level of the crossing left renal vein to the aortic bifurcation. Failure to visualize the left renal vein suggests that it may lie in a retroaortic position, an anomaly that occurs in approximately 1 percent of cases.[49–51] Iatrogenic venous injury and potentially significant intraoperative blood loss can occur if the retroaortic left renal vein or other major venous anomalies, are not correctly identified.[51]

Whereas the transperitoneal approach is performed with the patient in the supine position, the left retroperitoneal approach requires placing the patient in the lateral position with the left side up but with the hips free to allow access to the groins. An oblique incision is made from the left margin of the rectus muscle, just inferior to the umbilicus, and extended to the eleventh intercostal space. If suprarenal aortic control is necessary, the incision is carried into the tenth intercostal space. The muscles of the abdominal wall are divided, and the left kidney, ureter, and peritoneum are bluntly mobilized anteromedially. The lymphatic tissue over the aorta is ligated and divided, allowing exposure of the aorta from the left renal artery to the aortic bifurcation. A large descending lumbar branch of the left renal vein is easily exposed and divided to allow exposure of the left renal artery origin.

Irrespective of the operative approach, the principles of graft placement are the same. Tunnels from the aorta to the respective groins are developed by blunt dissection superficial to the iliac arteries and deep to the crossing ureters. The patient is administered intravenous heparin sodium (100 mg/kg). The femoral arteries are clamped initially to minimize the risk of distal embolization of intraaortic atheromatous debris. The distal abdominal aorta is then clamped, and finally, the proximal aortic clamp is placed just distal to the renal arteries. This clamp should be placed as close to the renal arteries as possible, since this segment of the infrarenal aorta should be least diseased. If there is dense, circumferential aortic mural calcification that precludes safe clamp application, or in the setting of a completely thrombosed infrarenal aorta, temporary suprarenal aortic control, usually at the supraceliac level, may be required to allow infrarenal aortic thromboendarterectomy.

An important technical issue is the method of proximal aortic anastomosis, i.e., end-to-end (EE) or end-to-side (ES). An EE anastomosis is absolutely indicated in the setting of aneurysmal dilatation of the aorta or in the patient with a complete infrarenal aortic occlusion. Conversely, an ES anastomosis may be preferable in the patient in whom important aortic branches must be preserved, such as a patent inferior mesenteric artery (IMA) or one or several accessory renal arteries, or to preserve antegrade arterial flow into the hypogastric arteries in the patient with critical bilateral external iliac artery occlusive disease in whom absent to minimal retrograde flow from the common femoral level is anticipated. Failure to maintain adequate pelvic blood flow via the hypogastric circulation in the patient undergoing an AFB graft may result in continued hip or buttock claudication, impotence in the male patient, an increased risk of postoperative colon ischemia, and a small but real risk of spinal cord ischemia.[52–55] In addition, an ES anastomosis may be preferable in the patient with a hypoplastic aortoiliac system,[4,5] while others have not demonstrated its superiority when compared with the EE anastomosis in this patient population.[9]

Exclusive of these specific indications, however, the method of proximal anastomosis depends on surgical preference and is somewhat controversial. There are several theoretical advantages of the EE anastomosis, including better hemodynamic flow characteristics, elimination of competitive aortoiliac flow, reduced risk of progressive atherosclerotic disease at the proximal anastomosis, minimal risk of distal atheroembolization, and easier retroperitoneal graft coverage and thus reduced risk of late aortoenteric fistula formation when compared to the ES anastomosis. It is difficult to confirm the superiority of the EE anastomosis with objective clinical data, however. For example, while some have reported superior graft patency with the EE proximal anastomosis as a reflection of its hemodynamic flow characteristics and elimination of competitive flow, these data have not been obtained in randomized, prospective trials,[56,57] and others have reported comparable graft patency with EE and ES anastomoses.[9] The EE approach does allow construction of the anastomosis close to the renal arteries, where the aorta is relatively less diseased in most cases. If an ES proximal anastomosis is elected, it should be performed as far cephalad as possible so as to avoid performing the anastomosis in an area of dense aortic atherosclerotic disease. Furthermore, when an ES proximal anastomosis is desirable, the left retroperitoneal approach will allow the graft to be anastomosed to a somewhat lateral aortotomy, thus minimizing contact between the graft and overlying bowel and reducing the risk of later aortoenteric fistula formation.

Whereas performance of the distal anastomosis to the common or external iliac arteries may be appropriate in the occasional patient undergoing operation to eliminate an embologenic aortic focus, in the overwhelming majority of cases, the graft limb should be carried to the groins, since there is convincing evidence that progressive iliac artery occlusive disease will compromise long-term graft patency in the former situation.[58,59] In the absence of significant femoropopliteal disease, the graft should be anastomosed to the common femoral artery in ES fashion, possibly extending the toe of the graft over the origin of the superficial femoral artery (SFA). Most patients undergoing aortoiliac reconstruction have multilevel disease, however, with coexistent SFA and/or profunda femoris occlusive lesions. In this situation, the toe of the graft should be carried over the origin of the profunda or, if the SFA is completely occluded, directly to the profunda femoris artery. There is considerable evidence that maximizing profunda outflow will enhance both early and late graft limb patency.[1,3,60,61] Prior to performance of each distal anastomosis, dilute heparin should be infused into the distal arterial tree, and prior to completing each distal anastomosis, the graft should be vigorously flushed and the distal arteries backbled, to min-

imize the risk of thrombosis in situ and/or distal thromboembolism.

An important decision the surgeon must make prior to closing the abdomen is whether to reimplant a patent IMA into the graft as a Carrell patch in the patient in whom an EE proximal aortic anastomosis was performed. Although the incidence of postoperative colon ischemia is low, it conveys substantial risk of mortality and can be avoided in most cases by preservation of IMA flow. While some have advocated routine reimplantation of the IMA,[62] this is clearly unnecessary in most cases. The patient's history, preoperative arteriogram, and intraoperative observations will help identify the patient in whom reimplantation of the IMA should be seriously considered (Table 11-3). One should have a low threshold for reimplantation in the patient with a patent IMA and severe coexisting celiac and/or SMA occlusive disease, especially if antegrade hypogastric flow is excluded through an EE proximal aortic anastomosis. A large meandering mesenteric artery with IMA to SMA flow provides further evidence of the need to reimplant the IMA. Likewise, prior colon resection may have compromised important mesenteric collateral channels so that exclusion of the IMA at the time of the AFB will increase the risk of colon ischemia without reimplantation of the IMA. Basing the decision to reimplant the IMA simply on intraoperative observations can be risky, particularly if one relies on the gross appearance of the bowel. Absence of a Doppler arterial flow signal in the mesenteric vessels with the IMA clamped and an IMA stump pressure of less than 40 mmHg are more objective indicators of the need for reimplantation of the IMA, especially if the aforementioned historical or angiographic signs are present.

Table 11-3. Guidelines for Reimplanting the IMA

History
  Prior colon resection
Arteriography
  Significant celiac/SMA occlusive disease
  Meandering mesenteric artery
Intraoperative
  Absent arterial doppler signal in mesentery
  IMA stump pressure < 40 mmHg
  Exclusion of internal iliac flow
  Colonic appearance

MEDICAL MANAGEMENT

While the fundamental principles of surgical management have been relatively constant, several aspects of the medical management of the patient during the performance of an AFB graft have changed in recent years and deserve mention. For example, while aortic surgery is routinely performed under general anesthesia, there is some evidence that the combination of epidural and general anesthesia may convey significant physiologic benefit for the patient undergoing aortic surgery, particularly with respect to reducing cardiac and pulmonary morbidity.[63,64] It appears that epidural anesthesia reduces the neuroendocrine response to surgical stress by blocking the afferent pain fibers, since a decrease in serum cortisol and catecholamine levels in the perioperative period has been reported.[65,66] In addition, the combination of general and epidural anesthesia has been associated with a reduction in the significant hemodynamic alterations associated with aortic clamping.[67] There may be a decrease in myocardial oxygen consumption and improvement in cardiac output in association with epidural anesthesia,[68] although other work has not confirmed this.[69] With respect to pulmonary complications, postoperative epidural analgesia reduces the need for narcotic medications, and this may promote earlier return of pulmonary function.[70,71] In a recent clinical trial, 144 consecutive patients underwent aortic surgery under general ($n = 67$) or general and epidural ($n = 77$) anesthesia. While operative mortality was not significantly different between the two groups, postoperative pulmonary complications occurred in 7.6 percent of the general and only 2.6 percent of the general/epidural anesthesia patients. Furthermore, more patients in the general anesthesia group required prolonged ventilatory support ($p < 0.05$). These findings were somewhat limited by the retrospective nature of the study, however.[72] Currently, a randomized, prospective trial is ongoing at the Johns Hopkins Hospital to address these issues.

Another increasingly important issue is reduction in the amount of banked blood received by patients undergoing aortic surgery. Preoperative donation and subsequent intraoperative transfusion of the patient's blood will clearly reduce the requirement for autologous transfusion and is appropriate for the patient undergoing elective aortic surgery.[73,74] Furthermore, recent improvements in rapid intraoperative salvage and autotransfusion systems have substantially reduced the requirement for banked blood in this patient population. In a series of aortic reconstructions reported by Ouriel et al.,[75] 100 patients undergoing autotransfusion of unwashed cells received a mean of 0.6 ± 0.1 units of banked blood intraoperatively versus 3.4 ± 0.1 units among patients in whom autotransfusion was not performed. In another series from the Mayo Clinic,[76] 86 percent of patients undergoing routine aortic surgery and intraoperative autotransfusion of washed cells did not require autologous blood transfusions perioperatively. Dilutional coagulopathy, a potential complication of autotransfusion of washed red cells, was not a problem in this study.[76] Furthermore, although air embolism was occasionally seen with earlier autotransfusion devices, this complication has largely been eliminated with modern systems.[75,76] In addition to reducing the risk of blood-borne infectious disease transmission, minimizing the transfusion of cold banked blood reduces the magnitude of hypothermia in the patient after aortic reconstruction.[75] Furthermore, in an era of increasing pressure for cost containment, the use of an autotransfusion system has resulted in an average savings of approximately $300 per patient in some series.[75,76]

RESULTS

Operative Mortality. Over the past 30 years, there has been a progressive and dramatic reduction in the operative risk of AFB, and operative mortality is less than 3 percent in many large centers today.[1,60,77–83] Cardiac complications are responsible for the majority of operative deaths, with renal failure, respiratory insufficiency, and stroke causing most of the remainder.[79] Adequate pre-angiography hydration and careful attention to intra- and postoperative fluid and hemodynamic management have substantially reduced the incidence of renal failure following aortic surgery over the past decade.[37,38] While it is not unreasonable for the patient with symptomatic carotid artery disease to undergo carotid endarterectomy prior to aortoiliac reconstruction, there are little data to support the performance of this operation prophylactically in the patient with asymptomatic carotid disease when one considers the relative infrequency of stroke among patients undergoing AFB.[84]

On the other hand, there is much less agreement on the indications for and benefits of aggressive cardiac evaluation of patients prior to major aortic surgery. An important study from the Cleveland Clinic[85] documented a 15 percent incidence of silent and surgically correctable coronary artery disease among patients with peripheral vascular disease. On this basis, some have advocated routine preoperative cardiac screening of patients scheduled to undergo aortic surgery.[86–89] Conversely, since the incidence of major cardiac complications following aortic surgery is quite low today, others have argued that aggressive preoperative cardiac evaluation is not a cost-effective utilization of health care resources because it is unlikely to substantially lower the rate of major cardiac morbidity,[90] which is under 5 percent in several institutions today.[90,91] On balance, it is difficult to document a significant difference in the incidence of perioperative myocardial infarction among series in which routine,[85,86] selective,[92] or no preoperative cardiac screening was performed.[90] These data clearly suggest that improvement in cardiac outcome in all likelihood largely reflects advances in intraoperative anesthetic and postoperative medical management of this patient population rather than the benefits of various screening protocols.[93,94] However, in the patient scheduled for aortic reconstruction, the clinical history should be carefully scrutinized for evidence of significant underlying coronary artery disease. In the older and/or diabetic patient in particular, there still may be a place for noninvasive cardiac evaluation with dipyridamole-thallium scanning.[90,95,96]

Patency. Precisely defining the long-term patency of the AFB graft is confounded by the fact that some series combine aortoiliac and aortofemoral reconstructions and/or aorto–unilateral femoral grafts, and earlier studies have not differentiated primary from secondary patency. Nevertheless, it is clear that the AFB graft is one of the most durable operations performed for arteriosclerotic occlusive disease at any anatomic location. In most

large centers, patency exceeds 85 percent at five years, 70 percent at 10 years, and 55 percent at 20 years.[1,77–79,97–100] As noted from the several representative series depicted on Table 11-4, there has been a remarkable consistency in overall patency over the last 15 years. The most important determinant of both early and long-term graft patency is the status of the infrainguinal vessels. Graft limb patency is somewhat compromised in the patient with multilevel disease including an SFA occlusion, although as noted earlier, ensuring adequate profunda runoff with the distal anastomosis will markedly enhance patency in this patient population.[61] For example, in a large series of patients undergoing AFB from 1978 to 1987, 5-year patency was approximately 98 percent in the absence of SFA occlusive disease and approximately 93 percent in the presence of significant SFA disease when the distal anastomosis was constructed to the profunda femoris artery. On the other hand, among patients with SFA occlusive disease in whom the distal anastomosis was performed to the common femoral artery, the 5-year patency was only approximately 83 percent. At 10 years, patency in this group was approximately 70 percent, while patency in the former two groups was still greater than 90 percent.[97]

There is little question that progressive infrainguinal arterial occlusive disease is the most important determinant of graft limb thrombosis during long-term follow-up. It is clear, however, that reoperation and distal anastomotic revision or infrainguinal bypass can salvage most of these AFB graft limbs. Aggressive reoperation will yield secondary AFB patency rates 10 to 20 percent better

Table 11-4. Aortofemoral Graft Patency

Source (Year)	No. of Patients	Patency (%)		
		5 yrs	10 yrs	15 yrs
Nevelsteen (1991)	912	93	83	77
Vantinnen (1991)	177	91	—	—
Rutherford (1986)	157	86	—	—
Szilagyi (1986)	1748	85	80	74
Crawford (1981)	949	87	—	—
Martinez (1980)	376	88	78	—
Brewster (1978)	464	88	75	—

than primary patency rates.[77,101–105] Conversely, graft material does not appear to significantly influence patency. Most series of AFB grafts reported to date have used knitted Dacron prostheses, although more recently woven and collagen-coated Dacron grafts have been introduced and are gaining popularity. At the present time, there are little objective patency data to support the preferential use of any of these conduits. Furthermore, while some type of Dacron prosthesis continues to be most frequently implanted by vascular surgeons in this country, recently there has been renewed interest in the use of large-diameter bifurcated PTFE grafts. Early results suggest comparable patency when compared with Dacron prostheses in the AFB position. For example, Cintora et al.[43] reported a 5-year cumulative patency of 90 and 97 percent for Dacron and PTFE AFB grafts, respectively. Further research will be required to establish whether the purported theoretical advantages of bacterial resistance and lower thrombogenicity of PTFE grafts are clinically significant in the surgical treatment of aortoiliac disease.[9,43,106–108]

Far more important than graft material is selecting the appropriate size match between the graft limb and native femoral artery to which the distal anastomosis is performed. Formerly, surgeons favored using larger grafts in order to minimize the potential harm of neointimal hyperplastic lesions developing at the femoral anastomoses. However, it is now clear that thrombus deposition leading to a thickened layer of pseudointima will occur in larger grafts as a result of reduced flow velocity in these larger conduits. Furthermore, Dacron prostheses have demonstrated the potential to progressively dilate over time.[109,110] These concerns suggest that one should err on the side of undersizing in selecting the appropriate size of a synthetic AFB conduit. Although there has been some concern that small bifurcation grafts are predisposed to an increased risk of early and late failure, this is not supported by the available data. For example, in a series of 79 patients undergoing AFB Dacron bifurcation grafts, 3-year primary patency was 84 and 87 percent for 14 × 7 and 16 × 8 mm grafts, respectively.[111]

Vascular Complications. Complications associated with the AFB graft may appear from a few hours to as long as several months or years post-

Table 11-5. Aortofemoral Bypass: Complications

Early
    Graft thrombosis
    "Trash foot"
    Lymph fistula
    Ischemic colitis
Late
    Graft infection
    Aortoenteric fistula
    Anastomotic aneurysms
    Graft thrombosis
    Sexual dysfunction
    Ureteral obstruction

operatively (Table 11-5). Acute thrombosis of a graft limb should occur in no more than 2 percent of cases.[12] Excluding the rare patient who may suffer from an underlying and undiagnosed hypercoagulability syndrome, early graft limb thrombosis usually results from either technical or anatomic problems for which immediate reexploration is indicated. An intimal flap at the distal anastomosis, kinking or twisting of the graft limb, and incomplete clot evacuation at the original operation are the most frequent etiologies. Since the specific cause usually can be identified at reexploration, and since arteriography will not be particularly informative while the graft limb is thrombosed, angiography is not necessary prior to reexploration. Intraoperative angiography and/or angioscopy can be quite helpful, however. In the occasional patient with an SFA occlusion in whom no technical problem is identified, graft limb thrombosis may have resulted from inadequate outflow, particularly if the profunda femoris artery is relatively small or diffusely diseased. In this situation, an infrainguinal bypass may be required to maintain patency of the AFB graft limb. This is a determination that ideally should be made preoperatively based on a careful analysis of the vascular laboratory hemodynamic data and arteriogram, as described earlier.[3]

On the other hand, distal limb ischemia in the setting of a patent graft typically results from microembolization of atherosclerotic debris from the diseased aortoiliac segment. The risk of developing this "trash foot" syndrome can be minimized by careful attention to intraoperative technical details such as avoiding unnecessary arterial manipulation prior to clamping, clamping the femoral arteries before clamping the aorta, and vigorously flushing each graft limb and backbleeding the distal vessels prior to completing the distal anastomoses.

As noted previously, ischemic colitis is one of the potentially more serious, albeit relatively infrequent, early complications associated with aortic reconstructive surgery. The incidence of this complication is about 2 percent, although it has ranged from 0.2 to 10 percent in several large series.[12–17] When the ischemic process is confined to the mucosa or muscularis, most patients will respond to conservative management, including cessation of an oral diet, nasogastric suction, intravenous antibiotics, and close physical and sigmoidoscopic follow-up. Late strictures may occur, however. On the other hand, transmural involvement and perforation have been associated with mortality in up to 50 percent of patients.[12–17] In most cases, this complication can be prevented through reimplantation of the IMA in the patient at risk (see Table 11-3).

A potentially serious wound complication is the development of a lymph fistula in the groin, since persistence of the serous leak may lead to graft infection. Conservative management of this problem has consisted of bed rest, pressure dressings, and prophylactic broad-spectrum antibiotic administration.[118] However, in view of the potential for deep infection to develop, others have advocated early reoperation and ligation of the responsible lymphatic channel.[114] Preoperative lymphangiography may define the precise site of leakage in some cases.[119]

The most serious complications of AFB grafts are septic. Frank graft infection occurs in approximately 2 percent of cases.[121–126] The conventional management of the infected AFB graft, including complete graft excision and extraanatomic revascularization, has been associated with operative mortality ranging from 30 percent to greater than 50 percent, as well as a significant risk of limb loss and delayed aortic stump rupture among survivors.[123,125–131] In view of the substantial morbidity associated with this conventional approach, alternative treatments have been pursued in recent years. Some have advocated excision of the infected graft and in situ replacement with freshly harvested cadaveric venous homografts.[132] Clagett et al.[133] recently have reported the use of deep and saphenous vein autografts for the in situ

replacement of infected aortic prostheses. When aortic graft infection is localized to one graft limb, aggressive local soft tissue debridement and coverage with a rotational muscle flap have been shown to be safe and highly efficacious is salvaging the graft.[134,135]

An equally serious late complication is the development of a secondary aortoenteric fistula, usually involving the duodenum. Like graft infection, the incidence of aortoenteric fistula formation is no more than 2 percent, and has been associated with a mortality rate approaching 50 percent.[131,136–139] There has been some recent experience suggesting that in situ graft replacement may be an acceptable, and significantly less morbid, solution than graft excision and extraanatomic bypass, which has been the conventional approach.[137,140]

While graft infection may present initially as an anastomotic false aneurysm, in most cases these lesions are unrelated to infection. The incidence of anastomotic aneurysms following AFB grafting varies widely from series to series, ranging from 0.5 to greater than 20 percent.[141–147] Obviously, the incidence will depend, in part, on the duration of follow-up. The vast majority occur at the femoral anastomoses and usually result from graft-artery suture line disruption. Etiologic factors include prior endarterectomy of the artery, suture fragmentation, suture line stress due to compliance mismatch between graft and artery, progressive arteriosclerotic disease at the suture line, hypertension, and as noted, infection.[145–148] Surgical repair, usually by placement of a short new interpositional segment to a more distal anastomotic site, is indicated to prevent progressive enlargement and the secondary complications of graft limb thrombosis or rupture.

As noted earlier, during long-term follow-up, at least 10 to 20 percent of patients will experience occlusion of at least one limb of an AFB graft, and in most cases, progressive infrainguinal arteriosclerotic occlusive disease is the etiology.[12,101] In contradistinction to graft thrombosis in the early postoperative period, however, an arteriogram is very useful prior to reoperating on the patient with a graft limb thrombosis. Crucial anatomic information includes the integrity of the proximal aortic anastomosis, the status of the contralateral patent graft limb, and most important, the status of the infrainguinal vessels on the side of the occlusion. While thrombectomy of the acutely occluded graft limb usually can be achieved easily at the time of groin exploration, if the outflow tract on the affected side was not adequately visualized angiographically in the setting of graft limb thrombosis, treatment of the thrombosed limb with a thrombolytic drug prior to operating will not only obviate the need for thrombectomy in many cases but, more important, also will allow a more complete and informative preoperative arteriogram to be obtained. In the majority of cases, progressive SFA and/or profunda femoris disease is responsible for the occlusion, and outflow can be enhanced, and graft patency maintained, by extending the original graft as a profundaplasty. In no more than one-third of cases, especially when the profunda is small and/or significantly diseased, a new infrainguinal bypass will have to be constructed to achieve satisfactory outflow.[101,103] If the occluded graft limb cannot be thrombectomized successfully with a conventional balloon catheter, suggesting a more chronic occlusive process, use of an endarterectomy loop instrument may facilitate removal of the occlusive plug.[149,150] In the occasional patient in whom the occluded graft limb cannot be thrombectomized, inflow can be restored by constructing a femorofemoral (FF) graft based on the contralateral graft limb.[101,151,152]

Finally, genitourinary problems also may complicate AFB surgery. One troublesome potential complication of aortic reconstruction in the male patient is sexual dysfunction, which occurs in 15 to 25 percent of cases and includes both retrograde ejaculation and impotence.[12] The former disturbance is related to disruption of sympathetic nerve fibers typically located at the aortic bifurcation and results in failure of the ureteral sphincter to closed during ejaculation. The patient should be fully apprised of the risk of this complication preoperatively, and the surgeon should keep dissection at the aortic bifurcation to a minimum to reduce the likelihood of its occurrence. On the other hand, impotence may result from exclusion of one or both internal iliac arteries during construction of the AFB graft.[153,154] In the sexually active male, therefore, the surgeon may elect to construct a separate graft limb to at least one internal iliac artery as part of the AFB procedure.[155] Alternatively, if adequate antegrade internal iliac artery flow is documented on the preoperative arteriogram, one may elect to perform the proximal aortic anastomosis in ES fashion to preserve that flow. Finally, while postoperative ureteral obstruction has been identified clinically in approximately 1 to 2 percent of cases, the true incidence may be two or three times greater if asymptomatic patients are routinely screened during long-term follow-up.[156–158]

Aortoiliac Endarterectomy

INDICATIONS/CONTRAINDICATIONS

Thirty years ago, endarterectomy was the most frequently performed surgical procedure for aortoiliac occlusive disease.[1,159] Over the past three decades, however, the number of aortoiliac endarterectomies performed has dramatically declined, and today this procedure is performed very infrequently by most busy vascular surgeons, for several reasons. First, as durable grafts became available and the fear of graft infection dissipated, the somewhat less technically demanding AFB procedure quickly gained in popularity. Second, analysis of the experience gained with endarterectomy more clearly elucidated the appropriate anatomic indications for this procedure. Specifically, aortoiliac endarterectomy is an operation for focal occlusive disease involving the distal infrarenal abdominal aorta and common iliac arteries. Contraindications to the procedure include occlusive disease extending proximally to the level of the renal arteries, since in this situation an AFB graft would require less dissection and potential intraoperative blood loss; disease extension involving the external iliac arteries, since the endarterectomy plane will not end satisfactorily distally; and aneurysmal aortic or iliac arteries, since endarterectomy will further weaken the artery wall. Perhaps one of the most important reasons for the near disappearance of this operation on most vascular surgery services in recent years is that the patient presenting today with the anatomic distribution of aortoiliac disease that is amenable to endarterectomy in many centers can be treated adequately by percutaneous transluminal angioplasty (PTA) and/or stent placement. Nevertheless, in the patient with focal aortoiliac disease that cannot be treated by PTA, aortoiliac endarterectomy avoids the potential complications associated with placement of a prosthetic graft while achieving comparable long-term results (see below).

TECHNICAL DETAILS

The operation may be performed either via the midline transperitoneal or via the left retroperitoneal approach, and operative dissection is somewhat more extensive than for performance of an AFB graft. The aorta just distal to the renal arteries, its middle sacral and lumbar branches, the IMA, and the proximal external and internal iliac arteries bilaterally should be exposed to allow clamp placement, since the endarterectomy must be performed in a relatively bloodless field. A longitudinal aortotomy is made proximal to the bifurcation and extended onto one common iliac artery, but it is ended proximal to the bifurcation. A second longitudinal arteriotomy is made in the contralateral common iliac artery.

An endarterectomy is begun in the aorta and completed circumferentially. The plaque is then endarterectomized distally along this arteriotomy into the common iliac artery and feathered to an endpoint in that vessel. In many cases, the distal ledge may have to be secured by placement of 5-0 polypropylene sutures. This is preferable to extending the endarterectomy into the external iliac artery, since the plaque is not likely to adequately end at that level, so one must then "tack down" the distal intima in the smaller external iliac artery. Any residual plaque at the aortic bifurcation is then everted through the contralateral common iliac arteriotomy and feathered to a suitable endpoint with or without distal tacking sutures in that vessel. In most cases, the arteriotomies are closed primarily with 5-0 polypropylene sutures, although if the vessels are unusually small and/or if some plaque was left in the common iliac arteries, it may be preferable to close each arteriotomy as a patch angioplasty.

RESULTS

Mortality/Patency/Complications. While technically somewhat more demanding, the acute operative risk of aortoiliac endarterectomy appears comparable with that of AFB grafting. For example, in a recent series of 57 patients undergoing aortoiliac endarterectomy, there were no operative deaths.[160]

Furthermore, in properly selected patients, early and late patency appears no different from what has been reported for the AFB graft procedure. For example, Naylor et al.[160] have reported a 4 percent incidence of acute postoperative aortoiliac thrombosis after endarterectomy. On occasion, even when the occlusive process appears quite focal angiographically, at operation one may find much more extensive disease, so the surgeon should be prepared to abort the endarterectomy and place a bifurcation graft to avoid early postoperative thrombosis. In properly selected patients, however, long-term patency is excellent. Five-year patency has exceeded 90 percent in several large series and has ranged from 68 to 85 percent at 10 years.[1,160–163] Most late failures result from recurrent or progressive occlusive disease in the external iliac arteries and much less frequently from disease in the proximal infrarenal aorta.[160,164–166]

In general, other early and late complications are similar to those seen in association with the AFB, with some exceptions.[163–167] In addition to eliminating the risk of graft infection, avoidance of a groin incision essentially eliminates the incidence of lymph fistula. On the other hand, since the periaortic dissection is more extensive, the incidence of retrograde ejaculation may be somewhat higher after endarterectomy than following AFB grafting.

Iliofemoral Bypass

INDICATIONS

While arteriosclerotic occlusive disease typically presents in a symmetrical fashion with bilateral involvement, on occasion a patient may present with unilateral symptoms due to unilateral occlusive disease. An alternative anatomic reconstruction for such a patient is the iliofemoral bypass (IFB) graft. This procedure has been performed infrequently not only because patients with the appropriate anatomic distribution of disease are seen relatively infrequently but also because prior experience with unilateral aortofemoral bypass

(AFB) grafts yields relatively disappointing results and may have prejudiced some within the vascular surgical community against unilateral IFB.[168–170] The unilateral AFB typically was anastomosed to the distal abdominal aorta in ES fashion so that progressive aortic arteriosclerotic disease contributed to eventual graft failure in a significant percentage of cases. It has therefore been assumed that progressive aortic and common iliac artery occlusive disease would have a comparably adverse impact on the long-term performance of the IFB graft. However, an expanding clinical experience has confirmed excellent long-term patency associated with IFB grafting so that when the aorta and contralateral iliac arteries are disease-free, IFB grafting can provide a durable result while avoiding the risks specifically associated with aortic reconstruction.

TECHNICAL DETAILS

With the patient in the supine position and the operative side elevated 30 degrees, after the femoral vessels are exposed and controlled in the usual fashion, an oblique incision is made extending from just inferior to the twelfth rib to the lateral rectus border below the umbilicus. The muscles of the abdominal wall are divided, the peritoneum is mobilized medially, and the ureter is identified and protected. While distal aortic exposure can be achieved through this approach, proximal control of the common iliac arteries is usually sufficient. Distal control is obtained either of the distal common iliac artery or of the external and internal iliac artery origins. While an ES proximal anastomosis is acceptable, I prefer an EE reconstruction either to the common iliac artery or to the proximal external iliac artery if the internal iliac artery is patent and its antegrade flow is to be preserved. A retrograde endarterectomy of the more proximal common iliac artery may be performed either by the eversion technique or by using the loop endarterectomy instrument. In most cases, an 8-mm graft, either Dacron or PTFE, is suitable. After the proximal anastomosis is completed, the graft is tunneled just superior to the distal artery and deep to the ureter to the groin. The inguinal ligament should be slightly incised to avoid constriction of the graft. After completion of the distal anastomosis, the incisions are closed in the usual fashion.

RESULTS

Mortality/Patency/Complications. Considerable experience has demonstrated the IFB graft to be a safe procedure. Operative mortality clearly depends on patient selection but has ranged from 0 to 6 percent in several recent series of isolated IFB reconstruction.[100,168,171–174] In fact, in the only prospective, randomized trial reported to date, the operative mortality of IFB and unilateral AFB (1.4 percent) was not significantly different from the mortality of femorofemoral bypass (FFB) (0 percent).[174]

In most series, the long-term patency of IFB grafts has been excellent (Table 11-6). Among six series including over 600 patients reported over the past two decades, primary patency has ranged from 48 to 93 percent and has been 75 percent or greater in four of these six reports.[100,168,171,173,175,176] Strict comparison of these series is difficult, since the indications for operation, case selection, and technical details differ from institution to institution. For example, Harrington et al.[175] reported that smoking, endarterectomy of the donor or recipient artery, prior surgery, and performing the distal anastomosis to the profunda femoris artery in the setting of an SFA occlusion adversely affected primary patency. Others also have noted somewhat poorer long-term patency when IFB is performed in the setting of multilevel disease and/or for limb-salvage indications.[100,172] However, progressive ipsilateral iliac artery occlusive disease has not adversely affected long-term results in the vast majority of cases. For example, in the experience of Piotrowski et al.,[100] only 1 (6 percent) of 17 IFB grafts failed due to progressive iliac artery occlusive disease.

While performance of an IFB graft does require a retroperitoneal dissection, perioperative morbidity has been consistently low. Cardiac complications have been most frequent. The incidence of postoperative myocardial infarction has ranged

Table 11-6. Iliofemoral Bypass: 5-Year Patency

Source	Year	No. of Patients	Patency (%)
Levinson	1973	65	52
Couch	1985	100	77
Piotrowski	1988	17	48
Perler	1991	22	93
Harrington	1992	82	75
Darling	1992	322	82

from 1 to 9 percent and arrhythmia from 3 to 5 percent in two recent series of IFB grafts.[171,173] Postoperative ileus has not been a significant problem. For example, in a comparative analysis of IFB and FFB grafts, patients in each group resumed an oral diet 1.1 days postoperatively, respectively.[173]

EXTRAANATOMIC RECONSTRUCTION

Femorofemoral Bypass

INDICATIONS

An alternative procedure for the patient with unilateral aortoiliac occlusive disease is the extraanatomic femorofemoral bypass (FFB) graft. Although first performed in this country more than 40 years ago, this procedure remains a somewhat controversial method of aortoiliac reconstruction.[177,178] This operation was introduced initially to provide inflow for the patient with multiple associated medical problems felt to be prohibitive for performance of an anatomic form of reconstruction,[174] and its more generalized acceptance has been limited by two fundamental reservations. First, there has been concern that new or progressive arteriosclerotic occlusive disease in the donor iliac artery might compromise graft patency. Second, it has been assumed that the graft would "steal" flow from the donor limb either acutely or later due to the development of new or progressive occlusive disease in the donor iliac artery and/or the ipsilateral infrainguinal vessels.[180] However, considerable clinical experience accumulated over the past four decades has provided little objective support for these hypothetical reservations, so the FFB graft can be expected to provide acceptable early and long-term results in properly selected patients and should be part of the therapeutic armamentarium of the busy vascular surgeon today.

The appropriate candidate is a patient with unilateral iliac artery occlusive disease. If the preoperative arteriogram demonstrates atherosclerotic lesions in the aorta or donor iliac artery, the hemodynamic significance of these lesions should be assessed with direct pressure measurements in the aorta and donor femoral artery at baseline and after administration of intraarterial papaverine.

Ideally, the hemodynamic gradient should be less than 25 mmHg to adequately support an FFB graft. However, FFB may be a reasonable option in the occasional patient with bilateral iliac artery disease if the stenotic/occlusive process in the proposed donor iliac artery can be treated successfully by PTA. The obvious appeal of the FFB graft is avoidance of a major intraabdominal reconstructive procedure and its associated potential morbidity. This approach is particularly appealing in the patient with limb-threatening ischemia due to multilevel disease who requires a synchronous infrainguinal bypass graft for limb salvage. General anesthesia is avoided. While in most cases the FFB graft is performed under spinal or epidural anesthesia, it can be performed under local anesthesia.[180]

The choice of IF versus FFB for the patient with unilateral iliac artery occlusive disease remains problematic. While the retroperitoneal dissection required to perform an IFB graft precludes performing the operation under local anesthesia, in most cases an epidural or spinal anesthetic will be adequate. Although it has been assumed that the retroperitoneal dissection necessary to perform an IFB graft would increase perioperative morbidity when compared with the FFB graft, this has not been confirmed in clinical studies.[173,174] The IFB graft obviates the risk of compromising flow by "steal" or technical fault in the donor extremity. On the other hand, a severely calcified iliac artery increases the technical difficulty of performing an IFB so that FFB reconstruction may be preferable. On balance, IFB graft patency appears somewhat superior to that reported for FFB (see below). In many cases, however, the ultimate factor in selecting IFB or FFB reconstruction is surgical preference.

TECHNICAL DETAILS

Although the operation is performed via bilateral groin incisions, the abdomen should be included in the operative field because if inflow at the donor femoral artery is unexpectedly found to be less than adequate, a more proximal dissection may have to be carried out. The femoral vessels are exposed and individually controlled on each side in the usual fashion, and prior to systemic anticoagulation with sodium heparin, a tunnel is created between the two groins. I prefer a suprafascial plane, although others have advocated tunneling the graft in a subfascial course.[169,178] The tunnel should be developed so that the graft will lie as a gentle inverted U as it traverses the lower quadrants of the abdomen. Saphenous vein has been displaced as the bypass conduit by synthetic grafts, since in most patients an 8- or 10-mm-diameter graft is most appropriate. The specific graft material, essentially either Dacron or PTFE, remains controversial. I prefer Dacron because it has less tendency to kink as it exits and enters the respective groins. There is also some evidence that anastomotic neointimal hyperplasia is more likely to occur in this setting when PTFE is the graft material.[180]

It is important to perform the anastomoses somewhat distal to the inguinal ligaments so as to avoid kinking or constriction of the graft by the ligament with wound closure. In the patient in whom the common femoral artery bifurcates unusually proximally, the inguinal ligament should be incised partially to allow the graft to lie properly. If the SFA is patent, the toe of the anastomosis should extend onto this vessel, whereas if the SFA is occluded and/or the profunda origin stenotic, the anastomosis is carried onto the profunda. The proximal (donor) anastomosis should be performed first. After the recipient femoral arteriotomy is made, the graft is clamped distally and the appropriate length measured while it is pulsatile so as to avoid redundancy. The graft must be vigorously flushed prior to completing the distal anastomosis to evacuate any fresh mural thrombus. The groin incisions are then closed in layers, taking care not to constrict the graft at the inguinal ligament on each side.

RESULTS

Mortality. In comparison with the "gold standard" procedure for aortoiliac occlusive disease, the AFB graft, FFB grafting is clearly a compromise operation. In many cases this is an operation reserved for the high-risk patient due either to advanced age or serious associated medical problems or to severe multilevel occlusive disease requiring multilevel revascularization.[173] However, in properly selected candidates, FFB grafting provides very satisfactory long-term patency and with a minimum of operative risk. Over the last two decades, operative mortality

has ranged from 0 to 6 percent in several large series.[100,173,180–185] These reports include a heterogeneous patient population. However, it seems clear that as an elective solitary procedure, FFB can be performed today with a mortality risk under 2 percent, even in an elderly, medically compromised patient population.[100,173,181–183]

Patency. There is some variability in long-term patency reported for the FFB graft, in part due to heterogeneous patient populations, methods of data reporting, and other factors. For example, most earlier studies have not stratified results into primary and secondary patency. Nevertheless, it is clear that this extraanatomic form of reconstruction provides reasonably durable results. Cumulative patency has ranged from 77 to 100 percent at 1 year, from 47 to 90 percent at 3 years, and from 45 to 80 percent at 5-years[13–100,173,175,180,181,184–186,188–190] (Table 11-7). Furthermore, it is clear that a significant number of failed FFB grafts can be salvaged through timely reoperation. For example, among 47 patients without a history of previous arterial reconstruction, primary and secondary 5-year FFB graft patency was 74 and 82 percent, respectively; among 13 patients who had undergone other prior vascular procedures, the primary and secondary patency rates were 39 and 51 percent, respectively.[191]

Based on these results, in recent years some have advocated extending the indications for FFB to include patients with bilateral iliac artery

Table 11-7. Femorofemoral Bypass: 5-Year Patency

Source	Year	No. of Patients	Patency (%)
Eugene	1977	33	45
Mannick	1977	53	80
Flanigan	1978	80	74
Livesay	1979	36	56
Dick	1980	133	73
Plecha	1984	119	72
Lamerton	1985	61	60
Piotrowski	1988	47	55
Hepp	1988	26	80
Perler	1991	50	57
Harrington	1992	130	60
Brener	1993	150	63

Source: Adopted from Brener BJ, et al: Extraanatomic bypasses. *In* Veith FJ, Hobson RW, Williams RA, Wilson SE (eds): Vascular Surgery: Principles and Practice, 2d ed. New York, McGraw-Hill, 1994, p. 489.

occlusive disease if inflow on the proposed do-nor side can be normalized by PTA.[173] The rationale for this approach is based, in part, on the excellent long-term results being reported for iliac PTA procedures.[192,193] At the Johns Hop-kins Hospital, 26 percent of the FFB grafts performed in recent years were preceded by do-nor iliac artery PTA. No statistically significant difference in patency has been documented at 3 and 5 years of follow-up between patients who did or did not undergo preoperative donor iliac artery PTA.[173] Several other reports also have confirmed satisfactory results when FFB was preceded by donor iliac artery PTA.[187,191,194]

This issue addresses one of the fundamental concerns about the FFB graft, namely, progres-sive donor iliac artery occlusive disease ulti-mately compromising long-term graft patency. If this were a valid concern, it would be most cogent in the patient who already has hemody-namically significant iliac artery disease that must be dilated prior to performance of an FFB graft. The clinical results reported to date seem to mitigate against this reservation. In fact, there is some evidence that by performing an FFB graft and enhancing flow velocity in the donor iliac artery, one may actually be retarding the pro-gression of disease in that donor iliac arterial system. In one recent study, for example, serial angiographic studies documented a generalized dilatation of the donor iliac artery system with time after FFB, most likely as a result of the increased flow in those vessels.[195] In fact, pro-gressive iliac artery disease rarely has been iden-tified among patients undergoing FFB recon-struction. In one report, for example, pro-gressive iliac artery occlusive disease requiring operation developed in only 2 (4 percent) of 45 patients who underwent FFB.[196] In a recent multicenter study of 317 patients who under-went FFB grafts, progressive iliac artery occlu-sive disease requiring either PTA or surgical intervention developed in only 6 percent, with a mean follow-up of 38 months.[197]

Furthermore, experience gained over the past two decades has provided scant evidence of a clin-ically significant "steal" phenomenon occurring af-ter FFB in properly selected candidates. In one report, no symptomatic deterioration developed in the donor limb of 51 patients after FFB, although a mean decline in the ankle-arm index of 0.12 was documented in 80 percent of the cases.[13] In an-other study of 44 patients who underwent FFB for claudication, there was no functional deterioration noted in the donor limb, although an asymptom-atic decline in the ankle-arm index may have oc-curred in 45 percent of the cases.[198] In a series of 133 patients who underwent FFB grafts over a 12-year period, clinical "steal" did not develop in any patients.[184] Interpretation of these reports and analysis of this issue are confounded by the fact that the improvement in functional status of the recipient limb may unmask symptoms in the do-nor limb or allow more vigorous exercise, which produces some decline of measurable Doppler pressures in the donor limb.[197] In a VA prospec-tive multicenter trial including 317 patients, a clin-ical "steal" was documented in 12 cases but ap-peared to reflect an unmasking of preexisting disease in the majority. In fact, a new clinical "steal" was documented in only 3 percent of the patients in this study.[197] These studies support several earlier experimental models in which the development of a hemodynamically significant "steal" after FFB was largely dependent on the presence of flow-limiting disease in the donor iliac and distal arterial tree.[199–201]

It is clear that early and long-term results after FFB depend, for the most part, on the variables that influence the results of other inflow revascu-larization procedures, such as the clinical presen-tation and status of the infrainguinal arterial tree. For example, long-term results are somewhat poorer among patients who have undergone pre-vious arterial bypass procedures when compared with those in whom the FFB graft is the initial intervention.[187,191] One can expect better results, at least early, among patients who undergo FFB for claudication versus limb salvage indications.[173] The influence of the recipient infrainguinal vessels on graft patency is somewhat controversial. In general, an occluded recipient SFA results in some-what poorer graft patency when compared with those in which the SFA is patent,[13,100,191] al-though this observation is not universal.[187] In my experience, FFB graft patency at 2-year follow-up was superior among patients in whom the SFA was patent when compared with those in whom the vessel was occluded, although by 3 years the results were comparable, suggesting possible progression of distal disease among patients in whom the SFA was initially patent.[173] This may in part explain the conflicting results noted in earlier studies. Finally, the influence of graft material on long-term patency is also undecided. In one report, long-term patency was superior among bypasses constructed with Dacron, although others have reported equally excellent results with PTFE grafts.[202]

Complications. The obvious advantages of FFB are brief operative duration, limited operative dissection, and minimal intraoperative blood loss when compared with an AFB, or even an IFB graft. The incidence of cardiac complications should be less than associated with the AFB graft, and in general, patients resume an oral diet and are discharged from the hospital earlier.[173] Perhaps most important, FFB reconstruction avoids a number of serious complications associated with a AFB, such as colon ischemia, aortoenteric fistula development, ureteral obstruction, impotence, and retrograde ejaculation.

The other vascular complications associated with FFB are comparable with those seen after AFB or IFB reconstruction and are managed in a similar fashion. Early postoperative graft thrombosis is uncommon and warrants immediate reexploration to rule out an easily correctable technical problem. It is particularly important to rule out redundancy of the graft, kinking of the graft at either groin, and twisting or compression of the graft by the groin closure. In the absence of technical error, and if outflow appears adequate, one must make certain that inflow is satisfactory to support the graft by measuring arterial systolic pressure in the donor common femoral artery. There is no evidence that the incidence of wound infection or lymphorrhea is significantly greater after FFB than AFB.[173] Furthermore, while the incidence of graft infection is low,[180] it represents a less formidable problem than when infection involves an AFB prosthesis. There is no evidence that femoral anastomotic aneurysms occur more frequently in association with FFB reconstruction. Long-term graft failure in most cases results from progressive infrainguinal occlusive disease in the recipient limb, and graft salvage and secondary

patency may be enhanced by construction of a new infrainguinal bypass after thrombectomy or thrombolysis of the FFB graft.[187,191] Finally, a relatively infrequent complication seen among patients undergoing FFB is the late development of an abdominal aortic aneurysm. In one series of 119 patients, 2 (1.8 percent) aortic aneurysms developed 22 and 38 months, respectively, after FFB, and each was repaired with placement of a unilateral AFB to the FFB graft.[180]

Axillofemoral Bypass

INDICATIONS

The extraanatomic axillofemoral (AXF) bypass was first reported by Blaisdell and Hall[203] as an emergency unilateral inflow procedure in 1963.[203] Subsequently, Sauvage and Wood[204] added a crossover femorofemoral graft to create the bilateral AXF reconstruction. Over the last three decades, considerable experience has accrued with this operation performed either as a unilateral or a bilateral procedure. There is general agreement that AXF bypass is a compromise operation for aortoiliac revascularization, and its indications are well-defined and limited (Table 11-8). One of the most important indications for AXF bypass is aortic sepsis, namely, to provide lower extremity arterial flow through clean tissue planes in the patient with either an infected aortic graft, a secondary (graft) aortoenteric fistula, or a primary mycotic aortic aneurysm in which the infected graft and/or aortic tissue must be resected and the infrarenal abdominal aorta oversewn. AXF bypass also may be required in the patient with a primary aortoenteric fistula, although in many of these cases in situ aortic reconstruction has been performed recently.[140] In the elective setting, AXF bypass is a reasonable alternative in the patient

Table 11-8. *Indications for Axillofemoral Bypass*

Aortic graft infection
Aortoenteric fistula
  Primary
  Secondary
Mycotic aortic aneurysm
"Hostile" abdomen
Poor-risk patient

with multilevel occlusive disease manifested in limb-threatening ischemia and in whom multiple associated medical problems and/or a limited life expectancy preclude performance of an AFB graft. I would disagree with those who support performance of AXF bypass purely for symptoms of intermittent claudication.[205] If the patient's overall clinical status is so precarious as to preclude performance of an AFB graft, one must question why operation is being contemplated for a non-limb-threatening indication. Finally, in the occasional patient with a "hostile" abdomen due to extensive previous intraabdominal surgery, AXF bypass reconstruction may potentially allow inflow revascularization with a minimum of risk, although in many of these patients today approaching the aorta via the left retroperitoneal incision will allow performance of an AFB graft while avoiding intraperitoneal adhesions.

Prior to performing an elective AXF bypass graft, it is important to make certain that there is no hemodynamically significant disease in the axillary artery selected for inflow. Since the incidence of brachiocephalic occlusive disease is relatively low, in the absence of symptoms, a normal upper extremity Doppler examination and/or symmetrical brachial artery systolic blood pressure measurements will effectively rule out significant disease precluding performance of an AXF bypass graft, although some have advocated formal arteriography preoperatively in the AXF bypass candidate.[206,207]

TECHNICAL DETAILS

The patient is placed in the supine position with the arm on the side of the donor axillary artery abducted approximately 90 degrees. The neck, shoulder, upper arm, chest, abdomen, and both lower extremities are prepared and included in the sterile field. After exposure of the femoral arteries in the usual fashion, the axillary artery is approached through a transverse incision approximately a finger breadth inferior to the distal two-thirds of the clavicle. The fibers of the pectoralis major are separated, and in most cases the origin of the pectoralis minor is divided to aid exposure. The brachial plexus is identified and carefully protected. After division of several branches, the axillary vein is usually mobilized inferiorly, allowing

exposure of the artery in a bed of adipose tissue, and the vessel is controlled proximally and distally with vascular tapes. The thoracoacromial trunk may require ligation and division to provide an adequate length of the artery for performance of the proximal anastomosis to its first or second portion. An important technical step is creation of the necessary tunnel to the ipsilateral groin. While some have advocated placing the graft in an intrathoracic plane,[208] this seems unnecessary and potentially meddlesome. Others have advocated a subfascial tunnel.[209] In most cases, however, a subcutaneous tunnel is adequate. The tunnel should course somewhat laterally toward the anterior axillary line, and in some cases, a short transverse incision is required to complete the tunnel to the ipsilateral groin. The tunnel to the contralateral groin is likewise created in a suprafascial plane as in performance of an FFB graft.

Either a PTFE or Dacron graft may be used, and in most cases, an 8- or 10-mm graft is appropriate. I favor PTFE because it obviates preclotting and the potential for a Dacron graft to ooze within the tunnel initially after unclamping. In order to resist external compression, most vascular surgeons today, including myself, prefer to use externally supported conduits.[178,205] After systemic anticoagulation, a longitudinal axillary arteriotomy is performed with the vessel rotated somewhat superiorly, and the proximal anastomosis is created in ES fashion. The graft is then clamped proximally, and the axillary artery is opened. The graft is tunneled to the ipsilateral groin, and after the appropriate length has been determined with the graft pulsating, it is cut and the femoral anastomosis performed in ES fashion. Prior to opening the AXF limb, however, one should perform the proximal anastomosis of the crossover graft to the hood of the AXF distal anastomosis. Formerly, some workers advocated anastomosing the crossover limb several centimeters proximal to the groin so that the graft assumed an inverted-Y configuration.[210] However, this leaves a relatively low-flow cul-de-sac in the main AXF limb distal to the takeoff of the femorofemoral limb and has largely fallen out of favor. By constructing the bifurcated graft as an inverted U with the crossover limb originating from the site of the AXF to femoral artery anastomosis, this relatively low-flow graft segment, which might predispose to thrombosis, is avoided. After completion of the graft-graft anastomosis, the femorofemoral limb is clamped and the AXF limb unclamped. The distal anastomosis of the crossover limb is then performed to the contralateral femoral artery, the graft is unclamped, and the incisions are closed in layers. In addition to assessing pedal flow by Doppler prior to leaving the operating room, one also must make certain that there has been no compromise of flow to the arm due to some technical fault at the site of the graft–axillary artery anastomosis.

RESULTS

Mortality. The AXF bypass graft is an operation performed through superficial tissue planes in selected patients with chronic occlusive disease because it is a minimally invasive procedure. Nevertheless, it is associated with a greater rate of operative mortality than other surgical reconstructive procedures for aortoiliac occlusive disease. Operative mortality has ranged widely, from 1.7 to 16 percent, over the last two decades.[188,209,211–222] This wide variability in operative mortality reflects the heterogeneity of the patient populations studied, the varied indications for the operation, and other factors. For example, Ward et al.[209] reported a 16 percent operative mortality, but 77 percent of the deaths occurred after emergency AXF bypass procedures. At the other extreme, Johnson et al.[214] reported a series of elective AXF bypass reconstructions, including 22 percent performed for claudication, and the mortality was only 1.7 percent. On balance, one can anticipate an operative risk of under 10 percent, and probably much closer to 5 percent, among the typically elderly patient population undergoing elective or semielective AXF bypass for limb-threatening chronic aortoiliac occlusive disease today.

Patency. There is also considerable variability in the reported patency rates associated with AXF bypass reconstruction for several reasons. In addition to case selection, most series include both axillounifemoral and axillobifemoral grafts, and in varying proportions. In addition, both Dacron and PTFE grafts are reported, including grafts that are and are not externally supported. Since most series are relatively small, stratifica-

tion for these potentially confounding variables is not feasible. Finally, most series have reported cumulative patency, without differentiating primary and secondary patency rates. Nevertheless, a review of series reported over the past two decades provides a reasonable context in which one can judge the performance of this extraanatomic operation. Cumulative patency has ranged from 30 to 98 percent at 1 year, from 36 to 92 percent at 3 years, and from 34 to 87 percent at 5 years[188–191,205,211–217,219–221,223–228] (Table 11-9). Although a significant percentage of AXF bypass grafts will experience thrombosis during follow-up, graft thrombectomy is a relatively uncomplicated procedure that typically can be performed rapidly under local anesthesia. Furthermore, where results are stratified into primary and secondary (cumulative) patency, it is clear that reoperation and thrombectomy have markedly enhanced long-term results. For example, Ascer et al.[207] have reported 5-year primary and secondary patency rates of 44 and 71 percent, respectively, for unilateral grafts and 50 and 75 percent, respectively, for axillobifemoral reconstructions.[207] Likewise, Rutherford et al.[191] have reported primary and secondary patency rates of 19 and 37 percent for unilateral grafts and 62 and 82 percent, respectively, for axillobifemoral grafts. These observations clearly justify aggressive reoperation to maintain graft patency in this patient population. There is less agreement on the long-term durability of unilateral versus axillobifemoral grafts. It has been assumed that since the crossover femorofemoral limb increases flow velocity in the main AXF conduit, early and long-term patency should be enhanced.[191,209,213,214,229] However, the superiority of the bilateral graft has not been consistently demonstrated.[188,207,211,220] A number of other variables that potentially influence graft patency may confound resolution of this issue.

As with most grafts performed for occlusive disease, the clinical indication for surgery will affect long-term patency. Specifically, AXF bypass grafts performed for claudication appear to have superior patency when compared with those performed for limb-salvage indications. For example, Donaldson et al.[212] have reported a 3-year primary patency rate of 46 percent for

Table 11-9. Axillofemoral Bypass: Cumulative Patency

Source	Year	No. of Patients	Patency (%)		
			1 year	3 years	5 years
Mannick	1970	37	—	80	—
Moore	1971	24	—	74	54
LoGerfo	1976	64	64	—	37
Johnson	1977	56	83	76	76
Eugene*	1977	24	60	36	36
De Laurentis	1978	42	62	—	—
Ray*	1979	21	90	85	77
Livesay	1979	14	—	75	—
Whittemore	1980	54	30	—	—
Burrell*	1982	38	—	97	—
Ascer*	1985	22	90	77	77
Chang*	1986	88	—	—	75
Donaldson*	1986	100	42	—	34
Savrin	1986	33	—	—	75
Christenson	1986	85	78	—	72
Rutherford*	1987	27	—	—	82
Hepp*	1988	22	85	73	73
Cina*	1988	24	—	—	72
Schneider	1992	34	92	74	74
El-Massry	1993	79	98	92	87

*Includes only axillobifemoral reconstructions
Source: Adopted from Brener BJ, et al: Extraanatomic bypasses. *In* Veith FJ, Hobson RW, Williams RA, Wilson SE (eds): Vascular Surgery: Principles and Practice, 2d ed. New York, McGraw-Hill, 1994, p 492.

AXF bypass grafts performed for claudication versus 28 percent when performed for limb-salvage indications. In a remarkable recent series, 5-year primary patency was 80 and 65 percent, respectively, for claudication and limb-salvage patients.[205] Likewise, Ray et al.[220] have reported secondary patency of 81 percent among claudicants versus 50 percent in limb-salvage cases. Conversely, there is less agreement with respect to the influence of infrainguinal arterial occlusive disease on AXF bypass graft patency. While most studies addressing this issue have reported superior patency in patients in whom the SFA was patent at the time of the AXF bypass graft,[191,214,220] others have not confirmed this observation.[205,207]

Furthermore, there is no consensus on the optimal graft material for AXF bypass. Specifically, an analysis of several retrospective studies has failed to document a significant difference in early or long-term results of Dacron and PTFE grafts. While one recent series reported superior results with PTFE grafts,[216] several other studies have not confirmed this observation.[209,215,223,227] One possible advantage of PTFE in this setting is the relative ease with which it may be thrombectomized. Likewise, while externally supported grafts are theoretically appealing, since they may resist external compression, and although in at least one study this characteristic was felt to be responsible for markedly improved results when compared with historical controls,[216] the efficacy of ringed grafts has not been demonstrated to date in a randomized, prospective trial.

Complications. In addition to its susceptibility to early and late thrombosis, there appears to be an increased incidence of graft infection associated with AXF bypass when compared with other vascular procedures performed for aortoiliac occlusive disease. The reported incidence of AXF bypass graft infection has ranged from 4 to 12 per cent.[205,215] In at least some cases, infection results from graft placement in patients with preexisting aortic infection. In one series, for example, there was a 29 percent incidence of AXF bypass graft infection when the procedure was performed for aortic sepsis.[212] The subcutaneous location of the graft and the performance of repeated thrombectomy procedures also may predispose to graft infection when the procedure is performed for chronic occlusive disease.

The most important complications specific to the AXF bypass graft involve the axillary artery anastomosis. In one comprehensive review, there was a 1.6 percent incidence of complications specifically related to the axillary artery.[230] Disruption of the proximal anastomosis is a rare but potentially serious complication. Disruption tends to occur when the patient fully extends and raises the arm. In one recent report, two patients experienced this complication 6 weeks postoperatively, although a different etiologic mechanism was postulated in each case.[231] In one case, the graft had been tunneled between the fibers of the pectoralis minor muscle, and it was presumed that the muscle may have "scissored" the graft with the arm fully abducted. It is preferable to perform the anastomosis medial to the insertion of the muscle, although whether or not one should completely transect or simply retract the muscle at the time of graft placement remains problematic.[230, 231] In the second case, the anastomosis had been performed too far laterally. It is clear that the graft should be performed either to the first or second portion of the axillary artery so that the patient may have full range of motion without creating tension at the anastomosis.[231] In other words, careful attention to technical detail at the time of AXF bypass graft placement should obviate this potential complication.

Other axillary artery complications include pseudoaneurysm formation, thrombosis, and peripheral embolism. In one series, 2 of 29 patients (6.9 percent) who underwent AXF bypass developed pseudoaneurysms within the first 22 months postoperatively.[232] It is likely that excessive tension at the anastomosis, as described above, may contribute to this relatively infrequent complication. Axillary artery thrombosis is also a relatively infrequent complication. In one report, 1 of 56 patients (1.8 percent) experienced an axillary artery thrombosis during 5 years of follow-up.[214] Broome et al.[224] observed two (3.3 percent) axillary artery thromboses among 61 patients during 3 years follow-up. In the largest series reported to date, only 1 (0.9 percent) of 106 patients followed for 3.5 years developed an axillary artery throm bosis.[215] Finally, ipsilateral upper extremity emboli, presumably related to perianastomotic thrombus, have been described in four patients following AXF bypass grafts.[233,234]

CONCLUSIONS

The increasing performance of PTA has had some impact on the surgical treatment of aortoiliac occlusive disease in recent years. Furthermore, in view of the excellent results associated with iliac artery PTA,[192,193] when the patient's disease process appears amenable to this endovascular modality, and if symptoms warrant intervention, it seems reasonable that PTA should be the initial therapeutic intervention. Nevertheless, and particularly in view of the aging of our population, there will continue to be a sizable number of patients with aortoiliac occlusive disease beyond the scope of endovascular intervention who will therefore require surgical reconstruction. The vascular surgeon has a wide variety of surgical options from which to select a method of reconstruction that is appropriate both to the patient's pathologic anatomy, and to his or her overall medical condition.

REFERENCES

1. Brewster DC, Darling RC: Optimal methods of aortoiliac reconstruction. Surgery 1978;84:739.
2. Darling RC, Brewster DC, Hallett JW Jr, et al: Aorto-iliac reconstruction. Surg Clin North Am 1979;59:565.
3. Brewster DC, Perler BA, Robison JG, et al: Aortofemoral graft for multilevel occlusive disease. Predictors of success and need for distal bypass. Arch Surg 1982;117:1593.
4. DeLaurentis DA, Friedman P, Wolferth CC Jr, et al: Atherosclerosis and the hypoplastic aortoiliac system. Surgery 1978;83:27.
5. Jernigan WR, Fallat ME, Hatfield DR: Hypoplastic aortoiliac syndrome: An entity peculiar to women. Surgery 1983;94:752.

6. Lallemond RC, Gosling RG, Newman DL: Role of the bifurcation in atheromatosis of the abdominal aorta. Surg Gyn Obstet 1973;737:987.

7. Palmaz JC, Carson SN, Hunter G, et al: Male hypoplastic infrarenal aorta and premature atherosclerosis. Surgery 1983;94:91.

8. Caes F, Cham B, Van den Brande P, et al: Small artery syndrome in women. Surg Gynecol Obstet 1985;161:165.

9. Burke PM Jr, Herrmann JB, Cutler BS: Optimal grafting methods for the small abdominal aorta. J Cardiovasc Surg 1987;28:420.

10. Darling RC: Medical progress: Peripheral arterial surgery. N Engl J Med 1969;280:84.

11. Malone JM, Moore WS, Goldstone J: Life expectancy following aorto-femoral arterial grafting. Surgery 1977;81:551.

12. Brewster DC: Clinical and anatomical consideration for surgery in aortoiliac disease and results of surgical treatment. Circulation 1991;83(suppl I):I-42.

13. Flanigan DP, Pratt DG, Goodreau JJ, et al: Hemodynamic and angiographic guidelines in selection of patients for femorofemoral bypass. Arch Surg 1978;113:1257.

14. Mannick JA, Maini BS: Femorofemoral grafting: Indications and late results. Am J Surg 1978;136:190.

15. Cronenwett JL, Davis JT Jr, Gooch JB, et al: Aortoiliac occlusive disease in women. Surgery 1980;88:775.

16. Weiss NS: Premature menopause and aortoiliac occlusive disease. J Chronic Dis 1972;25:133.

17. Lallemand RC, Brown KGE, Boulter PS: Vessel dimensions in premature atheromatous disease of aortic bifurcation. Br Med J 1972;2:255.

18. Johnston KW, Demorais D, Colapinto RF: Difficulty in assessing the severity of aortoiliac disease by clinical and angiographic methods. Angiology 1981;32:609.

19. Goodreau JJ, Creasy JK, Flanigan DP, et al: Rational approach to the differentiation of vascular and neurologic claudication. Surgery 1978;84:749.

20. Kempczinski RF: Lower extremity arterial emboli from ulcerating atherosclerotic plaques. JAMA 1979;241:807.

21. Perler BA, Kadir S, Williams GM: Aortic mural thrombus in young women: Premature arteriosclerosis or separate clinical entity? Surgery 1991;110:912.

22. Kavanaugh GJ, Svien HJ, Holman CB, et al: "Pseudoclaudication" syndrome produced by compression of the cauda equina. JAMA 1968;206:2477.

23. Silver RA, Schuele HL, Stack JK, et al: Intermittent claudication of neurospinal origin. Arch Surg 1969;98:523.

24. Evans JG: Neruogenic intermittent claudication. Br Med J 1964;2:985.

25. Blau JN, Logue V: Intermittent claudication of the cauda equina. An unusual syndrome resulting from central protrusion of a lumbar interverterbral disc. Lancet 1961;1:1081.

26. Brish A, Lerner MA, Braham J: Intermittent claudication from compression of cauda equina by a narrowed spinal canal. J Neurosurg 1964;21:207.

27. Verbeist H: A radicular syndrome from developmental narrowing of the lumbar vertebral canal. J Bone J Surg 1954:36B:230.

28. Verbiest H: Further experiences on the pathologic influences of a developmental narrowness of the bony lumber vertebral canal. J Bone J Surg 1955;37B:576.

29. Sumner DS, Strandness DE Jr: The relationship between calf blood flow and ankle blood pressure in patients with intermittent claudication. Surgery 1969;65:763.

30. Bruns-Slot H, Strijbosch L, Greep JM: Interobserver variability in single-plane aortography. Surgery 1981;90:497.

31. Flanigan DP, Ryan TJ, Williams LR, et al: Aortofemoral or femoropopliteal revascularization? A prospective evaluation of the papaverine test. J Vasc Surg 1984;1:215.

32. Langsfeld M, Neptune J, Hershey FB, et al: The use of deep duplex scanning to predict hemodynamically significant aortoiliac stenoses. J Vasc Surg 1988;7:395.

33. Moneta GL, Yeager RA, Antonovic R, et al: Accuracy of lower extremity arterial duplex mapping. J Vasc Surg 1992;15:275.

34. Cossman DV, Ellison JE, Wagner WH, et al: Comparison of contrast arteriography to arterial mapping with color flow duplex imaging in the lower extremities. J Vasc Surg 1989;10:522.

35. Edwards JM, Caldwell DM, Goldman ML, et al: The role of duplex scanning in the selection of patients for transluminal angioplasty. J Vasc Surg 1991;13:69.

36. Kohler TR, Andros G, Porter JM, et al: Can duplex scanning replace arteriography for lower extremity arterial disease? Ann Vasc Surg 1990;4:280.

37. Martin-Pavedero V, Dixon SM, Baker JD, et al: Risk of renal failure after major angiography. Arch Surg 1983;118:1417.

38. Mason RA, Arbeit LA, Giron F: Renal dysfunction after arteriography. JAMA 1985;253:1001.

39. Oudot J: La graffe vasculaire dan les thromboses du carrefour aortique. Presse Med 1951;59:234.

40. Blakemore AH, Voorhees AB: The use of tubes constructed from vinyon "N" cloth in bridging arterial defects—Experimental and clinical. Ann Surg 1954;170:324.

41. DeBakey ME, Crawford SE: Vascular prostheses. Transplant Bull 1957;4:2.

42. Ernst CB, Rutkow IM, Cleveland RJ, et al: Vascular surgery in the United States. Report of the Joint Society for Vascular Surgery-International Society for Cardiovascular Surgery Committee on vascular surgical manpower. J Vasc Surg 1987;6:611.

43. Cintora I, Pearle DE, Cannon JA: A clinical survey of aortobifermoal bypass using two inherently different graft types. Ann Surg 1988;208:625.

44. Williams GM, Ricotta JJ, Zinner M, et al: The extended retroperitoneal approach for the treatment of extensive atherosclerosis of the aorta and renal vessels. Surgery 1980;88:846.

45. Sicard GA, Freeman MB, VanderWonde JC, et al: Comparison between the transabdominal and retroperitoneal approach for reconstruction of the infrarenal abdominal aorta. J Vasc Surg 1987;5:19.

46. Leather RP, Shah DJ, Kaufman JL, et al: Comparative analysis of retroperitoneal and transperitoneal aortic replacement for aneurysm. Surg Gynecol Obstet 1989;168:387.

47. Nevelsteen A, Suy R, Daenen W, et al: Transabdominal or retroperitoneal approach to the aortoiliac track: Pulmonary function studies. Eur J Vasc Surg 1988;2:229.

48. Cambria RP, Brewster DC, Abbott WM, et al: Transperitoneal versus retroperitoneal approach for aortic reconstruction: A randomized prospective study. J Vasc Surg 1990;11:314.

49. Brener BJ, Darling RC, Frederick PL, et al: Major venous anomalies complicating abdominal aortic surgery. Arch Surg 1974;108:155.

50. Milloy FJ, Anson BJ, Cauldwell EW: Variations in the inferior vena caval veins and in their renal and lumbar communications. Surg Gynecol Obstet 1962;115:131.

51. Perler BA: Abdominal aortic replacement with a left-sided vena cava: Transperitoneal and retroperitoneal approaches. J Cardiovasc Surg 1989;30:236.

52. Weinstein MH, Machleder HI: Sexual function after aortoiliac surgery. Ann Surg 1975;181:787.

53. Flanigan DP, Schuler JJ, Keifer T, et al: Elimination of iatrogenic impotence and improvement of sexual function after aortoiliac revascularization. Arch Surg 1982;117:544.

54. Picone AL, Green RM, Ricotta JR, et al: Spinal cord ischemia following operations on the abdominal aorta. J Vasc Surg 1986;3:94.

55. Gloviczki P, Cross SA, Stansen AW, et al: Ischemic injury to the spinal cord or lumbosacral plexus after aorto-iliac reconstruction. Am J Surg 1991;162:131.

56. Pierce GE, Turrentine M, Stringfield S, et al: Evaluation of end-to-side v. end-to-end proximal anastomosis in aortobifemoral bypass. Arch Surg 1982:117:1580.

57. Dunn DA, Downs AT, Lye CR: Aortoiliac reconstruction for occlusive disease: Comparison of end-to-end and end-to-side proximal anastomosis. Can J Surg 1982;28:382.

58. Baird RJ, Feldman P, Miles JT, et al: Subsequent downstream repair after aorto-iliac and aorto-femoral bypass operations. Surgery 1977;82:785.

59. Crawford ES, Manning LG, Kelly TF: "Redo" surgery after operations for aneurysm and occlusion of the abdominal aorta. Surgery 1977;81:41.

60. Malone JM, Moore WS, Goldstone J: The natural history of bilateral aortofemoral bypass grafts for ischemia of the lower extremities. Arch Surg 1975:110:1300.

61. Goldstone J, Malone JM, Moore WS: Importance of the profunda femoris artery in primary and secondary arterial operations for lower extremity ischemia. Am J Surg 1978;136;215.

62. Seeger JM, Doe DA, Kaelin LD, et al: Routine reimplantation of patent inferior mesenteric arteries limits colon infarction after aortic reconstruction. J Vasc Surg 1992;15:635.

63. Christopherson R, Beattie C, Frank S, et al: Perioperative morbidity in patients randomized to epidural or general anesthesia for lower extremity vascular surgery. Anesthesiology 1993;79:422.

64. Sofwat A: Epidural anesthesia in abdominal vascular surgery: Pro: Epidural anesthesia is a valuable adjunct to general anesthesia for abdominal vascular surgery. J Cardiothorac Anesth 1989;3:505.

65. Hendoin H, Lahtinen J, Lansimies E: The effect of thoracic epidural analgesia on postoperative stress and morbidity. Ann Chir Gynecol 1987;76:234.

66. Kehlet H, Brandt MR, Hansen AP, et al: Effect of epidural analgesia on metabolic profiles during and after surgery. Br J Surg 1979;66:543.

67. Seeling W, Ahnefeld FW, Hamann H, et al: Aortofemoraler Bifurkations bypass. Der Einfluss des Anaesthesieverfahrens (NLA, Throakale Kontinuierliche Katheterperidual-anaesthesie) und Kraislauf, Atmung und Stoffwechsel Intraoperatives Kraislaufverhalten. Anaesthesist 1985;34:417.

68. Diebel LN, Lange MP, Schneider F, et al: Cardiopulmonary complications after major surgery: A role for epidural analgesia? Surgery 1987;102:660.

69. Bunt TJ, Manczuk M, Varley K: Continuous epidural anesthesia for aortic surgery: Thoughts on peer review and safety. Surgery 1987;101:706.

70. Raggi R, Dardik H, Mauro A: Continuous epidural anesthesia and postoperative epidural narcotic in vascular surgery. Am J Surg 1987;154:192.

71. Yeager MD, Glass DD, Neff RK, et al: Epidural anesthesia and analgesia in high risk surgical patients. Anesthesiology 1987;66;729.

72. Mason RA, Newton GB, Cassel W, et al: Combined epidural and general anesthesia in aortic surgery. J Cardiovasc Surg 1990;31:442.

73. Toy PTCY, Strauss RG, Stehling LC, et al: Predeposited autologous blood for elective surgery: A national multicenter study. N Engl J Med 1987; 316:517.

74. O'Hara PJ, Hertzer NR, Krajewski LP, et al: Reduction in the homologous blood requirement for abdominal aortic aneurysm repair by use of preadmission autologous blood donation. Surgery 1994:115:69.

75. Ouriel K, Shortell CK, Green DM, et al: Intraoperative autotransfusion in aortic surgery. J Vasc Surg 1993;18:16.

76. Hallet JW Jr, Popovsky M, Ilstrup D: Minimizing blood transfusion during abdominal aortic surgery: Recent advances in rapid autotransfusion. J Vasc Surg 1987;5:601.

77. Crawford ES, Bomberger RA, Glaeser DH, et al: Aortoiliac occlusive disease: Factors influencing survival and function following reconstructive operation over a twenty-five-year period. Surgery 1981;90:1055.

78. Szilagyi DE, Elliott JP Jr, Smith RF, et al: A thirty-year survey of the reconstructive surgical treatment of aortoiliac occlusive disease. J Vasc Surg 1986;3:421.

79. Baird RJ: Techniques and results of arterial prosthetic bypass for aortoiliac occlusive disease. Can J Surg 1982;28:476.

80. Szilagyi DE: Ten years experience with aorto-iliac and femoro- popliteal arterial reconstruction. J Cardiovasc Surg 1964;5:502.

81. Hangsteen V, Lorentsen E, Silvertssen E, et al: Long-term follow-up of patients with peripheral arterial obliterans treated with arterial surgery. Acta Chir Scand 1975;141:725.

82. Vanttirev E, Inberg MV: Aorto-iliofemoral arterial reconstructive surgery with special reference to profunda revascularization. Acta Chir Scand 1975;141:600.

83. Poulias GE, Polemis L, Skoutas B, et al: Bilateral aortofemoral bypass in the presence of aortoiliac occlusive disease and factors determining results. Experience and long-term follow-up with 500 consecutive cases. J Cardiovasc Surg 1985;26:527.

84. Barnes RW, Liebman PR, Marszalek PB, et al: The natural history of asymptomatic carotid disease in patients undergoing cardiovascular surgery. Surgery 1981;90:1075.

85. Hertzer NR, Beven EG, Young JR, et al: Coronary artery disease in peripheral vascular patients. A classification of 1000 coronary angiograms and results of surgical management. Ann Surg 1984;199:223.

86. Culter BS, Leppo JA: Dipyridamole–thallium 201 scintigraphy to detect coronary artery disease before abdominal aortic surgery. J Vasc Surg 1984; 1:190.

87. McEnroe CS, O'Donnell TF, Yeager A, et al: Comparison of ejection fraction and Goldman risk factor analysis to dipyridamole-thallium 201 studies in the evaluation of cardiac morbidity after aortic aneurysm surgery. J Vasc Surg 1990; 11:497.

88. McPhail N, Ruddy TD, Calvin JE, et al: A comparison of dipyridamole-thallium imaging and exercise testing in the prediction of postoperative complications in patients requiring arterial reconstruction. J Vasc Surg 1989;10:51.

89. Kresowick TF, Bower TR, Garner SA, et al: Routine preoperative cardiac screening with dipyridamole-thallium scans alters patient management. J Vasc Surg 1992;15:52.

90. Taylor LM Jr, Yeager RA, Moneta GL, et al: The incidence of perioperative myocardial infarction in general vascular surgery. J Vasc Surg 1991;15:52.

91. Cambria RP, Brewster DC, Abbott WM, et al: The impact of selective use of dipyridamole-thallium scans and surgical factors on the current morbidity of aortic surgery. J Vasc Surg 1992; 15:43.

92. Golden MA, Whittemore AD, Donaldson MC, et al: Selective evaluation and management of coronary artery disease in patients undergoing repair of abdominal aortic aneurysms. Ann Surg 1990; 212:415.

93. Rao TLK, Jacobs KH, El-Etr AA: Reinfarction following anesthesia in patients with myocardial infarction. Anesthesiology 1983;59:499.

94. Rivers SP, Scher LA, Gupta SK, et al: Safety of peripheral vascular surgery after recent acute myocardial infarction. J Vasc Surg 1990;11:70.

95. Eagle KA, Singer DE, Brewster DC, et al: Dipyridamole-thallium scanning in patients undergoing vascular surgery. JAMA 1987;257: 2185.

96. Eagle KA, Coley CM, Newell JB, et al: Combining clincal and thallium data optimizes preoperative assessment of cardiac risk before major vascular surgery. Ann Intern Med 1989;110:859.

97. Nevelsteen A, Wouters L, Suy R: Long-term patency of the aortofemoral Dacron graft. A graft limb related study over a 25 year period. J Cardiovasc Surg 1991;32:174.

98. Rutherford RB, Jones DN, Martin MS, et al: Serial hemodynamic assessment of aortobifemoral bypass. J Vasc Surg 1986;4:428.

99. Martinez BD, Hertzer NR, Beven EG: Influence of distal arterial occlusive disease on prognosis following aortobifemoral bypass. Surgery 1980; 88:795.

100. Piostrowski JJ, Pearce WH, Jones DN, et al: Aortobifemoral bypass: The operation of choice for unilateral iliac occlusion? J Vasc Surg 1988;8:211.

101. Brewster DC, Meier GH, Darling RC, et al: Reoperation for aortofemoral graft limb occlusion: Optimal methods and long-term results. J Vasc Surg 1987;5:363.

102. Szilagyi DE, Elliott JP, Smith RF, et al: Secondary arterial repair: The management of late failures in arterial reconstructive surgery. Arch Surg 1975; 110:485.

103. Malone JM, Goldstone J, Moore WS: Autogenous profundaplasty: The key to long-term patency in secondary repair of aortofemoral graft occlusion. Ann Surg 1978;188:817.

104. Behamou AC, Kieffer E, Tricot JF, et al: "Redo" surgery for late aortofemoral graft occlusive failures. J Cardiovasc Surg 1984;25:118.

105. Robbs JV, Wylie EJ: Factors contributing to recurrent lower limb ischemia following bypass surgery for aortoiliac occlusive disease and their management. Ann Surg 1981;193:346.

106. Corson JD, Baraniewski HM, Shah DM, et al: Large diameter expanded polytetrafluoroethylene grafts for infrarenal aortic aneurysm surgery. J Cardiovasc Surg 1990;31:702.

107. Schmidt DD, Bandyk DF, Peguet AJ, et al: Bacterial adherence to vascular prostheses: A determinant of graft infection. J Vasc Surg 1986;3:732.

108. Allen BT, Sicard GA, Welch MJ, et al: Platelet deposition in vascular grafts: The accuracy of in vivo quantification and the signifigance of in vivo platelet reactivity. Ann Surg 1986;203:318.

109. Nunn DB, Carter NM, Donohue MT, et al: Postoperative dilatation of knitted Dacron aortic bifurcation graft. J Vasc Surg 1990,12:291.

110. Blumberg RM, Gelfand ML, Barton EA, et al: Clinical significance of aortic graft dilatation. J Vasc Surg 1991;14:175.

111. Schneider JR, Zwolak RM, Walsh DB, et al: Lack of diameter effect on short-term patency of size-matched Dacron aortobifemoral grafts. J Vasc Surg 1991;13:785.

112. Ernst CB: Prevention of intestinal ischemia following abdominal aortic reconstruction. Surgery 1983;93:102.

113. Ernst CB, Haghara PF, Daugherety ME, et al: Incidence of ischemic colitis following abdominal aortic reconstruction. A prospective study. Surgery 1975;80:417.

114. Johnson WC, Nabseth DC: Visceral infarction following aortic surgery. Ann Surg 1974;180:312.

115. Ottinger LW, Darling RC, Nathan MJ, et al: Left colon ischemia complicating aorto-iliac reconstruction. Arch Surg 1972;105:841.

116. Smith RF, Szilagyi DE: Ischemia of the colon as a complication in the surgery of the abdominal aorta. Arch Surg 1960;80:806.

117. Young JR, Humphries AW, de Wolfe VG, et al: Complications of aortic surgery. II: Intestinal ischemia. Arch Surg 1963;86:51.

118. Sethi GK, Scott SM, Takaro T: Persistent lymphatic fistula: Unusual complicationof femoral arterial bypass. J Cardiovasc Surg 1978;19: 155.

119. Kwaan JHM, Bernstein JM, Connelly JE: Management of lymph fistula in the groin after arterial reconstruction. Arch Surg 1979;114:1416.

120. Perler BA, Kinnison ML: Therapeutic lymphangiography: A new solution to post-bypass lymphorrhea. Vasc Surg 1987;21:436.

121. Reilly LM, Altman H, Lusby RJ, et al: Late results following surgical management of vascular graft infection. J Vasc Surg 1984;1:36.

122. Conn JH, Hardy JD, Chavez CM, et al: Infected arterial grafts: Experience in 22 cases with emphasis on unusual bacteria and techniques. Ann Surg 1970;171:704.

123. Fry WJ, Lindenauer SM: Infection complicating the use of plastic arterial implants. Arch Surg 1967;94:600.

124. Hoffert PW, Gonsler S, Haimovici H: Infection complicating arterial grafts. Arch Surg 1965;90:427.

125. Szilagyi DE, Smith RF, Elliott JP, et al: Infection in arterial reconstruction with synthetic grafts. Ann Surg 1978;176:321.

126. Bunt TJ: Synthetic vascular graft infections: I. Graft infections. Surgery 1983;93:733.

127. Goldstone J, Moore WS: Infection in vascular prostheses: Clinical manifestations and surgical management. Am J Surg 1974;128:225.

128. Jamieson GG, DeWeese JA, Rob CG: Infected arterial grafts. Ann Surg 1975;181:850.

129. Liekwig WG Jr, Greenfield LS: Vascular prosthetic infections. Collected experience and results of treatment. Surgery 1977;81:335.

130. Yashar JJ, Weyman AK, Burnard RJ, et al: Survival and limb salvage in patients with infected arterial prostheses. Am J Surg 1978;135:499.

131. Buchbinder D, Leather R, Shah D, et al: Pathologic interactions between prosthetic aortic grafts and the gastrointestinal tract. Am J Surg 1980;140:192.

132. Snyder SO, Wheeler JR, Gregory RT, et al: Freshly harvested cadaveric venous homgrafts as arterial conduits in infected fields. Surgery 1987;101:283.

133. Claggett GP, Bowers BL, Lopez-Viego MA, et al: Creation of a neo-aortoiliac system from lower extremity deep and superficial veins. Ann Surg 1993;248:239.

134. Perler BA, Vander Kolk CA, Dufresne CR, et al: Can infected prosthetic grafts be salvaged with rotational muscle flaps? Surgery 1991;110:30.

135. Perler BA, Vander Kolk CA, Manson PM, et al: Rotational muscle flaps to treat prosthetic graft infection: Long-term follow-up. J Vasc Surg 1993;189:165.

136. Sheil AGR, Reeve TS, Little JM, et al: Aortointestinal fistulas following operation on the abdominal aorta and iliac arteries. Br J Surg 1969;56:840.

137. Thomas WEG, Baird RN: Secondary aorto-entericfistulae: Towards a more conservative approach. Br J Surg 1986;73:875.

138. Bunt TJ: Synthetic vascular graft infections: II. Graft-enteric erosions and graft enteric fistulas. Surgery 1983;94:1.

139. Salo J, Verkkala K, Ketonen P, et al: Graft enteric fistulas and erosions. Vasc Surg 1986;11:88.

140. Walker WE, Cooley DA, Duncan JM, et al: The management of aortoduodenal fistula by in situ replacement of the infected abdominal aortic graft. Ann Surg 1987;205:727.

141. Szilagyi DE, Smith RF, Elliott JP Jr, et al: Anastomotic aneurysms after vascular reconstruction: Problems of incidence, etiology, and treatment. Surgery 1975;78:800.

142. Schellack J, Salam A, Abouzeid MA, et al: Femoral anastomotic aneurysms: A continuing challenge. J Vasc Surg 1987;6:308.

143. McCabe CJ, Moneure AC, Malt RA, et al: Host artery weakness in the etiology of femoral anastomotic false aneurysms. Surgery 1984;95:150.

144. Ernst CB, Elliott JP Jr, Ryan CJ, et al: Recurrent femoral anastomotic aneurysms. A 30-year experience. Ann Surg 1988;208:401.

145. Christensen RD, Bernatz PE: Anastommotic aneurysms involving the femoral artery. Mayo Clin Proc 1972;47:313.

146. Stoney RJ, Albo RJ, Wylie EJ: False aneurysms occurring after arterial grafting operations. Am J Surg 1965;110:153.

147. van den Akker PJ, Bravd R, van Schilfgaarde R, et al: False aneurysms after prosthetic reconstructions for aortoiliac occlusive disease. Ann Surg 1989;210:658.

148. Gaylis H: Pathogeneses of anastomotic aneurysms. Surgery 1981;90:1055.

149. Ernst CB, Daugherty ME: Removal of a thrombotic plug from an occluded limb of an aortofemoral graft. Arch Surg 1978;113:301.

150. Hyde GL, McCready RA, Schwartz RW, et al: Durability of thrombectomy of occluded aortofemoral graft limbs. Surgery 1983;94:748.

151. Crawford ES, Sethi GK, Scott SM: Femorofemoral grafts for unilateral occlusion of aortic bifurcation grafts. Surgery 1975;77:150.

152. Knudson JA, Downs AR: Reoperation following failure of aortoiliofemoral arterial reconstruction. Can J Surg 1978;21:316.

153. May AG, DeWeese JA, Rob CG: Changes in sexual function following operation on the abdominal aorta. Surgery 1969;65:41.

154. Schwartz SI: Sexual dysfunction. Contemp Surg 1989;17:31.

155. Queral LA, Whitehouse WM Jr, Flinn WR, et al: Pelvic hemodynamics after aortoiliac reconstruction. Surgery 1979;86:799.

156. Wright DJ, Ernst CB, Evans JR, et al: Ureteral complications and aortoiliac reconstruction. J Vasc Surg 1990;11:29.

157. Sieunarine K, Goodman M, Bary PR: Bilateral ureteral obstruction following aortobifemoral bypass graft. J Cardiovasc Surg 1991;32:209.

158. Daune B, Batt M, Hassen-Khudja R, et al: Hydronephrosis after aortofemoral bypass graft: A prospective study. J Cardiovasc Surg 1991;32:447.

159. Wylie EJ: Thromboendarterectomy for atherosclerotic thrombosis of major arteries. Surgery 1992:32:275.

160. Naylor AR, Ah-See AK, Engeset J: Aortoiliac endarterectomy: An 11-year review. Br J Surg 1990;77:190.

161. Inahara T: Endarterectomy for atherosclerotic aortoiliac and aortofemoral occlusive disease. In Ernst CB, Stanley JC (eds): Current Therapy in Vascular Surgery, 2d ed. Philadelphia, BC Decker, 1991, pp 398–401.

162. Duncan WC, Linton RR, Darling RC: Aortoiliofemoral atherosclerotic occlusive disease: Comparative results of endarterectomy and Dacron bypass grafts. Surgery 1971;70:974.

163. Inahora T: Eversion endarterectomy for aortoiliofemoral occlusive disease: A 16-year experience. Am J Surg 1979;138:196.

164. Darling RC, Linton RR: Aortoiliofemoral endarterecotmy for atherosclerotic occlusive disease. Surgery 1964;55:184.

165. Szilagyi DE, Smith RF, Whitney DG: The durability of aortoiliac endarterectomy. Arch Surg 1964;89:827.

166. Pilcher DB, Barker WF, Cannon JA: An aortoiliac endarterectomy case series followed for 10 years or more. Surgery 1970;67:5.

167. Graspord DJ, Cohen JL, Gaspar MR: Aortoiliofemoral thromboendarterectomy versus bypass graft: A randomized study. Arch Surg 1972;105:898.

168. Levinson SA, Levinson HJ, Halloran G, et al: Limited indications for unilateral aorto-femoral or iliofemoral vascular grafts. Arch Surg 1973;107:791.

169. McCoughan JJ, Kahn SF: Crossover graft for unilateral occlusive disease of the iliofemoral arteries. Ann Surg 1960;151:26.

170. Eastcott HHG: Arterial grafting for the ischemic lower limb. Ann R Coll Surg Engl 1953;13:177.

171. Couch NP, Clowes AW, Whittemore AD, et al: The iliac-origin arterial graft: A useful alternative for iliac occlusive disease. Surgery 1985;97:83.

172. Kalman PG, Hosang M, Johnston DW, et al: Unilateral iliac disease: The role of iliofemoral bypass. J Vasc Surg 1987;6:139.

173. Perler BA, Burdick JF, Williams GM: Femorofemoral or ilio-femoral bypass for unilateral inflow reconstruction? Am J Surg 1991;161:426.

174. Ricco JB: Unilateral iliac artery occlusive disease: A randomized multicenter trial examining direct revascularization versus crossover bypass. Ann Vasc Surg 1992;6:209.

175. Harrington ME, Harrington EB, Haimov M, et al: Iliofemoral versus femoro-femoral bypass: The

case for an individualized approach. J Vasc Surg 1992;16:841.

176. Darling RC III, Leather RP, Chang JB, et al: Is the iliac artery a suitable inflow conduit for iliofemoral occlusive disease: An analysis of 514 aorto-iliac reconstructions. J Vasc Surg 1993;17:15.

177. Freeeman NE, Leeds FH: Operations on large arteries: Application of recent advances. Calif Med 1952;77:229.

178. Blaisdell FW: Extraanatomical bypass procedures. World J Surg 1988;12:798.

179. Foley WJ, Dow RW, Fry WJ: Crossover femoro-femoral bypass grafts. Arch Surg 1969;99:83.

180. Plecha FR, Plecha FM: Femorofemoral bypass grafts: Ten-year experience. J Vasc Surg 1984; 1:555.

181. Mannick JA, Baini BS: Femoro-femoral grafting: Indications and late results. Am J Surg 1978; 136:190.

182. Subram AN, Urrutia-S CO, Oh DA, et al: Femoro-femoral bypass prognostic factors. Texas Heart Inst J 1983;10:257.

183. Hill DA, Lord RSA, Tracy GD: Hemodynamic consequences of cross femoral bypass. *In* Greenlaush RM (ed): Extra-anatomic and Secondary Reconstruction. Bath, England, Pitman Press, 1982, pp 142–152.

184. Dick LS, Brief DK, Alpert J, et al: A 12-year experience with femorofemoral crossover grafts. Arch Surg 1980;115:1359.

185. Lamerton AJ, Nicolaides AN, Eastcott HH: The femorofemoral graft. Arch Surg 1985;120: 1274.

186. Brener BJ, Brief DK, Alpert J, et al: Femorofemoral bypass: A twenty-five year experience. *In* Yao JST, Pearce WH (eds): Long-term Results in Vascular Surgery. East Norwalk, Conn, Appleton & Lange, 1993, pp 388–389.

187. Kalman PG, Hosang M, Johnston KW, et al: The current role for femorofemoral bypass. J Vasc Surg 1987;6:71.

188. Eugene J, Goldstone J, Moore W: Fifteen-year experience with subcutaneous bypass grafts for lower extremity ischemia. Ann Surg 1977;186:177.

189. Livesay JJ, Altkinson JB, Baker B, et al: Late results of extra-anatomic bypass. Arch Surg 1979;114:1260.

190. Hepp W, de Jonge K, Pallua N: Late results following extra-anatomical bypass procedures for chronic aortoiliac occlusive disease. J Cardiovasc Surg 1988;29:181.

191. Rutherford RB, Patt A, Pearce WH: Extra-anatomic bypass: A closer view. J Vasc Surg 1987; 6:437.

192. Johnston KW, Rae N, Hogg-Johnston SA, et al: Five year results of a prospective study of percutaneous transluminal angioplasty. Ann Surg 1987;206:403.

193. Van Andel GH, Van Erp WFM, Krepel VM, et al: Percutaneous transluminal angioplasty of the iliac artery: Long-term results. Radiology 1985; 156:321.

194. Poerter JM, Eidenmiller LR, Pottes CT, et al: Combined arterial dilatation and femoro-femoral bypass for limb salvage. Surg Gynecol Obstet 1973;137:409.

195. Dinis DA, da Gama A: The fate of the donor artery in extra-anatomic revascularization. J Vasc Surg 1989;8:106.

196. Davis RC, O'Hara ET, Mannick JA: Broadened indications for femorofemoral grafts. Surgery 1972;72:990.

197. Veterans Affairs Cooperative Study: Donor limb vascular events following femoro-femoral bypass surgery. Arch Surg 1991;126:681.

198. Harris JP, Flinn WR, Rudo ND, et al: Assessment of donor limb hemodynamics in femoro-femoral bypass for claudication. Surgery 1981; 90:764.

199. Ehrenfeld WK, Harris JD, Wylie EJ: Vascular "steal" phenomenon: An experimental study. Am J Surg 1968;116:192.

200. Trimble IR, Stonesifer GL, Wilgis EFS, et al: Criteria for femoro-femoral bypass from clinical and hemodynamic studies. Ann Surg 1972: 175:985.

201. Sumner DS, Strandness DE. The hemodynamics of the femoro-femoral shunt. Surg Gynecol Obstet 1972;134:629.

202. Chang JB: Surgical treatment of aorto-iliac artery disease. Angiology 1981;32:73.

203. Blaisell FW, Hall AD: Axillary-femoral artery bypass for lower extremity ischemia. Surgery 1963; 54:563.

204. Sauvage LR, Wood SJ: Unilateral axillary bilateral femoral bifurcation graft: A procedure for the poor risk patient with aortoiliac disease. Surgery 1966;60:573.

205. El-Massvy, Saad E, Sauvage LR, et al: Axillofemoral bypass with externally supported, knitted Dacron grafts: A follow-up through 12 years. J Vasc Surg 1993;17:107.

206. Calligaro KD, Ascer E, Veith FJ, et al: Unsuspected inflow disease in candidates for axillofemoral bypass operations. J Vasc Surg 1990; 11:832.

207. Ascer E, Gupta SK, Veith FJ, et al: Comparison of axillofemoral and axillobifemoral bypass operations. Surgery 1985;97:169.

208. Tangpraphephorn V, Spenazzola A, King J: Axillofemoral bypass: Intra-pleural method. Ann Thoracic Surg 1979;27:80.

209. Ward RE, Holcroft JW, Contis S, et al: New conception in the use of axillofemoral bypass grafts. Arch Surg 1983;118:573.

210. Ludtke-Handjery A, Schumann L, Gref H, et al:

Are axillofemoral bypass grafts worthwhile? A 10-year review. Thorac Cardiovasc Surg 1983;31:76.

211. Moore WS, Hall AD, Blaisdell FW: Late results of axillary-femoral bypass grafting. Am J Surg 1971;122:148.

212. Donaldson MC, Louras JC, Bucknam CA. Axillofemoral bypass: A tool with limited role. J Vasc Surg 1986;3:757.

213. Lo Gerfo FW, Johnson WC, Corson JD, et al: A comparison of the late patency rates of axillobilateral femoral and axillounilateral femoral grafts. Surgery 1977;81:33.

214. Johnson WC, LoGerfo FW, Vollman RW, et al: Is axillobilateral femoral graft an effective substitute for aortic-bilateral iliac/femoral graft? An analysis of ten years experience. Ann Surg 1977;186:123.

215. Burrell MS, Wheeler JR, Gregory RT, et al: Axillofemoral bypass: A ten-year review. Ann Surg 1982;195:796.

216. Harris EJ Jr, Taylor LM, McConnell DB, et al: Clinical results of axillobifemoral bypass using externally supported polytetrafluoroethylene. J Vasc Surg 1990;12:416.

217. Mannick JA, Williams LE, Nabseth DL: The late results of axillofemoral grafts. Surgery 1970;68:1038.

218. Richardson Jr, McDowell HA Jr: Extra-anatomic bypass grafting in aortoiliac occlusive disease: A seven-year experience. South Med J 1977;70:1287.

219. DeLaurentis DA, Sala LE, Russell E, et al: A twelve-year experience with axillofemoral and femorofemoral bypass operations. Surg Gyencol Obstet 1978;177:881.

220. Ray LI, O'Connor JB, Davis CC, et al: Axillofemoral bypass: A critical reappraisal of its role in the management of aortoiliac disease. Surgery 1979;138:117.

221. Cina C, Ameli FM, Kalman P, et al: Indications and role of axillofemoral bypass in high-risk patients. Ann Vasc Surg 1988;2:737.

222. Naylor AR, Ah-See AK, Engeset J: Axillofemoral bypass as a limb salvage procedure in high risk patients with aortoiliac disease. Br J Surg 1990;77:659.

223. Whittemore KE, Billig DM, Paneides C: Special considerations in the revascularization for aortoiliac occlusive disease: Anatomic and extraanatomic bypass. Am Surg 1980;46:279.

224. Broome A, Christenson JT, Eklof B, et al: Axillofemoral bypass reconstruction in sixty-one patients with leg ischemia. Surgery 1980;88:673.

225. Chang JB: Current state of extraanatomic bypasses. Am J Surg 1986;152:202.

226. Savrin RA, Record GT, McDonnel DE: Axillofemoral bypass. Arch Surg 1986;121:1016.

227. Christenson JT, Broome A, Nogren L, et al: The late results after axillo-femoral bypass grafts in patients with leg ischemia. J Cardiovasc Surg 1986;27:131.

228. Schneider JR, McDaniel MS, Walsh DB, et al: Axillofemoral bypass: Outcome and hemodynamic results in high-risk patients. J Vasc Surg 1992;15:952.

229. Kalman PG, Hosang M, Cina C, et al: Current indications for axillounifemoral and axillobifemoral bypass grafts. J Vasc Surg 1987;5:828.

230. Bunt TJ, Moore W: Optimal proximal anastomosis/tunnel for axillofemoral grafts. J Vasc Surg 1986;3:673.

231. Sullivan LP, Davidson PG, D'Anna JA Jr, et al: Disruption of the proximal anastomosis of axillobifemoral grafts: Two case reports. J Vasc Surg 1989;10:190.

232. Alexander RH, Selby JH: Axillofemoral bypass grafts using polytetrafluoroethylene. South Med J 1980;73:1325.

233. Bandyk DF, Thiele BG, Radke HM: Upper extremity embolus secondary to axillofemoral bypass grafts. Arch Surg 1983;118:673.

234. Scheiner TM. Peripheral vascular surgery: Alternative anatomical pathways and the use of allograft veins as arterial substitutes. Curr Probl Surg 1978;15:1.

12

Femoropopliteal Bypass

DONALD L. JACOBS
JONATHAN B. TOWNE

HISTORY

The earliest reported use of arterial bypass for femoral-popliteal occlusive disease was by Kunlin in 1948.[1] By the late 1950s, the development of vascular surgical techniques resulted in more widely reported experience in arterial reconstruction of the lower leg. The techniques for in situ and reversed saphenous vein femoropopliteal bypass have been highly refined over the last 40 years. The use of prosthetic conduit for femoropopliteal bypass (FPB) also has progressed in the last 20 years. In our aging population, as more patients are presenting with symptomatic lower extremity occlusive disease, the number of patients in need of revascularization is rising.

CLINICAL PRESENTATION

Patients with superficial femoral occlusive disease may present with a range of symptoms from mild claudication to rest pain and/or gangrene. Individuals with claudication typically have only superficial femoral artery occlusion with patent popliteal and tibial flow to the foot. Ankle-brachial pressure ratios in such patients range from 0.45 to 0.75. Single-level occlusive disease in the superficial femoral artery will not usually cause limb-threatening ischemia. The potential is great for collateral circulation via the profunda branches to reconstitute the popliteal artery distal to an occluded superficial femoral artery. Therefore, superficial femoral occlusive disease is usually coupled with iliofemoral or tibiopopliteal occlusive disease before the degree of ischemia becomes limb-threatening.

Arterial reconstruction with an FPB graft in patients with intermittent claudication is highly successful at relieving symptoms. However, the risks of reconstruction must be balanced against the fairly benign natural history of the disease in most patients. A review and meta-analysis of the literature on the natural history of intermittent claudication by McDaniel and Cronenwett[2] revealed that patients will have stable to improved symptoms in 55 percent of cases managed conservatively. The need for operation in patients with intermittent claudication was approximately 25 percent and the amputation rate was 4 percent after 5 years of follow-up. Cessation of smoking and exercise have definite beneficial effects, allowing increased walking distances in claudication patients and a lower risk of progression of disease requiring intervention. Medical therapy including antiplatelet, rheologic, and metabolic agents also may provide some benefit to these patients. Stable claudication must significantly affect the patient's ability to work or lifestyle before bypass is considered. To clearly define the significance of claudication in an individual case is sometimes difficult. Following a patient's symptoms over a period of months allows for an adequate trial of nonsurgical therapy and facilitates patient education so that the patient is reasonable in his or her expectations of revascularization.

Patients with limb-threatening ischemia (i.e., nonhealing ulcer, severe rest pain, or gangrene) have more clearly defined indications for operation yet represent a relatively more difficult group of patients to treat because of their diffuse arterial disease and higher incidence of comorbid disease. The risk of significant morbidity or mortality in these patients with a revascularization procedure is high, with cardiac and cerebrovascular events comprising the vast majority of complications. The average life expectancy of patients who present with limb-threatening ischemia is also relatively short. These factors must be considered when evaluating such patients for lower extremity revascularization.[3] The history and physical examination must be thorough and note the presence of significant comorbid cardiac, pulmonary, and cerebrovascular disease.

In addition to clinical examination and noninvasive vascular laboratory testing, angiographic definition of the disease is needed to allow the surgeon to decide, first, if reconstruction is possible and, second, if pursuing reconstruction is appropriate in a given patient's clinical situation. The availability of an adequate autogenous vein also may affect the decision to recommend reconstruction due to the differential in the patency rates of vein grafts versus prosthetic grafts.

RESULTS

The expected outcome for an FPB graft is predicted by the indications, type of conduit, site of the distal anastomosis, and the condition of the tibial outflow vessels. Stratification of patients is critical when discussing results of FPB. Following is a discussion of the various clinical characteristics that affect success and are the key to appropriate patient selection and technique application.

INDICATIONS

Overall, FPB grafting for claudication has a reported primary patency of 88 percent at 5 years and a limb-salvage rate of 98 percent at 5 years in a series that included both autogenous vein and prostheses as conduits. When one evaluates the long-term patency in patients with limb-threatening ischemia, results generally are better with autogenous vein, especially in patients requiring below-knee popliteal bypasses.[4] Veith et al.[5] reported no difference in patency of above-knee grafts between prosthesis and autogenous veins at 4 years. This was compared with below-knee revascularizations, where there was a significant difference between prosthetic and autogenous grafts. DeWeese and Rob[3] reported a 5-year patency in vein grafts of 74 percent in patients with claudication compared with 42 percent in patients with rest pain and 50 percent in patients with gangrene. The effect of poor outflow on long-term patency is difficult to ascertain because of the conflicting reports in the literature. Blackshear et al.[6] noted a marked decrease in long-term patency in those patients who had poor outflow. Cutler et al.[7] noted improved 3-, 5-, and 8-year patency in patients with good runoff. On the other hand, Ramsburgh et al.[8] and Koontz et al.[9] and associates noted no effect of runoff on patency. In our own experience with more distal vein grafts, runoff has not been a determinate factor in long-term patency.[10]

The percentage of patients having claudication as their indication for operation is few in comparison with the number of patients having limb-threatening ischemia in most series of patients undergoing lower extremity revascularization. This is a reflection of the conservative approach to managing patients with claudication that exists in most centers. It could be inferred that the patients with claudication selected for bypass are patients with more severe occlusive disease than the average claudication patient. These patients are also selected based on their coexisting medical risk factors. This would mean that in utilizing a conservative approach, one would exclude more medically ill patients from operative therapy. It is important to take these selection factors into consideration when applying the success rates that are reported with claudication to the *average* patient who presents with claudication. The reported series of patients with limb-threatening ischemia are also subject to the same selection factors, yet their effect is less pronounced due to the more absolute nature of their operative indication. The type of conduits used is another important consideration when looking at the results from FPB grafting. Many surgeons believe that the ipsilateral saphenous vein is best saved for limb-salvage situations. This would result in a high percentage of prosthetic conduits in patients with claudication, particularly in those with an above-knee distal anastomosis.

AUTOGENOUS VERSUS PROSTHETIC CONDUCT

It is generally held that autogenous vein is preferable to prosthetic conduit when performing infrainguinal bypass. In a randomized, prospective trial of polytetrafluoroethylene (PTFE) versus saphenous vein graft, the results showed that the patency rates for PTFE grafts to the popliteal artery were equivalent to the patency of autogenous saphenous vein bypasses.[5] This was true for patients with claudication and for patients with limb-threatening ischemia when followed for up to 2 years. After 2 years, the patency of PTFE decreases significantly as compared with vein, but the limb-salvage rate remained equivalent for the two conduits when followed for 4 years. The choice of prosthetic graft as the initial bypass conduit and saving the autogenous vein for failure of the prosthetic bypass or for use in coronary artery grafting has been proposed. Additional benefits of prosthetic bypass are the shorter operative time and fewer wound problems than is seen with vein grafts. The differential in the patency of bypasses using autogenous versus prosthetic material is increased with a more distal location of the distal anastomosis.[5] Some authors recommend prosthetic bypasses as the first graft of choice only in the above-knee position and use autogenous vein for a below-knee FPB graft.[11] Likewise, the use of prosthetic to an isolated popliteal segment yields poorer patency than vein grafts to an isolated segment, and therefore, the first choice of conduit in such patients is autogenous vein.[11]

IN SITU VERSUS REVERSED VEIN BYPASS

Controversy over the superiority of the in situ versus the reversed vein bypass has existed in the literature for over 25 years. Though many studies have looked at the clinical outcome of both techniques, no conclusive data showing superiority of either technique have been forthcoming.[12,13] A surgeon's choice of technique usually depends on personal experience and familiarity more than on distinct advantages of one technique or the other. Reversed vein bypass is purported to require a shorter operative time and is technically easier than the in situ method. A potentially damaging step in preparing the reversed vein is when the smaller distal end of the saphenous vein is distended to allow for use in the proximal anastomosis. It has been shown that overdistension can severely injure the endothelium. Gentle distension and the use of papaverine to reduce vasospasm can minimize the damage to the endothelium. The primary difficulty with the in situ technique is rendering the valves incompetent. This requires mastering the unique aspects of valve lysis, and as with any other skill, a learning curve exists. Injury to the vein by the valvulotome can cause significant technical problems requiring modification of the vein, which may reduce the patency rate. Retained competent valve cusps or missed arteriovenous fistulas do occur and result in a higher reoperative rate with the in situ method. A primary advantage of the in situ technique is the better size match of the proximal greater saphenous vein to the femoral vessels and the size match of the distal saphenous vein to the distal vessels. This size-match advantage is more pronounced with tibial bypass than with popliteal bypass. Theoretical advantages of the in situ method are that the vein is left intact with its nutritive bed for the greatest portion of the bypass, and there is less chance of ischemic injury to the endothelium when oxygenated blood flow is maintained in the vein during most of the procedure. The lack of a need to distend the proximal in situ vein prior to construction of the proximal anastomosis and the use of physiologic arterial pressure to distend the remaining in situ vein eliminate the injury that can occur with manual distension in the reversed technique. Use of smaller-caliber veins, as small as 2 mm, is possible with in situ technique. This results in a significant increase in the number of patients who will have an adequate ipsilateral greater saphenous vein to complete a bypass using the in situ as compared with the reversed vein technique. As with the advantage of size match noted above, the advantage of being able to use a smaller saphenous vein with in situ grafting is more relevant when considering tibial bypass than popliteal bypass.

SURGICAL TECHNIQUE

Angiographic delineation of the popliteal artery and its runoff allows one to determine if the popliteal artery is suitable as the recipient vessel for a bypass. From the medial approach, the middle portion of the popliteal artery is relatively inaccessible, and one must select either the above-knee (AK) or below-knee (BK) portion of the artery for the distal anastomosis. Femoral to above-knee popliteal bypass (AK bypass) is the shortest length and simplest bypass possible to treat superficial femoral artery occlusion.

The incision is made from just above the medial femoral condyle and extends proximally. The adductor muscles are retracted medially, and the artery is identified at Hunters canal. The popliteal artery is identified as it courses from medial to lateral to lie in the midline behind the most distal portion of the femur. Exposure may require transection of some of the adductor magnus tendon to access the popliteal space. Exposure of the distal popliteal artery is through a medial incision that extends distally from the joint space. The popliteal artery is free of investing muscles at this level.

If the saphenous vein is to be used, the entire saphenous vein and the distal proximal arteries are exposed through a continuous skin incision. In patients in whom the caliber of the saphenous vein is of reasonable size, 4 to 5 mm, bridging incisions can be made to decrease the length of the incision. When the veins are less than 3.5 mm in diameter, it is important to use a continuous incision so that the entire vein can be visualized to avoid damaging it during the valve ablation procedure.

The saphenofemoral junction is completely dissected, and the venous tributaries at the fossa ovalis are ligated and divided. Following administration of 5000 units of heparin sodium, Derra clamps are applied to the saphenofemoral junction, incorporating a small rim of the common femoral vein. The saphenous vein is divided and the com-

mon femoral vein oversewn with a continuous 5-0 polypropylene suture. The proximal two or three valves are excised according to the technique of Leather et al.[14] To bring the saphenous vein into juxtaposition with the common femoral artery for anastomosis, 8 to 10 cm of proximal vein is mobilized. The end-to-side proximal anastomosis is then performed with a continuous 5-0 polypropylene suture. Occasionally, the vein will not quite reach to the relatively uninvolved area of the common femoral artery. Because of its large size, a slightly increased amount of tension on the anastomosis can be tolerated when compared with using the vein in the reversed fashion. Also, in cases in which the vein will not reach the common femoral artery without excessive tension, the proximal deep femoral artery can be used for the proximal anastomosis. On occasion, femoral endarterectomy is necessary to provide adequate inflow for the in situ graft. In these cases, endarterectomy of the proximal occluded superficial femoral artery can provide a site for the proximal anastomosis to avoid excessive tension of the proximal suture line.

Following construction of the proximal anastomosis, blood flow is restored to the graft, and all distal valves are incised with the Leather valvulotome inserted through a vein side branch or through a puncture in the vein made with an 18-gauge needle. When a puncture wound is required to insert the valvulotome, a 6-0 polypropylene suture is necessary to close the puncture hole.[15] The valves in the distal 40 cm are lysed by inserting the valvulotome through the distal transected end of the vein. In veins 3 mm or less in diameter, the vein is gently distended with a solution of heparin sodium, papaverine, and dextran to relieve any vein spasm. In small veins, the vein can develop spasm and constrict so tightly around the valvulotome that the intima and subjacent media may be incised by the valvulotome, providing a nidus for platelet aggregation and subsequent graft thrombosis when arterial flow is restored to the graft.

Following ablation of all valves, there should be a good jet of blood flow emanating from the cut end of the graft. Methylene blue dots are then placed on the distal saphenous vein to help maintain axial orientation. The posterior tibial and peroneal arteries are exposed by a medial incision. The anterior tibial artery is approached by an incision lateral to the tibia, and a tunnel is made through the interosseous membrane from the medial aspect of the leg. Because a pneumatic tourniquet is used to obtain distal vascular control, the arteries are not circumferentially dissected. Dissection is limited to that portion of the artery which is necessary for the construction of the distal anastomosis. This generally requires dissecting a 2.5-cm segment covering approximately 120 degrees of the circumference of the artery. A pneumatic tourniquet is placed around the leg at a site above the level of the distal anastomosis. Prior to construction of the distal anastomosis, the leg is elevated and exsanguinated with an elastic bandage. The tourniquet is inflated to between 250 and 300 mmHg, and the elastic bandage is removed. The distal anastomosis is performed using 2.5 × loupe magnification with a continuous 6-0 or 7-0 polypropylene suture.

After the tourniquet is released, side branches of the saphenous vein are ligated. An intraoperative Doppler probe with real-time spectral analysis is used to detect any remaining branches and to analyze the graft for incomplete valve incision and anastomotic technical defects. Operative arteriography is used to ensure ligation of arteriovenous fistulas and a technically satisfactory distal anastomosis. The skin over the graft is closed with interrupted nylon sutures, except in the groin, where two layers of subcutaneous closure are placed prior to skin closure. Meticulous attention is paid to delicate handling of the skin and to precise closure of the wound because the graft lies in the subcutaneous tissue just beneath the skin surface. Patients are examined in the perioperative period at 7 days and 1 month postoperatively and then at 3-month intervals to assess graft blood flow velocity and ankle-brachial pressure indices.[16]

Because of the long skin incision, use of the in situ technique is associated with a higher incidence of wound problems. In our initial report, wound complications occurred in 18 percent of patients, 78 percent of whom were diabetics.[15] Complications included small areas of skin necrosis, almost exclusively found in patients with diabetic vascular disease. Also noted were wound hematoma, lymphocele, and inflamed skin flaps, which are more likely to occur in the midthigh. Inflamed skin flaps have occurred in several instances and each time have led to concern that wound suppuration with subsequent graft involvement would occur, but in each case inflammation cleared spontaneously with administration of parenteral antibiotics. This condition is probably a lymphangitis caused by disruption of lymphatics by the long skin incision coupled with bacteria often present in lymph tissue because of coexisting ulceration and areas of gangrene of the foot. No graft infections and no occlusion secondary to wound complications have occurred.

Because the length of graft that is dissected free is short, the in situ vein is prone to twisting. This is a particular problem in veins less than 3 mm in diameter, when the empty vein appears quite small and is difficult to handle. The incidence of graft twist was 3.8 percent in our early experience with the first 78 grafts.[15] Twisting of the graft has not occurred recently because of recognition of the problem and the application of the methylene blue dots to maintain axial orientation.

The in situ technique can be implicated as the cause of graft problems that require operative revision within the first 30 days.[15] These consist mainly of retained competent valves and arteriovenous fistulas. Competent valves become obvious in the perioperative period. Valves can be in an open position intraoperatively, and the graft may function well, but sometime during the postoperative period the valves will float into a closed position. This phenomenon is usually manifest by a hemodynamic result that is less than one would expect for that type of conduit. Generally, this is easily detected and corrected. Arteriovenous fistulas also can be a problem in the postoperative period. A fistula can be missed at the initial operation. Also, the valve at the origin of many side branches may initially impede flow. With time, arterial pressure gradually dilates the conduit, making the valve incompetent and allowing an arteriovenous fistula to develop spontaneously postoperatively.

One advantage to using the in situ vein is increased vein utilization.[15] In our initial study, the vein utilization rate was 91 percent. The vein diameter was 4 mm or greater in 40 percent of patients, 3.5 to 4 mm in 11 percent, 3 mm in 22 percent, 2.5 mm in 14 percent, and 2.0 mm in 5 percent. Our experience shows that the in situ vein clearly lends itself to better patency rates in dealing with small-caliber veins.

As would be expected, there is a learning curve with use of the in situ technique. The average operative time for the first 10 procedures was 5 hours and 8 minutes, which subsequently decreased to an average time of 4 hours following the first year of experience. With increased familiarity with the technique, an in situ bypass can be done as quickly as a reversed vein bypass.

A saphenous vein diameter of 4 mm or greater is the generally accepted criterion for an adequate vein conduit. On the basis of this criterion, 53 percent of patients in our first study had inadequate veins, and poor graft patency rates would have been predicted.[15] Composite grafting with vein harvested from other sites may have been possible in many of these patients had the reversed vein method been chosen; however, this approach would limit the availability of vein for future arterial revascularization of the contralateral lower extremity or coronary arteries. In no instance was vein from the contralateral extremity required, but in one patient an upper extremity vein was used to obtain sufficient graft length. Of the vein bypasses with diameters of about 2.5 mm, none occluded in the early postoperative period and only two occluded during the follow-up period, at 56 and 84 days.[17] We believe that 2.5 mm is an adequate vein diameter; 2 mm is the absolute minimum. Veins less than 2 mm in diameter are susceptible to laceration of the intima and media when the valvulotome is manipulated for valve incision.

OPERATIVE GRAFT ASSESSMENT

After flow is established in the graft, intraoperative Doppler spectral analysis is used to identify patent vein side branches and to detect any unsuspected technical error.[18] Arterial flow pattern analysis is performed with a 20-MHz, direction-sensitive Doppler flow detector in a real-time fast Fourier transform spectral analyzer. Doppler spectral analysis of midstream flow is used to examine blood flow patterns in the region of the anastomosis and valve incision sites to locate patent vein side branches and to assess outflow resistance.

Outflow resistance was assessed from the Doppler velocity waveform configuration and the calculation of peak systolic and end-diastolic flow velocities. Graft flow velocity calculations are made on the basis of Doppler signals recorded from the distal graft segment. Calculation of flow velocity requires a normal arterial flow pattern without turbulence and the accurate measurement of the Doppler beam angle in a vessel diameter that does not vary over a short distance. Doppler flow analysis has been found to be an ideal screening test for assessing the technical adequacy of the in situ vein bypass. Incompletely incised valve cusps, anastomotic strictures, and arteriovenous fistulas are readily located, thereby reducing operative time and the need for multiple arteriograms. Using this technology, only one angiogram was required in 83 percent of operations. In the absence of technical error, graft flow velocity calculations are an accurate predictor of patency. Early graft occlusions were associated with low peak systolic flow velocities of less than 40 cm/s and absent diastolic forward flow. Completion angiograms were obtained routinely to verify technically satisfactory distal anastomoses and exclude the presence of thrombus or stricture in the outflow arteries.

POSTOPERATIVE GRAFT SURVEILLANCE

All patients underwent preoperative and serial postoperative noninvasive hemodynamic testing at 3-month intervals. The in situ bypasses were evaluated by resting limb pressure measurements and duplex scanning. Serial duplex examinations were used to measure changes in graft flow velocity and to identify flow abnormalities that increase the risk for sudden thrombosis, such as low graft flow velocity, peak systolic flow velocity less than 45 cm/s, or decrease in flow velocity greater than 30 cm/s compared with the previous examination. The criteria for interpretation of the duplex examination were based on the magnitude of flow velocity, changes in the velocity waveform configuration, and the presence and degree of spectral broadening and turbulence in the Doppler signal.

By careful postoperative evaluation of patients, it is possible to study the biology of the in situ conduit. Occlusions generally fall into three categories: those which occur in the first 30 days, those occurring 30 days to 2 years after operation, and those occurring more than 2 years later.[19] Occlusions occurring within the first 30 days are related to selection of patients, coagulation abnormalities, and technical errors in the performance of the bypass. In the evaluation of 192 consecutive in situ bypasses, 19 required revision within the first 30 days. Of these 19, 11 were related to problems associated with the in situ graft, such as retained valves, persistent arteriovenous fistulas, or graft torsion. In the interval between 30 days and 2 years, the prime cause of graft failure relates to fibrointimal hyperplasia, which takes two forms. The first is the development of sclerosis and scarring at valve incision sites, and the other is the development of narrowing of either the proximal or the distal anastomosis. Twenty-nine in situ bypass grafts required revision more than 1 month after the initial operation; 18 revisions were the result of either sclerosis at valve sites or fibrointimal hyperplasia at the proximal or distal anastomosis. Beyond 2 years, the causes of graft failure are related primarily to progression of atherosclerosis in the inflow or outflow tract.

With vigilant postoperative surveillance, it is possible to detect thrombosis-prone grafts prior to thrombosis, allowing elective revisions and preservation of in situ graft patency. Primary patency of FPB grafts was 48 percent at 36 months. This was improved to 89 percent secondary patency at 36 months, primarily as a result of detection of hemodynamically failing but not thrombosed grafts. Similarly, patency of tibial grafts was 58 percent at 36 months. This was improved to 80 percent at 36 months because of vigilant postoperative surveillance. When one analyzes the temporal distribution of bypass revision, as expected, 10 percent are revised 30 days to 2 years later. After the first 2 years, the revision rate is generally 3 percent.

Only 3 of the 29 grafts that required revision after the first 30 days were thrombosed. Durability of revised in situ vein grafts was demonstrated by a patency rate of the revised grafts of 83 percent at 48 months, compared with a rate of 84 percent for grafts that did not require revision.[13] It is important to note that, on occasion, veins require more than one revision in the postoperative follow-up period; occasionally, three or four different procedures are necessary. With meticulous operative technique, the perioperative revision and thrombosis rate can be reduced to a minimum, currently 5 percent in our series. With careful postoperative surveillance, the long-term graft failure rate can be reduced, resulting in excellent long-term results.

REFERENCES

1. Kunlin J: Le treatment de l'arterite obliterante par la grette venouse. Arch Mal Coeur 1949;42:371.
2. McDaniel MD, Cronenwett JL: Natural history of intermittent claudication. *In* Porter JM, Taylor LM (eds): Basic Data Underlying Clinical Decision Making in Vascular Surgery. St. Louis, Quality Medical Publishing, 1994, pp 129–133.
3. DeWeese JA, Rob CG: Autogenous venous grafts 10 years later. Surgery 1977;82:775.
4. Donaldson MC, Mannick JA: Femoropopliteal bypass grafting for intermittent claudication. Arch Surg 1980;115:724.
5. Veith FJ, Gupta SK, Ascer E, et al: Six-year prospective multicenter randomized comparison of autologous saphenous vein and expanded polytetrafluoroethylene grafts in infrainguinal arterial reconstructions. J Vasc Surg 1986;3:104.
6. Blackshear WM Jr, Thiele BL, Strandness DE Jr: Natural history of above- and below-knee femoropopliteal grafts. Am J Surg 1980;140:234.
7. Cutler BS, Thompson JE, Kleinsasser LJ, Hempel GK: Autologous saphenous vein femoropopliteal bypass: Analysis of 298 cases. Surgery 1976; 79:325.
8. Ramsburgh SR, Lindenauer SM, Weber TR, et al: Femoropopliteal bypass for limb salvage. Surgery 1977;81:453.
9. Koontz TJ, Stansel HC Jr: Factors influencing patency of the autogenous vein-femoropopliteal bypass graft: An analysis of 74 cases. Surgery 1972;71:553.
10. Plecha DJ, Seabrook GR, Bandyk DF, Towne JB: Determinants of successful peroneal artery bypass. J Vasc Surg 1993;17:97.
11. Patterson RB, Fowl RJ, Kempczinski RF, et al: Preferential use of ePTFE for above-knee femoropopliteal bypass grafts. Ann Vasc Surg 1990; 4:338.
12. Taylor, Jr LM, Edwards JM, Porter JM: Present status of reversed vein bypass grafting: Five-year results of a modern series. J Vasc Surg 1990; 11:193.
13. Bergamini TM, Towne JB, Bandyk DF, et al: Experience with in situ vein bypasses from 1981–1989: Determinant factors of long term patency. J Vasc Surg 1991;13:137.

14. Leather RP, Shah DM, Karmody AM: Intra-popliteal arterial bypass for limb salvage. Surgery 1981;90:1000.
15. Levine AW, Bandyk DF, Bonier PH, Towne JB: Lessons learned in adopting the in situ saphenous vein bypass. J Vasc Surg 1985;2:145.
16. Cato R, Vollrath K, Bandyk DF, Towne JB: Post-operative surveillance of in situ saphenous vein arterial grafts: Application of quantitative velocity waveform analysis. Bruit 1986;10:235.
17. Towne JB, Schmitt DD, Seabrook GR, Bandyk DF: The effect of vein diameter on patency of in situ grafts. J Cardiovasc Surg 1991;32:192.
18. Bandyk DF, Zierler RE, Thiele BL: Detection of technical error during arterial surgery by pulsed Doppler spectral analysis. Arch Surg 1984;119:421.
19. Towne JB: In situ saphenous vein graft for lower extremity occlusive disease. *In* Current Therapy in Vascular Surgery, 2nd ed. Philadelphia, B C Decker, 1991, pp 491–495

Bypasses to the Infrapopliteal Arteries

WILLIAM D. SUGGS
FRANK J. VEITH

The last two decades have produced enormous advances in the treatment of lower limb ischemia secondary to infrainguinal arteriosclerosis. Interventional management strategies have been developed to treat virtually all patterns of arteriosclerosis underlying limb-threatening ischemia.[1] Bypasses to the infrapopliteal arteries with autologous vein have become routine for limb salvage. As this technique has evolved, the distal limits of revascularization have been extended to include arteries near the ankle or in the foot for patients who have no patent arteries for a more proximal bypass. In addition, some patients presenting with patent popliteal arteries have three vessel distal occlusive disease and forefoot gangrene, requiring a bypass to a distal tibial or tarsal vessel.[2,3] Those patients who require very distal bypasses have frequently undergone previous vascular reconstructions, and they may be candidates for alternative approaches to the profunda, popliteal, or infrapopliteal arteries to permit access to previously unused arterial segments for performance of these secondary bypasses.

PATIENT EVALUATION

Careful history and physical examination should be directed toward correctly staging the extent of the patient's atherosclerotic disease. A thorough history should attempt to distinguish true rest pain from other pain, such as that from arthritis or neuritis. Significant ischemic pain is usually associated with decreased pulses as well as other manifestations of ischemia, such as atrophy, decreased skin temperature, marked rubor, and pain relief with dependency. Physical examination should detect the presence and extent of any underlying infection. Close observation for surgical scars will provide clues to the nature and extent of any previous vascular operations, including prior utilization of saphenous vein. A careful pulse examination should be performed to assess the baseline arterial status, which will provide a basis for comparison if subsequent disease progression occurs and give some indication of the approach that should be used to salvage a threatened limb. Noninvasive testing such as segmental pressures and pulse volume recordings is useful, since it gives a semiquantitative assessment of the circulation and helps to confirm the diagnosis made by the history and physical examination.

Careful assessment should look for evidence of other organ system disease, such as coronary artery disease, hypertension, renal disease, pulmonary disease, and cerebrovascular disease. Patients with severe angina should undergo cardiac evaluation prior to their vascular intervention. Patients with a history of congestive heart failure or recent myocardial infarction should be monitored with a pulmonary artery catheter during and after their operation to optimize their fluid replacement.[4,5]

Only patients with threatened limbs as manifested by disabling claudication, rest pain, frank gangrene, or nonhealing ulcers should be considered candidates for a distal arterial bypass for limb salvage. Those with gangrene extending into the deeper tarsal regions of the foot or a severe organic mental syndrome or those who do not ambulate are not candidates for limb-salvage surgery and should be treated with primary amputation.[6,7]

ANGIOGRAPHIC EVALUATION

High-quality angiograms are essential to make an accurate diagnosis of infrainguinal arteriosclerosis, to determine whether therapeutic intervention is possible, and to allow the surgeon to plan the optimal form that this intervention should take. The arterial tree from the groin to the forefoot should be well visualized in continuity. Oblique views may be required to visualize the origin and proximal portion of the deep femoral artery.[8] Visualization of the distal arteries is the key to performing bypass surgery to arteries in the foot and lower leg.

INFRAPOPLITEAL BYPASSES

Bypasses to arteries beyond the popliteal are done only when a femoropopliteal bypass is not possible. These distal bypasses are performed to the posterior tibial, anterior tibial, or peroneal artery. A tibial vessel is used if its lumen runs unobstructed to the foot. A peroneal artery is employed only when it is continuous with one or two of the terminal branches that run into the foot. Some patients require a bypass to an artery or arterial branch in the foot. Traditionally, the femoral artery has served as the inflow site of choice for infrainguinal bypasses. Over the last two decades, the superficial femoral, deep femoral, popliteal, and tibial arteries have been used as inflow sites when these vessels were relatively disease-free or there was limited available autologous vein. The superficial femoral and popliteal arteries are now preferentially used for primary bypasses when they are disease-free.[9]

When possible, all distal bypasses should be performed with autologous vein. The operations are performed under general or epidural anesthesia, and the vessels are occluded with minimum distortion and trauma. We have found tourniquet occlusion to be useful in constructing the distal anastomosis, since it eliminates the need for clamping the often small, fragile vessels and it reduces the requirement for extensive dissection.[10,11] Anastomoses are constructed with running 6-0 polypropylene sutures, and a completion angiogram is obtained in all cases. Details of the operative technique for distal bypasses have been described previously.[12] The approaches for bypasses to the infrapopliteal vessels are illustrated in Figures 13-1 through 13-3.

BYPASS RESULTS

A large retrospective study by Taylor and associates[13] noted a 5-year patency rate of 69 percent for bypasses to tibial arteries using the reversed vein technique. Limb salvage was greater than 90 percent.[13] In a similar review of cases employing the in situ vein bypass technique, Bergamini et al.[14] reported a 4-year patency rate of 63 percent (Fig. 13-4). A prospective, multicenter, randomized comparison of in situ and reversed vein grafts revealed a 30-month patency rate of 67 percent for reversed vein grafts versus 69 percent for in situ vein grafts.[15] Limb salvage was 76 percent or better for both techniques at 3 years. In addition, the results obtained using the in situ technique appeared better than those for the reversed technique when the vein was 3 mm or less in diameter. However, because of the small numbers, this difference was not statistically significant. Not all patients will have sufficient vein for a bypass employing the in situ technique. Furthermore, neither technique has proven superior except for the potential advantage of an in situ bypass when the saphenous vein is small. Therefore, surgeons will need to be proficient in both techniques because they will be applicable to varied clinical situations.

Bypasses to the pedal arteries have demonstrated results that approach those to more proximal tibial vessels above the ankle. Schneider and

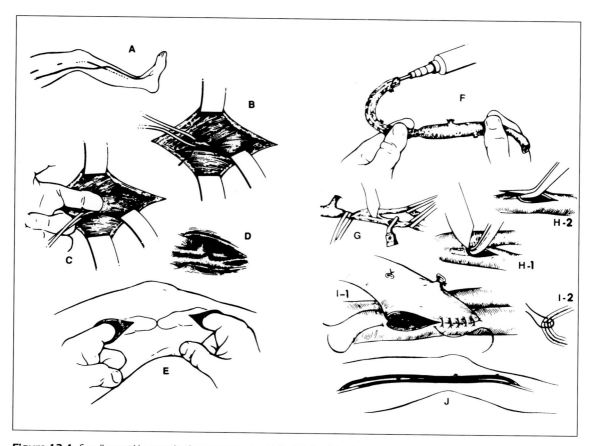

Figure 13-1. Small-vessel bypass in the upper and middle thirds of the leg. This may be performed to the tibioperoneal trunk, the posterior tibial artery, or the peroneal artery using a medial approach below the knee joint to gain access to these vessels. The anterior tibial artery requires an additional anterior incision (shown in Fig. 13-2). (**A**) In heavy lines, the position of the incisions required to perform bypasses from the femoral artery to the tibioperoneal trunk or the peroneal or posterior tibial arteries in the upper third of the leg. The upper incision provides access to the common or superficial femoral artery. The above-knee incision allows tunneling under the sartorius muscle and along the course of the popliteal vessels behind the knee. The dashed extension to the lower incision provides access to the posterior tibial and peroneal arteries in the middle third of the leg. If the saphenous vein is to be used, all incisions should be placed over the vein, as shown by the solid line, and access to deeper structures should be obtained when needed by raising thick flaps. (**B**) The below-knee incision opened through the skin, subcutaneous fat, and deep fascia of the popliteal space. The gastrocnemius muscle is retracted posteriorly. The more superficial popliteal vein is encircled with a Silastic loop to facilitate dissection of the underlying popliteal artery (*arrow*), which can be seen disappearing deep to the fibers of the soleus muscle. (**C**) A finger or right-angle clamp being placed deep to the soleus muscle prior to cutting it at its origin from the fibrous band that attaches to the back of the tibia. This exposes the origin of the anterior tibial artery and its accompanying vein or veins. (**D**) Division of these veins allows further retraction of overlying veins and exposure of the tibioperoneal trunk and its terminal branches. (**E**) Tunnels are fashioned by finger dissection. (**F**) Details of vein preparation using a long (6-in) cannula to permit the vein to be distended in segments so that leaks can be controlled and recanalized segments detected. (**G**) Elevation of the arteries by Silastic vessel loops and the beginning of the scalpel incision in the artery. In this view, except for the posterior tibial artery, which also has a microvascular clip applied to it, only the taut Silastic loops are required to control bleeding. (**H**) Placement of a mosquito clamp to facilitate extension of the initial opening in the artery (*1*). Alternatively, microvascular scissors may be used to extend the arteriotomy if the vessel is thin-walled and normal (*2*). (**I**) Details of the anastomotic suturing, which is begun at the distal end and continued to the midportion of each side of the anastomosis of the artery and the saphenous vein graft. Equal bites of all layers of each vessel are included in each stitch, which is always placed under direct vision. (**J**) Completed graft in place. If more distal exposure of the posterior tibial or peroneal arteries is required, further separation of the soleus muscle from the posterior surface of the tibia and its overlying muscles provides access to the neurovascular bundles. Careful dissection of the veins with ligation of crossing branches provides access to the more deeply placed arteries. These can be dissected free, taking great care to preserve all branches, so that an appropriate segment of artery can be elevated and controlled to perform the distal anastomosis. (Reprinted with permission from Veith FJ, Gupta SK: Femoral-distal artery bypasses. *In* Bergan JJ, Yao JST (eds): Operative Techniques in Vascular Surgery. New York, Grune & Stratton, 1980, p.141.)

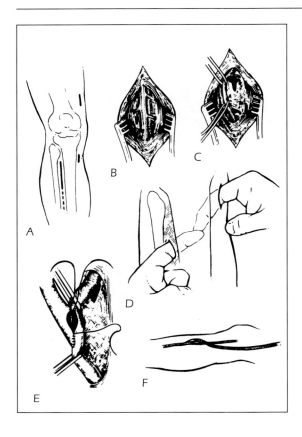

Figure 13-2. Bypass of the anterior tibial artery in the upper and middle thirds of the leg. (**A**) This requires an anterolateral incision in the leg midway between the tibia and fibula over the appropriate segment of patent artery. Additional small medial incisions are also required for tunneling. (**B**) The anterior incision is carried through the deep fascia, and the fibers of the anterior tibial muscle and the long extensors of the toes are separated to reveal the neurovascular bundle. Mobilization of accompanying veins with division of branches allows visualization of the anterior tibial artery, which can then be carefully mobilized. (**C**) After the artery is freed, it is elevated and retracted along with the accompanying veins by Silastic loops. This permits further posterior dissection, which allows the interosseous membrane to be visualized and incised in a cruciate fashion. (**D**) Careful, blunt finger dissection from this anterior approach and from the popliteal fossa via the medial incision facilitates creation of a tunnel without injuring the numerous veins in the area. Alternatively, the tunnel for the bypass may be placed lateral to the knee in a subcutaneous plane. (**E**) By elevating the anterior tibial artery, a meticulous distal anastomosis can be constructed, as already described. (**F**) The resulting graft in place. The anterior tibial artery also can be approached by a lateral incision with fibulectomy, but we believe this approach to be bloodier and more time-consuming than the one we have described. (Reprinted with permission from Veith FJ, Gupta SK: Femoral-distal artery bypasses. *In* Bergan JJ, Yao JST (eds): Operative Techniques in Vascular Surgery. New York, Grune & Stratton, 1980, p. 141.)

associates[16] reported a 59 percent 3-year primary patency rate for bypasses specific to the dorsalis pedis artery; these results were comparable with their results for more proximal bypasses to tibial vessels.[16] Using noninvasive graft surveillance and revision of graft-threatening lesions, the assisted primary and secondary patency rates for dorsalis pedis bypasses improved to 82 percent, and the limb-salvage rate at 3 years was 92 percent.[16] Similar results also were noted by Harrington et al.[17] with a 2-year primary patency rate of 59 percent for bypasses to the dorsalis pedis artery. In this review, those patients with intact pedal arches were found to have patency rates superior to those for patients who did not have intact pedal arches. However, the lack of visualization of the pedal arch on preoperative arteriogram did not preclude the performance of these bypasses for limb salvage (Fig. 13-5).

The strategy of using more distal inflow sources is particularly applicable to inframalleolar

bypasses when extensive vein length is required to reach the dorsalis pedis or branch arteries in the foot. Both Cantelmo et al.[18] and Rosenbloom et al.[19] noted that patency rates for bypasses originating from the superficial femoral and popliteal arteries were comparable with those which used the common femoral artery as the inflow site. In a review of our own experience with popliteal to distal vein bypasses, a life-table patency rate of 65 percent was noted at 4 years.[3] As stated previously, the patency rates for femorodistal grafts using the greater saphenous vein in either the reversed or the in situ position are similar to the 4-year patency rates, ranging between 63 percent and 69 percent, respectively.[13–15] Therefore, surgeons should not hesitate to employ the popliteal or superficial femoral artery as an inflow source, since the results obtained using these arteries have been quite good. Utilization of this technique will result in shorter bypasses

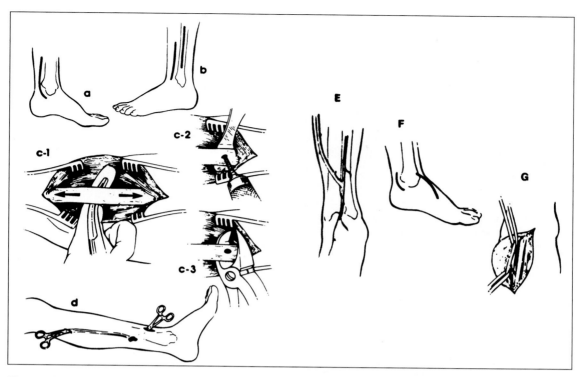

Figure 13-3. Bypasses to the distal third of the leg and the foot. Bypasses to the anterior tibial, posterior tibial, or peroneal arteries in the distal leg can be performed by techniques similar to those already described, with the exception of certain features illustrated here. (**A**) The distal posterior tibial artery can be approached by an incision along the posterior edge of the tibia. By deepening this incision along the tibialis posterior muscle and the posterior surface of the tibia, the distal peroneal artery also can be located and isolated just medial to the medial edge of the fibula. By dividing restraining fascia and fibers of the flexor hallucis longus muscle, it is possible to free this artery and elevate it into the wound so that a careful anastomosis can be constructed. However, in its distal third and particularly in patients with a stout calf and ankle, this vessel is approached by a lateral incision with excision of the fibula (**B**). (**C**) This is accomplished by freeing a long segment of fibula from its muscle attachments using a combination of blunt and sharp dissection. Particular care should be taken in the dissection along the medial edge of the bone, since the peroneal vessels are just deep to this edge and are easily injured by instruments. Once a finger has been passed around the fibula, this free edge of bone can be further developed by pushing a right-angled clamp forcefully inferiorly and superiorly. A right-angled retractor can then be passed behind the bone, and a hole drilled in it. Then the fibula can be divided easily and cleanly with a rib shears. The peroneal artery can be dissected free from surrounding veins so that it can be used for construction of a distal anastomosis. Gentle, blunt finger dissection is required to develop a tunnel from this lateral wound to the lower popliteal fossa. Great care is taken to avoid injury to the numerous veins in the area. From there, the tunneling to the femoral artery wound is performed in the previously described fashion. Because it is the least accessible of the three leg arteries and normally has the poorest connections with the arteries of the foot, we recommend use of the peroneal artery as a distal implantation site only when the anterior and posterior tibial arteries are not suitable for use. (**D**) The tunnel from the popliteal fossa to the distal posterior tibial artery is made just deep to the deep fascia. This is best accomplished with a long, gently curved clamp. The distal anterior tibial artery is approached by an anterior incision midway between the tibia and fibula (**B**). For bypass to this vessel, a tunnel is made from the distal popliteal fossa, deep to the deep fascia, to a point 5 to 7 cm above the medial malleolus. (**E**) From this point, the tunnel is made subcutaneously in a gentle curve across the tibia and adjacent tendons to reach the anterior tibial wound. The underlying tendons are those of the anterior tibial muscle and the long extensors of the toes. The tunnels are marked with umbilical tapes for subsequent identification. After completion of the distal anastomosis and drawing the graft through these tunnels, any tendons that distort or compress the graft in its course around the tibia are divided. This is usually required in low anterior tibial bypasses. (**F,G**) When no more proximal procedure is possible, bypasses to the ankle region or foot can be used to salvage limbs. The dorsalis pedia artery can easily be approached via an incision on the dorsum of the foot. We place this incision laterally, curve it, and raise a flap so that the incision will not be directly over the anastomosis. If this artery must be approached at the ankle, it is necessary to divide the extensor retinaculum. Otherwise, the operation is performed as already described for distal anterior tibial bypasses. The posterior tibial artery can be approached down to a point several centimeters below the medial malleolus. (Reprinted with permission from Veith FJ, Gupta SK: Femoral-distal artery bypasses. *In* Bergan JJ, Yao JST (eds): Operative Techniques in Vascular Surgery. New York, Grune & Stratton, 1980, p.141.)

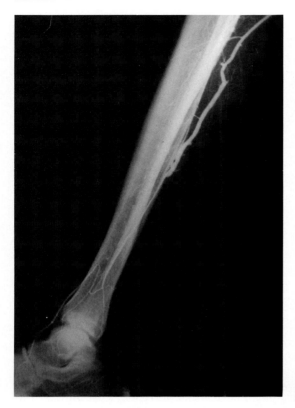

Figure 13-4. A completion angiogram following a common femoral to peroneal artery bypass with in situ saphenous vein. The dorsalis pedis artery is visualized via collaterals from the peroneal artery.

and allow for the preservation of portions of the saphenous vein for later use.

BYPASSES TO PLANTAR ARTERIES

An extended approach to limb salvage has led to the performance of bypasses below the ankle joint. These bypasses are required when the more proximal tibial vessels are occluded and are frequently secondary to a failed more proximal bypass. The technique involved in performing bypasses to secondary branches in the foot is essentially the same as that required for reconstruction to major infrapopliteal vessels. The arteries of the foot are illustrated in Figure 13-6.

Optimal illumination with the use of head lamps is an important factor in obtaining technical success with these bypasses, and loupe magnification is helpful when the vessel is less than 1.5 mm in diameter. Whenever the recipient branch is in communication with an isolated tibial segment, the anastomosis should be constructed directly across its origin. In a previously reported group of patients, the primary graft patency rates for these grafts at 1 and 2 years were 74 percent and 67 percent, respectively, and the limb salvage rate was 78 percent at 2 years.[2] Similar success was achieved by Andros et al.[20] with vein bypasses to the paramalleolar arteries. An illustration of a plantar bypass is shown in Figure 13-7. These techniques offer a clear alternative to a major amputation. The

Figure 13-5. A completion angiogram of a superficial femoral to dorsalis pedis artery bypass performed with reversed greater saphenous vein. Note the patent arch with visualization of the posterior tibial artery.

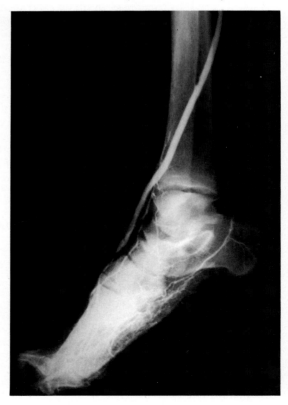

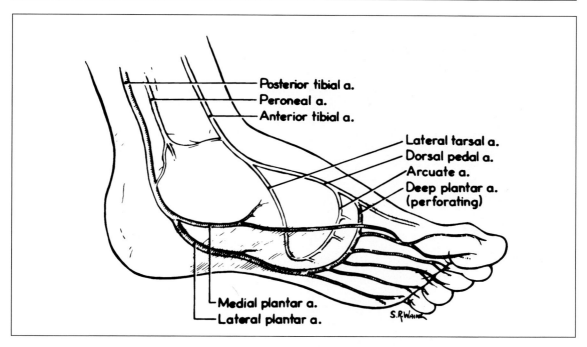

Figure 13-6. Diagram of named arteries in the ankle region and foot. Any of the main arteries or their branches, if patent, may be approached surgically and used as the distal outflow for a limb salvage bypass. (Reprinted with permission from Ascer E, Veith FJ, Gupta SK: Bypasses to plantar arteries and other tibial branches: An extended approach to limb salvage. J Vasc Surg 1988;8:434.)

anatomic approaches to these distal branch vessels are outlined below.

EXPOSURE OF THE LATERAL AND MEDIAL PLANTAR BRANCHES

The lateral and medial plantar branches are the continuation of the posterior tibial artery in the foot (see Fig. 13-6). The lateral plantar artery forms the main plantar arch, and it is larger than the medial branch. If the lateral branch is occluded, the medial branch may enlarge and feed the plantar arch through collaterals. The initial skin incision is made over the terminal end of the posterior tibial artery below the malleolus. After the artery is isolated, the incision is extended inferiorly and laterally onto the sole. A direct approach to the individual branches is difficult for several reasons. Since the skin of the sole is not easily retracted, adequate exposure of these branch vessels is hard to obtain when the inci-

sion does not follow their exact course. In addition, the plantar branches lie deep within the foot, and coupled with their small diameter, they can be difficult to locate. Finally, dissection of the terminal end of the posterior tibial artery can aid in distinguishing the lateral from the medial plantar branch. When the foot is externally rotated on the operating table, the lateral branch is usually located inferiorly. Exposure of the proximal 2 to 3 cm of the plantar branches is accomplished by incision of the flexor retinaculum and adductor muscle of the great toe. More distal exposure of these branches can be obtained by division of the medial border of the plantar aponeurosis and the short flexor muscles of the toes (Fig. 13-8).

The deep plantar arch and lateral tarsal artery are branches of the dorsalis pedis artery, which originates at the metatarsal level. It descends into a foramen that is bounded proximally by the dorsal metatarsal ligament, distally by the dorsal interosseous muscle ring, and medially and laterally by the base of the first and second metatarsal

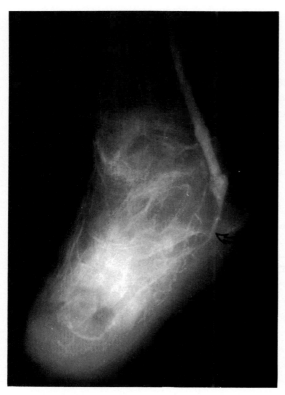

Figure 13-7. Intraoperative angiogram of a below-knee popliteal to lateral plantar artery bypass after a failed tibial to dorsalis pedis artery bypass. (Arrow points to the lateral plantar artery below the anastomosis.)

THE FAILING GRAFT

Intimal hyperplasia, progression of proximal or distal disease, or lesions within the graft itself can produce signs and symptoms of hemodynamic deterioration in patients with a prior arterial reconstruction without producing concomitant thrombosis of the bypass graft.[21-27] We have referred to this condition as a *failing graft* because, if the lesion is not corrected, graft thrombosis will almost certainly occur.[23] The importance of this failing graft concept lies in the fact that many difficult lower extremity revascularizations can be salvaged for protracted periods by relatively simple interventions if the lesion responsible for the circulatory deterioration and diminished graft blood flow can be detected before graft thrombosis occurs.

Over the last 10 years, we have been able to detect approximately 87 failing vein grafts and have corrected the lesions before graft thrombosis

Figure 13-8. Diagram showing exposure of the distal portion of the posterior tibial artery. The lateral and medial plantar branches are deep to the flexor retinaculum and the abductor hallucis muscle, which can be incised. (Reprinted with permission from Ascer E, Veith FJ, Gupta SK: Bypasses to plantar arteries and other tibial branches: An extended approach to limb salvage. J Vasc Surg 1988;8:434.)

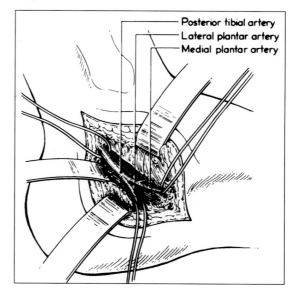

bones. The deep plantar branch connects with the lateral plantar branch as it exits from this tunnel, forming the deep pedal arch (Fig. 13-9).

A slightly curvilinear, longitudinal, 3- to 4-cm incision over the dorsum of the mid-portion of the foot permits dissection of the dorsalis pedis artery down to its bifurcation into the deep plantar and first dorsal metatarsal branches. The short extensor muscle of the great toe is retracted laterally or transected, if necessary, and the dorsal interosseous muscle ring is split to allow better exposure of the proximal portion of the deep plantar branch. The periosteum of the proximal portion of the second metatarsal bone is then incised and elevated. A fine-tipped rongeur is used to excise enough of the metatarsal shaft to permit ample exposure of the deep plantar branch (Fig. 13-10).

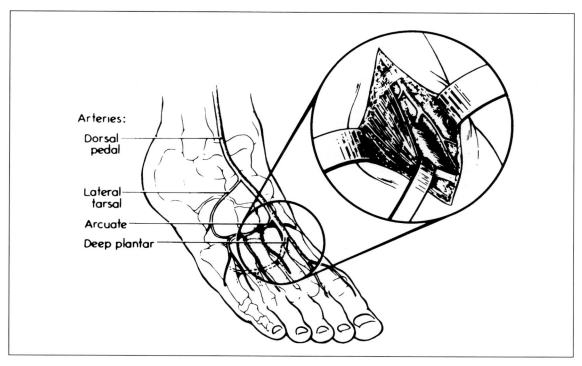

Figure 13-9. Diagram showing the deep plantar arch as the main terminal branch of the dorsalis pedis artery. Insert highlights the origin of the deep plantar branch and its downward course between the first and second metatarsal bones. This exposure is facilitated by the lateral retraction of the short extensor muscle of the great toe. (Reprinted with permission from Ascer E, Veith FJ, Gupta SK: Bypasses to plantar arteries and other tibial branches: An extended approach to limb salvage. J Vasc Surg 1988;8:434.)

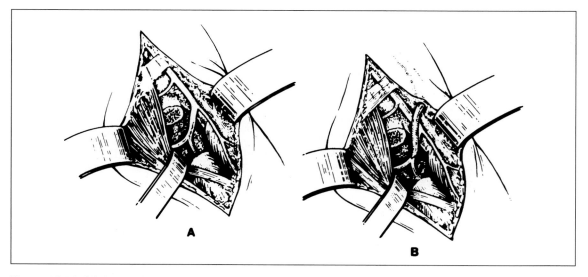

Figure 13-10. (A) Entire exposure of the deep plantar or deep metatarsal branch after partial resection of the second metatarsal bone. **(B)** Placement of an anastomosis can be accomplished easily through this exposure. (Reprinted with permission from Ascer E, Veith FJ, Gupta SK: Bypasses to plantar and other tibial branches: An extended approach to limb salvage. J Vasc Surg 1988;8:434.)

has occurred.[26,28] Invariably, the corrective procedure is simpler than the secondary operation that would be required if the bypass went on to thrombose. Vein grafts tend to fail as the result of hyperplastic lesions associated with the body or anastomotic areas of the graft. Solitary vein graft lesions of 15 mm or less in length can be treated by percutaneous transluminal angioplasty. Longer or multiple vein graft lesions should be treated by an interpositional graft or a proximal or distal graft extension depending on the lesion location. Some transluminal angioplasties of these lesions fail and require a second reintervention; others remain effective in correcting the responsible lesion, as documented by arteriography, more than 2 to 5 years later. If the failing graft is a vein bypass, detection of the failing state permits accurate localization and definition of the responsible lesion by arteriography as well as salvage of any undiseased vein. In contrast, if the graft is allowed to thrombose, the responsible lesion may be difficult to identify, the vein may be difficult or impossible to thrombectomize, and the patient's best graft—the ipsilateral greater saphenous vein—may have to be sacrificed, rendering the secondary operation even more difficult and more likely to fail with associated limb loss. More important, the results of reinterventions for failing grafts in terms of both continued cumulative patency and limb salvage rates have been far superior to the results of reinterventions for grafts that have thrombosed and failed.[23–33]

The improved results associated with reintervention for failing grafts mandate that surgeons performing bypass operations follow their patients closely in the postoperative period and indefinitely thereafter. Ideally, noninvasive laboratory tests, including duplex studies, should be performed with similar frequency.[25–28,30,31] If the patient has any recurrence of symptoms, or if the surgeon detects any change in the peripheral pulse examination or other manifestations of ischemia, the circulatory deterioration must be confirmed by noninvasive parameters and urgent arteriography.

REOPERATION

All patients whose bypasses thrombose in the first month after operation undergo reoperation.[1] The techniques employed have been described elsewhere.[32,33] Intraoperative angiographic examination is used routinely after graft thrombectomy. Vein grafts that fail immediately after operation usually require interposition of a segment of polytetrafluoroethylene (PTFE) or total replacement with this material, although in our experience an occasional thrombectomized vein graft will remain patent if no etiologic lesion is present.

Patients whose bypasses thrombose after the first postoperative month are considered for aggressive reoperation, and femoral angiography is usually performed; however, these patients are subjected to reoperation only if the bypass failure is associated with a renewed threat to limb viability. If the patient has originally undergone operation elsewhere and details of the first operation are not known or the distal anastomosis is to an infrapopliteal artery, a totally new bypass is performed. This is best accomplished using a variety of unusual approaches that permit access to infrainguinal arteries via unscarred, uninfected tissue planes.[33,34] These unusual approaches include a direct approach to the distal two zones of the deep femoral artery,[35] lateral approaches to the popliteal artery above and below the knee,[36] and medial or lateral approaches to all three of the infrapopliteal arteries.[37] In addition to permitting dissection in virginal tissue planes, these unusual access routes facilitate use of shorter grafts, which enable the surgeon to use the patient's remaining segments of good vein when the ipsilateral greater saphenous vein has been used or injured by the primary operation.[33]

NEWER TECHNIQUES

An increasing number of the procedures performed for limb salvage are secondary interventions. These secondary procedures are generally more difficult to perform because the access routes to arteries have been dissected previously and there is a scarcity of good autologous vein. Some patients will present with gangrene below a functioning bypass or after a previous failed bypass. Often they will need only a short distal extension of their functioning bypass or have only enough vein for a short bypass. In these situations, a tibiotibial bypass may provide an effective alternative revascularization.

Over the past decade, our group has performed 42 tibiotibial artery bypasses. The majority of these were performed because of a limited amount of available autologous vein. Ten of these bypasses were below previously performed bypasses. Approximately 50 percent of the bypasses were to pedal or tarsal vessels. The 5-year patency rate for these grafts was 65 percent, with a limb-salvage rate of 73 percent.[38,39]

SUMMARY

Patients with threatened limbs and distal tibial occlusive disease present an ongoing challenge to the vascular surgeon. Often they have had previous surgery and now have limited amounts of autologous vein. Careful attention to high-quality preoperative angiograms and a willingness to use alternative approaches should yield good results for limb salvage.

REFERENCES

1. Veith FJ, Gupta SK, Wengerter KR, et al: Changing arteriosclerotic disease patterns and management strategies in lower-limb-threatening ischemia. Ann Surg 1990;212:402.
2. Ascer E, Veith FJ, Gupta SK: Bypasses to plantar arteries and other tibial branches: An extended approach to limb salvage. J Vasc Surg 1988;8:1434.
3. Wengerter KR, Yang PM, Veith FJ, et al: A twelve-year experience with the popliteal-to-distal artery bypass: The significance and management of proximal disease. J Vasc Surg 1992;15:143.
4. Veith FJ, Gupta SK, Ascer E, et al: Alternative approaches to the deep femoral, the popliteal, and infrapopliteal arteries in the leg and foot. *In* Bergan JJ, Yao JST (eds): Techniques in Arterial Surgery. Philadelphia, WB Saunders Company, 1990, p 145.
5. Whittemore AD, Clowes AW, Hechtman HB, Mannick JA: Aortic aneurysm repair: Reduced operative mortality associated with maintenance of optimal cardiac performance. Ann Surg 1980;192:414.
6. Rivers SP, Scher LA, Gupta SK, Veith FJ: Safety of peripheral vascular surgery after recent acute myocardial infarction. J Vasc Surg 1990;11:70.
7. Veith FJ, Gupta SK, Samson RH, et al: Progress in limb salvage by reconstructive arterial surgery combined with new or improved adjunctive procedures. Ann Surg 1981;194:386.
8. Sprayregen S: Principles of angiography. *In* Haimovici H (ed): Vascular Surgery: Principles and Techniques. New York, McGraw-Hill, 1976, p. 39.
9. Veith FJ, Gupta SK, Samson RH, et al: Superficial femoral and popliteal arteries as inflow site for distal bypasses. Surgery 1981;90:980.
10. Bernhard VM, Boren CH, Towne JB: Pneumatic tourniquet as a substitute for vascular clamps in distal bypass surgery. Surgery 1980;87:709.
11. Wagner WH, Treiman RL, Cossman DV, et al: Tourniquet occlusion technique for tibial artery reconstruction J Vasc Surg 1993;18:637.
12. Veith FJ, Gupta SK. Femoral-distal artery bypasses. *In* Bergan JJ, Yao JST (eds): Operative Techniques in Vascular Surgery. New York, Grune & Stratton, 1980, p 141.
13. Taylor LM, Edwards JM, Porter JM: Present status of reversed vein bypass grafting: Five-year results of a modern series. J Vasc Surg 1990;11:193.
14. Bergamini TM, Towne JB, Bandyk DF, et al: Experience with in situ saphenous vein bypasses during 1981 to 1989: Determinant factors of long-term patency. J Vasc Surg 1991;13:137.
15. Wengerter KR, Veith FJ, Gupta SK, et al: Prospective randomized multicenter comparison of in situ and reversed vein infrapopliteal bypasses. J Vasc Surg 1991;13:189.
16. Schneider JR, Walsh DB, McDaniel MD, et al: Pedal bypass versus tibial bypass with autogenous vein: A comparison of outcome and hemodynamic results. J Vasc Surg 1993;17:1029.
17. Harrington EB, Harrington ME, Schanzer H, et al: The dorsalis pedis bypass: Moderate success in difficult situations. J Vasc Surg 1992;15:409.
18. Cantelmo NL, Snow JR, Menzoian JO, LoGerfo FW: Successful vein bypass in patients with an ischemic limb and a palpable popliteal pulse. Arch Surg 1986;121:217.
19. Rosenbloom JS, Walsh JJ, Schuler JJ, et al: Long-term results of infragenicular bypasses with autogenous vein originating from the distal superficial femoral and popliteal arteries. J Vasc Surg 1988;7:691.
20. Andros G, Harris RW, Salles-Cunha SX, et al: Bypass grafts to the ankle and foot. J Vasc Surg 1988;7:785.
21. Szilagyi DE, Smith RF, Elliot JP, et al: The biologic fate of autogenous vein implants as arterial substitutes: Clinical, angiographic and histopathologic observations in femoropopliteal operations for atherosclerosis. Ann Surg 1973;178:232.
22. O'Mara CS, Flinn WR, Johnson ND, et al: Recognition and surgical management of patent but hemodynamically failed arterial grafts. Ann Surg 1981;193:467.

23. Veith FJ, Weiser RK, Gupta SK, et al: Diagnosis and management of failing lower extremity arterial reconstructions. J Cardiovasc Surg 1984;25:381.

24. Whittemore AD, Clowes AW, Couch NP, et al: Secondary femoropopliteal reconstruction. Ann Surg 1981;193:35.

25. Berkowitz HD, Hobbs CL, Roberts B, et al: Value of routine vascular laboratory studies to identify vein graft stenosis. Surgery 1981;90:971.

26. Sanchez LA, Gupta SK, Veith FJ, et al: A ten-year experience with one hundred fifty failing or threatened vein and polytetrafluoroethylene arterial bypass grafts. J Vasc Surg 1991;14:729.

27. Sanchez LA, Suggs WD, Veith FJ, et al: Is surveillance to detect failing polytetrafluoroethylene bypasses worthwhile? Twelve-year experience with ninety-one grafts. J Vasc Surg 1993;18:981.

28. Sanchez LA, Suggs WD, Marin ML, et al. Is percutaneous balloon angioplasty appropriate in the treatment of graft and anastomotic lesions responsible for failing vein bypasses? Am J Surg 1994;168:97.

29. Smith CR, Green RM, DeWeese JA: Pseudoocclusion of femoropopliteal bypass grafts. Circulation 1983;68(suppl II):88.

30. Bandyk DF, Cata RF, Towne JB: A low flow velocity predicts failure of femoropopliteal and femorotibial bypass grafts. Surgery 1985;98:799.

31. Bandyk DF, Bergamini TM, Towne JB, et al: Durability of vein graft revision: The outcome of secondary procedures. J Vasc Surg 1991;13:200.

32. Veith FJ, Gupta SK, Daly V: Management of early and late thrombosis of expanded polytetrafluoroethylene (PTFE) femoropopliteal bypass grafts: Favorable prognosis with appropriate reoperation. Surgery 1980;87:581.

33. Veith FJ, Gupta SK, Ascer E, et al: Improved strategies for secondary operations on infrainguinal arteries. Ann Vasc Surg 1990;4:85.

34. Veith FJ, Ascer E, Nunez A, et al: Unusual approaches to infrainguinal arteries. J Cardiovasc Surg 1987;28:58.

35. Nunez A, Veith FJ, Collier P, et al: Direct approach to the distal portions of the deep femoral artery for limb salvage bypasses. J Vasc Surg 1988;8:576.

36. Veith FJ, Ascer E, Gupta SK, et al: Lateral approach to the popliteal artery. J Vasc Surg 1987;6:119.

37. Dardik H. Dardik I, Veith FJ: Exposure of the tibial-peroneal arteries by a single lateral approach. Surgery 1974;75:372.

38. Ascer E, Collier P, Gupta SK, et al: Reoperation for PTFE bypass failure: The importance of distal outflow site and operative technique in determining outcome. J Vasc Surg 1987;5:298.

39. Lyon RT, Veith FJ, Marsan BU, et al: Eleven-year experience with tibiotibial bypass: An unusual but effective solution to distal tibial artery occlusive disease and limited autologous vein. J Vasc Surg 1993;17:1128.

ACKNOWLEDGMENTS

This work was supported by grants from the U.S. Public Health Service (HL 02990-01), the James Hilton Manning and Emma Austin Manning Foundation, The Anna S. Brown Trust, and the New York Institute for Vascular Studies.

CHAPTER

14

Free-Tissue Transfer
in Lower Extremity Ischemia

JOSEPH M. SERLETTI
KENNETH OURIEL

Atherosclerosis of the lower extremity may lead to limb-threatening ischemic soft tissue wounds. Successful arterial bypass alone may be insufficient for complete lower extremity reconstruction in patients with exposed tendon or bone proximal to the metatarsophalangeal joints. Before the advent of free-tissue tranfer, these severely ischemic wounds of the distal leg, ankle, and proximal foot were treated with amputation. Combined vascular reconstruction with free-tissue tranfer for coverage of these wounds has permitted extended limb salvage.[1–6]

PATIENT SELECTION

The goal of any technique for lower extremity reconstruction must be to improve or restore function. Patient selection should be directed toward meeting this goal, which includes the preservation of limb length and ambulatory abilities. Patients generally have been selected by an interdisciplinary team of plastic surgeons, vascular surgeons, and orthopedic surgeons. Patients who were felt to be unable to live and ambulate independently, particularly if they had currently lived alone, have been considered for limb reconstruction. Other considerations have included a prior contralateral below knee amputation, the presence of diabetes, and avoiding the psychological stress of a major amputation. Contralateral amputation has been a strong parameter for selection because of the high functional demands of the bilateral amputee. Diabetes was selected as a consideration because of its propensity for bilateral lower extremity problems. In reconstructing one diabetic lower extremity, one can prolong or avoid the potential bilateral amputee.[1–6,9,10]

SITE OF SOFT TISSUE DEFECT

All patients have presented with limb-threatening soft tissue wounds of the lower extremity with significant bone, tendon, or joint exposure. No pattern of distal tissue necrosis has excluded patients from consideration for reconstruction. Vascular reconstruction and minor amputation or split-thickness skin grafting would not have resulted in stable lower extremity reconstruction in these selected patients. Approximately one-third of patients have had a concomitant diagnosis of osteomyelitis confirmed by bone biopsy. Preference for the treatment of osteomyelitis has been given to surgical debridement and soft tissue coverage over prolonged antibiotics.[4]

Soft tissue defects have been caused by advanced ischemia and diabetes in 50 percent of selected patients. One-third of the patients have had athersclerosis alone as the underlying pathophysiology. The remaining patients have had athersclerosis, diabetes, and renal failure. Some of these patients have been on diaylsis, whereas some have had functioning renal transplants.

Soft tissue defects have been grouped by their anatomic site and are divided into dorsal wounds, plantar wounds, and distal tibial and malleolar wounds. The sites of soft tissue involvment have been equally distributed in these selected patients, with no particular area having increased prevelance. Dorsal foot wounds have typically resulted in exposure of the midfoot skeleton and anterior compartment tendons (Fig. 14-1). Plantar wounds have been the most problematic and have occurred on all the weight-bearing surfaces of the foot. Most plantar wounds have occurred in diabetic patients with significant sensory neuropathy (Fig. 14-2). Wounds around the malleoli and distal tibia have resulted in bone or significant tendon exposure that could not be covered by local techniques[4] (Figs. 14-3 and 14-4).

TIMING OF SOFT TISSUE RECONSTRUCTION

Some patients have had primary soft tissue reconstruction at the time of the vascular reconstruction, and some have undergone delayed soft tissue reconstruction. Preference has been given whenever possible to simultaneous vascular and free soft tissue reconstruction. The preference for combined reconstruction has been to limit the number of significant operative procedures and associated anesthetic risks. The patients who underwent delayed reconstruction have usually had unrecognized or unapparent limb-threatening soft tissue wounds at the time of revascularization.[1–6,9,10]

VASCULAR RECONSTRUCTION

After a patient has been selected for reconstruction, an arteriogram is obtained if a recent study is not already available. Autogenous venous bypass has been performed to both the popliteal and the infrapopliteal arteries. No patient series has required a prosthetic reconstruction, although the possibility did not exclude any patient for potential reconstruction. Some patients have had inadequate outflow for complete vascular reconstruction and

have been treated with proximal vein grafts directed into the free flap.

Review of the arteriogram has been done not only to determine the type of vascular reconstruction but also to aid in flap selection and recipient vessel site selection. Preference has been given to performing infrapopliteal reconstructions (femoral to tibial artery bypass) and placing the bypass graft as close to the site of the soft tissue defect as possible. In some patients, this has resulted in placing the distal anastomosis of the vein graft at a site considerably more distant than would have been required for arterial reconstruction alone. This preference developed because it allowed use of a nondiseased, relatively soft recipient vessel (saphenous vein graft) for the microarterial anastomosis. When popliteal reconstructions (femoral to popliteal artery) have been performed, the preoperative arteriogram typically has shown good-quality reconstituted tibial vessels. These tibial vessels have been the recipient vessels for the free flap in these popliteal reconstructions. Microanastomoses to these vessels have been particularly difficult, requiring changes in technique, because of the presence of arterial wall disease. The degree of arterial wall disease has not been predicted by angiography because it has revealed only luminal defects. The diseased tibial arteries have been thickened, stiff, and friable with friable initima. The presence of vessel wall disease, however, has not affected outcome. All free flaps performed to the tibial arteries in our series survived, and none had thrombosis requiring reexploration. In general, we have continued to perform infrapopliteal reconstructions, despite the absence of distal disease using the nondiseased vein graft and avoiding the diseased tibial artery for the microarterial anastomosis.[4]

The technique for performing the microarterial anastomoses to both a diseased tibial artery and the saphenous bypass graft has been altered from the typical technique used in free-flap surgery. End-to-side microanastomoses for routine free flaps are first begun by placement of the apical sutures. The back wall is usually closed next by placement of individual sutures that are tied immediately. This is followed by similar closure of the front wall. The microarterial anastomosis in

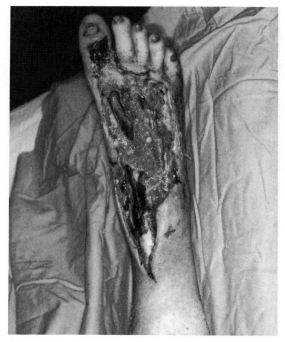

A

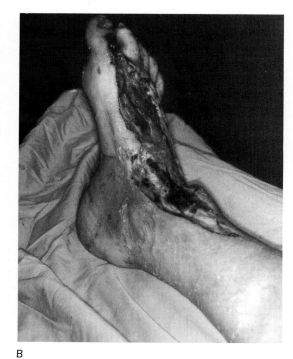

B

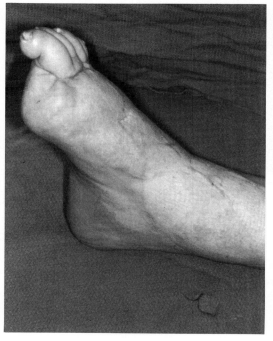

C

Figure 14-1. (**A,B**) Soft tissue defect after diabetic foot infection with exposure of dorsal skeleton and anterior compartment tendons. (**C**) Postoperative result after femoral to dorsalis pedis bypass and free rectus abdominis transfer with skin graft.

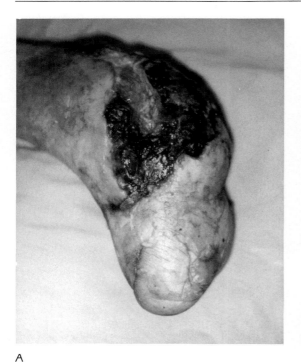

A

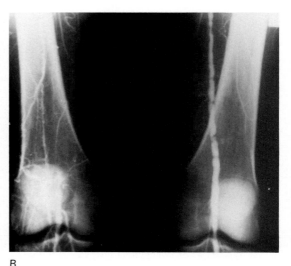

B

Figure 14-2. (A) *Severe necrosis of plantar surface of heel with osteomyelitis of calcaneus in a diabetic patient. **(B)** Preoperative angiogram showed superficial femoral occlusion. **(C)** Healed postoperative result at 2 years after femoral to popliteal bypass and free scapular fasciocutaneous flap to the weight-bearing surface of foot.*

C

these patients has begun with the normal placement of the apical sutures, which are tied. Because of the thickness and stiffness of the diseased tibial arteries and some saphenous veins, the individual sutures placed next are in the back wall, but they are placed without tying. By not tying each individual suture, better visualization of each vessel wall has been achieved in these diseased vessels. After placement of all back wall sutures, they are tied sequentially. The front wall is then similarly sutured.[4]

FREE-FLAP SELECTION

The free-flap tissues used in these lower extremity reconstructions have included the rectus abdominis muscle, the latissimus dorsi muscle, the radial forearm flap, the scapular flap, and the omentum. Specific flaps have been selected for the quality of the donor vessels, the length of reliable soft tissue, and to minimize contour deformity.[1–6,9,10]

A successful free-tissue transfer requires both inflow (the microarterial anastomosis) and

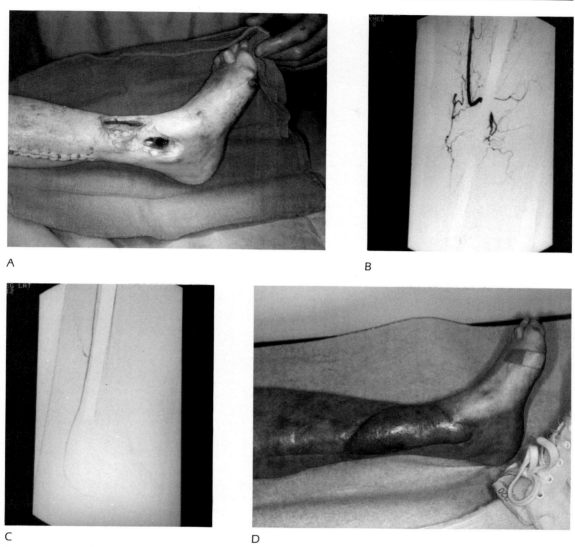

Figure 14-3. (A) Malleolar wound with exposure of intramedullary rod after simultaneous ankle and knee fusion in a patient with rheumatoid arthritis. Rod extends from ankle to greater trochanter. **(B)** Preoperative angiogram showed popliteal artery occlusion with **(C)** reconstitution of posterior tibial artery extending to foot. **(D)** Postoperative result 1 year after femoral to posterior tibial bypass and free rectus abdominis transfer.

outflow (the venous anastomosis). Inflow to the flap, or the microarterial anastomosis, has been from the bypass graft in patients undergoing an infrapopliteal vascular reconstruction. In patients with more proximal vascular reconstructions, the reperfused anterior or posterior tibial artery closest to the wound has been used. In patients with nonreconstructable distal vascular disease, an end-to-end microarterial anastomosis to a proximal vein graft has been performed. Anastomoses in patients with complete vascular reconstruction have been performed end-to-side with the use of an operating microscope or 3.5× optical loupe magnification. Either a segment of vein graft or arterial wall has been excised to match the circumference of the donor artery. Microanastomoses

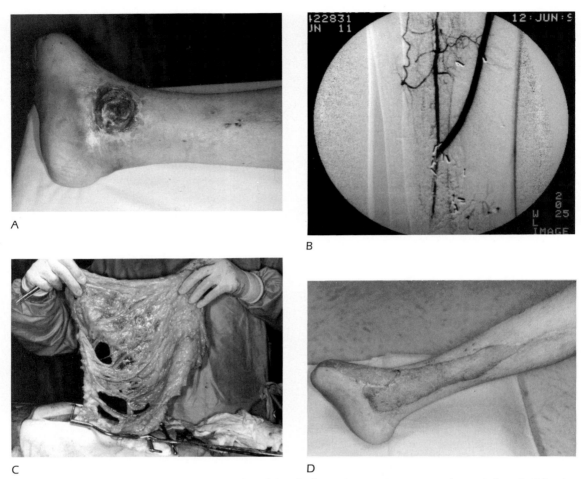

Figure 14-4. (**A**) Open wound with exposure of medial malleolus and open transmetatarsal amputation site following prior (**B**) femoral to peroneal bypass with high proximal crossover of the graft. (**C**) Because of the proximal position of the graft, omentum was selected as donor tissue, extending from just below knee to the end of the transmetatarsal amputation. (**D**) Postoperative result after free omentum transfer and skin graft.

are usually performed with interrupted 8-0 or 9-0 nylon sutures. Posterior wall sutures were left untied until all have been placed; the anterior wall is then sutured similarly.

Outflow for the flap, or the venous anastomosis, has been from the closest tibial vein to the soft tissue defect. Anastomoses are usually performed end-to-side after making a venotomy in the recipient vein. Anastomoses have been sutured with interrupted 9-0 nylon.

Patients have been followed by monitoring independent Doppler signals for both the bypass graft and the free flap. Aspirin (325 mg) has been given to all patients 1 day before surgery and continued throughout the follow-up period. Patients who underwent infrapopliteal bypasses have been treated with heparin during surgery and given an infusion for 5 days postoperatively. Graft patency rates, flap survival, and limb-salvage rates have been calculated from direct observation. Patient follow-up has averaged 2 years.

Nondiseased donor arteries, contour, skin thickness, and flap length were important initial considerations in donor tissue selection. We thought that arteries would be less affected by atherosclerosis in the upper extremity compared with the lower trunk and selected the latissimus dorsi muscle over the rectus abdominis muscle for our first reconstructions. Harvesting the latissimus dorsi required the decubitus position and rarely permitted simultaneous vascular and plastic surgery. In addition, changes in patient position were required to complete the surgery, thereby adding to the operative time. The necrosis of the distal 2 cm of the latissimus dorsi in most of our patients prompted our switch to the rectus abdominis. Harvest with a simultaneous two-team approach was simplified with the rectus abdominis because the patient was positioned supine and no patients required a position change during surgery. Atheroma was identified by palpation more frequently in the inferior epigastric artery compared with the thoracodorsal artery, however, no rectus flap was considered unusable because of the presence of arterial disease. The disease in the inferior epigastric artery was always variable along its length, with areas of increased or decreased involvement. A relatively soft area of artery was selected by palpation and loupe examination for the anastomosis. Despite the presence of arterial disease, all rectus abdominis flaps in our series survived completely without the distal necrosis seen with the latissimus dorsi muscle.[4]

Muscle flaps around the foot and ankle have tended to remain bulky for many months following surgery, necessitating alterations in footwear. This contour problem has been partially corrected by having the patient fitted with a custom pressure stocking. Contour difficulties with muscle flap reconstructions have persisted for 9 to 12 months, after which enough muscle atrophy has occurred. Most scapular flap reconstructions have had persistent contour abnormalities without any involution over time. Several of these patients have had a secondary debulking procedure. These patients have required custom-fitted footwear for protected ambulation. The radial forearm flap has provided thin, pliable skin with minimal contour problems for reconstructions around the foot and ankle. If the soft tissue defect permits, the radial forearm flap is the flap of choice when contour is a potential problem.[4]

For large defects on the weight-bearing plantar surface, the scapular fasciocutaneous flap has been used. It has been selected because of its increased skin thickness, which is felt to be important for plantar reconstructions. Despite the permanent contour problems with the scapular flap, it has demonstrated durablity on the plantar surface of the foot. The scapular flap remains a consideration for reconstruction of large plantar defects[4] (see Fig. 14-2).

Flap length has obviously been an important consideration, since good-quality recipient vessels cannot be found reliably next to the site of the soft tissue defect. One way of limiting potiential length problems has been to place the bypass graft (recipient artery for the free flap) as close to the soft tissue defect as possible. This has resulted in placing the distal anastomosis of the vascular bypass graft at a more distal site than would have been required to treat the more proximal arterial occlusion. This has required prior dialogue with the vascular surgeon and has been dependent on enough usable saphenous vein graft. When the bypass graft can be placed near the soft tissue defect, the length of the flap has not been an important factor in donor tissue selection. When the bypass graft cannot be placed near the soft tissue defect, flap length becomes a consideration.

The omentum has provided considerable length and has been used from just below the knee to an open transmetatarsal amputation site in several patients. For these extreme length requirements, the omentum has remained our first choice for donor tissue[4,8] (see Fig. 14-1). The entire rectus abdominis, including the portion overlying the anterior chest wall, has been used successfully to fulfill intermediate length requirements. The latissimus dorsi also has remained a consideration for intermediate length requirements, particularly when the soft tissue defect has involved a large surface area. The fanning shape of the distal latissimus has been particularly useful for these large surface area defects.

The following summarizes our current approach to donor tissue selection. Flap length is the most important first decision because it is determined by the most appropriate recipient vessel site. When extreme length is required, the omentum is used. For intermediate length requirements, the rectus abdominis, followed by the latissimus dorsi, is used. If no length requirements exist, the site of the defect is the next most important factor directing flap selection. For superficial defects of limited surface area, the radial forearm flap is used because it avoids contour problems. For deeper, larger defects, particularly with heavy bacterial contamination, muscle is used, with preference given to the rectus abdominis (see Figs. 14-1 and 14-3). For large plantar defects, the scapular flap is considered, with skin-grafted muscle also a possibility (see Fig. 14-2). The last consideration in flap selection is patient position during surgery. We try to select appropriate donor tissues that also allow the patient to remain supine throughout the entire procedure. This permits multiple teams working simulateously and has reduced operative times.

HOSPITALIZATION AND PERIOPERATIVE MORBIDITY AND MORTALITY

All series have reported very low operative morbidity and mortality. In our own series, there were no operative mortalities or mortalities during hospitalization. Postoperative morbidities included congestive heart failure in 20 percent of patients, treated successfully with diurectics. There were no postoperative myocardial infarctions during hospitalization.[1–6,9,10]

Hospitalizations for these patients have generally been lengthy but comparable with the lengths required for amputation, including rehabilitation. In our series, hospitalization for all patients from the day of admission to the day of discharge averaged 50 days. Hospitalization after free flap reconstruction was 33 days. Because these patients had cellulitis or severe tissue necrosis, there was frequently a considerable delay before free-tissue reconstruction. Often the need for combined vascular and free tissue reconstruction was apparent only after debridement and angiography. Length of hospitalization was examined for the varying subgroups within these patients. Mean hospitalization for the patients with a prior contralateral below-knee amputation was the longest at 77 days. Mean hospitalization was next longest in the group with an ASA classification IV or V at 56 days. Patients with ASA classes I to III had the shortest mean stay at 18 days. In patients with flap

and graft failures, a below-knee amputation was performed within 5 days of failed free-tissue transfer. These few patients had the longest mean hospitalization stay at 78 days (53 days after below-knee amputation).[1–7,9,10]

SUCCESSFUL INDEPENDENT AMBULATION

Most series reporting combined vascular and soft tissue reconstruction have demonstrated excellent functional results. The average follow-up in these series has been 2 years, with the longest follow-ups at 4 to 5 years. Approximately 70 percent long-term independent ambulation has been achieved with this combined technique. Graft patency and free-flap success have been achieved in 90 percent of patients, but this has not always resulted in independent ambulation. Approximately 20 percent of patients with successful reconstructions have developed ongoing infection and ischemia in the adjacent (nonflap) soft tissues. The bypass graft has remained patent in these patients. These patients have required a delayed below-knee amputation, and few have regained ambulation.[1–6,9,10]

Fifty percent of the independent ambulators have required minor secondary procedures. These have included recipient-site hematoma evacuation, donor-site hematoma evacuation, redebridement of osteomyelitis, limited repeat skin grafts, delayed toe amputations, and flap debulking.

Over one-third of patients have had a concomitant diagnosis of osteomyelitis established by bone biopsy and culture. These patients have been treated with radical bone debridement and antibiotics in addition to vascular reconstruction and coverage with well-vascularized soft tissue. The majority of these patients have maintained a stable lower extremity and independent ambulation without recurrent osteomyelitis.[4]

NONRECONSTRUCTABLE DISTAL VASCULAR DISEASE

Some patients have had inadequate distal lower extremity vascular outflow for arterial reconstruction. These patients have been treated with a proximal vein graft directly into the free flap. The specific free flaps in these patients were the radial forearm, the latissimus dorsi, and the rectus abdominis. The radial forearm flaps failed insidiously over a 5-day period characterized by blistering of the skin and diminishing Doppler signals. The remaining patients, each with a muscle flap, have had successful reconstructions without evidence of further lower extremity ischemia. Vascular bypass grafts fail when there is inadequate outflow in the distal vascular bed. We believe this principle applies to the failures seen with the radial forearm flap in this setting. The outflow or vascular bed in the radial forearm flap is probably inadequate to support the high flow from a femoral vein graft directed only into the flap. In contrast, larger muscles (latissimus dorsi and rectus abdominis) probably have adequate outflow to support this directed blood supply. A vein graft directed into a larger muscle flap has given excellent functional results and has become our primary method for patients with nonreconstructible distal vascular disease and a limb-threatening soft tissue wound.

There is some evidence that free-tissue transfer to ischemic wounds in the lower extremity that were not also reconstructed with an arterial bypass demonstrated neovascularization on follow-up angiography. In addition, these reports indicate that rest pain and claudication improved after this soft tissue only transfer. The soft tissue reconstruction acting as a nutrient flap may provide added vascularity and durability to these lower extremities so reconstructed.[9,10] We believe that the overall lower extremity reconstruction has a better chance of success when the arterial inflow is normal and we continue to use adjunctive arterial reconstruction in this setting.

AMPUTATION VERSUS RECONSTRUCTION

The appropriate management of critical ischemia of the lower extremity is still a matter of debate. While amputation is a universally accepted form of treatment, the notion that it is least costly and most effective has been challenged successfully. Vascular reconstruction has been shown to be comparable with amputation in terms of both overall success and total costs. In fact, including the subsequent costs of rehabilitation and a prosthesis, several studies have demonstrated that vascular reconstruction is slightly less expensive than amputation in the treatment of limb-threatening ischemia.[11–14]

These patients generally have more critically threatened limbs, including significant bone, tendon, and joint exposure, than those reported in studies comparing amputation with vascular reconstruction alone. These patients also have had more frequent and severe manifestations of comorbid disease, including diabetes, renal failure, contralateral amputation, and osteomyelitis. It might seem implicit that these patients are most prone to surgical complications and should, therefore, be managed conservatively with amputation. These are several important reasons why this conclusion is flawed and that these patients are especially appropriate candidates for aggressive management with combined vascular reconstruction and free-tissue transfer.

Most of the patients have been deemed poor candidates for rehabilitation. The basis for this has been multifactorial. Factors limiting the likelihood of successful rehabilitation following amputation included diabetes, advanced age, and existing contralateral amputation. In addition, many of these patients were living alone. It was felt that these patients would be unable to regain ambulation with a prosthesis and would no longer be capable of living independently. Many of these patients might require nursing home placement subsequent to lower extremity amputation. A report by High et al.[15] found that only 45 percent of amputation patients used a prosthesis successfully. Even studies[16] that have made very aggressive attempts at rehabilitation and prosthesis fitting have reported that only 73 percent of good candidates for rehabilitation achieved their ambulation goals. In our series, only one patient who underwent amputation following reconstructive failure was ambulating successfully with a prosthesis.

One of the most important considerations favoring aggressive strategies for lower extremity salvage is the likelihood of developing bilateral amputation in the future. Most of these patients are diabetic with a proven significant chance of developing eventual bilateral limb loss. Bodily and Burgess[17] demonstrated that 50 percent of patients undergoing amputation will develop severe limb-threatening contralateral disease requiring amputation within 2 years. These patients will have a greatly reduced likelihood of maintaining ambulation even if they are able to ambulate successfully with one below-knee amputation and a prosthesis.

Ouriel et al.[12] performed a retrospective study of 362 patients matched for age and severity of disease using ASA classification who underwent either amputation or revascularization. They found that patients treated with amputation experienced greater mortality rates than those patients undergoing revascularization. This difference was greatest in patients with the most severe disease. Only 29 percent of amputation patients with ASA classification IV or V were alive after 3 years as compared with 76 percent of the revascularization patients of the same risk classification.[12] Other studies also have found significantly elevated mortality rates in patients undergoing amputation as compared with revascularization, although these data do not reflect matching for general medical status of the patients.

In the most medically compromised patients, hospitalizations have been found to be significantly longer in those patients undergoing amputation than in matched patients undergoing revascularization. The mean length of hospitalization of amputation patients with ASA classification IV or V was 31 days, more than twice the hospitalization for revascularization patients of the same risk classification. We believe that in our severely ill patients, hospitalizations would have been correspondingly complicated and prolonged had those patients been treated with amputation.

Finally, it has been shown that revascularization can be performed safely and successfully in medically compromised patients of advanced age.[18–20] Even severely compromised diabetic patients with renal failure and large gangrenous defects are surgical candidates for combined reconstruction. Taylor et al.[14] found that a disporportionate number of attempts at limb salvage failed in these patients even though revascularization was successful because of a lack of concomitant soft tissue reconstruction. A success rate of only 67 percent limb salvage at 3 years in renal failure patients was attributed by this group to a lack of sufficiently aggressive wound management with free-tissue transfers.[14]

CONCLUSION

The combined application of vascular and free-flap soft tissue reconstruction for the threatened ischemic lower extremity has produced excellent functional results in the majority of patients. This combined technique has permitted extended limb salvage without significant mortality or morbidity. The overall success in these patients has been due to the interdisciplinary participation by plastic surgery, vascular surgery, and orthopedic surgery. These patients must continue to be followed for ongoing flap durability, graft patency, and the development of associated diseases.

REFERENCES

1. Chowdary RP, Celani VJ, Goodreau JJ, et al: Free-tissue transfers for limb salvage utilizing in situ saphenous vein bypass conduit as the inflow. Plast Reconstr Surg 1991;87:529.
2. Cronenwett JL, McDaniel MD, Zwolak RM, et al: Limb salvage despite extensive tissue loss: Free tissue transfer combined with distal revascularization. Arch Surg 1989;124:609.
3. Greenwald LL, Comerota AJ, Mitra A, et al: Free vascularized tissue transfer for limb salvage in peripheral vascular disease. Ann Vasc Surg 1990; 4:244.
4. Serletti JM, Hurwitz SR, Jones, JA, et al: Extension of limb salvage by combined vascular reconstruction and adjunctive free-tissue transfer. J Vasc Surg 1993;18:972.
5. Shenaq SM, Dinh TA: Foot salvage in arteriolosclerotic and diabetic patients by free flaps after vascular bypass: Report of two cases. Microsurgery 1989;10:310.
6. Shestak KC, Fitz DG, Newton ED, Swartz WM: Expanding the horizons in treatment of severe peripheral vascular disease using microsurgical techniques. Plast Reconstr Surg 1990;85:406.
7. Dripps RD, Lamont A, Eckenhoff JE: The role of anesthesia in surgical mortality. JAMA 1961; 178:261.
8. Herrera HR, Geary J, Whitehead P, Evangelisti S: Revascularization of the lower extremity with omentum. Clin Plast Surg 1991;18:491.
9. Shestak KC, Hendricks DL, Webster MW: Indirect revascularization of the lower extremity by means of microvascular free-muscle flap: A preliminary report. J Vasc Surg 1990;12:581.
10. Mimoun M, Hilligot P, Baux S: The nutrient flap: A new concept of the role of the flap and application to the salvage of arteriosclerotic lower limbs. Plast Reconstr Surg 1989;84:458.

11. Mackey WC, McCullough JL, Conlon TP, et al: The costs of surgery for limb-threatening ischemia. Surgery 1986;99:26.

12. Ouriel K, Fiore WM, Geary JE: Limb-threatening ischemia in the medically compromised patient: Amputation or revascularization? Surgery 1988; 104:667.

13. Raviola CA, Nichter LD, Baker D, et al: Cost of treating advanced leg ischemia: Bypass graft vs primary amputation. Arch Surg 1988;123:495.

14. Taylor LM Jr, Hamre D, Dalman RL, Porter JM: Limb salvage vs amputation for critical ischemia: The role of vascular surgery. Arch Surg 1991;126: 1251.

15. High RM, McDowell DE, Savrin RA: A critical review of amputation in vascular patients. J Vasc Surg 1984;1:653.

16. Harris KA, van Schie L, Carroll SE, et al: Rehabilitation potential of elderly patients with major amputations. J Cardiovasc Surg 1991;32:463.

17. Bodily KC, Burgess EM: Contralateral limb and patient survival after leg amputation. Am J Surg 1983;146:280.

18. Cogbill TH, Landercasper J, Strutt PJ, Gundersen AL: Late results of peripheral vascular surgery in patients 80 years of age and older. Arch Surg 1987;122:581.

19. Friedman SG, Kerner BA, Friedman MS, Moccio CG: Limb salvage in elderly patients: Is aggressive surgical therapy warranted? J Cardiovasc Surg 1989;30:848.

20. O'Mara CS, Kilgore TL Jr, McMullan MH, et al: Distal bypass for limb salvage in very elderly patients. Am Surg 1987;53:66.

Interventional Angiographic Techniques

JACOB CYNAMON

This chapter is meant as an overview of the techniques of percutaneous intervention for peripheral arterial occlusive disease. In the past few years vascular surgeons have come to recognize the value of the percutaneous intervention that angiographers have been performing for the past 30 years. As early as 1964, Dotter[1] reported on the use of coaxial catheters to restore flow to a gangrenous extremity. In 1974, Gruntzig[2] introduced a double lumen balloon catheter which revolutionized the field of interventional radiology. Many vascular surgeons have become more liberal with the use of these techniques. Patients of vascular surgeons who developed a close working relationship with their interventional radiologists benefited by these advances. Interventional radiologists can treat most lesions amenable to angioplasty at the time of the diagnostic arteriogram. In addition, these procedures can be used during vascular surgery to improve inflow and/or outflow while limiting the time and morbidity involved with extending the operation.

Although percutaneous intervention is more accepted by the surgical community, we must guard against its overuse. Vascular intervention should be limited to patients with severe claudication only after an attempt at conservative therapy (i.e., smoking cessation and an exercise program). Rest pain, non-healing ulcers or gangrene are clear indications for therapy.[3] Many of these patients present with multilevel disease. Often in these patients, percutaneous therapy can be performed at the time of the diagnostic arteriogram as an adjunct to surgery, especially to improve inflow.

Usually a good history, physical exam, and noninvasive studies will confirm the presence of vascular disease. If the indications for intervention are met, then an angiogram should be performed.

TECHNIQUE

In our institution, we choose to access the vascular system when possible via the common femoral artery contralateral to the symptomatic extremity. This approach facilitates angioplasty and/or thrombolysis using the original puncture and does not preclude performing a second percutaneous puncture of the symptomatic extremity once the pathology is defined. Seldinger technique,[4] using either a double wall or single wall needle, is used to enter the common femoral artery. It is extremely important to enter the common femoral artery below the inguinal ligament and above its bifurcation so as to limit complications such as retroperitoneal hematomas, pseudoaneurysms, and arteriovenous fistulae.[5] Using fluoroscopy, the common femoral artery is entered in its course over the lower half of the femoral head. The inferior epigastric artery and the deep circumflex iliac artery are good anatomic landmarks for the position of the inguinal ligament. It has been well documented that the position of the inguinal ligament cannot accurately be determined by external landmarks. However, it is safe to assume that the inguinal ligament does not dip below the mid femoral head in almost all cases.[6] If a prior angiogram is available, it should be reviewed to note the position of the inferior epigastric and circumflex iliac arteries.

In most cases, a bilateral femoral arteriogram is performed from the level of the renal arteries to the foot. Appropriate oblique views of the pelvis and groin must be obtained to exclude lesions at the bifurcations of the common iliac artery and common femoral artery. When evaluating the angiogram, one must take into consideration the patient's history, physical exam, and noninvasive studies. If the angiogram does not correlate with these other studies, additional views must be obtained to rule out lesions which may not be clearly evident on the original arteriogram. Thrombolysis for acute and subacute arterial occlusions is discussed in other chapters. The remainder of this chapter will cover interventional therapy for chronic atherosclerotic disease.

ILIAC ANGIOPLASTY

If an iliac lesion is identified or suspected, pressures must be obtained above and below the lesion to document its hemodynamic significance. Any resting gradient is considered significant. If no resting gradient is present, a vasodilator such as 60 mg of papaverine or 100 to 200 micrograms of nitroglycerine should be administered intra-arterially in the affected extremity. A peak systolic gradient of greater than 10 to 15 mm of mercury is considered significant. When the outflow is markedly obstructed (such as in the presence of both superficial femoral artery and profunda femoral artery disease), there may not be a demonstrable gradient despite the presence of a high grade stenosis. These lesions should be identified and treated preoperatively, otherwise the femoral popliteal reconstruction may be compromised due to inadequate flow. Although iliac angioplasty can be performed around the aortic bifurcation using the puncture site of the diagnostic arteriogram,[7] in most circumstances we choose to puncture the ipsilateral common femoral artery in a retrograde fashion. This approach allows for simultaneous arterial pressure measurements and also facilitates stent placement, if necessary.

Lesions that are ideally suited for angioplasty are short focal stenoses of the common iliac artery.[8] Tight stenoses should ideally be crossed using road mapping. The best guidewire catheter combination is dependent on the lesion and the operator. All intervention should be performed through a vascular sheath. The sheath usually facilitates the intervention, allows for easier postprocedure evaluation and is associated with a lower incidence of complications. All patients are pretreated with aspirin as an antiplatelet agent. Although many physicians use intraprocedural anticoagulation with heparin, its value is unconfirmed. Excessive use of heparin may lead to higher incidence of local complications such as hematomas and pseudoaneurysms.

Long lesions, external iliac artery lesions, and occlusions can also be treated. The optimal percutaneous therapy for iliac occlusions has not yet been determined. These lesions have been treated with initial lysis and angioplasty with or without stents of underlying lesions. Other successful treatments include primary stenting of iliac occlusions.[9] The response to balloon angioplasty of longer lesions may be less than ideal, however, if a suboptimal angioplasty or an occlusive dissection occurs. A stent—either a Palmaz balloon expandable stent (Johnson and Johnson) or a Wallstent (Schneider)—can be placed which will almost invariably convert a suboptimal angioplasty to a successful angioplasty. (This is also true for suboptimal angioplasty of ideal lesions.) After intervention, pressures must again be obtained to hemodynamically assess the adequacy of the intervention.

Most complications of angioplasty can be managed nonoperatively. The most common complication is a hematoma, which is usually self-limited. Pseudoaneurysms can be definitely treated using ultrasound guided compression.[10] In situ thrombosis during angioplasty can be treated with intra-arterial thrombolysis. Obstructing flaps can be stented.[11,12] Iliac rupture is the feared complication because these patients will require surgery to prevent exsanguination. Iliac rupture is suggested by the presence of continued pain after the angioplasty balloon is deflated and the presence of free extravasation of contrast after angioplasty. The angioplasty balloon should be immediately reinflated across the lesion to tamponade the rupture and the patient should be transferred to the operating room for repair of the vessel. Alternatively, a covered stent (if available) can be delivered via the femoral access to effectively exclude the rupture.

SUPERFICIAL FEMORAL AND POPLITEAL ARTERY INTERVENTION

Stenoses and/or occlusions of the superficial femoral artery and popliteal artery up to 10 cm in length are considered amenable to balloon angioplasty.[13,15,19] These lesions can be approached from the contralateral extremity using the common femoral artery access created during the diagnostic arteriogram.[7] Using an "over the corner" sheath markedly facilitates the advancement of balloon catheters across lesions using the contralateral approach. Alternatively, an antegrade puncture can be performed. An antegrade puncture can be technically challenging, especially in obese patients. One must be careful to enter the common femoral artery below the inguinal ligament and above its bifurcation. The guidewire must then be advanced into the superficial femoral artery. There have been several techniques developed to redirect the wire that preferentially advances into the profunda femoral artery. Once the wire is in place in the superficial femoral artery, a vascular sheath is introduced. Most physicians will anticoagulate patients during the procedure to prevent thrombus formation during the catheter manipulations and balloon inflation. Using road mapping, a directional catheter and floppy guidewire (choice of guidewire and catheter is operator- and lesion-dependent) are used to cross the lesion. The catheter is then exchanged for a balloon of appropriate size and length. The post-angioplasty result is evaluated by a repeat angiogram. Less than a 30 percent residual stenosis without embolic complication constitutes a successful result. If there is an obstructing flap or a residual stenosis, a prolonged dilatation can be attempted to improve this initial result. If an obstructing flap or a residual stenosis persists, a directional atherectomy device can be used to remove the residual plaque or obstructing flap.[15] In these circumstances, atherectomy may be useful in converting a failed angioplasty into a successful intervention. Alternatively, stents can be used to bridge obstructing flaps post-angioplasty,[1] however, the long-term patency of femopopliteal stents in this location is not well documented.

INFRAPOPLITEAL ANGIOPLASTY

The availability of low profile catheters and thinner wires has made tibial angioplasty technically feasible; additionally the results have been shown to be quite durable.[18,19] The indications for infrapopliteal angioplasty are primarily limb salvage. These patients require straight line flow to the foot by at least one of the three tibial vessels.[19] The challenge in these patients is to reestablish straight line flow in at least one of the three tibial vessels.

Infrapopliteal angioplasty should be performed by an antegrade puncture of the ipsilateral common femoral artery. The patient should be anticoagulated systemically throughout the entire procedure to prevent clot formation in the tibial vessels during catheter manipulation. The lesions should be crossed using road mapping. An 0.18 in platinum tip guidewire or glidewire (Turumo, Tokyo, Japan) should be used to cross the stenosis or occlusions. Low profile angioplasty balloons should be used. As opposed to iliac and femoral angioplasty, where the use of vasodilators may be helpful but nonessential, vasodilators in the tibial distribution are extremely helpful to avoid spasm in these small vessels.

The presence of long superficial femoral artery (SFA) occlusive disease requiring bypass and focal tibial lesions is not uncommon. An approach to be considered in this group of patients is an above knee bypass and an intraoperative angioplasty of the tibial vessels.[20] This combined approach can save limbs while preserving vein and reducing the morbidity associated with a distal bypass.

Revascularizing ischemic extremities is the goal of both interventional radiologists and vascular surgeons. This goal should be achieved with the lowest morbidity and mortality possible. Combining the techniques of the radiologist and surgeon will assure the best outcome in these challenging cases.

REFERENCES

1. Dotter CT, Judkins MP: Transluminal treatment of arteriosclerotic obstruction: Description of a new

technic and a preliminary report of its application. Circulation 1964;30:654.

2. Grüntzig A: Die perkutane rekavalisation chrovischer artelieller verschlusse (Dotter-Privzip) mit einem nemen doppellumingen dilatationskatheter. Rofo 1976;124:80.

3. Veith FJ, Gupta SK, Samson RH, et al: Progress in limb salvage by reconstructive arterial surgery combined with new or improved adjunctive procedures. Ann Surg 1981;194:386.

4. Seldinger S: Catheter replacement of needle in percutaneous arteriography: New technique. Acta Radiol (Stockh) 1953;39:378.

5. Gardiner GA, Meyerovitz MF, Stokes KR, et al: Complications of transluminal angioplasty. Radiology 1986;159:201.

6. Rupp SB, Vogelzang RL, Nemcek AA Jr, et al: Relationship of the inguinal ligament to pelvic radiographic landmarks: Anatomic correlation and its role in femoral arteriography. J Vasc Interv Radiol 1993;4:409.

7. Kashdan BJ, Trost DW, Jagust MB, et al: Retrograde approach for contralateral iliac and infrainguinal percutaneous transluminal angioplasty: Experience in 100 patients. J Vasc Interv Radiol 1992;3:515.

8. Guidelines for Percutaneous Transluminal Angioplasty. Standards of Practice Committee of the Society of Cardiovascular and Interventional Radiology. Radiology 1990;177:619.

9. Vorwerk D, Guenther RW, Schürman K, et al: Primary stent placement for chronic iliac artery occlusions: Follow-up results in 103 patients. Radiology 1995;194:745.

10. Coley BD, Roberts AC, Fellmeth BD, et al: Post-angiographic femoral artery pseudoaneurysms: Further experience with US-guided compression repair. Radiology 1995;194:307.

11. Becker GJ, Palmaz JC, Res CR, et al: Angioplasty-induced dissections in human iliac arteries: Management with Palmaz balloon-expandable intraluminal stents. Radiology 1990;176:31.

12. Gunther RW, Vorwerk D, Antonucci F, et al: Iliac artery stenosis or obstruction after unsuccessful balloon angioplasty: Treatment with a self-expandable stent. AJR 1991;156:389.

13. Standards of Practice Committee of the Society of Cardiovascular and Interventional Radiology: Guidelines for percutaneous and transluminal angioplasty. Radiology 1990;177:619.

14. Capek P, McLean GK, Berkowitz HD: Femoropopliteal angioplasty: Factors influencing long-term success. Circulation (suppl. I) 1991;83:I-70.

15. Becker GJ, Katzen BT, Dake MD: Noncoronary angioplasty. Radiology 1989;170:921.

16. Maynar M, Reyes R, Cabrera V, et al: Percutaneous atherectomy as an alternative treatment for post-angioplasty obstructive intimal flaps. Radiology 1989;170:1029.

17. Sapoval MR, Long AL, Raynaud AC, et al: Femoropopliteal stent placement: Long-term results. Radiology 1989;172:961.

18. Schwarten DE, Cutcliff WC: Arterial occlusive disease below the knee: Treatment with percutaneous transluminal angioplasty performed with low-profile catheters and steerable guidewires. Radiology 1988;169:71.

19. Bakal CW, Sprayregen S, Scheinbaum K, et al: Percutaneous transluminal angioplasty of the infrapopliteal arteries. AJR 1990;154:171.

16

Endovascular Imaging Techniques

RODNEY A. WHITE

Endovascular imaging techniques, including angiography, angioscopy, and intraluminal ultrasound, are evolving rapidly as the devices and techniques for endovascular procedures develop. Although arteriography was addressed in detail in the preceding chapter, a brief description of its role and interface with other endovascular imaging methods is included in this chapter.

ANGIOGRAPHY

Angiography is the "gold standard" for imaging the distribution and severity of vascular lesions. Uniplanar angiography can be quite accurate in defining vessel luminal dimensions and cross-sectional area if the luminal profile is circular, as it is in most normal and mildly diseased arteries. The method is also very useful to demonstrate the distribution and continuity of patent vessels.

In severe disease, arteriography yields limited information regarding the morphology or extent of disease in the arterial wall, aside from demonstrating visible calcification and the topography of the luminal surface. Clinically significant atherosclerosis is usually eccentrically positioned in the arterial lumen, and the lumen may be either circular or elliptical in shape. In instances where the lumen is elliptical, biplanar angiograms more accurately define luminal cross-sectional areas and allow better calculation of percentage area stenosis than do conventional uniplanar views.[1] The cross-sectional area of the vessel lumen is estimated using vessel diameters measured from the angiograms.

Unless the lumen is circular, the accuracy of this method can be limited.

The quality of equipment available for radiologic imaging during vascular procedures varies from traditional C-arm fluoroscopes to sophisticated high-resolution intensifiers and television monitoring systems. Conventional angiographic techniques often lack good spatial and contrast resolution and may require multiple reinjections of contrast material to visualize the entire field of interest. Digital subtraction techniques have increased contrast sensitivity, allowing detection of low levels of iodinated contrast material. Many digital units have freeze-frame and "road-mapping" features that permit superimposition of a subtracted contrast image of the stenotic or occluded vessel on a live fluoroscopic image. The real-time image of the manipulation of guidewires or angioplasty instruments can then be viewed overlying the retained angiographic road map of the lesion, enhancing the safety and accuracy of the intervention by constant visual guidance.

ANGIOSCOPY

Angioscopy, the endoscopic examination of the luminal anatomy of blood vessels, is being used to establish the diagnosis and etiology of vascular diseases, to evaluate the technical accuracy of vascular reconstructions, and to visualize intraluminal instrumentation. Available devices range from 0.5 to 3.3 mm in diameter and have high-quality fiberoptic imaging systems and light sources that enable intraluminal inspection of small-diameter vessels.

Angioscopy Equipment

For angioscopy of peripheral vessels larger than 3 mm in diameter, a multichannel endoscopic catheter that incorporates a fluid channel for irrigation of the vessel lumen to keep the field of view and lens free of blood is recommended. Angioscopes which include a fluid channel are approximately 2.5 mm in diameter. This channel or additional channels in larger devices can be used for passage of guidewires, snares, laser fibers or other instruments. The larger angioscopes (2.5 to 3.3 mm in diameter) are suited for most peripheral vascular procedures, while 0.5- to 1.7-mm-diameter instruments are required for smaller vessels, such as the coronary or tibial arteries. The smaller designs sacrifice the fluid lumen to provide a narrower catheter diameter.

Angioscopic visualization is enhanced by coupling the scopes to a video camera that enlarges the image. In this way, the field of view can be projected on a television monitor and is magnified 40 to 200 times. Permanent recordings of the procedure can be made using an on-line video recorder. Using the improved angioscopes and video display, intravascular detail with greater than 0.2-mm spatial resolution at 5 mm is achieved, and the minimum focus distance ranges from 2.0 to 6.5 mm.[2] A high-power light source of at least 300 W is required to provide sufficient illumination to obtain adequate images through the fiberoptics in most devices. Light sources that are available in hospitals for gastrointestinal and surgical endoscopy are usually about 100 to 150 W power.

Blood is cleared from the field of view by infusion of fluid, usually heparinized saline, under pressure either through a channel in the scope or through a catheter placed coaxial to the angioscope. A pressure bag at 300 mmHg is satisfactory to deliver the irrigant at a rate of 30 to 75 ml/min, although roller pump systems with foot-pedal controls to regulate the rate of fluid irrigation are the best alternatives.

Reusable angioscopes, video camera, and cables are all gas sterilizable and are set up on a sterile field on a sidetable prior to procedures. At all times these instruments must be handled with care be-

cause of the fragility of the optical fibers. Immediately following use, blood is cleared from the tubing and internal channels of the devices to avoid deterioration of the optics. Ethylene oxide gas sterilization and airing procedures take 12 to 18 hours, so each angioscope usually can be used in only one procedure each day. Disposable angioscopes are also available and can be used as an alternative when reusable scopes are being sterilized.

Angioscopy Technique

PERCUTANEOUS ANGIOSCOPY

To provide access to the vessel being evaluated, Seldinger technique is used for puncture and for guidewire insertion into the lumen. A dilatation catheter is inserted over the guidewire, and this is followed by an introducer catheter. A number of hemostatic introducer sheaths are available for this purpose.

There are several problems in achieving good images with percutaneous angioscopes. Some currently available systems are relatively stiff, which makes control and centering of the devices difficult. To aid manipulation of the tip of the scope, a steering mechanism in at least one plane is desirable. Control of proximal blood flow in the area being examined is achieved by inflation of a balloon on the tip of the catheter. A rapid flow of irrigating solution through the delivery catheter is then required to control blood from collateral vessels. Back-bleeding from the distal circulation also can be limited by having an assistant apply a tourniquet around the distal point of an extremity.

Percutaneous angioscopy is currently being used as a method to inspect the vessel lumen before procedures and to define the mechanisms and accuracy of interventions. In these procedures, angioscopy is performed before the angioplasty device is inserted. Using the percutaneous technique, the angioscope and delivery catheter must be removed during an intervention, since both the angioscope and the angioplasty device will not fit simultaneously through the percutaneous access. Following completion of the angioplasty, which is performed using fluoroscopic monitoring, the angioscope is reinserted to inspect the recanalized vessel. Small intimal flaps, mural thrombus, laser-thermal damage to the vessel wall, and balloon dilatation cracks in the wall are all easily visualized if blood can be cleared adequately from the arterial lumen (Fig. 16-1).

Percutaneous angioscopy has been particularly useful for studying the pathogenesis of vascular diseases and for determining the appropriate treatment modality. For example, angioscopy performed during cardiac catheterization has been shown to be useful in redefining the role of complex atheroma and thrombosis in myocardial ischemia where no lesion was apparent or one was misinterpreted on coronary angiography.[3]

INTRAOPERATIVE ANGIOSCOPY

Angioscopy can be performed intraoperatively in approximately 10 minutes or less through an opening in the vessel. To perform the intraluminal inspection, vascular occlusion is obtained by conventional operative means or by a balloon on the end of the angioscope. Infusion of saline under approximately 300 mmHg pressure (30 to 75 ml/min) through an irrigation channel in the angioscope or by a coaxial catheter clears the intraluminal blood and enables visualization in approximately 80 to 90 percent of cases.

Figure 16-1. Intimal flaps (I) that remain following a balloon angioplasty of the superficial femoral artery lesion.

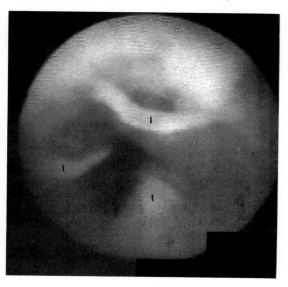

Clinical Applications of Angioscopy

MONITORING OF SURGICAL PROCEDURES

Several investigators have reported that angioscopy reveals clinically important information that is not apparent by extraluminal inspection, probing, or angiography in 15 to 30 percent of vascular procedures.[4-6] The angioscopic findings have altered the surgical therapy in a significant number of these cases. In my own prospective evaluations, angioscopic findings differed significantly from preoperative or intraoperative angiograms in 24 percent of cases, resulting in an alteration in the operation in 17 percent.[6]

ANGIOSCOPIC THROMBECTOMY

I have found that performing embolectomy and thrombectomy of peripheral vessels is greatly enhanced by angioscopy.[7] Unless the whole length of vessel is occluded, the angioscope may be introduced initially through the arteriotomy to inspect the lumen and define the exact site and extent of thrombosis or embolism and to determine whether there is preexisting atherosclerotic disease. Fogarty catheters may then be passed beside the angioscope if the arterial lumen is large enough to accommodate both devices. Balloon inflation and detachment and removal of thrombus and debris can then be monitored visually.

Direct visual observation of the degree of inflation of the balloon is quite important because it allows determination of the amount of balloon distension necessary for adequate removal of the lesion without causing injury to the vessel related to overinflation. Frequently, balloon catheters slide over thrombus that is adherent to the wall, leaving large fragments which may or may not be removed with repeated passes of the catheter and which are frequently not adequately demonstrated by completion arteriograms. When adherent thrombus is observed, further attempts at retrievel may be made by positioning the balloon just distal to the clot and by then oscillating the balloon back and forth over the site. If this is not successful, a decision must be made as to whether or not it is warranted to attempt extraction by other instruments such as flexible grasping forceps, rotatory atherectomy devices, or vascular brushes. A further possible alternative is the intraoperative use of fibrinolytic agents.

When thromboembolectomy is considered complete, a final angioscopic inspection of the entire artery is made. Angiographic examination of the smaller runoff vessels may be obtained by injection of contrast medium through the fluid channel of the angioscope before the scope is withdrawn and the arteriotomy is closed. One of the advantages offered by angioscopy is that complications and technical errors such as retained thrombus or intimal flaps can be corrected while the arterial lumen is still open and before blood flow is restored. The angiogram usually fails to demonstrate the smaller irregularities of the wall caused by intimal flaps or adherent thrombus and may underestimate larger lesions as well. These aspects are seen quite easily with the three-dimensional intraluminal view provided by the angioscope.

Transfemoral thromboembolectomy of the iliac artery is performed by initially clearing blindly about 80 percent of the length of occlusion with the Fogarty catheter and then introducing the angioscope to inspect the lumen for retained thrombus, mural defects, and atherosclerotic plaque. After the remainder of the iliac segment has been reopened, the Fogarty catheter is inflated at the level of the aortic bifurcation to impede blood flow and enable inspection of the thrombectomized vessel. If there is good collateral flow through branches of the iliac artery, it may be quite difficult to overcome the blood in the field to obtain an adequate view. Similar techniques are used for thromboembolectomy in an occluded limb of an aortobifemoral graft (Fig. 16-2). In this case, the absence of blood flow from branch vessels ensures a relatively blood-free field.

Femoral-popliteal-tibial thromboembolectomy is performed through a groin incision and by obtaining exposure and control of the common femoral, profunda, and superficial femoral arteries. An arteriotomy is performed, and the angioscope is first inserted into the profunda femoris artery, where it will usually pass easily to a distance of 20 to 25 cm. Because of the narrow diameter of this artery, the Fogarty catheter cannot be inserted at the same time, so angioscopic monitoring of throm-

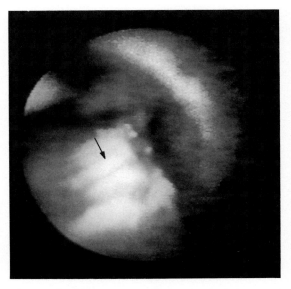

Figure 16-2. Angioscopic examination of a segment of the iliac limb of an aortoiliac graft near the femoral anastomosis. There is a kink (*arrow*) in the posterior wall of the prosthesis that was easily corrected by extension of the graft by an additional segment of prosthetic material. (Reproduced with permission from White RA, White GH: Angioscopic endovascular surgical techniques. *In* Color Atlas of Endovascular Surgery. London, Chapman & Hall, 1990, p 116.)

boembolectomy of the profunda is limited to inspection before and after passage of the balloon.

In the superficial femoral artery and within prosthetic bypass grafts in this position, the Fogarty catheter will pass comfortably alongside the angioscope so that the whole procedure can be monitored visually. At the distal popliteal level, the orifices of each of the tibial arteries can be identified, and selective cannulation with the Fogarty catheter is often possible. This is achieved by slightly bending the catheter tip to enhance cannulation. It is more difficult to achieve access to the anterior tibial artery because of the severe angle. On occasion, selective cannulation of the tibial artery can avert exposure of the vessels below the knee to retrieve embolic or thrombotic material.

In prosthetic grafts, extensive buildup of neointimal hyperplasia may be difficult to differentiate from chronic thrombus. Use of alternative instruments such as forceps, curettes, and brushes is probably safer here than in the native vessels.

Inspection of the distal anastomosis is important, since this is often the site of hyperplastic stenosis. Twists or kinks of the graft also can be identified by angioscopic inspection.

Thrombectomy of the iliac and femoral veins is challenging because tenacious adherence of clot to the vein wall and the physical barrier of the valves make angioscopy difficult. Vollmar et al.[7] have reported the results of more than 200 endoscopic procedures in the venous system and note that angioscopy was superior to venograms for demonstration of residual thrombus, poor operative result, and the presence of venous spurs in the left common iliac vein. When incomplete thrombectomy was demonstrated endoscopically, this group constructed a temporary peripheral arteriovenous fistula as a means of improving patency rates.

In a preliminary series, my colleagues and I[8] reported that residual thrombus was identified angioscopically within arteries and grafts after standard thromboembolectomy procedures in approximately 80 percent of cases. The direct three-dimensional view obtained provided significantly more information regarding luminal compromise than did contrast radiologic imaging. Further experience in more than 60 cases of thromboembolectomy has revealed some residual thrombus after passage of the balloon in almost every treated vessel or graft. This was an unexpected finding, since angiograms of the same site often have appeared relatively normal. In many cases, the missed clot is quite small and probably would not significantly jeopardize the outcome. This is most likely with soft mural thrombus that is closely attached to the wall and is not stenotic. In such instances, the balloon catheter has been observed to pass between the vessel wall and the clot without dislodging it.

With lesser amounts of thrombus, especially nonobstructing mural thrombus, it is difficult to judge whether further attempts at removal are indicated. It is likely that many of these minor defects would normally be resolved by the natural fibrinolytic and healing processes. During angioscopic thrombectomy, infusion of the irrigating fluid simulates blood flow, thus giving a dynamic representation of potential flaps and loose debris.

In general, I have observed that balloon thromboembolectomy often results in only partial removal of the obstructing material. I have also noted that mural thrombus often simulates spasm on angiograms and that good backflow does not necessarily correlate with a satisfactory result. I have elected to attempt removal of as much of this material as possible by further passes of the balloon catheter, as well as by other instruments if the residual thrombus is considered significant. In other cases, severe dissections or atherosclerotic stenosis or occlusion that could not be treated has led me to proceed immediately to vascular bypass rather than persist with unproductive attempts at thrombectomy.

ANGIOSCOPY-ASSISTED IN SITU VEIN BYPASSES

Observing the completeness of valvulotomy in in situ vein bypasses has improved the technical accuracy of the procedure and reduced the operative time by ensuring complete incompetence of valve cusps. The valvulotome is inserted through a side branch of the upper segment of the saphenous vein or through the vein lumen at the distal end. The valulotome is passed proximally from the distal vein through the most proximal valve, and the angioscope is inserted proximally and passed distal until the valvulotome can be visualized at the valve site. I prefer to perform the valvulotomy using a Mills valvulotome because this device can be visualized and controlled easily by angioscopic inspection and does not obstruct the field of vision. Incompetence of valve cusps is easily tested under direct vision by distending the vein with saline infusion and compressing the vein lumen by external pressure (Fig. 16-3). As valve cusps are serially disrupted, the valvulotome and angioscope are advanced distally to the next valve.

Intraluminal identification of tributary veins during the procedure helps limit dissection and isolation of the vein and prevents tears in the vein caused by hooking a side branch with the valvulotome. Microinstruments that can be passed through a lumen in an angioscope or coaxial to the scope to enhance accurate and expedient valvulotomy under direct vision are also available. During the procedure, extreme care must be taken to prevent damaging the vein with the intraluminal instruments. Angioscopes too small to pass easily through the lumen can produce severe trauma.

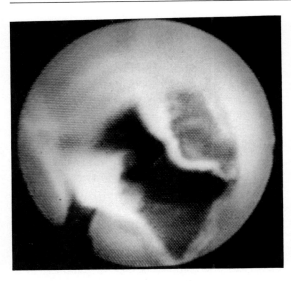

Figure 16-3. Division of the valve cusps after a single pass of a Mills valvulotome. The cusp is seen to be torn and shredded, and flow of fluid through the valve shows it to be incompetent. (Reproduced with permission from White RA, White GH: Angioscopy. *In* Color Atlas of Endovascular Surgery. London, Chapman & Hall, 1990, p 109.)

ANGIOSCOPIC MONITORING OF ANGIOPLASTY PROCEDURES

Angioscopy has an appealing theoretically advantage over arteriography for monitoring angioplasty procedures in that it helps reduce the hazards of radiation exposure and contrast reactions and allows immediate detection and correction of technical complications. Arteriography tends to underestimate wall irregularities and stenosis. Angioscopic inspection under magnification and video control has enabled placement of the intraluminal devices without deviation into collateral vessels. Proximal stenotic lesions or tapering of the vessel near the site of an occlusion limits angioscopic inspection and prevents clear visualization of the occlusion. Angioscopy following angioplasty has been extremely helpful in determining the adequacy of recanalizations, inspecting the surface for fragments, and helping to determine the mechanism of action of recanalization devices. An example of the utility of angioscopic monitoring of angioplasty procedures is the evaluation of laser angioplasty in patients with long or multisegmental

arterial occlusions who have been treated by laser thermal–assisted balloon angioplasty in the operating room.[9] Inspection of the recanalized segment frequently showed charring of the walls after plaque vaporization, with some fragmentation and mural thrombus typical of balloon-dilated arteries.[10]

Another benefit of intraoperative angioscopy is that the examination is conducted before restoration of blood flow and may help prevent embolization of fragments of arterial wall or thrombus. Angioscopy examinations are limited in that assessment of distal smaller vessels is usually not possible because of the angioscope diameters. Examination of normal vessels beyond the treated segment may cause intimal lesions or induce spasm. Angiography of the distal vasculature can be performed by injecting contrast material through a channel in the scope. This allows direct correlation of the angiogram and angioscopic image.

I have not found angioscopy to be very beneficial during the angioplasty procedure itself, since in most cases one cannot see the probe once it has entered an occlusion. Angioscopy has therefore been of only partial help in preventing perforations. This experience parallels that of Abela and Seegar,[11] who found that with angioscopy used to control the position of the laser fiber, perforation was still a frequent occurrence in early cases but was avoided in later patients as improved techniques were developed. These authors concluded that the use of angioscopy as a method of positioning the laser fiber appeared to be associated with a lower rate of vessel perforation than previously reported for laser angioplasty. An obvious limitation of current angioscopic equipment is that there is no way to evaluate the vessel thickness or concentricity of lesions. In the future, combining angioscopy with transmural intraluminal ultrasound imaging may provide a complete perspective on vessel morphology.

Angioscopic monitoring of angioplasty procedures has broadened the ability to treat intimal flaps or dissections detected after thrombectomy or angioplasty by enabling intraluminal removal of lesions using flexible grasping forceps and other instruments. Removal of thrombogenic arterial dissections and flaps of the iliac, femoral, and popliteal arteries by flexible forceps introduced remotely by means of the femoral artery under angioscopic control has been performed in 8 patients with traumatic intimal flaps (5 iatrogenic, 3 external trauma). In addition, tightly occlusive arterial thrombi were removed with flexible biopsy forceps in 10 of 64 (16 percent) patients.[12]

Overview of the Utility of Angioscopy

At present, angioscopy provides an alternative to angiography with the advantage of providing repeatable three-dimensional intraluminal views before blood flow is restored. Potential complications of angioscopy include vessel perforation and fluid overload from excessive administration of irrigant fluid, producing intimal trauma and embolization. Fluid overload can be averted by occlusion of both the vessel being inspected and its collateral branches or by performing the procedures with a tourniquet on the extremity. Inspecting vessels that approximate or are smaller than the diameter of the angioscope can produce spasm and possible thrombosis. The clarity of angioscopic images is usually excellent, but adequate cleaning of blood flow from collateral and distal vessels by fluid infusion and centering of the device for examinations require an initial learning curve. These are frequently the factors that limit visualization, although adequate examinations can be performed in approximately 85 percent of cases.

Future developments may lead to a combination of angioscopy and intraluminal ultrasound technologies to provide an accurate assessment of the three-dimensional anatomy of the vessel wall. Small diameter catheters (nos. 3 to 8 Fr) with an ultrasound transducer on the distal end are under development and have been shown to provide an accurate delineation of vessel wall thickness and consistency while also demonstrating areas of vessel wall dissection and intimal flaps.[13] The combination of the luminal anatomy and surface topography supplied by angioscopy and the information regarding the vessel wall provided by ultrasound may solve a current limitation of intraluminal angioplasty devices: precise recanalization and debulking of lesions.

At present, angioscopy is finding widespread acceptance in the vascular surgical community, with benefits being demonstrated in preliminary studies using this technology to evaluate the technical accuracy of repairs and for improving the speed and completeness of thrombectomies and valvulotomies in in situ vein bypasses. The role of the device in guidance of angioplasty devices is yet to be determined, although the device is of significant benefit for inspecting lesions prior to intervention and determining the mechanism and adequacy of recanalizations following the procedure.

INTRAVASCULAR ULTRASOUND IMAGING

Intravascular ultrasound (IVUS) has developed rapidly in the last few years. By providing an accurate luminal and transmural image of vascular structures, IVUS displays vascular pathology and illustrates immediate results of interventions. In addition to obvious diagnostic applications, the potential significance of IVUS has become even more apparent due to the simultaneous development of minimally invasive catheter-based therapeutic techniques, including balloon angioplasty, atherectomy, laser angioplasty, and intravascular stents. The thrust of current development is to incorporate IVUS as an adjunct to peripheral and coronary angioplasty procedures. It is probable that IVUS will become a critical component of future interventional devices, and an understanding of the technique will be essential for individuals involved in the management of patients with cardiovascular disease.

Device Development and Imaging Configurations

A major advantage of diagnostic ultrasound is that it avoids ionizing radiation and intravenous contrast agents. Conventional transcutaneous ultrasound has limited ability to assess structures obscured by bone or air and to obtain fine resolution of deep-lying tissues. By attaching the ultrasound transducer to an intraluminal catheter and increasing the frequency of the ultrasound energy, there is enhanced interrogation and resolution of organs that are poorly accessible to transcutaneous ultrasound.

IVUS CATHETER DESIGN

The first IVUS prototypes were used to measure intracardiac dimensions and cardiac motion in the

1950s, utilizing A-mode transducers fixed to large intraluminal catheters.[14,15] Various devices (A-, B-, and M-mode) were developed for both intravascular and transesophageal imaging of vascular structures, but it was not until early 1970s that true intraluminal cross-sectional imaging of vessels was reported using a multielement array transducer.[16–19] In order to obtain a 360-degree cross-sectional image, the ultrasound beam must be scanned through a full circle, and the beam direction and deflection on the display must be synchronized. This can be achieved by mechanically rotating the imaging elements or by using electronically switched phased arrays (Fig. 16-4).

Current multiple-element IVUS catheters utilize frequencies in the range of 10 to 30 MHz. The plane of imaging is perpendicular to the long axis of the catheter and provides a full 360 degree image of the blood vessel. A problem of the early phased array devices was the electronic noise caused by the multiple wires within the catheter itself, since each of the 32 elements was an independent minitransducer needing its own connections. This problem was later overcome by the incorporation of a miniature integrated circuit at the tip of the catheter which provided

Figure 16-4. (A) Schematic diagram of a mechanical ultrasound device with rotating (1) and fixed (2) elements. Either the transducer or the mirror may be fixed with the other element in a rotating position. (B) Schematic diagram of a phased-array device with the elements arranged circumferentially around the tip of the catheter. (Reproduced with permission from White RA: Indications for fiberoptic angioscopy and intraluminal ultrasound. Compr Ther 1990;16:23.)

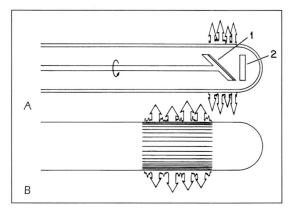

sequenced transmission and reception without the need for numerous electric circuits traveling the full length of the catheter. In addition to reducing the electronic noise, this modification simplified the manufacturing complexity and improved the flexibility of the catheter. A problem of these imaging catheters, common to all high-frequency ultrasound devices to some extent, is the inability to image structures in the immediate vicinity of the transducer, i.e., in the "near field." Because the imaging crystals in a phased-array configuration are in almost direct contact with the structure being imaged, a bright circumferential artifact known as the *ring down* surrounds the catheter. The ring-down artifact can be removed electronically, but structures within the masked region will not be seen.

Mechanical transducers are the most frequently used type of IVUS catheters and are one of two basic configurations; either the transducer itself or an acoustic mirror is rotated at the tip of the catheter using a flexible, high-torque cable that extends the length of the device. Some catheters use a transducer that is angled slightly forward of perpendicular, which produces a cone-shaped ultrasound beam resulting in an image of the vessel slightly forward or in front of the transducer assembly. Devices that utilize a rotating acoustic reflector have the mirror set at a 45-degree angle to the rotating shaft, producing an image that is perpendicular to the axis of the catheter. In both rotating-transducer and rotating-mirror devices, ultrasound frequencies between 12.5 and 30 MHz are generally used, although some experimental devices using frequencies up to 45 MHz have produced excellent images of human arteries in vitro.[20]

In the rotating-mirror devices, the ultrasound energy produced by the fixed transducer at the distal tip of the catheter is directed toward an angled mirror placed a short distance proximally. In addition to avoiding the need for rotating the transducer, an advantage of this configuration is afforded by the necessary distance between the transducer and the rotating mirror, partially eliminating the ring-down image artifact and the poor resolution near field of the scan. Both these problems are substantially reduced by allowing the ultrasound energy to travel a short distance in the imaging chamber filled with saline. The scan converter in the image-processing unit compensates for this nonimaging portion of the beam and generates images beginning at the surface of the catheter. In the rotating-transducer and multiple-array devices, a part of the ring-down region and near-field zone of the beam occurs outside the catheter, so it is not possible to image clearly in this area. However, both types of mechanical imaging catheters suffer less from image loss due to these problems than the phased-array trans ducers.[21] In devices with a distally placed transducer and proximal rotating mirror, it is necessary for an electrical connecting wire to pass along the side of the imaging assembly. This wire produces an artifact that occupies approximately 15 degrees of the image cross section. A similar artifact is generated in any device where a wire passes along the side of the imaging element. An interesting modification of the mechanical catheter design involves rotation of both the transducer and the mirror, offering the advantage of no electrical wire artifact. Current disposable mechanical catheters use a saline- or water-filled imaging chamber that must be rendered and maintained bubble-free to allow adequate imaging.

Miniaturization of the moving parts of the mechanical systems is a major limitation that may ultimately separate these devices from phased-array catheters in their utility in smaller-caliber vessels. On the other hand, as phased-array catheters are used in progressively smaller vessels, the problems of ring down and near-field imaging become more apparent. The smallest currently available mechanical catheters (no. 2.9 Fr or 0.9 mm diameter) approximate the size of diseased coronary arteries and, when used with higher-frequency ultrasound, may prove to be superior in most applications.

COMPUTERIZED THREE-DIMENSIONAL IMAGE RECONSTRUCTION

Three-dimensional (3D) intravascular ultrasound imaging has developed as a result of advances in digital computer graphics technology and mass data storage capabilities of personal computers. Algorithms of 3D image reconstruction can be classified as either surface or volume rendering; currently available 3D IVUS imaging utilizes surface rendering. Object surfaces are explicitly formed prior to creating their depiction on a 2D screen using techniques such as hidden-part removal, shading, translucency, dynamic rotation, and stereo projection.[22] With this technology, a longitudinally aligned set (up to 300 images per set) of consecutive 2D images obtained during a "pullback" through a vessel segment is assembled in sequence to produce the 3D image (Image Comm, Inc., Santa Clara, Calif.)[23] (Fig. 16-5). The pullback is performed by withdrawing the imaging catheter at a uniform rate using a mechanical device at a rate of 1 cm every 4 s. The 2D intravascular ultrasound data set from a 5-cm vessel segment is therefore represented by a 20-s pullback, which can be recorded on videotape or reconstructed on-line. The images are then sampled in digital format, following analogue-to-digital conversion, at rates of up to 7.5 frames per second (150 frames for a 20-s pullback). Currently, most processing is accomplished using data sets recorded on magnetic videotape. Preacquisition of these data provides the advantage of selection of the most suitable segments for reconstruction and allows the user to adjust screen cropping parameters to electronically eliminate the artifact of the IVUS catheter and other unwanted image data.

Computer processing time of approximately 12 s is required for the initial reconstruction of a high-resolution gray-scale longitudinal 2D view of the vessel segment. Prior to final 3D reconstruction, the image-density threshold is adjusted to optimize differentiation of structures. This step is particularly important when it is necessary to separate tissues of similar echodensity, i.e., soft plaque and thrombus. The 3D image is then displayed in multiple orientations to allow inspection of the arterial segment in all possible projections, both from within the lumen and from the adventitial surface. Other parameters such as image sharpness, contrast, and ambient light can be altered to improve the resolution of particular features being examined in the reconstructions. Images of the luminal volume alone also can be produced by removing vessel wall signals.

Although it has been shown that 2D cross-sectional intravascular ultrasound and longitudinal gray-scale reconstructions provide accurate

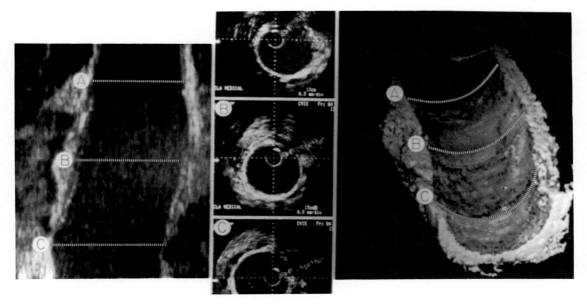

Figure 16-5. The 2D images labeled A, B, and C (*center panel*) are "stacked" by the computer and correspond to the sites labeled with the same letters on the 3D image (*right*) and longitudinal section of the 3D image (*left*). The longitudinal section of the 3D image is displayed on the computer monitor to allow optimal adjustments of the image density threshold and viewing orientation. (Reproduced with permission from Cavaye DM, Tabbara M, Kopchek G, et al: Three-dimensional vascular ultrasound imaging. Am Surg 1991;57:751.)

luminal and transmural dimensions, the accuracy of currently available 3D imaging has not been established. By viewing all three image formats simultaneously on a screen, however, the location of the 2D image site along the length of the 3D image can be identified using a linear cursor, and dimensions of a site on the 3D image can be estimated. A continuing problem associated with many 3D imaging techniques is the near-field effect of the ultrasound imaging catheters at frequencies of 20 to 30 MHz, resulting in bright imaging of the blood immediately surrounding the catheter. As the 3D imaging software has improved, it has allowed manipulation of the image data to reduce the blood artifact, but this problem still remains in some images because of the inherent features of the imaging catheter.

FORWARD-LOOKING INTRAVASCULAR ULTRASOUND

An exciting recent advance is the development of forward-looking IVUS, utilizing acoustic beams that radiate in the shape of a cone from the front of a no. 7.5 Fr catheter (Echo Cath, Ltd., Princeton, N.J.).[24] A 27-MHz transducer fills a 60-degree divergent cone with 2000 sequential beams each comprised of 64 axially aligned acoustic measurements. The result is a 3D image of a volume shaped like a truncated cone, with the near surface located 5 mm from the catheter tip and extending forward 9 mm to the most distant surface (Fig. 16-6). Although this system is experimental, it provides new and unique imaging data that may be critical for guidance of endoluminal devices in treating occlusive vascular lesions.

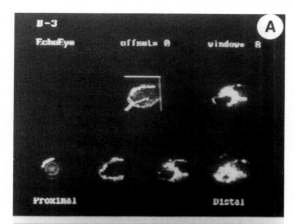

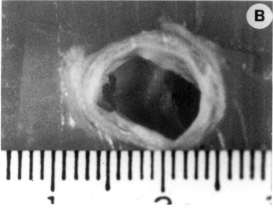

Figure 16-6. (**A**) FL-IVUS images and (**B**) gross specimen of an arterial bifurcation. Serial cross-sectional images show branching of main lumen into two distal branch vessels and structure of the prominent flow divider. (Reproduced with permission from Back M, et al: Forward-looking intravascular ultrasonography: In vitro imaging of normal and atherosclerotic human arteries. Am Surg 1994;60:738.)

An additional forward-looking IVUS prototype also has been evaluated in vitro in canine and human arteries.[25] The system consists of a 4-mm-diameter catheter (Cardiovascular Imaging Systems, Sunnyvale, Calif.) that provides B-mode cross-sectional ultrasound data for a distance of up to 2 cm distal to the catheter. The initial evaluations confirm that the device provides forward-viewing images corresponding to the arterial geometry and vascular landmarks and atherosclerotic lesions. Further utility of the forward-looking prototypes awaits additional in vivo evaluation.

IVUS Imaging Techniques

Intravascular ultrasound catheters can be introduced either percutaneously or through a standard arterial access sheath (no. 7 Fr to no. 9 Fr) or through an opening in a vessel during a surgical procedure. If large vessels proximal to the arteriotomy are imaged (e.g., iliac artery imaging via a femoral cutdown), a hemostatic access device should be used to reduce blood loss and prevent catheter damage during insertion. Most devices can be passed over a guidewire, which allows more controlled maneuvering of the device within the lumen of the vessel from a remote introduction site, particularly in tortuous or tightly stenotic vessels.

It is important to orientate the IVUS catheter within the vessel so that anteroposterior accuracy can be achieved. The best methods to maintain orientation are to use the image artifact produced by the transducer connecting wires and by establishing correct initial alignment at the point of catheter insertion. For example, when imaging the aortoiliac segments via a femoral puncture site, rotational alignment can be confirmed by the relative position of anatomic landmarks such as the aortic and iliac bifurcation. Because the catheters are rotationally rigid, there is very little loss of orientation with torquing and manipulation during imaging. Careful positioning of the catheter tip within the vessel and appropriate size matching of the device to the artery caliber are essential to optimize visualization. Image quality is best when the catheter is parallel to the vessel wall (i.e., the ultrasound beam is directed at 90 degrees to the luminal surface), while minor angulations may affect the luminal shape and dimensional accuracy. Eccentric positioning causes the vessel wall nearer the imaging chamber to appear more echogenic than the distant wall, producing an artifactual difference in wall thicknesses. Positioning the catheter in the center of the lumen is especially difficult in tortuous vessels and is often best achieved as the catheter is withdrawn rather than during advancement. Luminal flushing with saline or a radiographic contrast agent has been reported to improve delineation of acoustic interfaces in medium- and small-sized vessels.[26,27]

Clinical Utility of Intravascular Ultrasound

DISEASE DISTRIBUTION AND CHARACTERIZATION

Several studies have reported that IVUS is accurate in determining the luminal and vessel wall morphology of normal or minimally diseased arteries both in vitro and in vivo.[28-33] In muscular arteries, distinct sonographic layers are visible with the media, appearing as an echolucent layer sandwiched between the more echodense intima and adventitia (Fig. 16-7). The precise correlation between the ultrasound image and the microscopic anatomy of the muscular artery wall is still uncertain. The internal and external elastic laminae and adventitia are considered to be the backscatter substrates for the inner and outer echodense zones.[28,34] Precise measurements of the adventitia may be difficult to obtain unless the vessel is surrounded by tissues of differing echogenicity, e.g., echolucent fat. Even small intimal lesions such as flaps or intimal tears are well visualized because of their high fibrous tissue content and the difference in echoic properties of these structures when compared with surrounding blood. The three-layer appearance of muscular arteries is not readily seen in larger vessels (e.g., aorta) because of the increased elastin content in the media.

Intravascular ultrasound devices are sensitive in differentiating calcified and noncalcified vascular lesions. Because the ultrasound energy is strongly reflected by calcific plaque, it appears as a bright image with dense acoustic shadowing behind it (see Fig. 16-7). For this reason, the exact location of the media and adventitia cannot be seen in segments of vessels containing heavily calcific disease, and dimensions must be estimated by interpolation of adjacent size data. Gussenhoven et al.[34] have described four basic plaque components that can be distinguished using 40-MHz IVUS in vitro[34]: echolucent (lipid deposit, lipid "lake"), soft echoes (fibromuscular tissue or intimal proliferation, including varying amounts of diffusely dispersed lipid), bright echoes (collagen-rich fibrous tissue), and bright echoes with acoustic shadowing (calcified tissue).

Numerous investigations have compared angiography and IVUS for determining luminal and transmural dimensions of normal and moderately

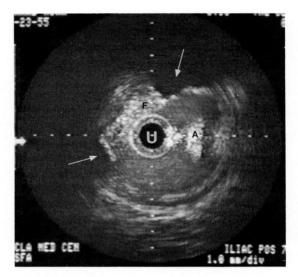

Figure 16-7. Intravascular ultrasound image of atherosclerotic human iliac artery. A large calcified plaque (*arrows*) produces a bright luminal line with acoustic showing behind it (*f*, fibrous plaque; *u*, ultrasound catheter void; *a*, imaging artifact). (Reproduced with permission from Tabbara M, White R, Cavaye D, et al: In vivo human comparison of intravascular ultrasound and angiography. J Vasc Surg 1991;14:496.)

atherosclerotic human arteries.[33,35,36] The cross-sectional areas calculated from biplanar angiograms and measured from IVUS correlate well for normal or minimally diseased peripheral arteries in vivo. Most studies reveal that IVUS and angiography also correlate well when used to image mildly elliptical lumens, but when used to derive dimensions from severely diseased vessels, the angiogram tends to underestimate the severity of disease. By offering a method to define the luminal and transmural morphology and dimensions, IVUS provides a new perspective from which to investigate arterial disease.

Recent studies have compared 2D and 3D IVUS with angiography and 3D computed tomography (CT) for images of abdominal aortic aneurysms.[37] Each modality provides unique information regarding the anatomy of the aorta and the distribution of components of the aneurysm (Figs. 16-8 and 16-9). In the case illustrated in the figures, the aortogram confirmed that the aneurysm was confined to the infrarenal aorta and

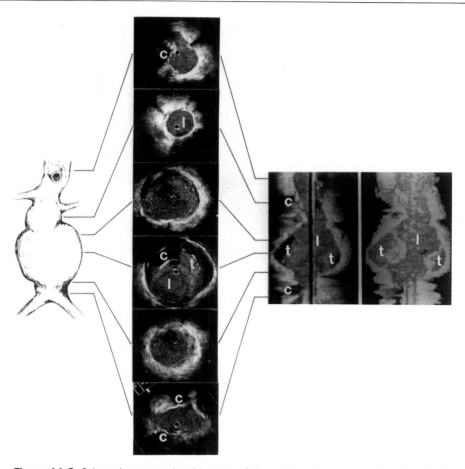

Figure 16-8. Selected cross-sectional images of the aorta and aneurysm at various levels (*center*) compared with a schematic diagram of the lesion (*left*) and the longitudinal gray-scale and 3D IVUS images (*right*) of the aneurysm. Note the evidence of thrombus (*t*) and calcification (*c*) at several levels throughout the length of the vessel (*l*, lumen). (Reproduced with permission from White RA, Scocerant M, Back M, et al: Innovations in vascular imaging: Angiography, 3D CT and 2D and 3D intravascular ultrasound of an abdominal aortic aneurysm. Ann Vasc Surg 1994;8:285.)

documented patency of adjacent branch arteries. The luminal morphology imaged on angiogram underestimated the size of the aneurysm, although displacement of the right ureter suggested a larger dimension. In addition, the angiogram did not provide precise cross-sectional and volumetric data regarding the dimensions of the neck of the aneurysm, quantity of thrombus, aortic wall characteristics, etc. that were apparent on CT and IVUS.

Tomographic views of cross sections of the aneurysm acquired by CT and IVUS enabled ac-

curate sizing of luminal and wall dimensions and correlated closely at various levels along the aorta. Surrounding anatomic structures and characteristics of the vessel wall were highlighted using each method. The IVUS images demonstrated the origin of visceral vessels (superior mesenteric and renal arteries) in relation to the aneurysm and displayed areas of calcification compared with thrombus and fibrous wall components. Calcification was clearly identified by IVUS as hyperechoic areas with shadowing beyond the lesion. Calcification of the wall of the aorta

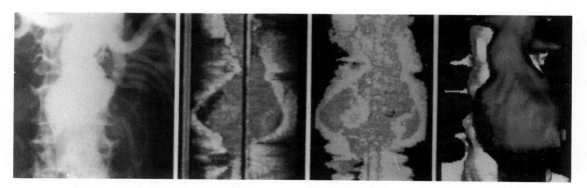

Figure 16-9. (*Left to right*) Aortogram, longitudinal gray-scale IVUS, surface rendered 3D IVUS, and 3D CT scan of the external surface of the aortic aneurysm. The images are of comparable lengths of the aorta with similar magnification to enable comparison of the methods. (Reproduced with permission from White RA, Scoccianti M, Back M, et al: Innovations in vascular imaging: Angiography, 3D CT and 2D and 3D intravascular ultrasound of an abdominal aortic aneurysm. Ann Vasc Surg 1994;8:285.)

was more readily apparent on IVUS compared with angiography or CT. Although the 2D cross-sectional CT and IVUS images corresponded closely for determining the luminal and vessel wall dimensions, the 3D IVUS reconstructions demonstrated some variation in the shape and topography of the wall surface along the longitudinal axis of the aneurysm compared with the 3D CT. The 3D CT scan outlined the external surface of the aorta, while the IVUS visualized the lumen and transmural wall characteristics. Development of future interventional methods, such as intravascular graft deployment, will utilize specific applications of each method to enhance precision of endovascular repairs. In particular, IVUS is being used to size and assess the characteristics of the aortic wall and aneurysm prior to deployment, to precisely place the device during the procedure, and to assess the accuracy of graft positioning.

Conventional angiography has been unable to provide adequately sensitive data regarding the effects of endovascular therapies. For meaningful critical assessment of these new methods, plaque consistency and distribution of residual lesions following intervention must be known. IVUS imaging provides the ability to accurately measure percentage stenoses produced by comparing luminal dimensions with normal-appearing adjacent reference vessels. This is due in part to the

restrictions of single or biplanar arteriography but also to the fact that an angiogram is a luminal silhouette rather than a transmural image.

Three-dimensional IVUS can be used to demonstrate atherosclerotic lesion volume, distribution, and tissue characteristics and is particularly relevant to investigation of the natural history of atherosclerotic disease and to the development volumetric plaque studies before and after endovascular interventions. Lesion volume is measurable using 3D IVUS imaging, but data regarding its accuracy are not currently available. Plaque volume estimation is based on the concept of differing cylindrical volumes, where the inner (smaller) cylinder is represented by the vessel lumen and the outer (larger) cylinder is confined by the adventitia. By creating a surface-rendered luminal image and a complete cylindrical adventitial reconstruction of a vascular segment, these two volumes can be displayed. The difference between the two cylinders represents the "volume" occupied by the arterial wall elements, either normal or pathologic. If this volume is measured before and after intervention, such as atherectomy, the difference in the volumes represents the amount of actual lesion removed. This information is required to delineate the mechanisms of angioplasty failure, since the roles of residual stenosis and recurrent stenosis have not been defined adequately using currently available angiographically determined data.

IVUS provides essential information in the investigation of arterial wall dissections by determining the size, location, and extent of intimal flaps. Because IVUS imaging is a dynamic, real-time imaging modality, the movement of arterial flaps with systolic-diastolic blood flow can be seen. The precise location and orientation of the flap are important, since they may determine the need for excision and grafting, stenting or repair. IVUS has been used to identify the location and severity of dissections and flaps and may enable endovascular assessment and treatment alone.[38–41] Three-dimensional IVUS imaging is especially useful in this role because aortic dissection commonly results in a spiral or complex-shaped flap that is difficult to appreciate in three dimensions using alternative imaging modalities. Three-dimensional reconstruction allows identification of the dissection entry site, extent of the flap, and relation of the false lumen to major visceral branches and plays a vital role in experimental endoluminal stenting of aortic dissections.

IVUS AS AN ADJUNCT TO ENDOVASCULAR INTERVENTIONS

Recent studies have indicated that percutaneous transluminal angioplasty (PTA) balloon size is often underestimated when selection is made using quantitative angiography and that optimal balloon size is determined more accurately by IVUS.[42] Additional findings suggest that angiographic success of balloon angioplasty is more likely when hard lesions are disrupted with dissections extending into the media of the vessel, while angiographic failure is seen in lesions that are nondisplaceable or when circumferential dissections or intimal flaps occur.[43] Angiographic success in soft lesions is associated with superficial fissures or fractures of the luminal surface, while vessel recoil and luminal disruption or thrombosis at sites of plaque rupture lead to failure. IVUS is capable of imaging all these features and may be invaluable in providing information that will be used to choose lesions suitable for balloon therapy. By combining information about plaque and vessel wall consistency with lesion location data such as eccentricity, and by quantitating residual stenosis and dissections, IVUS is ideally suited to act as a screening and guidance method to improve results from balloon angioplasties.[44,45] The balloon ultrasound imaging catheter (BUIC, Boston Scientific, Watertown, Mass.) has been used clinically with promising results. It has been confirmed that single-plane images can be obtained through the midsection of the angioplasty balloon at all times during the course of the angioplasty procedure, and preinflation, inflation, and postinflation luminal features such as plaque fracture and elastic recoil can be monitored with real-time IVUS.[46,47] Peripheral balloon angioplasty has been monitored with IVUS and has been especially useful in identifying and assessing the effect of intimal flaps.[22]

Preliminary studies have used IVUS to localize and treat coarctation of the aorta both experimentally and clinically.[48] IVUS clearly shows the coarctation and accurately measures the adjacent normal aortic lumen for balloon sizing. Following dilation, IVUS displays the appearance of the dilatation, including documentation of dissections.

IVUS has been used as a method to study the mechanism of action and function of atherectomy devices, lasers, and stents.[49–53] For each type of interventional device, the combination of the guidance and lesion-assessment capabilities of IVUS with an interventional technique may produce specific benefits for a particular type of approach.

IVUS also provides a method to guide deployment and assess the effect of intravascular stents in peripheral vessels. It allows selection of the correct stent size for a particular vessel and is useful in identifying the most appropriate site for stenting. Two- and three-dimensional IVUS are ideally suited to assessing vascular segments before and after stent deployment. Also, unique information regarding adequacy of deployment and changes in morphology produced by the stent can be seen (Fig. 16-10).

REAL-TIME IVUS ASSESSMENT OF INTRAVASCULAR GRAFT DEPLOYMENT

Candidates for surgical repair of vascular lesions are selected using physical examination, transcutaneous ultrasound, angiography, CT, and magnetic resonance imaging (MRI) to characterize the size and extent of the pathology and to plan operative

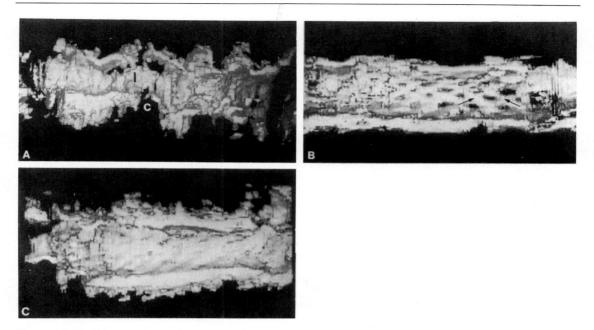

Figure 16-10. (**A**) After laser recanalization, the vessel lumen is irregular with evidence of intimal debris. Calcified plaque (c) is seen protruding into the lumen (I) with acoustic shadowing behind it. (**B**) Following initial stent deployment, the plaque is displaced from the lumen, and the intimal surface appears smoother. The typical "lattice" appearance of the incompletely expanded stent is seen (arrows). (**C**) Following final expansion, the stent is fully deployed with all struts against the vessel wall, and a smooth luminal contour is seen. (Reproduced with permission from Cavaye DM, Dicthrich EB, Santiago O, et al: Intravascular ultrasound imaging: An essential component of angioplasty assessment and vascular stent deployment. Int Angiol 1993;12:214.)

strategy. New intraluminal approaches to deploy vascular prostheses additionally require accurate assessment of factors such as the diameter of the proximal and distal neck of aneurysms, the length of the lesions, the position and volume of thrombus in relation to adjacent arteries, the characteristics of the vessel wall, and other variables. For these reasons, multiple diagnostic modalities are required to properly select patients and ensure adequate imaging and precise device deployment during the intervention.

Comparison of the various imaging modalities demonstrates that each provides information that may be useful for preinterventional selection of patients, for sizing of the vessel lumen and ensuring accurate deployment of devices during interventions, and for follow-up assessments. Some information is complementary to that acquired by other methods, and some is unique to a particular modality. Angiog-

raphy is useful for defining the continuity and morphology of vascular anatomy and for determining the presence of associated vascular abnormalities. Two- and three-dimensional CT scans and MRI are useful for determining both luminal and wall characteristics in a noninvasive manner, in addition to providing anatomic information on the location of surrounding structures. The CT and MRI examinations are limited to pre- and postintervention studies and cannot be used intraoperatively. They are especially important for selecting patients who are appropriate for a particular device and for determining vessel lumen dimensions of the proximal and distal fixation sites.

IVUS enables catheter-based interrogation of vascular segments during interventional angiographic or operative procedures and provides unique information regarding luminal and vessel wall cross-sectional dimensions and the distribution of arterial disease in the vessel wall. IVUS is useful for detecting the presence of calcium and for inspecting the morphology and distribution of intraluminal thrombus. IVUS is particularly helpful in assessing the relationship of branch artery ostia as well as determining the total length and diameters along the lesion.

Experimental laboratory studies have shown that IVUS is useful for choosing the site of graft deployment and for determining the appropriate device size by accurately measuring the luminal dimensions of the aorta.[37] IVUS interrogation of the aortic lumen before device deployment enables accurate identification of the branch arteries and selection of the appropriate site for proximal stent placement. During placement of an intraluminal graft, IVUS is the most accurate way to determine full stent expansion and to obtain information regarding the continuity and alignment of the graft material in the aortic lumen. Using certain devices, it is possible to place prostheses by IVUS guidance alone. Although cinefluoroscopy and IVUS are complementary in enabling expedient placement of intraluminal grafts, an additional important aspect supporting the use of IVUS in this application is that fluoroscopy time can be significantly reduced during the procedures, minimizing the exposure of both personnel and the patient.

In approximately 20 percent of graft deployment in an experimental series,[54] incomplete proximal stent expansion was determined by IVUS when there was no apparent abnormality on angiography. This is an important observation because it averted potential migration of the devices by enabling further expansion of the stent before completing the procedure. The implications of secure proximal stent positioning are obvious. The improved accuracy of IVUS in determining stent deployment has been confirmed by other investigators who document that IVUS examination leads to repositioning of intravascular stent devices in approximately 20 to 30 percent of cases when cinefluoroscopy suggests that the deployment is adequate.[53] The implications of these observations on the development of future deployment devices and the effect that IVUS will have on enhancing the success of procedures are yet to be determined.

Developing Applications of IVUS

IVUS is an invasive technique requiring intravascular puncture and catheter insertion. The diagnostic applications are useful when combined with invasive studies such as peripheral angiography or cardiac catheterization or as a guidance method during therapeutic procedures, including angioplasty stent deployment and intraluminal graft placement. Developing potentials of the method range from improved localization of vascular tumors before surgery[55] or imaging the long-term function of vena caval filters[56] to possible application as the primary guidance method for laser angioplasty.[57]

A priority in the development of IVUS technology is the need for further miniaturization and cost-effective manufacturing. Current devices are relatively expensive, and if the technique is to be of clinical benefit as a component of a disposable catheter system for diagnostic or therapeutic intervention, the price of individual units must be justified by the benefits of IVUS imaging.

Future angioplasty guidance devices may combine the benefits of angioscopy and IVUS in a single delivery system suitable for incorporating mechanical or laser ablation devices. Angioscopy would allow visual inspection of the lumen, with ultrasound determining the vessel wall characteristics and dimensions. An added benefit of this type of guidance device would be the ability to select an appropriate ablation method for particular plaque types or volumes. Tissue characterization by analyzing the raw radiofrequency ultrasound signal shows promise for differentiating plaque types.

IVUS also provides exciting opportunities for vascular research, including investigation of blood vessel compliance, dynamic changes in the vascular wall caused by disease or pharmacologic intervention, and the natural history of atherosclerosis.

REFERENCES

1. Sumner DS, Russel JB, Miles RD: Pulsed Doppler arteriography and computer assisted imaging of carotid bifurcation. *In* Bergan JJ, Yao JST (eds): Cerebrovascular Insufficiency. New York, Grune & Stratton, 1983, pp 115–135.

2. Grundfest WS, Litvack F, Hickey A, et al: The current status of angioscopy and laser angioplasty. J Vasc Surg 1987;5:667.

3. Sherman CT, Litvack F, Grundfest WS, et al: Coronary angioscopy in patients with unstable angina pectoris. N Eng J Med 1986;315:913.

4. Towne JB, Bernhard VM: Vascular endoscopy: Useful tool or interesting toy. Surgery 1977;82:415.

5. Grundfest WS, Litvack F, Sherman CT, et al: Delineation of peripheral and coronary detail by intraoperative angioscopy. Ann Surg 1985;202:394.

6. White GH, White RA, Kopchok GE: Intraoperative video angioscopy compared to arteriography during peripheral vascular operations. J Vasc Surg 1987;6:488.

7. Vollmar JF, Loeprecht H, Hutschenreiter S: Advances in vascular endoscopy. Thorac Cardiovasc Surg 1987;35:334.

8. White GH, White RA, Kopchok GE, Wilson SE: Angioscopic thromboembolectomy: Preliminary observations with a recent technique. J Vasc Surg 1988;7:318.

9. White RA, White GH: Angioscopic monitoring of laser angioplasty. *In* White GH, White RA (eds): Angioscopy: Vascular and Coronary Applications. Chicago, Year Book Medical Publishers, 1989, pp 104–113.

10. White GH, White RA, Colman PD, Kopchok GE: Experimental and clinical applications of angioscopic guidance for laser angioplasty. Am J Surg 1989;158:495.

11. Abela GS, Seegar JM, Barbieri E, et al: Laser angioplasty with angioscopic guidance in humans. J Am Coll Cardiol 1986;8:184.

12. White GH, White RA, Kopchok GE, Wilson SE: Endoscopic intravascular surgery removes intimal flaps, dissections and thrombus. J Vasc Surg 1990;11:280.

13. Kopchok GE, White RA, Guthrie C, et al: Intraluminal vascular ultrasound: Preliminary report. Ann Vasc Surg 1990;4:291.

14. Bom N, ten Hoff H, Lancee CT, et al: Early and recent intraluminal ultrasound devices. Int J Cardiac Imaging 1989;4:79.

15. Cieszynski T: Intracardiac method for the investigation of structure of the heart with the aid of ultrasonics. Arch Immunol Ther Exp (Warsz) 1960;8:551.

16. Kossof G: Diagnostic applications of ultrasound in cardiology. Australas Radiol 1966;10:101.

17. Carleton RA, Sessions RW, Graettinger JS: Diameter of heart measured by intracavitary ultrasound. Med Res Engng 1969;May:28.

18. Frazin L, Talano JV, Stephanides L, et al: Esophageal echocardiography. Circulation 1976;54:168.

19. Bom N, Lancee CT, Van Egmond FC: An ultrasonic intracardiac scanner. Ultrasonics 1972;10:72.

20. Lockwood GR, Ryan LK, Foster FS: High frequency intravascular ultrasound imaging. *In* Cavaye

DM, White RA (eds): Arterial Imaging: Modern and Developing Technologies. London, Chapman & Hall, 1993, pp 125–129.

21. Yock PG, Linker DT, Angelsen BAJ: Two-dimensional intravascular ultrasound: Technical development and initial clinical experience. J Am Soc Echocardiol 1989;2(4):296.

22. Heffernan PB, Robb RA: A new method for shaded surface display of biological and medical images. IEEE Trans Med Imaging 1985;MI-4:26.

23. Cavaye DM, Tabbarra MR, Kopchok GE, et al: Three-dimensional vascular ultrasound imaging. Am Surg 1991;57:751.

24. Back M, Kopchok G, White R, et al: Forward-looking intravascular ultrasonography: In vitro imaging in normal and atherosclerotic human arteries. Am Surg 1994;60:738.

25. Evans JL, Ng Hwee-kok, Vonesh MJ, et al: Arterial imaging with a new forward-viewing intravascular ultrasound catheter: I. Initial studies. Circulation 1994;89:712.

26. van Urk H, Gussenhoven WJ, Gerritsen GP, et al: Assessment of arterial disease and arterial reconstructions by intravascular ultrasound. Int J Cardiac Imaging 1991;6:157.

27. Burns PN, Goldberg BB: Ultrasound contrast agents for vascular imaging. *In* Cavaye DM, White RA (eds): Arterial Imaging: Modern and Developing Technologies. London, Chapman & Hall, 1993, pp 61–67.

28. Gussenhoven WJ, Essed CE, Lancee CT: Arterial wall characteristics determined by intravascular ultrasound imaging: An in vitro study. J Am Coll Cardiol 1989;14:947.

29. Kopchok GE, White RA, Guthrie C, et al: Intraluminal vascular ultrasound: Preliminary report of dimensional and morphologic accuracy. Ann Vasc Surg 1990;4:291.

30. Kopchok GE, White RA, White G: Intravascular ultrasound: A new potential modality for angioplasty guidance. Angiology 1990;41:785.

31. Mallery JA, Tobis JM, Griffith J, et al: Assessment of normal and atherosclerotic arterial wall thickness with an intravascular ultrasound imaging catheter. Am Heart J 1990;119:1392.

32. Nissen SE, Grines CL, Gurley JC, et al: Application of new phased-array ultrasound imaging catheter in the assessment of vascular dimensions. Circulation 1990;81:660.

33. Nissen SE, Gurley JC, Grines CL, et al: Intravascular ultrasound assessing of lumen size and wall morphology in normal subjects and patients with coronary artery disease. Circulation 1993;88:1087.

34. Gussenhoven WJ, Essed CE, Frietman P, et al: Intravascular echographic assessment of vessel wall characteristics: A correlation with histology. Int J Cardiac Imaging 1989;4:105.

35. Tabbara MR, White RA, Cavaye DM, Kopchok GE: In vivo human comparison of intravascular ultrasound and angiography. J Vasc Surg 1991; 1991;14:496.

36. Tobis JM, Mahon D, Lehmann K, et al: The sensitivity of ultrasound imaging compared to angiography for diagnosing coronary atherosclerosis (abstract). Circulation 1990;82(suppl III):439.

37. White RA, Scoccianti M, Back M, et al: Innovations in vascular imaging: Angiography, 3D CT and 2D and 3D intravascular ultrasound of an abdominal aortic aneurysm. Ann Vasc Surg 1994;8:285.

38. Cavaye DM, French WJ, White RA, et al: Intravascular ultrasound imaging of an acute dissecting aortic aneurysm: A case report. J Vasc Surg 1991;13:510.

39. Pandian NG, Fries A, Broadway B, et al: Intravascular high-frequency two-dimension detection of arterial dissection and intimal flaps. Am J Cardiol 1990;65:1278.

40. Neville RF, Yasuhara H, Watanabe BI, et al: Endovascular management of arterial intimal defects: An experimental comparison by arteriography, angioscopy and intravascular ultrasonography. J Vasc Surg 1991;13:496.

41. Cavaye DM, White RA, Lerman RD, et al: Usefulness of intravascular ultrasound for detecting experimentally induced aortic dissection in dogs and for determining the effectiveness of endoluminal stenting. Am J Cardiol 1992;69:705.

42. Cacchione J, Nair R, Hodson J: Intracoronary ultrasound is better than conventional methods for determining optimal PTCA balloon size (abstract). J Am Coll Cardiol 1991;17:112A.

43. Leon M, Keren G, Pichard A, et al: Intravascular ultrasound assessment of plaque responses to PTCA helps to explain angiographic findings (abstract). J Am Coll Cardiol 1991;17:47A.

44. Davidson CJ, Sheikh KH, Kisslo K, et al: Intracoronary ultrasound evaluation of interventional procedures (abstract). Circulation 1990;82(suppl III):440.

45. Gurley J, Nissen S, Grines C, et al: Comparison of intravascular ultrasound following percutaneous transluminal coronary angioplasty (abstract). Circulation 1990;82:90.

46. Crowley RJ, Hamm MA, Joshi SH, et al: Ultrasound guided therapeutic catheters: Recent developments and clinical results. Int J Cardiac Imaging 1991;6:145.

47. Isner JM, Rosenfield K, Losordo DW, et al: Combination balloon-ultrasound imaging catheter for percutaneous transluminal angioplasty. Circulation 1991;84:739.

48. Sanzobrino B, Gillam L, McKay R, et al: A direct clinical role for intravascular ultrasound: Utility in the assessment of coarctation of the aorta (abstract). J Am Coll Cardiol 1991;17:68A.

49. Smucker ML, Scherb DE, Howard PF: Intracoronary ultrasound: How much "angioplasty effect" in atherectomy? (abstract). Circulation 1990;82(suppl):676.

50. Mintz G, Potkin B, Keren G, et al: Intravascular ultrasound evaluation of the effect of rotational atherectomy in obstructive athererosclerotic coronary disease. Circulation 1992;86:1383.

51. Cavaye DM, Tabbara MR, Kopchok GE, et al: Intravascular ultrasound assessment of vascular stent deployment. Ann Vasc Surg 1991;5:241.

52. Cavaye DM, Diethrich EB, Santiago OJ, et al: Intravascular imaging: An essential component of angioplasty assessment and vascular stent deployment. Int Angiol 1993;12:212.

53. Katzen BT, Benenati JF, Becker GJ, Zemel G: Role of intravascular ultrasound in peripheral atherectomy and stent deployment. Circulation 1991;84(suppl II):2152.

54. White RA, Verbin C, Scoccianti M, et al: Role of cinefluoroscopy and intravascular ultrasound in the deployment and healing of endoluminal vascular prostheses in normal canine aortas. J Vasc Surg (in press).

55. Barone GW, Kahn MB, Cook JM, et al: Recurrent intracaval renal cell carcinoma: The role of intravascular ultrasonography. J Vasc Surg 1990;13:506.

56. Greenfield LJ, Tauscher JR, Marx V: Evaluation of a new percutaneous stainless steel Greenfield filter by intravascular ultrasonography. Surgery 1991;109:722.

57. White RA, Kopchok GE, Tabbara MR, et al: Intravascular ultrasound-guided holmium:YAG laser recanalization of occluded arteries. Lasers Surg Med 1992;12:239.

CHAPTER

17

Endovascular Aortoiliac Reconstruction for Occlusive Disease

MICHAEL L. MARIN
FRANK J. VEITH

Prosthetic arterial reconstructions represent the "gold standard" for bypass of the aortoiliac segment.[1–4] Such reconstructions have been effective in the treatment of lower extremity ischemia and have proven to be durable. Unfortunately, aortoiliofemoral bypass grafting is not perfect. Between 10 and 20 percent of all aortofemoral bypass grafts may be expected to develop at least one graft limb thrombosis over a 10-year period. Such failures frequently necessitate reoperation, which is often associated with an increased morbidity over primary procedures.[5,6] Reoperative aortoiliac surgery in patients who also have significant comorbid medical illnesses, including renal, pulmonary, and cardiac insufficiencies, results in an increased risk of developing a perioperative complication.

Alternative treatments to open aortic reconstruction include the use of percutaneous transluminal angioplasty and intravascular stenting.[7–13] These procedures may be performed without major anesthesia and have been shown to be effective for treating short-segment occlusive disease of the iliac arteries. However, balloon angioplasty has not proven to be a durable form of treatment for multiple and long segment arterial occlusive diseases in the aortoiliac segment.[14]

An alternative method for treating long segment aortoiliac disease without the use of standard open aortofemoral grafting employs endovascular stented grafts to bridge the vascular pathology. Stented grafts represent a blending of intravascular

stent, angioplasty, and prosthetic graft technologies to produce a new device that may be inserted under minimally invasive conditions. These devices can be inserted under general, regional, or local anesthesia, require less operative dissection, minimize local tissue trauma, and are associated with reduced blood loss and a more rapid postprocedure recovery. This chapter reviews the development of the field of endovascular stented grafts and their potential for the treatment of aortoiliac occlusive disease.

Intravascular stents were first proposed in 1969 by Charles Dotter,[15] the father of percutaneous angioplasty. At the time of this important report, Dotter also suggested that stents could be used for the treatment of a variety of arterial lesions, including aneurysms and arteriovenous fistulas. Feasibility studies that showed the potential utility of stented graft devices were carried out in experimental animals using a variety of stent and graft materials.[16–18] Recent clinical applications of endovascular stented grafts have included the treatment of abdominal and peripheral artery aneurysms.[19,20] In addition, endovascular stented grafts have been used effectively and safely to treat penetrating arterial injuries.[21,22] One of the first clinical applications of endovascular stented grafts for the treatment of arterial occlusive disease was performed by Volodos et al.,[23] who used a self-expanding, spring-type stent device covered with a Dacron

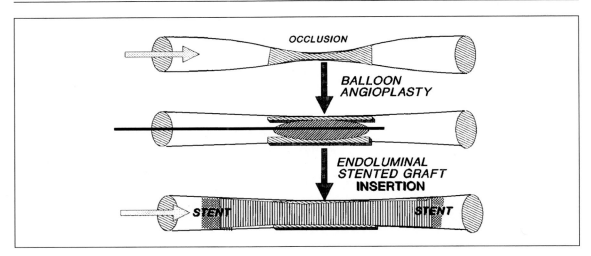

Figure 17-1. This is an illustrated summary of the steps involved in transluminal stented graft repair for arterial occlusive disease. A stenotic or narrowed segment within the arteries is first crossed with an angiographic wire. The entire stenosis is then balloon dilated. Next, the endovascular stented graft composed of a prosthetic conduit coupled with two intraarterial stents is inserted within a guiding sheath and is placed into the arterial system. Following balloon expansion of the individual stents, the new endovascular graft relines the diffusely dilated arterial segment.

graft material to treat an aortoiliac obstruction. This device was used effectively to treat a long segment of occluded artery by dilating and relining the vessel. Following this report, several devices have been used to treat a variety of occlusive arterial lesions within the aortoiliac and femoropopliteal arteries.[24,25] While the applications of endovascular stented grafts may extend to markedly different arterial pathologies, the same general principles and techniques of graft insertion are preserved in all. These include remote arterial access site, less trauma to the surrounding artery, minimal anesthetic requirements, and repair of arterial pathology from within the vessel lumen.

TECHNIQUE

Stented graft procedures for the treatment of arterial occlusive disease employ three basic techniques for endovascular reconstruction (Fig. 17-1).

Arterial Access

The arterial pathology to be treated with a stented graft is usually approached from a remote site. Direct access is obtained by one of two methods: If the access vessel is patent, it may be approached through a percutaneous puncture technique. However, many patients with extensive limb-threatening aortoiliac occlusive disease have occluded access arteries. The presence of an occluded vessel at the site of arterial access does not preclude the ability to perform an endovascular stented graft procedure. When occluded vessels are present, they can be approached by open surgical exposure of the access artery (Fig. 17-2A). Once the occluded vessel is identified, recanalization wires (often with hydrophilic coatings) are inserted directly into the central axis of the occluded vessel and guided in their course cephalad through the patent artery by means of directional catheters (Fig. 17-2B).

Arterial Dilation

Once the recanalization wires have established a connection between the remote access site and the patent segment of the proximal artery, diffuse arterial dilation is performed using angioplasty balloons inserted over the guidewire (Fig. 17-2C). Such dilation permits the formation of a widened tract through the atheromatous arterial wall and facilitates insertion of the new endovascular graft within this tract.

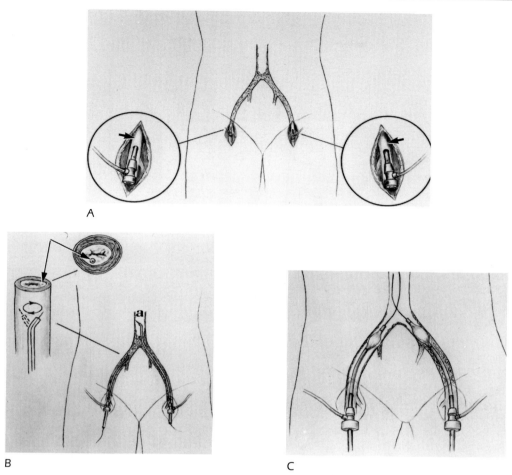

Figure 17-2. This series of illustrations details the individual steps required to perform an endovascular stented graft repair for aortoiliac occlusive disease. (**A**) Bilateral femoral cutdowns are performed, and introducer catheters are inserted into the exposed common femoral arteries (*arrows*). It is through these introducer catheters that all subsequent interventions on the occluded segment of the vascular system are accomplished. (**B**) By way of the previously placed introducer catheters, directional catheters then guide hydrophilic wires through the arterial stenoses into the patent artery above (*a* = aorta). As illustrated in the adjacent drawing, the ideal plane of dissection is in the intraintimal segment (*arrow*). Recanalization in the deep portions of the media may make reentry into the patent abdominal aorta difficult. (**C**) Following recanalization, balloon dilation is then performed over the wire along the entire length of the occluded or diseased arterial segment.

Illustration continued on following page.

Stent Graft Insertion

When a neoarterial tract has been created within the wall of the occluded or diseased artery, a carrier system composed of a guiding catheter or sheath containing an endovascular stented graft is inserted over the previously placed wire and advanced under fluoroscopic control to the patent proximal arterial segment. After angiographic confirmation of the position of the stented graft, it is fixed into position by a stent attachment device (Fig. 17-2D). The attachment device provides a watertight seal between the

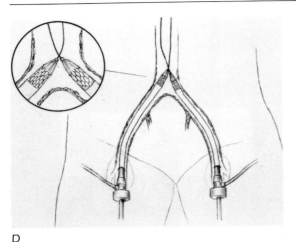

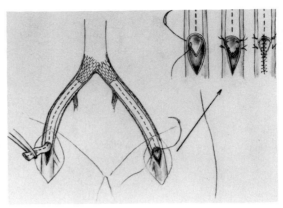

D   E

Figure 17-2 *continued.* (**D**) Following balloon dilation, endovascular stented grafts are simultaneously inserted through both newly dilated iliac systems. Their final proximal position is confirmed using fluoroscopy. (**E**) The proximal stents of both endovascular iliac grafts are dilated, creating a watertight seal between the graft, the stent, and the aortic wall. The distal end of each graft is then endovascularly anastomosed to the common femoral artery, as illustrated in the side drawing. An endovascular anastomosis consists of a series of 6-0 prolene tacking sutures placed within the prosthetic graft.

proximal end of the graft and the patent portion of the proximal artery. The distal end of the endovascular graft is then ready for suture anastomosis or stenting to the patent portion of an outflow artery. When performed with sutures, this may be accomplished by a standard end-to-side or end-to-end arterial anastomosis. Alternatively, the endovascular stented graft may be sutured to the patent portion of the outflow artery using an endovascular anastomotic technique (Fig. 17-2E).

All procedures must be followed by a completion arteriogram to inspect for technical adequacy of the procedure and patency of the outflow arteries without embolization.

CASE EXAMPLES

Case 1

This patient had undergone three previous left lower extremity revascularizations for limb-threatening ischemia. The last revascularization was 4 years prior to the present admission and was associated with a deep left groin and retroperitoneal infection that resolved but was followed 3 years later by graft occlusion. Laboratory analysis

for a hypercoagulable state was negative. The patient's current admission was for an acute anterior wall myocardial infarction. At the time of admission to the coronary care unit, severe left foot ischemia with gangrene and infection was present in conjunction with absent femoral and pedal pulses in both lower extremities. Arteriography demonstrated an occlusion of the distal left external iliac artery with reconstitution of the distal superficial femoral artery (SFA) (Fig. 17-3A). Because of the risks associated with a complex peripheral revascularization within 10 days of an acute myocardial infarction, as well as the extreme urgency associated with the pedal sepsis and gangrene, a stented graft was inserted through a mid-SFA arteriotomy under local anesthesia. After balloon dilation of an endovascular tract created between the external iliac and superficial femoral arteries, a 6-mm thin-walled polytetrafluoroethylene (PTFE) graft was inserted and fixed to the external iliac artery with a 30-mm-long Palmaz stent. Preservation of terminal external iliac artery collateral branches was achieved by placing that portion of the stent which was not covered by prosthetic graft across the ostia of these collaterals (Fig. 17-3B). This permitted continued circulation to the branches through the uncovered interstices of the stent. The distal portion of the graft was

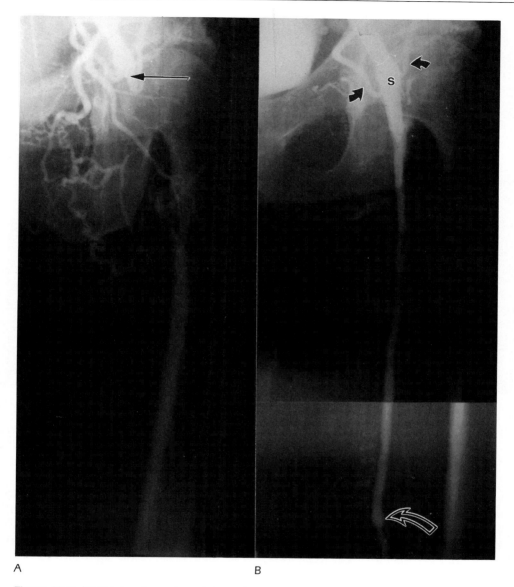

A   B

Figure 17-3. (A) This is a femoral arteriogram demonstrating occlusion of the external iliac artery at its junction with the common femoral artery. Multiple, terminal collateral branches can be seen (*arrow*). **(B)** Following insertion of an endovascular stented graft through the distal superficial femoral artery, this arteriogram demonstrates continuity between the previously occluded external iliac artery (*s* = stent) and the distal superficial femoral artery (*open arrow*). The collateral branches at the terminal portion of the external iliac artery remain patent (*curved arrows*). Reproduced with permission from Marin ML, Veith FJ et al. Transfemoral stented graft treatment of occlusive arterial disease for limb salvage. Circulation 1993;88:1.

anastomosed end-to-side to the distal SFA using a standard technique. Restoration of pedal pulses was associated with complete resolution of the gangrene, and the graft has remained patent for 11 months (Fig. 17-4).

Case 2

This patient was transferred to our institution with bilateral lower extremity ischemia, gangrene of the left foot, and severe rest pain in the right leg. He had previously had seven arterial reconstructions

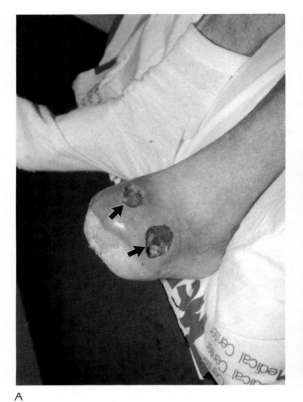 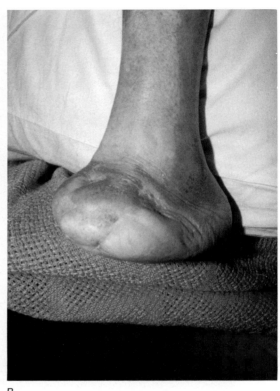

A   B

Figure 17-4. (A) This is a photograph of the previously healed transmetatarsal amputation site for the patient illustrated in Fig. 17-3. There are two gangrenous ulcers (*arrows*) and significant forefoot swelling. **(B)** Following endovascular stented graft insertion from the external iliac artery to the superficial femoral artery, full healing of the pedal remnant is achieved in 6 weeks.

for lower extremity ischemia. These included two aortofemoral, one left iliofemoral, one left femoropopliteal, and three femorofemoral bypasses. All had failed, leaving the arteriographic anatomy shown in Figure 17-5A. Evaluation for a hypercoagulable state, including analysis of antithrombin III, protein C, and protein S deficiencies, was negative.

Because of the risks associated with reoperative aortic and femoral surgery, a transfemoral route was elected and performed under general anesthesia. Through a distal left SFA arteriotomy, a guidewire tract between the mid-SFA and the distal aorta was created and dilated. A 6-mm PTFE graft was inserted and secured at the aortoiliac junction using a 30-mm-long Palmaz stent (Fig. 17-5B). The distal graft was sutured to the left SFA. For the right leg ischemia, a 6 mm × 40 cm PTFE graft was endovascularly inserted via the

right SFA through a similar predilated tract and secured with a 30-mm stent to the origin of the external iliac artery (Fig. 17-5C). The distal end of the right-sided graft was suture anastomosed to the midportion of the right SFA (Fig. 17-5D). Patency of both grafts for 14 months has been confirmed by arteriography and duplex ultrasonography. The left foot gangrene healed completely, and the right lower extremity is normally perfused.

DISCUSSION

Preliminary studies have shown that endovascular stented grafts are effective for the treatment of a variety of arterial lesions, including aneurysms, occlusions, and penetrating traumatic

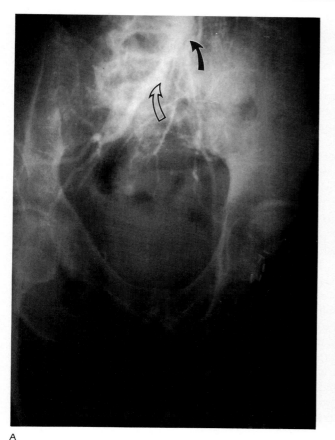

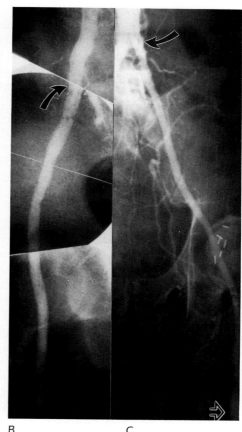

A

B   C

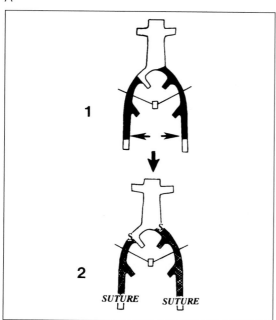

D

Figure 17-5. (A) This is a femoral arteriogram of a patient who has a total iliofemoral occlusion on the left (*closed arrow*) and an external iliac occlusion on the right (*open arrow*). **(B)** Following endovascular insertion of an aorto-superficial femoral artery stented graft, vascular continuity is reestablished through the left lower extremity. (*Open arrow* = site of distal, hand-sewn anastomosis; *curved arrow* = proximal stent anastomosis.) **(C)** Following endovascular insertion of a second stented graft through the right superficial femoral artery, this composite angiogram demonstrates the reestablishment of arterial flow from the distal common iliac artery (*arrow*) to the superficial femoral artery. **(D)** This is a summary of the endovascular arterial reconstructions for this patient. Illustration 1 is a depiction of the preoperative anatomy with the occlusions in black. The superficial femoral artery stent graft insertion sites are indicated by the arrows. Illustration 2 demonstrates the regions of the iliofemoral system that have been relined with endovascular grafts (*patched area* = graft; *s* = stent). Suture anastomoses were performed at the level of both superficial femoral arteries. Reproduced with permission from Marin ML, Veith FJ et al. Transfemoral stented graft treatment of occlusive arterial disease for limb salvage. Circulation 1993;88:1.

injuries.[19-25] While the pathology of these three arterial lesions varies dramatically, the principles behind the techniques for endovascular stented graft repair of these lesions are very similar. Endovascular stent graft procedures permit remote access to the vascular system, intravascular insertion of a stent and graft combination, and repair of the arterial pathology from within the arterial lumen. Using this technique, treatment of aortoiliac occlusions requires a long segment angioplasty of the arterial segment. Following diffuse arterial dilation, an endovascular stented graft may be inserted to reline the diffusely dilated arterial segment.

There are several theoretical advantages to using endovascular stented grafts. Because the procedures are performed from a remote arterial access site using minimal operative dissection, less anesthesia is required. In addition, there is no need for extensive incisions or periarterial dissection in the area of arterial occlusion, which may result in significant trauma to surrounding tissues. The occlusion is repaired in an "anatomic" fashion so that axillary arteries or the contralateral femoral artery will not be jeopardized, as might be the case with extraanatomic bypasses. Dissections in scarred or infected groins may be avoided. In the case of aortoiliac reconstruction, the avoidance of a transabdominal or retroperitoneal incision eliminates the potential for prolonged intestinal dysfunction, pulmonary complications, and large fluid shifts within the circulatory system, which may be responsible for cardiac and pulmonary failure. Preservation of sexual function in younger patients also can be anticipated with the avoidance of aortic dissection.

There are many unknowns with this new approach. The long-term behavior of the extrinsic portion of the dilated native arteries remains unclear. The potential for arterial recoil, disease progression, and a hyperplastic response in the atheromatous plaque that is extrinsic to the endovascular graft is of concern. While these problems have not been encountered during our preliminary clinical applications of this technique, their potential remains.

Endovascular stented grafts appear to be an important advance in the management of complex aortoiliac occlusive disease and may have particular merit in the treatment of patients with significant comorbid medical illnesses or those with failed, previous aortoiliac reconstructions. In these situations, stented grafts represent a way to reestablish arterial continuity without extensive operative procedures and associated morbidities. Long-term follow-up and careful comparisons with standard operative and endovascular techniques will be needed before widespread application of this technique can be advocated.

REFERENCES

1. Rutherford RB: Aortobifemoral bypass, the gold standard: Technical considerations. Semin Vasc Surg 1994;7:11.
2. Brewster DC, Darling RC: Optimal methods of aortoiliac reconstruction. Surgery 1978;84:739.
3. Brothers TE, Greenfield LJ: Long-term results of aortoiliac reconstruction. J Vasc Intervent Radiol 1990;1:49.
4. Poulias GE, Doundoulakis N, Prombonas E, et al: Aorto-femoral bypass and determinants of early success and late favourable outcome. Experience with 1000 consecutive cases. J Cardiovasc Surg 1992;33:664.
5. Szilagyi DE, Elliott JP Jr, Smith RF, et al: A thirty-year survey of the reconstructive surgical treatment of aortoiliac occlusive disease. J Vasc Surg 1986;3:421.
6. Nevelsteen A, Wouters L, Suy R: Long-term patency of the aortofemoral Dacron graft. A graft limb related study over a 25-year period. J Cardiovasc Surg 1991;32:174.
7. Martin EC: Percutaneous therapy in the management of aortoiliac disease. Semin Vasc Surg 1994;7:17.
8. Tegtmeyer CJ, Hartwell GD, Selby JB, et al: Results and complications of angioplasty in aortoiliac disease. Circulation 1991;83(suppl 1):I-53.
9. Johnston KW, Rae M, Hogg-Johnston SA, et al: 5-Year results of a prospective study of percutaneous transluminal angioplasty. Ann Surg 1987;206:403.
10. Liermann D, Strecker EP, Peters J: The Strecker stent: Indications and results in iliac and femoropopliteal arteries. Cardiovasc Intervent Radiol 1992;15:298.
11. Palmaz JC, Laborde JC, Rivera FJ, et al: Stenting of the iliac arteries with the Palmaz stent: Experience from a multicenter trial. Cardiovasc Intervent Radiol 1992;15:291.
12. Hausegger KA, Cragg AH, Lammer J, et al: Iliac artery stent placement: Clinical experience with a Nitinol stent. Radiology 1994;190:199.
13. Vorwerk D, Gunther RW: Stent placement in iliac arterial lesions: Three years of clinical experience with the Wallstent. Cardiovasc Intervent Radiol 1992;15:285.

14. Johnston KW: Iliac arteries: Reanalysis of results of balloon angioplasty. Radiology 1993;186:207.

15. Dotter CT: Transluminally-placed coilspring endarterial tube grafts. Long-term patency in canine popliteal artery. Invest Radiol 1969;4:329.

16. Mirich D, Wright KC, Wallace S, et al: Percutaneously placed endovascular grafts for aortic aneurysms: Feasibility study. Radiology 1989; 170:1033.

17. Laborde JC, Parodi JC, Clem MF, et al: Intraluminal bypass of abdominal aortic aneurysm: Feasibility study. Radiology 1992;184:185.

18. Balko A, Piasecki GJ, Shah DM, et al: Transfemoral placement of intraluminal polyurethane prosthesis for abdominal aortic aneurysm. J Surg Res 1986;40:305.

19. Parodi JC, Palmaz JC, Barone HD: Transfemoral intraluminal graft implantation for abdominal aortic aneurysms. Ann Vasc Surg 1991;5:491.

20. Marin ML, Veith FJ, Panetta TF, et al: Transfemoral endovascular stented graft repair of a popliteal artery aneurysm. J Vasc Surg 1994;19:754.

21. Marin ML, Veith FJ, Panetta TF, et al: Percutaneous transfemoral insertion of a stented graft to repair a traumatic femoral arteriovenous fistula. J Vasc Surg 1993;18:299.

22. Marin ML, Veith FJ, Panetta TF, et al: Transluminally placed endovascular stented graft repair for arterial trauma. J Vasc Surg 1994;20:466.

23. Volodos NL, Shekhanin VE, Karpovich IP, et al: Self-fixing synthetic prosthesis for endoprosthetics of the vessels. Vestn Khir (Russia) 1986;137:123.

24. Marin ML, Veith FJ, Panetta TF, et al: Transfemoral stented graft treatment of occlusive arterial disease for limb salvage: A preliminary report. Circulation 1993;88(4):I-11.

25. Cragg AH, Dake MD: Percutaneous femoropopliteal graft placement. J Vasc Intervent Radiol 1993;4:455.

ACKNOWLEDGMENTS

This work was supported by grants from the U.S. Public Health Service (HL 02990–01), the James Hilton Manning and Emma Austin Manning Foundation, The Anna S. Brown Trust, and the New York Institute for Vascular Studies.

Infected Aortic Grafts

DOUGLAS L. JICHA
RONALD J. STONEY

Aortic graft infection is the most serious complication of aortic grafting. Successful management usually has required an aggressive removal of infected tissue and revascularization. While these basic principles are simple, successful execution requires careful planning, flexibility, and adaption to the individual clinical situation. The formidable morbidity and mortality of aortic graft infection highlight the complexity of the problem.

The incidence of graft infection in the aortic position is fortunately low and appears increased with grafts that extend to the femoral level.[1] Estimates suggest an incidence of approximately 2.5 percent.[1-3] Mortality rates of 25 percent and amputation rates of 25 percent are still reported in contemporary series.[1,4-6] This chapter outlines the clinical problem and strategies to address this serious complication of aortic grafting.

ETIOLOGY OF GRAFT INFECTION

Graft incorporation involves ingrowth of surrounding tissue into and around grafts that is principly mediated by fibroblast activity. The period of time to graft incorporation is variable and depends on host and graft factors. Typically, graft incorporation is complete in 1 year. Graft infection is signaled by a disruption in the process of incorporation, which can occur in the acute or chronic phase. The acute phase is generally defined as within 30 days of a procedure. Acute-phase infection generally manifests as a wound problem. This is especially common at the groin, which is the most superficial portion of the graft. Chronic graft infection manifests months to years after initial graft placement. Bleeding from an aortoenteric fistula or anastomotic disruption, pseudoaneurysms, abscesses, and sinus tracts may accompany the nonincorporation that signals infection.

Most graft infections presumably occur at the time of implantation. Minor breaks in surgical technique can occur when the graft contacts the skin or wound edge, is exposed to unsterile instruments, or is not properly sterilized prior to use. Contact with infectious agents also can occur when concomitant procedures are performed, such as appendectomy or cholecystectomy. Organisms already in the field also come in contact with grafts. Prior groin manipulation by arteriogram, infected arterial walls, lymph nodes colonized by organisms from more distal infected areas, and colonized aneurysm contents can all be sources of contamination. The significance of culture-positive thrombus or aneurysm wall as the etiologic agent in graft infection is unclear. While positive cultures of thrombus and/or aneurysm wall occur in over 30 percent of patients, subsequent graft infection does not appear inevitable.[7] It is clear that the vascular prosthesis, as a foreign body, provides an environment that allows for enhanced bacterial survival.

Hematogenous seeding as a cause of graft infections is also possible. Bacteremias have been shown in animal models to result in graft infection when significant inocula are delivered following graft implantation.[8] Grafts appear especially vulnerable prior to graft incorporation. Presumably, the graft incorporation by surrounding tissues helps protect the graft from these bacteremias. Further work has demonstrated a decrease in the ability of bacteremias to cause graft infection over the life of the graft.[9] It is notable that this incorporation is never complete and may be disrupted, allowing for graft infection long after implantation.

The pathogenicity of infecting organisms is in part dependent on the integrity of host defenses. Host defenses can be compromised by malnutrition, immunosuppressive agents, and comorbid systemic disorders. Intact host defenses also may be compromised by perioperative complications, including hematomas and seromas. Reilly et al.[10] reported an association of graft infection with multiple vascular procedures, postoperative wound problems, intraoperative technical problems, and emergent procedures for ruptured abdominal aortic aneurysms or limb ischemia. Further demonstration of the importance of host factors is made by Phillips et al.,[11] who reported a 21 percent incidence of prosthetic graft infection in highly irradiated tissues. They recommend use of autogenous conduit or extraanatomic bypass to avoid irradiated fields and the complications of prosthetic infection.

BACTERIOLOGY

The majority of graft infections are due to grampositive cocci, including *Staphylococcus aureus* and *Staphyloccus epidermidis*. The infectivity of staphylococcal organisms is facilitated by their production of extracellular mucins that allow for adherence to graft material.[12] Gram-negative rods, including *Escherichia coli, Proteus, Pseudomonas,* and *Klebsiella* organisms, comprise most of the remaining pathogens. The variable presentation of graft infections is in part reflective of the variable natures of these infecting organisms.

S. epidermidis has been associated with "slime" production, resulting in a surface deposition of glycocalyx surrounding the graft. The "slime" protects bacteria from the immunologic functions of

the host[13] and results in the chronic nonincorporation of grafts that one sees in the operating room. Bergamini et al.[14] have shown that more aggressive culture techniques can lead to the increased recovery of *S. epidermidis* in aortic graft infections. This difficulty in culturing *S. epidermidis* probably accounts for the majority of "culture-negative" graft infections.

S. aureus infections are generally less indolent than *S. epidermidis* infections. The production of destructive extracellular enzymes results in perigraft tissue destruction and a more marked inflammatory response. The clinical result is abscess formation and erythema, as opposed to the chronic sinus formation that characterizes *S. epidermidis* infections. Gram-negative organisms produce the same inflammatory characteristics as *S. aureus* and generally present with more local tissue reaction and greater systemic manifestations.

The individual nature of different pathogenic organisms is further highlighted by *Pseudomonas aeruginosa,* which has been characterized in a dog model. The virulent and tissue-destructive nature of *Pseudomonas* was contrasted with *S. epidermidis.* This work suggests that *Pseudomonas* may be associated with arterial wall infection and resultant anastomotic disruption.[15]

PRESENTATION AND SYMPTOMS

The mean time from initial procedure to presentation with aortic graft infection is variable. In one large series, the mean time was 25 months, with a range of 3 days to 12 years.[10] Some variability may be associated with different organisms. *S. aureus* infections tend to present earlier than *S. epidermidis* infections. With all organisms, the majority of patients present with some evidence of infection usually related to the graft at the groin. A swelling mass, erythema, spontaneous drainage, and pain are common complaints. Graft limb occlusion also may be associated with graft infection, and in cases where no other etiology of graft occlusion is evident, graft infection should be considered.

Patients with only retroperitoneal components to their grafts may present with more subtle findings of prosthetic infection. Bleeding, fever, and leukocytosis, while supportive, are distinctly

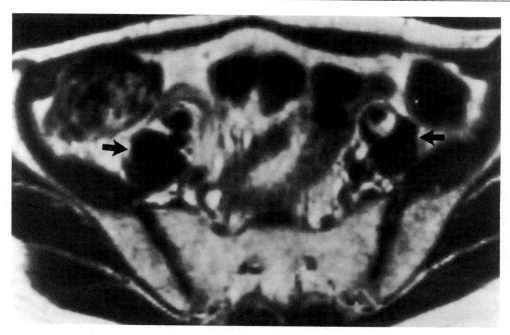

Figure 18-1. This MRI scan shows evidence of aortic graft infection with poor incorporation and perigraft fluid.

unusual symptoms. More subtle symptoms of back pain, malaise, and failure to thrive may be the only signs. A high index of suspicion for graft infection in any patient presenting with a nonspecific illness will assist in making the diagnosis.

DIAGNOSIS

Initial evaluation should include a careful history with attention to prior operative problems and perioperative complications. Previous operative records should be obtained and reviewed. Comorbid illnesses should be documented and evaluated. Physical examination should include careful inspection of all wounds, documentation of pulses, evaluation of extremities for septic emboli, and stool guaiac examination. Notably, stool guaiac examinations are positive in approximately two-thirds of patients with aortoenteric fistulas.

Laboratory evaluation should include a white blood cell count with differential and an erthrocyte sedimentation rate. Blood cultures also should be

obtained if suspicion of a graft infection exists. All draining material should be cultured to help direct subsequent antibiotic therapy. All these tests will be normal in a substantial number of patients, and this should not preclude further investigation in the correct clinical setting.

Further evaluation is directed at visualization of the graft to assess perigraft incorporation and perigraft tissues. Perigraft fluid, perigraft air, and/ or anastomotic breakdown with pseudoaneurysm all substantiate graft infections (Fig. 18-1). Ultrasound has been employed,[16] but has been supplanted by computed tomography (CT scan) and magnetic resonance imaging (MRI). Olofsson et al.[17] highlighted the use of MRI in prosthetic aortic infections. They studied 18 patients with a suspicious clinical history for infection. Perigraft infection was substantiated by MRI in 14 of 16 patients and was excluded in 2 patients. CT scan was performed in 12 patients and provided the correct diagnosis in only 5. Newer-generation MRI scanners and increased application of T2-weighted sequences may further heighten the specificity.

Radionucleotide-labeled leukocyte scans also can be employed in the assessment of graft infections. Their advantage may be their direct demonstration of the inflammation surrounding the graft without reliance on the anatomic changes resulting from the inflammation (including perigraft fluid, etc.). While leukocytes labeled with gallium-67, indium-111, and technetium-99m hexametazime localize to grafts with a high suspicion of infection, their use in distinguishing low-probability infection from uninfected grafts needs further evaluation, but some results are promising.[18,19] False-positive results have been noted, especially with pseudoaneurysms. We currently do not employ scintographic methods routinely to screen patients for graft infection.

Needle aspiration of fluid in the perigraft space also may be employed in the diagnosis of graft infections. Guidance for aspiration can be provided by ultrasound or CT scan. Aspirated material is Gram stained and cultured. The special methods sometimes necessary to recover *S. epidermidis* are an obvious limitation to this technique, which should not be employed alone to rule out graft infection.

In cases where wound sinuses exist, sinograms may be employed to help demonstrate communication to graft material and delineate the extent of graft infection. Some caution should be employed, however, since aggressive instillation of contrast material during a sinogram may result in further graft contamination. Furthermore, injecting contrast material under high pressure may result in a significant bacteremia and clinical deterioration of the patient.

Fiberoptic gastrointestinal endoscopy should be employed in patients with suspected aorto-enteric fistulas. Upper endoscopy can visualize the area of aortoenteric fistula in many cases and should be performed carefully to the fourth segment of the duodenum in any patient in whom this diagnosis is suspected. Lower gastrointestinal studies also may provide information substantiating graft erosion into large bowel in rare situations where this is suspected. In general, barium upper and lower gastrointestinal studies are of little value in patients suspected of prosthetic-enteric erosion or fistula.

Aortography should be employed in antero-posterior and lateral views in patients with graft infection. Views of the pelvis and groin arteries should be obtained, with emphasis on the iliacs, femoral arteries, and the profunda and superficial femoral artery patency, to plan the revascularization of the extremities. The study should define the location and configuration (end-to-end versus end-to-side) of proximal and distal anastomoses, as well as any evidence of pseudoaneurysm and disruption, to assist in operative planning.

Even with extensive preoperative evaluation, graft infection may be a diagnosis made only by direct operative inspection. Exploration of patients with high clinical suspicion for infection is justified. The diagnosis may be firmly established by noting poor graft incorporation and perigraft inflammation and obtaining positive intraoperative Gram stains (and cultures).

GENERAL MANAGEMENT STRATEGIES

The general principles of graft infection treatment are removal of all infected prosthetic material, administration of broad-spectrum antibiotics, and revascularization. The accomplishment of these goals in any one patient must be individualized. Traditional treatment combines removal of infected graft material and revascularization at the same sitting. Extended operative times with prolonged limb ischemia and concomitant metabolic demands make this approach less favorable. Sequential repair involves extraanatomic bypass prior to removal of infected material. Although this reduces ischemia to the lower extremities, it still results in long operative times. We advocate a "staged" approach with extraanatomic bypass followed by removal of the infected graft several days later or a "synchronous" approach with in-line autogenous revascularization.[6]

RECONSTRUCTION MATERIALS

In planning operative reconstruction, alternatives are in part dictated by the available material for revascularization. Prosthetic materials are prone to contamination by the initial infecting organism and are only safely used outside the infected field. In general, extraanatomic reconstruction with axillofemoral bypass circumvents the infected aortic graft.

When revascularization necessitates contact with the infected field, autogenous materials are used.[20,21] Several autologous options are possible in most patients. Arterial autografts may be obtained from the occluded superficial femoral artery, which is disobliterated by endarterectomy. Eversion or oscillating-loop techniques are suitable. The native iliac arteries previously bypassed by the infected prosthesis can be opened by endarterectomy or harvested for use as arterial autograft.

Venous autograft can be obtained from saphenous vein or deep veins of the lower extremity.[22] Deep (superficial femoral) vein should be harvested with care to preserve the profunda femoris vein and common femoral vein. Further, the greater saphenous and deep vein should not be harvested from the same leg to avoid lower extremity venous stasis.

Arterial or venous autograft can be used as a conduit or as material for patch angioplasty of the native arterial system.

GENERAL STRATEGY FOR AORTOBIFEMORAL GRAFT INFECTION

Patients with aortobifemoral graft infection commonly present with groin sepsis manifested by abscess or chronic draining sinus tracts. Following initial patient resuscitation, intravenous antibiotics, and careful patient evaluation, a staged reconstruction is undertaken.

In the first stage, axillofemoral bypass, preferably originating from the right axillary artery if normal flow is present, is performed. Careful exclusion of infected fields should precede any prosthetic procedure. A standard transverse infraclavicular incision is made to expose the area of subsequent proximal anastomosis. The distal anastomotic site is dictated by the preoperative arteriogram and the extent of groin sepsis. In most cases, the distal axillofemoral anastomosis should be below the groin to the superficial femoral or distal profunda femoral artery. Exposure of this area in a previously operated groin requires an incision lateral to the sartorius mus-

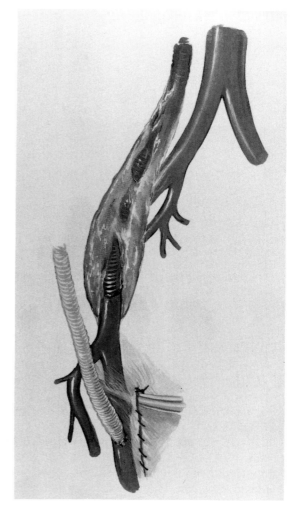

Figure 18-2. In treatment of generalized aortobifemoral graft infection, the axillofemoral prosthetic bypass is anastomosed to the distal superficial femoral artery in an incision remote from infected material. (Reprinted with permission from Stoney RJ, Effeney DJ: Complications requiring reoperation. *In* Wylie's Atlas of Vascular Surgery. Philadelphia, Lippincott, 1991.)

cle. Dissection is performed to identify the superficial femoral or profundus artery without exposing the prior aortobifemoral anastomotic limb. A tunnel is then made, and a prosthetic graft (generally externally supported PTFE) is employed in end-to-side configuration at both sites (Fig. 18-2). The native artery is then occluded proximal to the distal anastomosis to stop

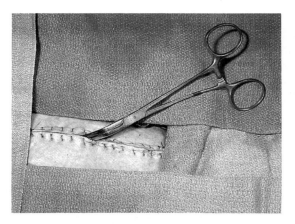

Figure 18-3. This intraoperative photograph shows the femoral wound closed around a vascular clamp left in place to prevent competative flow. (Reprinted with permission from Stoney RJ, Effeney DJ: Complications requiring reoperation. *In* Wylie's Atlas of Vascular Surgery. Philadelphia, Lippincott, 1991.)

antegrade flow from the native system and prevent axillofemoral conduit thrombosis because of competitive flow. These incisions are then closed and sealed to avoid later contamination from the subsequent groin exposure of the infected femoral graft limbs (Fig 18-3).

Both groins are then opened, and the infected prosthesis is detached at the anastomotic sites. The ligated prosthetic limbs are freed and displaced caudally above the inguinal ligament, and the perigraft tissue is closed. Cross-femoral flow is reestablished with autogenous material (vein or artery), at which time the occluding clamp preventing competitive flow is removed. Aggressive debridement is performed to remove the infected and colonized soft tissue in the groin area. Deep tissues are partially closed, but the groins are packed open (Fig. 18-4).

The second stage of the procedure (aortic graft removal) is typically performed at a later time (3 to 5 days later). The abdomen is entered through a midline incision. Proximal aortic mobilization above the prosthetic graft should be obtained early, and if the proximal aortic anastomosis is juxtarenal, it is safest at the suprarenal level. The perigraft tissue is then opened over the aortic bifurcation, and the graft limbs are withdrawn from

their tunnels (Fig. 18-5). Next, proximal aortic clamp control is established, and the proximal graft is removed from the aortic stump. Meticulous debridement of the proximal aortic stump is performed until healthy, noninfected aorta is achieved. The aortic stump is closed with a two-layer closure using monofilament suture (Fig. 18-6). The aortic clamp is removed and hemostasis verified. Aggressive retroperitoneal debridement of all infected and compromised tissue is then performed, and the retroperitoneum

Figure 18-4. Completion of the first stage of the procedure is schematized with the axillofemoral flow to the superficial femoral artery and femorofemoral flow established with autogenous saphenous vein. The distal limbs of the infected graft have been disconnected. (Reprinted with permission from Stoney RJ, Effeney DJ: Complications requiring reoperation. *In* Wylie's Atlas of Vascular Surgery. Philadelphia, Lippincott , 1991.)

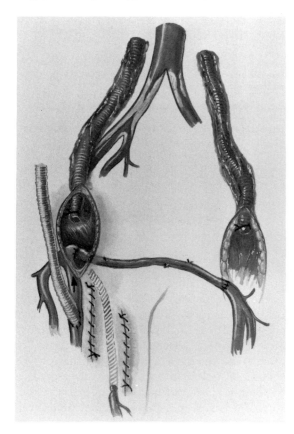

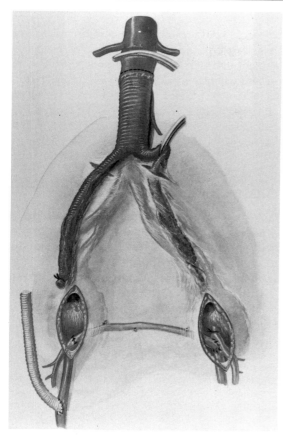

Figure 18-5. At a staged procedure, the infected aortobifemoral graft is removed. Proximal control is obtained and the graft limbs are freed from their tunnels. (Reprinted with permission from Stoney RJ, Effeney DJ: Complications requiring reoperation. In Wylie's Atlas of Vascular Surgery. Philadelphia, Lippincott, 1991.)

is closed, if possible. The abdominal wound is closed, but skin is packed open if gross infection is present.

This two-step approach, as outlined above, can be modified to revascularize patients with aortobi-iliac and aortic tube grafts. After institution of a right axillofemoral bypass, contralateral flow on the left is restored. Prosthetic crossfemoral bypass is a direct method, or revascularization via the native iliac arterial system using iliac-iliac anastomosis will provide cross-pelvic blood flow to the left leg.

IN SITU REVASCULARIZATION

In situ autogenous reconstruction was first described by Ehrenfeld et al.,[21] who employed the combination of endarterectomized native iliac arteries as well as venous and arterial autografts. The advantages include avoiding ectopic prosthetic occlusion and infection (both with limb-threatening consequences), as well as eliminating aortic stump dehiscence. All patients with aortic graft infection are not necessarily candidates, but a recent report by Clagett et al.[22] describes employment of the superficial femoral veins for in situ reconstruction of the aortoiliac system. This technique further expands the number of patients with adequate autogenous conduit for in situ reconstitution following infected graft removal.

Figure 18-6. The proximal aortic anastomosis is resected with some native arterial wall to ensure removal of all infected material. Aortic stump closure is secured with monofilament sutures placed under no tension in two layers. (Reprinted with permission from Stoney RJ, Effeney DJ: Complications requiring reoperation. In Wylie's Atlas of Vascular Surgery. Philadelphia, Lippincott, 1991.)

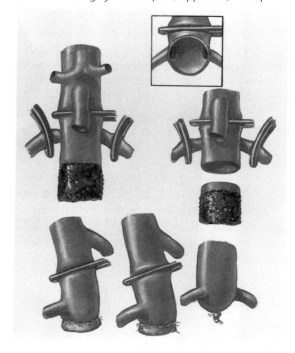

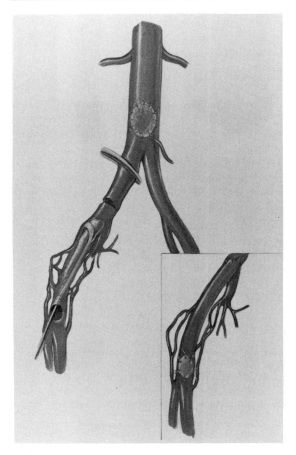

Figure 18-7. In-line revascularization can be performed with infected end-to-side aortobifemoral grafts as shown. Loop stripping thromboendarterectomy and patch angioplasty with autograft material is employed. (Reprinted with permission from Stoney RJ, Effeney DJ: Complications requiring reoperation. *In* Wylie's Atlas of Vascular Surgery. Philadelphia, Lippincott, 1991.)

In situ reconstruction following removal of an infected aortic prosthesis also should be considered in all cases where the proximal aortic anastomosis is end-to-side. In these patients, the native arterial system can be disobliterated with in situ thrombo-endarterectomy. Aortic lumen patency is maintained by patch aortoplasty with a variety of arterial or venous choices. Similarly, autogenous patch angioplasty also can be employed at the distal femoral anastomotic sites (Fig. 18-7).

Delayed conversion to an in-line aortofemoral prosthetic bypass also has been employed 6 months to 1 year after staged repair of aortic graft infection using extraanatomic revascularizations (Fig. 18-8). In these patients, conversion and subsequent graft removal may be precipitated by axillofemoral infection, occlusion, and/or inadequate circulation to the legs. In-line conversion may be a preferable option to axillofemoral or femorofemoral revision with their disappointing late failure rates.

PROSTHETIC ENTERIC FISTULA

Aortic prosthetic enteric fistulas (also known as *secondary aortoenteric fistulas*) most commonly occur with erosion into the adjacent duodenum but may occur with any portion of the small or large bowel in proximity with aortic graft. Two basic configurations of aortic prosthetic communications exist. Paraprosthetic enteric fistulas (Fig.

Figure 18-8. Late conversion of an aortic stump to part of an in-line revascularization requires control of the proximal aorta and branches. Left renal vein division, as shown, is often helpful in facilitating exposure. (Reprinted with permission from Stoney RJ, Effeney DJ: Complications requiring reoperation. *In* Wylie's Atlas of Vascular Surgery. Philadelphia, Lippincott, 1991.)

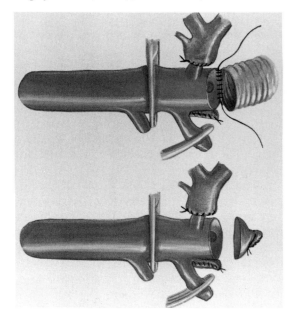

the duodenum may be overlooked. Caution should be employed if clot is seen in the duodenum during endoscopy. Disruption of clot may result in rapid life-threatening bleeding in patients with anastomotic prosthetic enteric fistulas.

In the treatment of massively bleeding anastomotic prosthetic enteric fistulas, the patient's abdomen should be emergently explored if the diagnosis is suspected. At exploration, control of the proximal aorta, if necessary, at the supraceliac level should be followed by detachment of the duodenum from the graft with the surrounding inflammatory tissue. The proximal graft anastomosis is explored, and if a fistula is found, the graft anastomosis is excised. The graft is replaced with a new graft, and the bowel erosion

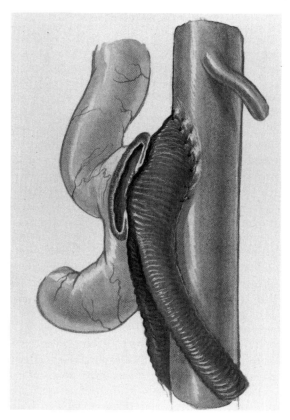

Figure 18-9. Lateral view of a paraprosthetic aortoenteric fistula. (Reprinted with permission from Stoney RJ, Effeney DJ: Complications requiring reoperation. *In* Wylie's Atlas of Vascular Surgery. Philadelphia, Lippincott, 1991.)

Figure 18-10. Lateral view of an anastomotic aortoenteric fistula with a false aneurysm. The potential for life-threatening hemorrhage exists in this case. (Reprinted with permission from Stoney RJ, Effeney DJ: Complications requiring reoperation. *In* Wylie's Atlas of Vascular Surgery. Philadelphia, Lippincott, 1991.)

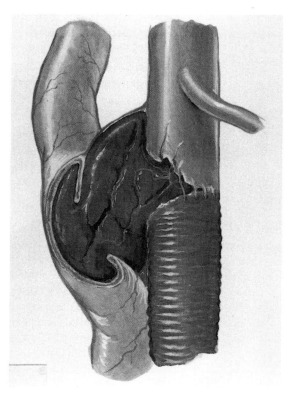

18-9) are remote from the anastomotic site and are the result of bowel erosion by the adjacent pulsatile prosthetic device. Anastomotic prosthetic enteric fistulas (Fig. 18-10) are at the anastomotic site and are often associated with false aneurysms that compress and erode the duodenum. Both types of prosthetic enteric communications present formidable obstacles to treatment, but anastomotic prosthetic enteric fistulas present the additional problem of life-threatening hemorrhage.

As mentioned previously, upper gastrointestinal endoscopy is extraordinarily helpful in identifying an aortoenteric fistula, but a negative study does not exclude the diagnosis. Fistulas located more distal in the small bowel or small lesions in

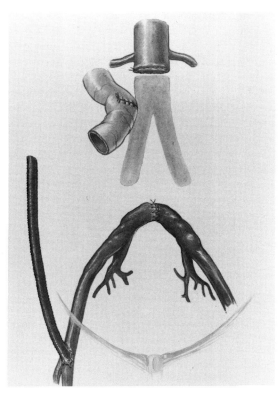

Figure 18-11. A schematic of repaired aortoenteric fistula with cross-femoral flow provided by iliac-iliac anastomosis. (Reprinted with permission from Stoney RJ, Effeney DJ: Complications requiring reoperation. In Wylie's Atlas of Vascular Surgery. Philadelphia, Lippincott, 1991.)

is repaired. In this way, the life-threatening situation is averted, and the patient can be subsequently stabilized prior to planned extraanatomic revascularization and graft reexcision in a more elective, controlled setting.

Bowel repair in aortoenteric fistula correction should be undertaken with careful attention to the size of the defect. Small defects are closed in standard two-layer fashion. Larger defects may require short segmental bowel resections or occasional roux-en-Y loop jejunoduodenostomy. In all cases, careful and complete debridement of the margin of the bowel wall should be employed to avoid anastomotic breakdown and recurrent fistula. In addition, retroperitoneal tissues should be debrided aggressively to avoid ongoing infection (Fig. 18-11).

AORTIC STUMP MANAGEMENT

Management of the aortic stump created following removal of an infected aortic prosthesis and prior extraanatomic revascularization requires special consideration. Impaired stump healing can result in stump disruption with attendant bleeding and a high mortality.[4,10] The etiology of aortic stump disruption is usually a combination of persistent infection of the aortic wall and tension on the closure. Two-layer tension-free monofilament suture closure following aggressive debridement of the infected aortic wall and surrounding tissues is essential to avoid aortic stump dehiscence. In some instances, this will require resection of pararenal aorta above the renal artery level. Proximal renal artery reimplantation or hepatic artery to right renal artery and splenic artery to left renal artery anastomoses allow blood flow from a more proximal level. Aortic closure is then performed at a level just below the origin of the superior mesenteric artery.

Avoidance may be the best solution to aortic stump dehiscence, and this implies in situ autogenous repair. Persistent infection of an aortic anastomosis will result in disruption and life-threatening hemorrhage. Aggressive aortic debridement is essential, even with autogenous in situ repairs. Others have suggested aortic stump reinforcement with omentum, anterior spinal ligament, and jejunal serosal patches.[23] These methods of protection are unproven and unlikely to provide healing if inadequate debridement and significant tension persist at the site of an aortic repair.

LOCALIZED GRAFT LIMB INFECTION

In general, prosthetic graft infections are relentless in their progressive involvement of the entire graft. Occasionally, bacterial spreading in the potential space between the graft and the surrounding fibrous tissue is limited, and a localized graft limb infection results. Bacterial infection is limited to a portion of one graft limb, perhaps because of late contamination (e.g., a groin reoperation) when there is good proximal graft incorporation. While selection of these patients is difficult, MRI and

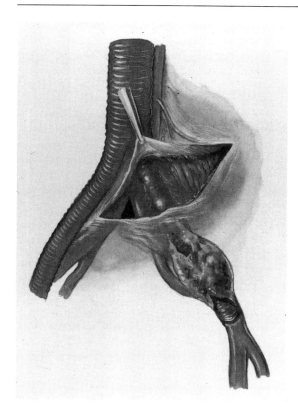

Figure 18-12. Retroperitoneal approach to the proximal limb of a localized graft infection. (Reprinted with permission from Stoney RJ, Effeney DJ: Complications requiring reoperation. *In* Wylie's Atlas of Vascular Surgery. Philadelphia, Lippincott, 1991.)

other imaging studies may help confirm localized prosthetic graft infection.

Definitive treatment requires an extraperitoneal approach to the ipsilateral graft limb below the bifurcation to confirm that the graft limb infection does not extend to the prosthetic bifurcation (Fig. 18-12). At this level, the graft should be well incorporated with no evidence of surrounding inflammation. When these findings are confirmed, the graft limb is divided near its origin, the proximal stump is oversewn, and a short segment of graft is resected. The distal perigraft capsule is closed over the residual graft limb, and the flank wound is subsequently closed and sealed. During the subsequent groin exploration, the distal graft is removed, and limb viability is determined. If collaterals are inadequate, autogenous femorofemoral

bypass is performed with care so as not to expose the contralateral graft limb (Fig. 18-13).

While localized graft infections can be treated effectively by local graft excision and cross-femoral bypass, in our experience, the majority of patients suspected of harboring a localized infection prove to have a diffuse aortofemoral graft infection requiring standard treatment.[3]

PREVENTION

Prevention of aortic graft infection remains the most important strategy in any discussion of the treatment of graft infections. Strict adherence to aseptic technique with protection of the graft from

Figure 18-13. Final repair of a localized graft infection. Cross-femoral flow is provided by an endarterectomized segment of autogenous superficial femoral artery. (Reprinted with permission from Stoney RJ, Effeney DJ: Complications requiring reoperation. *In* Wylie's Atlas of Vascular Surgery. Philadelphia, Lippincott, 1991.)

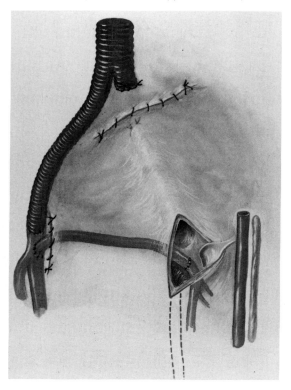

skin and wound contact should be pursued. Adhesive plastic drapes can be used to assist in protection of the graft. Skin preparation should include shaving patients only in the immediate preoperative period.

Meticulous surgical technique also can decrease the incidence of graft infection with attention to intraoperative hemostasis, careful ligation of lymphatics, and complete retroperitoneal placement of grafts. Wound and retroperitoneal hematomas as well as lymphatic leaks and lymphoceles must be avoided. Groin wounds deserve special attention. Careful three-layer anatomic closure and precise skin approximation should be performed.

Prophylactic antibiotics were first suggested to decrease graft infections by Goldstone and Moore.[3] Their work suggested a decrease in the prosthetic infection rate from 4.1 to 1.5 percent with perioperative antibiotics. Standard prophylaxis with cefazolin administered immediately preoperatively and continued perioperatively is the current preferred therapy. Intraoperative dosing at shorter (q4h) intervals also may be beneficial.[24]

Postoperatively, the prevention of graft infections should continue with the aggressive treatment of any suspected septic source with appropriate antibiotics as well as elimination of any proven septic source. Prompt removal of central venous lines and urinary catheters is essential. Careful wound surveillance is important, particularly in the vulnerable groin region. All these measures are critical to ensure a successful healing (incorporation) of the prosthetic graft.

CONCLUSIONS

Aortic prosthetic graft infections remain a challenging surgical problem with significant mortality and morbidity. The poor prognosis of some patients is signaled by persistent infection, which is associated with retained graft material and aortic stump disruption.[6] Recurrent sepsis can also develop within the prosthetic extraanatomic bypass and lead to late failure and amputation.[5] While autogenous materials have been employed in extraanatomic reconstruction[6,10] and with in situ repairs,[21] the durability of autogenous material needs further evaluation. Continued study of treatment options is needed to decrease the mortality and morbidity of managing infected aortic grafts and better understand the critical features associated with successful treatment outcome.

REFERENCES

1. Lorentzen JE, Nielsen OM, Arendrup H, et al: Vascular graft infection: An analysis of sixty-two graft infections in 2411 consecutively implanted synthetic vascular grafts. Surgery 1985;98:81.
2. Poulias GE, Polemis L, Skoutas B, et al: Bilateral aortofemoral bypass in the presence of aorto-iliac occlusive disease and factors determining results: Experience and long term follow up with 500 consecutive cases. J Cardiovasc Surg 1985;26:527.
3. Goldstone J, Moore WS: Infection in vascular prosthesis: Clinical manifestations and surgical management. Am J Surg 1974;128:225.
4. Bacourt F, Koskas F: Axillofemoral bypass and aortic exclusion for vascular septic lesions: A multicenter retrospective study of 98 cases. Ann Vasc Surg 1992;6:119.
5. Quinones-Baldrich WJ, Hernandez JJ, Moore WS: Long-term results following surgical management of aortic graft infection. Arch Surg 1991;126:507.
6. Reilly LM, Stoney RJ, Goldstone J, et al: Improved management of aortic graft infection: The influence of operation sequence and staging. J Vasc Surg 1987;5:421.
7. Farkas JC, Fichelle JM, Laurian C, et al: Long-term follow-up of positive cultures in 500 abdominal aortic aneurysms. Arch Surg 1993;128:284.
8. Moore WS, Rosson CT, Hall AD, et al: Transient bacteremia: A cause of infection in prosthetic vascular grafts. Am J Surg 1969;177:342.
9. Moore WS, Malone JM, Keown K, et al: Prosthetic arterial graft material: Influence in neointimal healing and bacteremic infectability. Arch Surg 1980;115:1379.
10. Reilly LM, Altman H, Lusby RJ, et al: Late results following surgical management of vascular graft infection. J Vasc Surg 1984;1:36.
11. Phillips GR, Peer RM, Upson JF, et al: Late complications of revascularization for radiation-induced arterial disease. J Vasc Surg 1992;16:921.
12. Schmitt DD, Bandyk DF, Pequet AJ, et al: Bacterial adherence to vascular prostheses: A determinant of graft infectivity. J Vasc Surg 1986;3:732.
13. Bandyk DF, Berni GA, Thiele BL, et al: Aortofemoral infection due to Staphylococcus epidermidis. Arch Surg 1984;119:481.
14. Bergamini TM, Bandyk DF, Govostis D, et al: Identification of Staphylococcus epidermidis vascular graft infections: A comparison of culture techniques. J Vasc Surg 1989;9:665.

15. Geary KJ, Tomkiewicz ZM, Harrison HN, et al: Differential effects of a gram-negative and gram-positive infection on autogenous and prosthetic grafts. J Vasc Surg 1990;11:339.

16. Gooding GAW, Effeney DJ, Goldstone J: The aortofemoral graft: Detection and identification of healing complications by ultrasonography. Surgery 1981;89:94.

17. Olofsson PA, Auffermann W, Higgins CB, et al: Diagnosis of prosthetic aortic graft infection by magnetic resonance imaging. J Vasc Surg 1988;8:99.

18. Sedwitz MM, Davies RJ, Pretorius HT, et al: Indium 111–labeled white blood cell scans after vascular prosthetic reconstruction. J Vasc Surg 1987; 6:476.

19. Fiorani P, Speziale F, Rizzo L, et al: Detection of aortic graft infection with leukocytes labeled with technetium-99m hexametazime. J Vasc Surg 1993;17:87.

20. Stoney RJ, Wylie EJ: Arterial autograft. Surgery 1970;67:18.

21. Ehrenfeld WK, Wilbur BG, Olcott CN, et al: Autogenous tissue reconstruction in the management of infected prosthetic grafts. Surgery 1979;85:82.

22. Clagett GP, Bowers BL, Lopez-Viego MA, et al: Creation of a neoaortoiliac system from lower extremity deep and superficial veins. Ann Surg 1993;218:239.

23. Shah DM, Buchbinder D, Leather RP, et al: Clinical use of the seromuscular jejeunal patch for protection of the infected aortic stump. Am J Surg 1983;146:198.

24. Edwards WH, Kaiser AB, Kernodle DS, et al: Cefuroxime versus cefazolin as prophylaxis in vascular surgery. J Vasc Surg 1992;15:35.

ACKNOWLEDGMENT

This work was supported in part by the Pacific Vascular Research Foundation.

19

Infected Infrainguinal Grafts

KEITH D. CALLIGARO
DOMINIC A. DeLAURENTIS
FRANK J. VEITH

Infection involving an arterial graft is arguably the most devastasting complication in vascular surgery. Purulent drainage from a sinus tract overlying a peripheral arterial graft uniformly provokes anxiety and dread among vascular surgeons. These complications are associated with significant amputation and mortality rates, prolonged hospitalization, and extremely high costs. Even if they survive their initial treatment, these patients may be plagued by recurrent, delayed complications.

Management of peripheral arterial graft infections requires a well-designed treatment plan with consideration of all available options. Only massive hemorrhage resulting in hypotension prohibits a careful and thorough preoperative evaluation. Diagnosis and management of aortic graft infections frequently differ from those of infections involving an extracavitary or peripheral graft. Similarly, infections involving prosthetic grafts occasionally require different treatment than infections involving autologous vein grafts.

We will address the etiology, diagnosis, and management of prosthetic and autologous vein grafts involving peripheral arteries. Traditional treatment of these complications will be considered along with new, controversial, and hopefully improved methods of management.

ETIOLOGY OF PERIPHERAL ARTERIAL GRAFT INFECTIONS

Several factors have been documented to predispose to arterial graft infections. Prolonged operative time, repeated dissections through previous operative sites, groin dissections, and obesity correlate with increased chance of infection.[1,2] We believe that multiple prior dissections at the site of the vascular surgery is probably the most common avoidable factor associated with infection, and accordingly, we generally favor using different inflow or outflow arterial sites for secondary bypasses when hostile wounds are encountered. Of approximately 140 extracavitary prosthetic and vein graft infections that we have treated at Montefiore Medical Center in New York and Pennsylvania Hospital in Philadelphia (approximately one-third referred), the average number of previous dissections at the operative site was greater than 2 (range 1 to 11).

We especially try to avoid groin incisions, which are the most common site of wound infections.[1,2] In our combined series, approximately two-thirds of all extracavitary graft infections involved the common, deep, or superficial femoral arteries in the groin. We frequently choose the external iliac artery, approached retroperitoneally through a small suprainguinal or larger flank incision, as an inflow site if the groin has been dissected two or more times. The distal superficial or deep femoral arteries are preferred arterial inflow sites of a femorodistal bypass if a proximal stenosis is not present.[3] When surgery is performed for aortoiliac occlusive disease, we prefer to anastomose the distal limbs of the aortic graft to the distal external iliac arteries to avoid a groin dissection if these arteries and the common and deep femoral arteries are free of disease.

Several prospective, randomized trials have documented the benefit of appropriate prophylactic intravenous antibiotics administered within 1 hour of the time of incision to decrease the incidence of wound and arterial graft infections.[4,5] We continue to use cephazolin (Ancef) as the prophylactic drug of choice before peripheral arterial graft surgery. For prolonged operations, an additional dose of cephazolin is given every 4 hours to maintain adequate antibiotic tissue levels.[6] Although irrigation of the wound with antibiotic solution is of questionable additive benefit when intravenous antibiotics are also given, we frequently flush the operative site before closure of the wound.[5] If lower extremity revascularization is indicated for an infected ischemic foot ulcer or wet gangrene and the patient is already receiving broad-spectrum antibiotics, we do not add cephazolin if it does not provide additional, appropriate bacterial coverage. In these cases, we continue administration of appropriate broad-spectrum antibiotics until final cultures return or the infection resolves.

If surgery is planned at a site of several previous dissections and we are particularly concerned about future wound complications and possible infection, we recently have not been using a first-generation cephalosporin for prophylaxis. Because of the greater chance of wound infection associated with repeated operative dissections, we favor giving one preoperative dose of vancomycin and gentamycin or a third-generation cephalosporin to cover Staphylococcus and Enterobacteriaceae, respectively. Some of these organisms are not covered adequately by cephazolin. However, there are no prospective, randomized studies proving a definite benefit of this strategy.

Most series of peripheral graft infections have documented gram positive bacteria as the predominant causative organism of these complications.[1,7]

In our experience and that of others, S. aureus and S. epidermidis and Streptococcus viridans and S. faecalis are the most common gram-positive bacteria associated with peripheral graft infections.[1,7,8] Pseudomonas aeruginosa, Proteus mirabilis, and Escherichia coli are the most frequently cultured gram-negative bacteria.[1,7,8] Infections involving groin wounds are more commonly associated with gram-negative bacteria than more peripheral wounds, most likely because of the proximity of the perineum.

More recent series of arterial graft infections have documented increasing prevalence of methicillin-resistant S. aureus (MRSA), coagulase-negative (slime-producing) S. epidermidis (CNS), and P. aeruginosa compared with reports in the 1970s and early 1980s.[1,8,9] This represents an important epidemiologic finding, because S. aureus and Pseudomonas are probably more virulent than other bacteria.[8,10] We and others have documented that these organisms are more likely to cause disrupted arterial anastomoses and systemic sepsis.[8,10] We also have documented that peripheral graft infections due to these bacteria are less likely to be treated successfully by attempted graft preservation.[8] S. epidermidis is a relatively benign, indolent organism that may exist as a slime layer on arterial prosthetic grafts for years without overt manifestations of infection.[9] Bandyk and associates[9] reported that if coagulase-negative S. epidermidis is found to be the sole causative organism of a graft infection, replacement of the infected graft with a new polytetrafluoroethylene (PTFE) graft is safe and associated with excellent mortality and limb-salvage rates. We will further discuss management of arterial graft infections in more detail later in the chapter.

DIAGNOSIS

Diagnosis of peripheral arterial graft infections is frequently obvious. Patients usually present with purulent drainage or with erythema surrounding an infected wound.[11] Other signs and symptoms of peripheral arterial graft infections include fever and malaise and frequently warmth and tenderness at the infected site. A pulsatile mass suggests an infected pseudoaneurysm, which most commonly occurs at a disrupted anastomotic site.

Frank hemorrhage and hypotension can occur with rupture of the graft and represent a surgical emergency.

In addition to clinical findings, ultrasound can support the diagnosis of a peripheral prosthetic or vein graft infection. As opposed to aortic graft infection, duplex ultrasonography can be highly suggestive of a graft infection because of the relatively superficial location of peripheral bypasses. Perigraft fluid and air or arterial flow within a pseudoaneurysm can be visualized with this study. If an adequate image cannot be obtained or doubt exists as to the presence of an inflammatory reaction around the graft, a computed tomographic (CT) scan or magnetic resonance imaging (MRI) is highly accurate. Presence of air or fluid around a graft after 4 to 6 weeks almost always implies a graft infection,[12] although perigraft fluid occasionally can be associated with sterile graft reactions. MRI may be more helpful to diagnose aortic graft infections than CT scan, but this technique has not yet been proven to be more accurate for peripheral graft infections.[13] For a definitive diagnosis, we continue to prefer CT scan as the test of choice if an ultrasound yields equivocal results.[14–16] If fluid around the graft is visualized with either technique, we favor ultrasound- or CT-guided needle aspiration of the fluid to confirm the diagnosis and to obtain a culture specimen.

Indium-labeled white blood cell scans are helpful to rule out graft infections but may result in a high incidence of false-positive findings.[16,17] Indium-labeled immunoglobulin G scans are also highly diagnostic but have been used primarily to diagnose aortic graft infections and are not widely available.[18] A sinogram is a simple test to perform and can diagnose the presence and extent of a peripheral graft infection. We perform this study using fluoroscopic imaging after inserting a catheter as far into the wound or along an exposed graft as possible and injecting 20 to 30 cc of contrast material with a hand-held syringe. Flouroscopic images may show tracking of dye along the graft and confirm lack of graft incorporation by surrounding tissues.

An arteriogram is essential to plan a secondary revascularization procedure when graft excision proves necessary. The only instance when a preoperative arteriogram is not obtained is when a patient presents with bleeding and requires emergent surgery. We also obtain an arteriogram of the aortic arch if the axillary artery may be used as a potential inflow source.[19] Distal outflow arteries must be imaged to plan the secondary bypass and perform unusual approaches to avoid the infected wound. If a patient presents with a groin infection involving an extracavitary arterial graft and the contralateral femoral pulse is weak or absent, the translumbar approach can be used to obtain the arteriogram. This technique has been shown to be safe and effective, although very distal outflow arteries are frequently not visualized if the lower extremity graft is occluded.[19] With use of smaller catheters, the brachial artery approach has been associated with few complications by our angiographers.

MANAGEMENT

We have proposed a modified classifications scheme of infected grafts and determine our management based on the presentation of the infection.[20] Patients with infected peripheral or extracavitary grafts can present with (1) anastomotic bleeding or sepsis, the most virulent type of graft infection, (2) occluded grafts, or (3) patent grafts without bleeding or sepsis. For purposes of the following discussion, we will refer to this classification, which we have been using routinely to treat infected peripheral arterial grafts for 20 years.

Disadvantages of Routine Total Graft Excision to Treat Infected Peripheral Arterial Grafts

Traditional treatment of infected peripheral grafts includes excision of the entire graft. However, there are primarily three disadvantages of this strategy. First, graft excision is technically difficult and time-consuming. If any part of the graft is well incorporated, it is usually encased in dense scar tissue, and it may be technically challenging not to injure important arterial collaterals or adjacent veins. Significant hemorrhage can result if surgical misadventure occurs.

Second, additional revascularization procedures are frequently required to prevent limb loss when the graft is excised. Even for patients with infected occluded grafts, important patent collaterals may be injured during graft excision with limb-threatening consequences unless a secondary revascularization procedure is performed. It is not uncommon for patients with peripheral graft infections to have limited arterial inflow and outflow sites. Also, autologous vein may not be available for use as a secondary bypass if patients have undergone multiple previous bypasses. In such cases, the vascular surgeon will have to resort to a prosthetic graft, with relatively inferior patency rates, to avoid a major amputation. Finally, the safest method to prevent recurrent hemorrhage at the infected site after the graft is excised is proximal and distal ligation of the involved artery. This technique will obviously exclude any important collaterals originating from the vessel. If the artery is oversewn in an attempt to maintain patency, arterial stenosis and subsequent thrombosis frequently result.

A third disadvantage of routine graft excision to treat patients with infected peripheral grafts is that these patients are usually high-risk patients with multiple medical problems who may not tolerate graft excision and revascularization. These operations are frequently time-consuming and associated with significant blood loss.

Supporting these concerns are reports that routine excision of infected peripheral arterial grafts is associated with mortality rates ranging between 10 and 30 percent and amputation rates of 10 to 70 percent.[1,7,11,21–23] The group of patients with the highest *mortality* rate in our series of patients with infected peripheral prosthetic and vein grafts was those individuals presenting with anastomotic *hemorrhage* or systemic *sepsis*. The mortality rate in these patients was approximately 20 percent despite immediate graft excision. Patients presenting with infected *occluded* grafts in our series had the highest *amputation* rate (approximately 20 percent) compared with patients presenting with one of the other manifestations of graft infection, i.e., infected patent grafts or bleeding or sepsis.

Despite these concerns, total graft excision to treat infected peripheral arterial grafts remains the gold standard against which other techniques must be compared. Graft excision remains the most widely accepted method to treat these complications.

Selective Graft Preservation to Treat Infected Peripheral Arterial Grafts

Because of the significant disadvantages of routine graft excision to treat all infected extracavitary grafts, Veith[14] proposed *selective complete or partial graft preservation* to treat these complications. He first began cautiously using this approach over 20 years ago.[14] DeLaurentis and associates[24] also have applied this technique to treat patients since the 1970s. Other groups with smaller series of patients also have recently reported excellent results using selective graft preservation.[25–27]

INFECTED PERIPHERAL GRAFTS PRESENTING WITH BLEEDING OR SEPSIS

We agree with others that *graft excision* is mandatory when patients present with anastomotic *bleeding* or systemic *sepsis*. The entire graft must be removed when the patient is septic to eradicate any source of persistent infection. However, if a patient presents with anastomotic disruption and further evaluation reveals that the infection is confined only to that part of the graft, we do not routinely excise the entire graft if it is found to be well incorporated at distant sites. Indeed, we frequently use a remaining segment of functioning, noninfected graft as an inflow or outflow source.

Patients who present with frank hemorrhage must be treated by control of the bleeding first and then revascularization, if necessary. However, patients who present with a stable infected pseudoaneurysm or with sepsis usually can undergo a secondary revascularization procedure before undergoing graft excision. Prolonged ischemia of the threatened extremity, which is usually poorly tolerated in these poor-risk patients, is thereby avoided.

INFECTED OCCLUDED PERIPHERAL ARTERIAL GRAFTS

When patients present with infected *occluded* grafts and intact anastomoses, we routinely perform *subtotal excision* of the graft.[20,28] Almost all the graft is removed except for 2- to 3-mm *remnants that are oversewn at both anastomoses* (Figs. 19-1 and 19-2). These graft remnants function as patches to maintain patency of the underlying arteries.

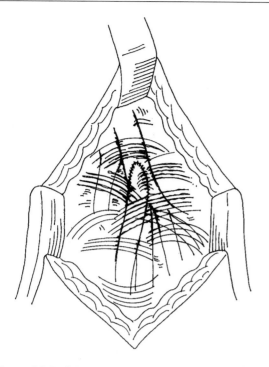

Figure 19-1. Schematic illustration of an infected occluded prosthetic graft anastomosed to the common femoral artery. The common and deep femoral arteries in this case are patent, and maintaining patency of the deep femoral artery may be vital in order to achieve limb salvage.

When an infected graft is totally excised and the involved artery is not ligated, the artery must be oversewn or a patch angioplasty performed to maintain patency of the artery and important collaterals. Several authorities recommend placing an autologous tissue patch or graft in the wound in these cases.[29] We have noted a high rate of rupture when we have placed new autologous tissue patches or grafts in an infected field.[20] We believe that totally excising the original graft and suturing a new patch will cause weakening of the artery wall and more likely will result in future arterial disruption. An advantage of this technique of leaving a small oversewn remnant of graft is that weakening of the arterial wall does not result. Even if the entire involved segment of artery is excised and a new graft is sutured to an uninvolved segment of artery, it is impossible to immediately sterilize an infected wound. Proliferation of bacteria into the

new autologous tissue graft can result in graft weakening and rupture. Subtotal graft excision with oversewing of a small stump of graft has proven especially useful for groin infections by maintaining patency of the deep femoral artery and potentially avoiding the need to perform a secondary bypass.[28] We have found that this technique resulted in successful wound healing achieved by delayed secondary intention in approximately three-quarters of cases after long-term follow-up.

REVASCULARIZATION AFTER TOTAL OR SUBTOTAL GRAFT EXCISION

When total or subtotal graft excision proves necessary for patients who present with bleeding or sepsis or with infected occluded grafts, we favor revascularization of the threatened limb by performing an extraanatomic secondary bypass

Figure 19-2. Schematic illustration of the same wound after subtotal graft excision, extensive wound debridement, and oversewing of a 2- to 3-mm graft remnant on the underlying common femoral artery. This technique maintains patency of the common and deep femoral arteries without requiring placement of a new patch or graft in the infected field.

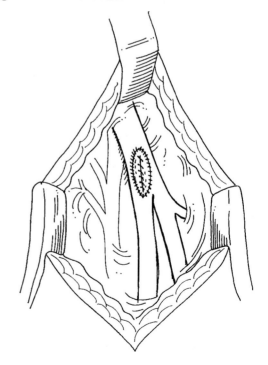

tunneled through sterile fields away from the infected area.[20,28] Detailed knowledge of the anatomy to perform unusual approaches to outflow arteries is essential to achieve limb salvage.[3,30] If the groin wound is extensive after operative debridement, we do not hesitate to tunnel the new graft lateral to the anterosuperior iliac spine.

We prefer to use a nondiseased iliac artery as the inflow source but also will use the thoracic or infrarenal aorta in low-risk patients and the axillary artery in high-risk patients[14,15,31] (Fig. 19-3). As mentioned previously, other alternatives include placing an autologous bypass using autologous vein or a segment of occluded, endarterectomized artery in the infected field.[29] Another option includes placing a new graft as an obturator bypass.[32] We have found that placing an extraanatomic bypass lateral or medial to the infected wound is quicker and simpler than performing an obturator bypass.

When coagulase-negative *S. epidermidis* is the only bacteria cultured from the wound and there is no evidence of gross infection such as pus or grossly infected tissue, Bandyk et al.[9] have reported that replacing the infected graft with a new polytetrafluoroethylene (PTFE) graft may yield acceptable results. However, in these cases, we would simply attempt complete graft preservation, which we will now discuss.

SELECTIVE COMPLETE GRAFT PRESERVATION

One of the more controversial aspects of our management scheme is to treat infected peripheral grafts using complete graft preservation under appropriate circumstances. This method should only be attempted when (1) the graft is patent, (2) the anastomoses are intact, and (3) the patient is not septic.[14,20,28] If all three conditions are not fulfilled, the graft must be excised, as discussed previously.

Several aspects of this technique are critical to achieve a successful outcome. Repeated, aggressive operative wound debridement and excision of all infected tissue are essential. Lack of adequate debridement is probably the most important factor in why selective graft preservation fails for those inexperienced with this technique. Any exudate on the graft or artery must be gently peeled away or

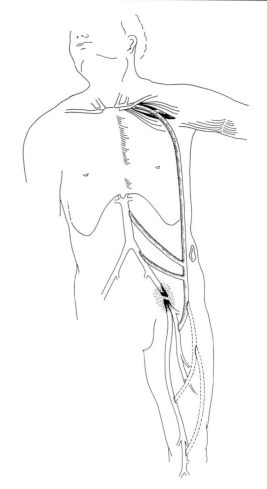

Figure 19-3. Schematic illustration of possible routes for secondary bypasses associated with excision of an infected graft in the groin. Potential inflow sources include the axillary artery, the infrarenal aorta, and the iliac artery. Potential outflow sources include the distal deep and superficial femoral arteries and the popliteal artery. We prefer tunneling the new graft lateral to the wound and do not hesitate to bring the graft lateral to the anterior superior iliac spine if the groin wound is extensive after operative debridement.

else this film may continue to harbor bacteria and result in failure of the technique. The wound is generally much larger after extensive debridement compared with when the patient first presents with a peripheral graft infection, but aggressive excision of any infected surrounding tissue is essential to achieve a healed wound and graft preservation. In addition, a larger segment of exposed graft after wound debridement, compared with the initial presentation, frequently results if wound debridement is performed adequately.

Appropriate intravenous antibiotics are administered for at least 6 weeks when complete graft preservation is attempted. We frequently do not provide any further antibiotic coverage after this time for fear of development of resistant organisms, although occasionally we administer an additional 6-week course of oral antibiotics for patients we consider at especially high risk of recurrent infection. Patients are not necessarily hospitalized during the 6 weeks of intravenous antibiotics, but instead the drugs are administered through an indwelling central venous catheter as an outpatient.

Wet-to-moist dressing changes are performed three times a day in an intensive care unit until the anastomosis is covered by granulation tissue or by a muscle flap. We use an antibiotic or dilute povidone-iodine solution to moisten gauze dressings packed into the open wound. A dilute Betadine solution has been shown to be toxic to bacteria but not to fibroblasts.[33] We do not routinely use continous irrigation catheter flushing of the wound.

Alternatively, a muscle flap can be placed over the graft after all infected tissue has been excised and granulation tissue has formed. During the last 20 years, we have used muscle flaps in less than a quarter of our cases when complete graft preservation was attempted and have not found a difference in terms of successful graft preservation.[34] However, we recently have been favoring this technique compared with secondary-intention wound healing in good-risk patients who can tolerate another major operation.

We have used selective complete graft preservation over the last 20 years at Montefiore Medical Center in New York and Pennsylvania Hospital in Philadelphia to treat approximately 140 infected extracavitary prosthetic and vein grafts. Total or subtotal graft excision was required in over half the patients because they presented with bleeding, sepsis, or occluded grafts. Our results treating the other 69 grafts using attempted complete graft preservation yielded a hospital mortality rate of 13 percent (9 of 69), a hospital amputation rate in

survivors of 5 percent (3 of 60), and a successful long-term complete graft preservation rate of 73 percent (44 of 60).

We determined that long-term graft preservation was equally successful whether the infection involved an autologous vein or a prosthetic graft.[35] We and others favor early coverage of an exposed vein graft with autologous tissue using either a muscle flap or a skin graft because a vein graft is more likely to become desiccated and either thrombose or rupture than a prosthetic graft.[35,36]

Successful graft preservation was accomplished in only approximately 40 percent of cases when *Pseudomonas* was cultured from the wound and about 60 percent of cases when *S. aureus* was cultured.[8] All other gram-negative and gram-positive infections had greater than 70 percent successful graft preservation if the graft was patent, the anastomoses were intact, and the patient was not septic.

Our overall results represent a significantly improved amputation rate and possibly an improved mortality rate compared with traditional routine total graft excision to treat infected peripheral grafts. In the future we hope to establish even more selective criteria to identify patients who can be treated successfully by graft preservation. Although our strategy of treating these complications is controversial, we believe it represents a simpler and improved method of managing infected peripheral arterial grafts.

REFERENCES

1. Bunt TJ: Synthetic vascular graft infections: I. Graft infections. Surgery 1983;93:733.
2. Cruse PJE, Foord R: A five-year prospective study of 23,649 surgical wounds. Arch Surg 1973;107:206.
3. Nunez AA, Veith FJ, Collier P, et al: Direct approaches to the distal portions of the deep femoral artery for limb salvage bypasses. J Vasc Surg 1988;8:576.
4. Kaiser AB, Clayson KR, Mulherin JL, et al: Antibiotic prophylaxis in vascular surgery. Ann Surg 1978;188:283.
5. Pitt HA, Postier RG, MacGowan WAL, et al: Prophylactic antibiotics in vascular surgery: Topical, systemic, or both? Ann Surg 1980;192:356.
6. Guglielmo BJ, Salazar TA, Rodondi LC, et al: Altered pharmacokinetics of antibiotics during vascular surgery. Am J Surg 1989;157:410.

7. Szilagyi DE, Smith RF, Elliott JP, Vrandecic MP: Infection in arterial reconstruction with synthetic grafts. Ann Surg 1972;176:321.

8. Calligaro KD, Veith FJ, Schwartz ML, et al: Are gram-negative bacteria a contraindication to selective preservation of infected prosthetic arterial grafts? J Vasc Surg 1992;16:337.

9. Bandyk DF, Bergamini TM, Kinney EV, et al: In situ replacement of vascular prostheses infected by bacterial biofilms. J Vasc Surg 1991;13:575.

10. Geary KJ, Tomkiewica AM, Harrison HN, et al: Differential effects of a gram-negative and a gram-positive infection on autogenous and prosthetic grafts. J Vasc Surg 1990;11:339.

11. Yeager RA, McConnell DB, Sasaki TM, Vetto RM: Aortic and peripheral prosthetic graft infection: Differential management and causes of mortality. Am J Surg 1985;150:36.

12. O'Hara PJ, Borkowski GP, Hertzer NR, et al: Natural history of periprosthetic air on computerized axial tomographic examination of the abdomen following abdominal aortic aneurysm repair. J Vasc Surg 1984;1:429.

13. Olofsson PA, Auffermann W, Higgins CB, et al: Diagnosis of prosthetic aortic graft infection by magnetic resonance imaging. J Vasc Surg 1988;8:99.

14. Veith FJ: Surgery of the infected aortic graft. In Bergan JJ, Yao JST (eds): Surgery of the Aorta and Its Body Branches. New York, Grune & Stratton, 1979, pp 521–533.

15. Calligaro KD, Veith FJ: Diagnosis and management of infected prosthetic aortic grafts. Surgery 1991;110:805.

16. Mark AS, McCarthy SM, Moss AA, Price D: Detection of abdominal aortic graft infection: comparison of CT and indium-labelled white blood cell scans. AJR 1985;144:315.

17. Serota AI, Williams RA, Rose JG, Wilson SE: Uptake of radiolabeled leukocytes in prosthetic graft infection. Surgery 1981;90:35.

18. LaMuraglia GM, Fischman AJ, Strauss HW, et al: Utility of the indium 111–labeled human immunoglobulin G scan for the detection of focal vascular graft infection. J Vasc Surg 1989;10:20.

19. Calligaro KD, Ascer E, Veith FJ, et al: Unsuspected inflow disease in candidates for axillofemoral bypass operations: A prospective study. J Vasc Surg 1990;11:832.

20. Samson RH, Veith FJ, Janko GS, et al: A modified classification and approach to the management of infections involving peripheral arterial prosthetic grafts. J Vasc Surg 1988;8:147.

21. Liekweg WG, Greenfield LJ: Vascular prosthetic infections: Collected experience and results of treatment. Surgery 1977;81:335.

22. Lorentzen JE, Nielsen OM, Arendrup H, et al: Vascular graft infection: an analysis of sixty-two graft infections in 2411 consecutively placed implanted synthetic vascular grafts. Surgery 1985;98:81.

23. Kikta MJ, Goodson SF, Bishara RA, et al: Mortality and limb loss with infected infrainguinal bypass grafts. J Vasc Surg 1987;5:566.

24. Calligaro KD, Westcott CJ, Buckley M, et al: Infrainguinal anastomotic arterial graft infections treated by selective graft preservation. Ann Surg 192;216:74.

25. Cherry KJ, Roland CF, Pairolero PC, et al: Infected femorodistal bypass: Is graft removal mandatory? J Vasc Surg 1992;15:295.

26. Kwaan JH, Connolly JE: Successful management of prosthetic graft infection with continuous povidone-iodine irrigation. Arch Surg 1981;116:716.

27. Miller JH: Partial replacement of an infected arterial graft by a new prosthetic polytetraflouroethylene segment: A new therapeutic option. 1993;17:546.

28. Calligaro KD, Veith FJ, Gupta SK, et al: A modified method for management of prosthetic graft infections involving an anastomosis to the common femoral artery. J Vasc Surg 1990;11:485.

29. Ehrenfeld WK, Wilbur BG, Olcott CN, Stoney RJ: Autogenous tissue reconstruction in the management of infected prosthetic grafts. Surgery 1979;85:82.

30. Veith FJ, Ascer E, Gupta SK, Wengerter KR: Lateral approach to the popliteal artery. J Vasc Surg 1987;6:119.

31. DeLaurentis DA: The descending thoracic aorta in reoperative surgery. In Bergan JJ, Yao JST (eds): Reoperative Arterial Surgery. Orlando, Fla, Grune & Stratton, 1986, pp 195–203.

32. Guida PM, Moore WS: Obturator bypass technique. Surg Gynecol Obstet 1969;128:1307.

33. Lineaweaver W, Howard R, Soucy D, et al: Topical antimicrobial toxicity. Arch Surg 1985;120:267.

34. Calligaro KD, Veith FJ, Sales CM, et al: A comparison of muscle flaps and delayed secondary intention wound healing in the management of infected lower extremity arterial grafts. Ann Vasc Surg 1994;8:31.

35. Calligaro KD, Veith FJ, Schwartz ML, et al: Management of infected lower extremity autologous-vein grafts by selective graft preservation. Am J Surg 1992;164:291.

36. Ouriel K, Geary KJ, Green RM, DeWeese JA: Fate of the exposed saphenous vein graft. Am J Surg 1990;160:149.

ACKNOWLEDGMENTS

This work was supported by grants from the John F. Connelly Foundation, the U.S. Public Health Service (HL 02990-01), the James Hilton Manning and Emma Austin Manning Foundation, the Anna S. Brown Trust, and the New York Institute for Vascular Studies.

Thrombolysis

Techniques of Percutaneous Intraarterial Thrombolysis (PIAT)

THOMAS McNAMARA
KELLY R. GARDNER

Thrombolysis is a tremendous therapeutic tool. High success rates with low patient morbidity and/or mortality can be achieved using the basic principles described herein. Use of a coaxial system makes the procedure easier to perform and decreases overall infusion times. Tailoring the specifics of the coaxial system to the occlusion also can facilitate lysis and minimize complications.

Thrombolysis is used increasingly as an alternative to surgery for arterial and graft occlusions in the peripheral circulation. Reduced mortality rates are testimony to its efficacy in instances of acute lower limb ischemia.

In our recent report[1] of the results of 72 high-dose urokinase infusions for acute lower limb ischemia (ALLI), the mortality rate was 1.6 percent and the amputation rate among the survivors was 8.5 percent. These results compare favorably with historical controls reported in the two largest reviews of the results of surgical treatment for ALLI.[2,3]

A review of surgical series published between 1963, the year of the introduction of the Fogarty catheter, and 1978 encompassed 3350 cases treated with immediate thromboembolectomy for ALLI with a cumulative mortality rate of 27 percent and an amputation rate of 39 percent.[2] A 1986 review of similar surgical series published between 1978 and 1984 encompassed 2495 cases with a cumulative in-hospital mortality rate of 18 percent and an amputation rate of 16 percent.[3]

This reduced mortality associated with use of the high-dose urokinase regimen for percutaneous intraarterial thrombolysis (PIAT) in patients with ALLI also has been demonstrated during use of the low-dose streptokinase regimen. Our review of reports in the surgical literature of the role of thrombolysis for low-dose streptokinase infusions for ALLI encountered a similarly low cumulative mortality rate of 1.9 percent in the 160 infusions performed.[4–11]

These lower mortality rates may reflect the less stressful nature of thrombolysis as compared with surgery. They also may reflect the beneficial effect of medical stabilization associated with not immediately rushing the patient to the operating room. Most of these patients are elderly and have associated cardiac, pulmonary, cerebrovascular, and renal diseases due to chronic smoking, hypertension, and/or diabetes. Given the fragility of such patients, it is not surprising that the most common cause of in-hospital mortality associated with the surgical treatment of ALLI is acute myocardial infarction within a few days of the procedure.

Although our improved mortality results were similar to prior reports of the use of PIAT for ALLI, other outcome parameters were different. We experienced a lower amputation rate of 8.5 versus 16 percent, a lower major bleeding rate of 2.8 versus 11 percent, and a higher thrombolysis success rate of 85 versus 53 percent, with a shorter mean infusion duration of 18 versus 42 hours.[1] We ascribe these differences to our use of the high-dose urokinase regimen rather than the low-dose streptokinase regimen used in the prior series. Similar differences suggesting greater efficacy with urokinase have been reported previously.[12–18]

Another possible explanation for our improved rates is the more rapid advancement of the catheter through the clot at 2-hour intervals with the high-dose urokinase regimen rather than at 6- to 12-hour intervals with the low-dose streptokinase regimen. These differences in technique may be particularly important when treating the acutely ischemic limb.

It seems axiomatic that this more aggressive approach to exposing the clot to the thrombolytic agent would lead to more rapid and complete clearing of the occlusion with a beneficial shortening of the period of ischemia. However, accomplishing this with the standard endhole catheter is arduous. It requires trundling the patient from the intensive care unit or ward to the angiography suite and then on and off the angiography table. It is labor-intensive for the interventional radiologist, nurses, and radiology technologists. It ties up the angiography suite for extended periods of time for careful repositioning of the infusion catheter.

A method of continuously depositing the thrombolytic agent throughout much or all of the clot from the outset without the need for frequent manipulations of the infusion catheter was therefore needed. A multiport system to deliver the thrombolytic agent was conceived as one solution. Our experience, however, indicated several features in addition to multiple ports that should be incorporated into an infusion system to make infusions easier and faster.

The design and specifications that we arrived at were based on the following empirical tenets: We continue to view it as desirable to have clot dissolution gradually progress from proximal to distal. This appears to minimize the risk of clot fragmentation that can result in distal embolization occurring prior to effectively clearing the initial occlusion. That event yields tandem lesions, which invariably make the patient more ischemic. The operator then has to contend with a more difficult pain-management situation; increased anxiety of the patient, nurse, staff, family, and attending vascular surgeon; and the added difficulty of trying to lyse occlusions at separated sites even more rapidly without increasing the risk to the patient. Risk may be increased when the dose of thrombolytic agent is markedly increased or intervention within the vessel becomes more vigorous.

The dissolution pattern we seek is more difficult to accomplish with a multisidehole than with an endhole-only catheter. We and others[19] have noted an increased incidence of distal migration of lysing clot with the use of some multiport systems. This seems particularly true if either the loci of the ports or the dosing regimen results in widely separated sites of high drug concentration in the clot. Nonetheless, the increased ease of performing the procedure with the multiport systems warrants design efforts to combine the best features of both approaches, however.

Our approach to effecting progressive proximal to distal thrombolysis of an easily penetrable occlusion is to have the emission volume gradually decrease from proximal to distal. Our experiments have demonstrated that most or all of the fluid exits via the first sidehole, at the low flow rates used during continuous infusions, if the standard-size sideholes are used. The holes must be much smaller than the standard angiographic sidehole so as to present increased resistance. This forces the fluid down the length of the catheter, regardless of whether or not it is in clot.

Additionally, close spacing of the sideholes effectively functions as a larger sidehole by more rapidly reducing the pressure in the catheter such that its distal portion emits much less fluid per centimeter than the proximal portion. Thus the flow pattern is controlled by the size, number, and spacing of the sideholes. Each of the available infusion systems has a unique emission volume per centimeter of infusion segment. The McNamara system has a gradually decreasing curve, the Mewissen and Katzen systems have sharply decreasing curves, and the EDM system has a flat curve.[20]

A straight catheter configuration is considered most desirable, since the catheter "memory" of a curved tip often makes it more difficult to advance the catheter over the guidewire through tortuous vessels. This configuration also can result in the re-forming of the curve during infusion such that

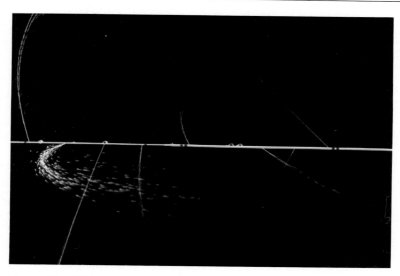

Figure 20-1. With use of a 10-cc or smaller-volume syringe, a jet of fluid can be easily expressed out of sideholes in both inner and outer portions of the McNamara coaxial infusion system. Tip occluder is not required as outer no. 5.5 French catheter has endhole occluded by the inner no. 3 French catheter. Endhole of inner no. 3 French catheter is occluded by 0.015-in guidewire.

the tip withdraws from the occlusion and enters an adjacent collateral, incurring the cost and risk of the drug without providing the benefit. The straight catheter configuration does require, however, that the system have an endhole through which a torquable wire can pass so as to affect direction during advancement. It is desirable for both the inner and outer portions to have these characteristics in a coaxial system.

The patent endholes that permit use of torquable guidewires must be able to be occluded during the infusion so as to force fluid to exit through the sideholes. We have demonstrated in our laboratory and clinical research that this can be simply and effectively obtained by occluding the endhole of the outer catheter with the inner catheter and the endhole of the inner catheter with the directable guidewire.

This occlusion of the endhole must be accompanied by retained ability to infuse slowly (0.4 to 1.6 ml/min) to achieve a gradually decreasing emission pattern over the length of the catheter(s). The system also must be able to emit jets of fluid through each sidehole (Fig. 20-1) when using the pulsed-spray technique.[21]

It is also desirable for the inner portion of the system to be smaller than the proximal outer portion to match the progressive distally decreasing caliber of the arteries. The smaller the system, the less it will dampen flow, and flow is a great potentiator of thrombolysis. It is therefore preferable to keep both portions of the system as small as possible.

The outer catheter should be no. 5 to 6 French in size in a coaxial system. A larger size than no. 5 French provides a tighter seal between the catheter and the arteriotomy margin following removal of the diagnostic catheter, even when a no. 5 French rather than our preferred no. 4 French size has been used. A catheter smaller than no. 6 French provides for adequate space around the catheter when placed through a no. 6 French sheath, if a sheath is required. These considerations led us to size the outer catheter of the McNamara coaxial infusion system at 5.5 French (Fig. 20-2).

Both portions of the system should provide for enough flow during hand injections (Fig. 20-3) to obtain adequate digital subtraction arteriography (DSA) images during rechecks following periods of infusion. Optimally, this should be accomplished without disassembling the system.

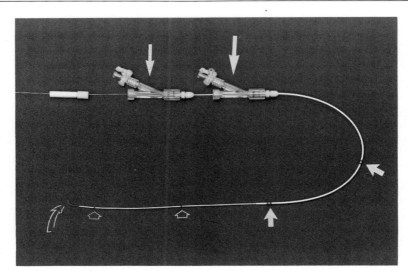

Figure 20-2. This coaxial infusion system consists of an outer straight no. 5.5 French catheter plus an inner straight no. 3 French catheter. Paired black rings (*short closed arrows*) demarcate proximal and distal ends of infusion segment of outer catheter. Single black rings (*open arrows*) demarcate ends of infusion segment. System includes 0.015-in directable guidewire and torque device (*curved arrow*). It also includes clear plastic Touhy-Borst Y-adapters to secure watertight seals around both the no. 3 French catheter and the 0.015-in guidewire (*long closed arrows*). Two three-way stopcocks are attached to the adapters to provide access for hand injections during follow-up DSA imaging without the need to break these connections between the infusion pumps and catheter lumens.

Figure 20-3. Three-way stopcock can be turned off to pump (*arrow*) allowing access to lumen of infusion catheter for hand injections of contrast material or medications without disassembling system.

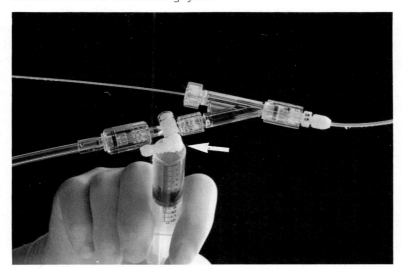

We, therefore, use three-way stopcocks at the junction of the infusion catheter and the tubing leading into the infusion pump (see Fig. 20-3).

Varying lengths should be available to fit the different needs of the ipsilateral, contralateral, and upper extremity approaches to an infrainguinal occlusion. It should be possible to vary the infusion length by telescoping or separating the infusion segments of a coaxial system in response to the changing length and location of the clot during lysis.

We have developed a system that incorporates these features (Figs. 20-2 and 20-3). Radiodense markers at both ends of the infusion segments facilitate fluoroscopically controlled positioning. The markers of the outer and inner portions of the system should be distinguishable (Fig. 20-4). Others have developed infusion systems that also incorporate many of these features. Further clinical testing and experience are required to determine the specific instances in which a particular system is the best choice.

ARTERIOGRAPHY

We prefer a retrograde contralateral femoral approach for arteriography but use a high left brachial approach as an alternative. We prefer to do the procedure with a no. 4 French pigtail catheter. We commonly use Conray 60 for hand injections and Hexabrix for large-volume injections.

We obtain an anteroposterior (AP) projection of the abdominal aorta to evaluate the renal artery origins and the infrarenal aorta. We also obtain oblique views of the aortic bifurcation and distal vessels because most of the plaque formation is posterior in the iliac, common femoral, and popliteal arteries, and AP views often underestimate it.

CONTRALATERAL ACCESS

The no. 4 French pigtail catheter often can be manipulated to obtain the contralateral access, as previously described.[22] A no. 4 French horseshoe hook catheter (Cook) (Fig. 20-5) frequently can

Figure 20-4. A, Double radiodense ringlike markers on outer catheter (*arrows*) are clearly visible for aid in positioning proximal portion of thrombus occluding right limb of an aortobifemoral graft (ABF). **B,** Single radiodense rings (*open arrows*) facilitate fluoroscopically controlled positioning of inner catheter as it extends beyond outer catheter into distal portion of thrombus. Radiodensity of distal portion of 0.015-in guidewire facilitates visualization during selection maneuvers and positioning of tip just beyond the tip of no. 3 French inner catheter to effect significant occlusion of the endhole and force infusate out of sideholes (*white arrow*).

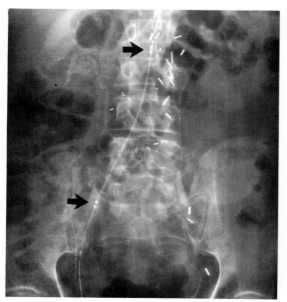

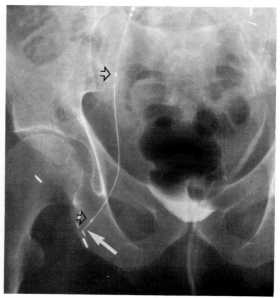

A   B

select the contralateral iliac orifice if the pigtail catheter will not. This curve is easier to manipulate into the orifice and the radiodense tip facilitates visualization. The no. 4 French size does not resist deformity and therefore follows readily over the wire (0.035-in outside diameter).

A no. 4 French modified shepherd's hook catheter (McNamara contralateral catheter) also readily selects the opposite iliac orifice and follows easily over an 0.035-in guidewire through even a tortuous iliac system (see Fig. 20-9). This catheter curve is usually re-formed in the proximal portion of the descending thoracic aorta.

After re-forming the curve, an 0.035-in Bentson guidewire (Cook) is advanced through it to

Figure 20-5. Horseshoe hook catheter is available in no. 4 and no. 5.5 French sizes. No. 4 French size (*left*) is usually used for initial catheterization. No. 5.5 French size (*right*) with 0.038-in endhole is usually used for definitive arteriography following thrombolysis or angioplasty, while 0.035-in guidewire remains across site of occlusion or angioplasty.

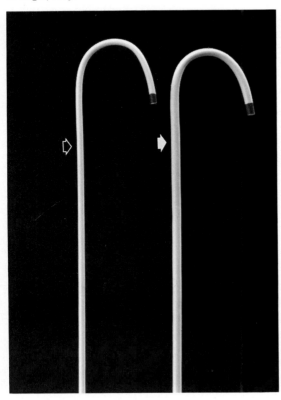

extend 3 to 5 cm beyond the catheter tip. This soft guidewire does not straighten out the curve and points straight distally. This prevents the curved catheter tip from inadvertently selectively entering intercostal, visceral, renal, or lumbar branches during withdrawal maneuvers used to position the tip in the contralateral iliac artery.

The catheter is modeled after the Motarjeme catheter (Mallinckrodt) but is no. 4 French and has a radiodense tip and two sideholes near the tip. The sideholes prevent catheter recoil during diagnostic arteriography injections and enable the no. 5.5 French version to function as the proximal part of a coaxial system.

The 0.035-in Bentson will then be used to traverse the iliac system. If it cannot be advanced to the opposite common femoral artery, a 0.035-in angled Glidewire (Medi-tech) will be used. This can almost always be manipulated through even the most tortuous iliac arteries.

Despite the lack of rigidity of the regular Glidewire (not the Stiff version), any of these no. 4 French catheters will usually readily advance over it. The no. 5 French curved catheters are more likely to resist and do not readily advance over the Glidewire through a tortuous iliac system. They often buckle and form a loop in the distal aorta, causing the guidewire to withdraw from the iliac system. We therefore prefer the no. 4 French catheters for this portion of the procedure.

ANTEGRADE APPROACH

We have found that the antegrade puncture of the common femoral artery is facilitated by visualization of this artery via a diagnostic angiographic catheter that was introduced in a retrograde manner from the contralateral side. Contrast material can be injected through either the pigtail catheter in the distal abdominal aorta or the selective catheter in the proximal segment of the iliac artery on that side. This provides for direct fluoroscopic visualization of the common femoral artery. Advancing the needle under fluoroscopic control during such an injection incurs a small radiation dose to the operator's hands but greatly facilitates precise needle placement.

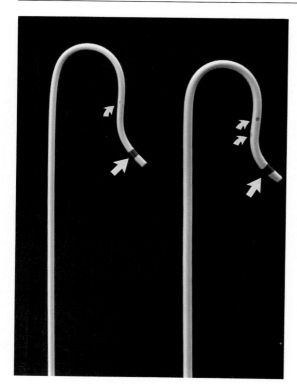

Figure 20-6. Black rings on no. 4 French modified shepherd's hook catheter (*large arrows*) are radiodense markers. Two small sideholes (*small arrows*) prevent recoil during injection through either catheter and allow infusion around inner no. 3 French catheter when using no. 5.5 French size.

We prefer the no. 4 French micropuncture sets (Cook) for the antegrade punctures because we believe they are safer than the standard needle and guidewires. With the former, the initial puncture is made with a 21-gauge needle. Consequently, abandonment of a misplaced initial artery puncture is less worrisome as a site for bleeding during subsequent thrombolysis.

COMMON ILIAC OCCLUSIONS

A coaxial system is to be used for a common iliac artery occlusion if the occlusion is penetrable. We use the no. 5.5 French McNamara contralateral as the outer catheter (Fig. 20-6). The 0.040-in (inner diameter) endhole allows the passage of a no. 3

French infusion catheter or guidewire of one's choice (Fig. 20-7). Two small sideholes near the tip allow easy egress of fluid during slow infusions. They also allow for adequate injections of contrast material for DSA images without removal of the inner infusion catheter or guidewire during thrombolysis (Fig. 20-8).

The outer catheter is situated in the proximal 2 cm of the clot by pulling down on the catheter after the curve has been re-formed and a guidewire advanced into the clot (Fig. 20-9), as previously described.[22] An inner infusion guidewire or catheter is introduced through the O-ring of a Touhy-Borst type of adaptor attached to the hub of the outer catheter. When an endhole-only catheter or infusion guidewire is used, it is advanced until the tip is at or just beyond the midportion of the occlusion (see Fig. 20-8). When a multisidehole system is used, it is advanced until the proximal sidehole is just distal to the tip of the outer catheter.

The inner endhole systems we use are the Cook rendition of the SOS wire (Cook and Bard), the Cragg wire (Medi-tech), the Tracker II catheter (Target Therapeutics), and the Cook no. 3

Figure 20-7. No. 3 French endhole infusion catheter with radiopaque tip has been advanced through no. 5.5 French McNamara contralateral catheter. This combination can serve as coaxial system for short iliac occlusions, as seen in Fig. 20-8.

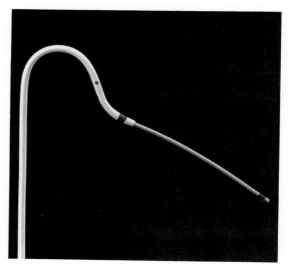

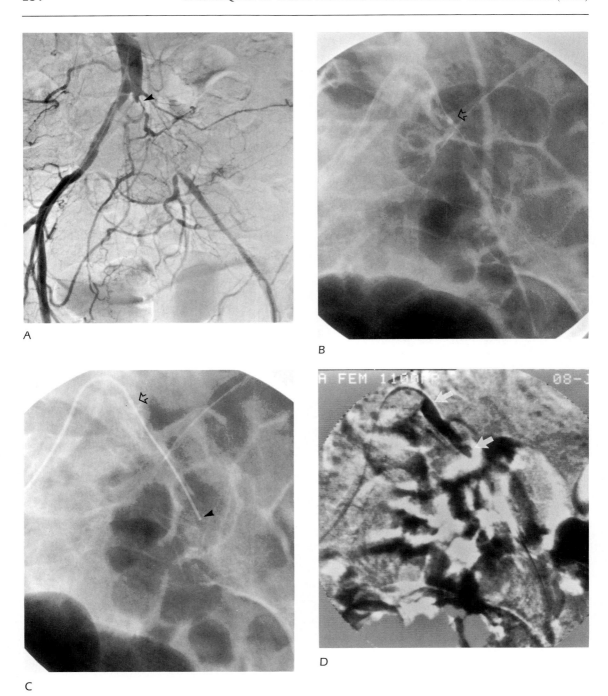

Figure 20-8. A 62-year-old woman with a 12-hour history of acute ischemia involving left lower extremity. **A**, Left common iliac artery (*arrowhead*) is occluded. **B**, No. 5.5 French McNamara contralateral catheter has been positioned with radiodense tip (*arrow*) in the proximal portion of clot. **C**, 0.038-in endhole-only SOS infusion guidewire (*arrowhead*) is advanced until it is positioned beyond tip (*open arrow*) of no. 5.5 French catheter. **D**, Injection through side arm of Y-adapter connected to a no. 5.5 French catheter without removal of infusion wire provides sufficient contrast material for digital subtraction angiographic image to confirm proximal to distal progression of clot lysis following 2 hours of infusion.

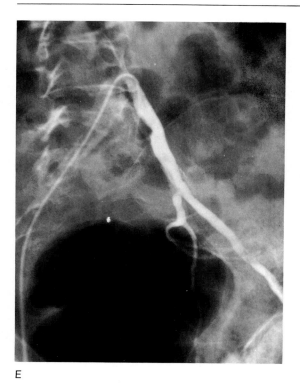

E

Figure 20-8 *continued.* **E,** Removal of inner (infusion) guidewire or catheter provides for rapid flow infections of contrast material through no. 5.5 French catheter for cut film arteriography following thrombolysis.

French endhole infusion catheter with a radio-paque tip (see Fig. 20-7). The inner multisidehole systems we employ are the no. 3 French inner catheter of the McNamara coaxial infusion set and the Katzen infusion guidewire. The former allows a 0.015-in torque wire through the endhole for directability. This also occludes the endhole, forcing fluid out of the sideholes during either continuous or pulse-spray infusions (see Fig. 20-1). The Katzen guidewire does not have an endhole but can be directed by curving the tip of a removable mandril.

A long common iliac occlusion also can be treated by positioning the outer portion of the multisidehole coaxial system in the occlusion and effecting occlusion of the tip with the passage of an endhole no. 3 French catheter. When the clot is not penetrable, it is necessary to employ a single-port system. We use the no. 5 French endhole-only Motarjeme catheter or the no. 4 or no. 5.5 French endhole-only horseshoe hook catheter. Both types are positioned with the catheter tip in contact with the clot. Both these endhole systems also can be used when there is flow through the occlusion at the outset of the infusion, since there is no need to penetrate the clot to have the entire surface exposed to the drug (Fig. 20-10).

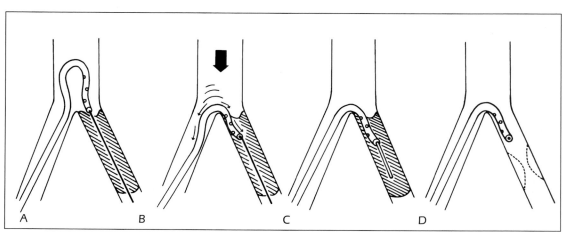

A   B   C   D

Figure 20-9. A, B, Steps in seating McNamara no. 5.5 French contralateral catheter within an occluded common iliac artery. **C,** Substitution of an infusion guidewire no. 3 French catheter for angiographic guidewire creates a coaxial infusion system. Occlusion of the endhole of no. 5.5 French catheter by inner guidewire/catheter forces infusate out of sideholes of no. 5.5 French catheter. **D,** High-flow-rate injections can be made through the no. 5.5 French catheter by removal of the inner guidewire/catheter.

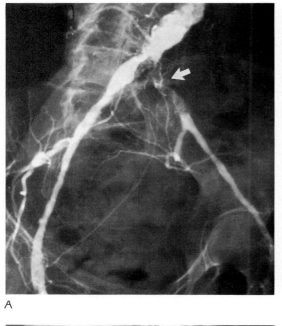

A

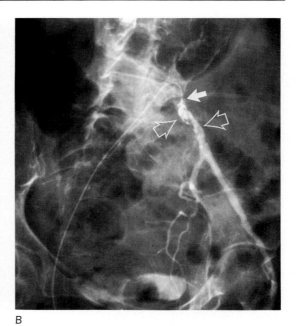

B

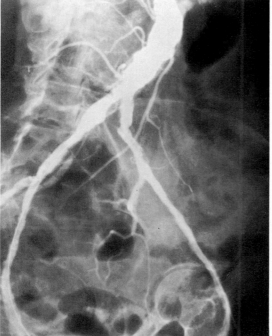

C

Figure 20-10. A 78-year-old woman with an 18-hour history of sudden onset of cold, pale, painful left lower extremity. **A**, Small amount of contrast material trickles through occlusion of left common iliac artery (*arrow*) on initial arteriogram. **B**, Radiodense tip (*closed arrow*) of no. 4 French horseshoe hook catheter is positioned at proximal margin of occlusion. There is almost complete clot lysis (*open arrows*) following 2 hours of high-dose urokinase regimen (4000 IU/min). **C**, After 2 more hours of continuous infusion of urokinase at 4000 IU/min, complete clot lysis was accomplished and PTA performed to clear underlying stenosis.

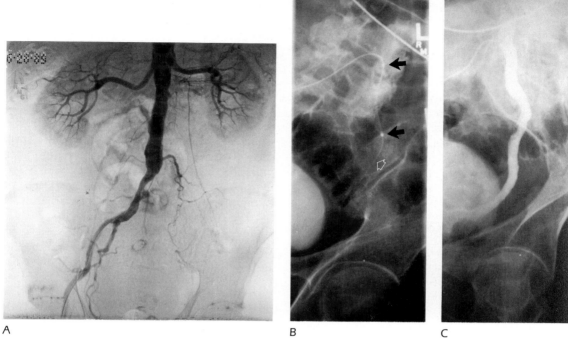

Figure 20-11. An 82-year-old man with a 36-hour history of acute onset of cold, pale, painful left lower limb. **A,** Occlusion of left common, internal, and external iliac arteries. **B,** Early version of McNamara coaxial system with single-ring radiodense markers. Outer system is positioned throughout common iliac occlusion (*black arrows*). Inner catheter extends beyond into proximal half of external iliac occlusion (*open arrow*). **C,** Following 4 hours of a high-dose continuous infusion (4000 IU/min) of urokinase, there is restoration of flow and almost complete clot lysis.

COMBINED ILIAC OCCLUSIONS

We prefer to introduce more sideholes for the longer combined common and external iliac artery occlusions. We usually attempt to introduce both portions of the McNamara infusion system (see Figs. 20-2 and 20-11). This consists of an outer no. 5.5 French catheter that emits fluid out of sideholes for 12 cm and then out of the partially occluded 0.038-in (inner diameter) tip for an effective length of 15 cm. It also includes a no. 3 French inner catheter that emits fluid through sideholes over a distance of 9 cm as well as from the partially occluded 0.018-in (inner diameter) tip for an effective distance of 12 cm.

We also have used other multisidehole systems. The Mewissen (Medi-tech) infusion catheter has either a 0.035- or 0.038-in endhole. It is no. 5 French and has infusion segment lengths of 5 and 10 cm. The EDM (Peripheral Systems Group) infusion catheter is no. 4.8 French and has four sideholes distributed over 6-, 9-, 12-, or 15-cm infusion lengths. It also has an 0.018-in endhole.

The Katzen infusion guidewire is a closed end multisidehole system that has sideholes distributed over 3-, 6-, 9-, or 12-cm distances. It is available in 0.035 and 0.038-in. The Katzen and Mewissen systems have closely spaced sideholes. They therefore emit most of the fluid in the proximal portion of the infusion segment. The EDM catheter has only four sideholes, each of which is supplied by a separate channel and emits about the same amount of fluid from each sidehole.

SUPRAINGUINAL GRAFT OCCLUSIONS

Aortoiliac or aortofemoral graft occlusions are always long clots. The same principles apply to these occlusions as to the combined common and external iliac artery occlusions (see Fig. 20-4). One important distinction, however, is that the bilateral aortoiliac occlusions usually need to be approached from a high brachial artery access, since the occluded aortoiliac system precludes initial placement from the common femoral artery.

Even a unilateral common iliac artery or aortoiliac graft limb occlusion occasionally requires a brachial artery puncture because of a difficult-to-traverse acute angulation at the junction with the contralateral iliac artery graft limb or severe iliac artery tortuosity (Fig. 20-11).

FEMORAL OCCLUSIONS

Proximal superficial femoral artery (SFA) occlusions that are fresh are easily penetrable. A coaxial multisidehole system is usually used. The proximal sidehole is positioned just within the orifice of the SFA.

Distal SFA occlusions are also usually treated with a coaxial system, but the outer portion does not need to be long. It can be a simple angiographic catheter that has a few sideholes near the tip to allow emission of fluid into the proximal SFA when the endhole is occluded by the inner part of the system.

This positioning bathes the slow-flowing blood with either the thrombolytic agent or heparin to reduce the chance of pericatheter clot formation around the inner catheter. The inner portion is then advanced into the distal clot. The tip of an endhole-only system or the proximal sidehole of a multisidehole inner system is positioned in the proximal 1 cm of the occlusion.

We occasionally use the antegrade approach for infrainguinal occlusions. We use a triaxial system when treating a long combined supra- and infrageniculate occlusion. The third component and port is a no. 6 French sheath.

INFRAINGUINAL GRAFT OCCLUSIONS

The coaxial system is again the preferred method of treatment for infrainguinal graft occlusions. The femoral origin of the graft site is usually best

profiled in an oblique position with the same side up. Gentle probing with a wire and catheter is then done in that projection to enter the graft. One must be careful not to traumatize the profunda femoris artery, which is usually the only good collateral pathway.

We place the most proximal sidehole just within the proximal aspect of the occluded graft. A long segment of sideholes allows more of the clot to be exposed to the lytic agent. The distal graft is gently traversed with a guidewire, creating a small channel throughout the graft. We position the multisidehole inner catheter in the middle to distal third of the graft, thereby optimizing the area of thrombus simultaneously exposed to the drug.

We are careful not to make vigorous, large-volume test injections into the thrombosed graft as that may dislodge thrombus downstream and worsen the acute ischemia. We usually infuse at twice the flow rate through the outer catheter as through the inner, to effect a gradually decreasing dose to promote proximal to distal clot lysis without fragmentation.[20]

Prompt reestablishment of flow usually occurs. Experience has taught us that residual thrombus can be difficult to distinguish from underlying fixed stenosis. When in doubt, we withdraw the inner catheter from the body and position the tip of the outer catheter just within the orifice of the graft for a prolonged low-dose infusion (6 to 12 hours). Using this approach, we have frequently been surprised to see complete resolution or a considerable decrease in the size of what we had thought was an atherosclerotic stenosis (Fig. 20-12).

Prematurely dilating within residual thrombus can lead to distal embolization with worsening of symptoms and the need for vigorous thrombolysis efforts or emergency surgery. We thus tend to err on the side of a longer than necessary infusion if we are uncertain about the nature of a residual stenosis after only a few hours' infusion.

POPLITEAL ARTERY

In cases in which we successfully enter the occluded segment, we place an inner catheter with a short infusion segment well into the thrombus.

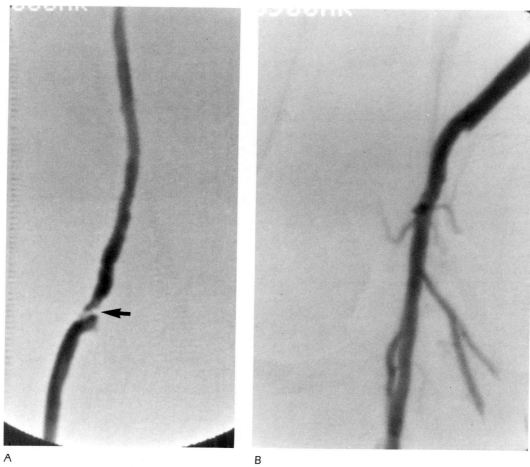

A   B

Figure 20-12. A 48-hour-old occlusion of PTFE femoropopliteal graft. **A,** Flow has been reestablished after 2 hours of continuous infusion of urokinase at a dose of 4000 IU/min. Severe stenosis is demonstrated at the junction of the graft and the popliteal artery (*arrow*). This was believed to represent stenosis due to either myointimal hyperplasia or atherosclerosis. Mild irregularity of the graft lumen indicated the presence of some residual thrombus. Therefore, overnight infusion of urokinase at 1000 IU/min was performed. **B,** Stenosis completely cleared, indicating that it was residual thrombus. This is an example of the difficulty in distinguishing between fixed stenosis and residual thrombus on the initial images obtained following rapid reestablishment of flow.

We then advance a short infusion segment outer catheter into the occlusion, leaving the most proximal sidehole just above the occluding thrombus. This provides for stability of the system but can occlude flow if the vessels are small. If the SFA is small or has very slow flow, we leave the larger outer catheter at the origin of the SFA so as not to impede flow. This bathes the low-flow SFA segment with lytic agent to prevent new clot from forming around the inner catheter.

Use of a no. 5 French outer catheter to reduce flow impedance should be considered. The inner portion of the McNamara catheter system as well as the Katzen infusion guidewire will fit through no. 5 French catheters with a 0.038-in endhole. Infusion around these inner catheters can be accomplished as long as the no. 5 French catheter has sideholes and a 0.038-in (inner diameter) endhole.

If one cannot enter the occlusion, an endhole catheter may be placed directly against the occlusion for infusion, or a very short segment outer multisidehole catheter may be placed directly on the clot. If the catheter position cannot be maintained directly on the thrombus or, preferably, within it, the likelihood of successful lysis decreases substantially.

The inner infusion system is frequently dislodged if a patient bends his or her knee. The softest inner systems will sometimes loop or kink as they move up and down with knee movement (Fig. 20-13). This requires repositioning or replacement of the inner catheter, since the pumps may register occlusion and repeatedly alarm. The Tracker II catheter is more susceptible to this problem with popliteal infusions than other infusion catheters or guidewires. It may be too soft in this application.

INFRAPOPLITEAL ARTERY

Occlusions in these small vessels may be long or short. We carefully advance a small 0.018-in guidewire through the occlusion. A small no. 3 French inner system is then advanced into the occluded segment. The selection of multisidehole versus endhole depends on the length of the occlusion. We do not use the larger outer infusion catheters in the infrapopliteal vessels because they restrict flow. The outer catheter is placed either in a large popliteal artery or in the proximal SFA if the vessels are small.

Occlusions at the level of the ankle or more distally are treated with endhole inner catheters (Fig. 20-14). We commonly use the Tracker II catheter in these locations because it is the softest and least likely to cause spasm.

PUMPS AND CONNECTIONS

We deliver the thrombolytic agent via Travenol IVAC infusion pumps (Baxter). The rotating device on the pumps accurately delivers the prescribed volume of medicine only if there is minimal resistance to flow. Unfortunately, most of the coaxial systems have a fair amount of resistance to flow and usually deliver only 70 to 90 percent of the actual prescribed amount.[20]

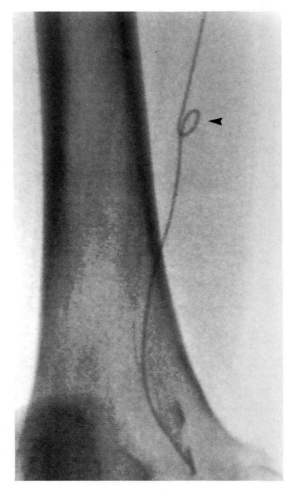

Figure 20-13. Loop (*arrowhead*) has formed in Cragg infusion guidewire used for overnight infusion of popliteal occlusion. In our experience, infusate can still traverse this infusion system. A similar loop in a Tracker catheter will usually result in a kink that will obstruct flow.

Checking the volume infused with a given flow rate is the only way to be certain how well a pump performs. Other pumps are available that deliver the exact amount regardless of resistance in the system. These are preferred over the IVAC delivery system but are not as readily available in many hospitals.

Appropriate connecting tubing is important to ensure patient safety and to facilitate patient transfer to and from the angiography suite. We use

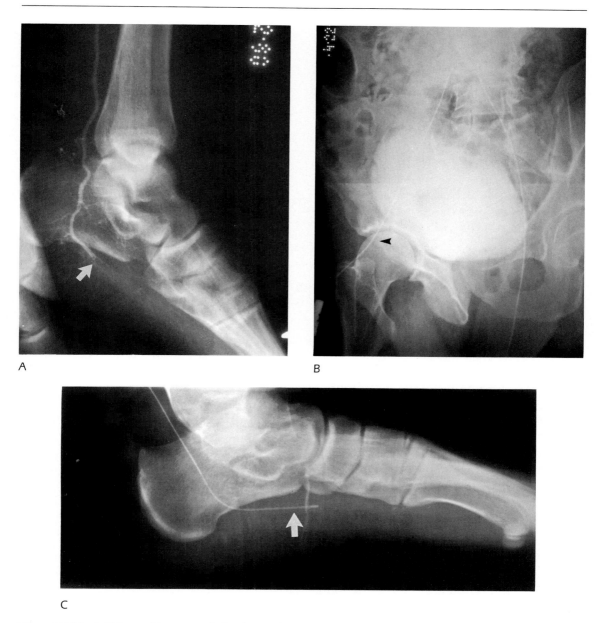

Figure 20-14. A 16-hour-old acute embolization to the plantar arteries. **A**, Distal portion of posterior tibial artery is occluded (*arrow*). **B**, Contralateral femoral artery (*arrowhead*) was used for access to perform diagnostic arteriography and subsequent thrombolytic infusion. **C**, SOS infusion guidewire has been advanced into thrombus (*arrow*).

Illustration continued on the following page

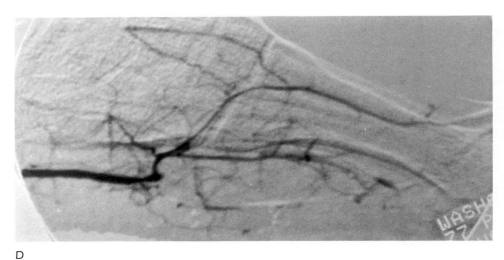

D

Figure 20-14 *continued.* **D,** Flow has been reestablished through most branches of plantar artery following high-dose urokinase continuous in infusion (4000 IU/min).

extralong connecting tubing (8-ft clear pressure monitoring line from Medex) so that the tubing is not pulled or stretched during transport. Additionally, we no longer use the typical slip-tip type of connecting junctions. We use only tubing that has Luer-locs at both ends. This protects against inadvertent separation at the connections with resulting blood loss.

TAILORING SPECIFICS

Thrombolysis is a tremendous tool, and lytic therapy can be enjoyable and rewarding. High success rates with low morbidity and/or mortality can be achieved using the basic principles we have described. Use of a coaxial system makes the procedure easier to perform and decreases overall infusion times.[23]

Tailoring the specifics of the coaxial system to the occlusion also can facilitate lysis and minimize complications. In the setting of acute ischemia we use UK at 4,000 u/min until flow has been reestablished. This usually can be accomplished within 2 to 4 hours. We concomitantly heparinize and use a dose that will maintain the aPTT in the range of 80–120 sec. Once flow has been restored

we drop the UK dose to 1,000–2,000 u/min and reduce the heparin dose to obtain an aPTT time of 60 sec.

REFERENCES

1. McNamara TO, Bomberger RA, Merchant RF: Intraarterial urokinase as the initial therapy for acutely ischemic lower limbs. Circulation 1991; 1991;83(suppl 1):106.
2. Blaisdell FW, Steele M, Allen RE: Management of acute lower extremity ischemia due to embolism and thrombosis. Surgery 1978;84:822.
3. Jivegard L, Holm J, Schersten T: The outcome in arterial thrombosis misdiagnosed as arterial embolism. Acta Chir Scand 1986;152:251.
4. Fong H, Downs A, Lye C, Morrow I: Low-dose streptokinase infusion therapy of peripheral arterial occlusions and occluded vein grafts. Can J Surg 1986; 29:259.
5. Kakkasseril JS, Cranley JJ, Arbouth JJ, et al: Efficacy of low-dose streptokinase in acute arterial occlusion and graft thrombosis. Arch Surg 1985;120:427.
6. Seeger JM, Flynn TC, Quintessenza JA: Intra-arterial Streptokinase in the treatment of acute arterial emboli. Surg Gynecol Obstec 1987;164: 303.
7. Battey PM, Fulenwider JT, Smith RB, et al: Intraarterial thrombolysis for acute limb ischemia: A three year experience. South Med J 1987; 80:479.

8. Berni GA, Bandik DF, Zierler RE, et al: Streptokinase treatment of acute arterial occlusion. Ann Surg 1983;198:185.

9. Gregg RO, Chamberlain BE, Myers JK, Tyler DB: Embolectomy or heparin therapy for arterial emboli. Surgery 1982;93:377.

10. Rush DS, Gewertz BL, Lu CT, et al: Selective infusion of streptokinase for arterial thrombosis. Surgery 1983;93:828.

11. Hargrove WC, Barker CF, Berowitz HD, et al: Treatment of acute peripheral arterial and graft thromboses with low-dose streptokinase. Surgery 1982;92:981.

12. McNamara TO, Fischer JR: Thrombolysis of peripheral arterial and graft occlusions: Improved results using high-dose urokinase. AJR 1985; 144:769.

13. McNamara TO: Technique and results of "higher-dose" infusion. Cardiovasc Intervent Radiol 1988; 11:548.

14. Tennant SN, Dixon J, Venable TC, et al: Intracoronary thrombolysis in patients with acute myocardial infarction: Comparison of the efficacy of urokinase with streptokinase. Circulation 1984; 69:756.

15. Belkin M, Belkin B, Bucknam CA, et al: Intraarterial fibrinolytic therapy: Efficacy of streptokinase vs. urokinase. Arch Surg 1986;121:769.

16. Gardiner GA, Koltun W, Kandarpa K, et al: Thrombolysis of occluded femoropopliteal grafts. AJR 1986;147:621.

17. Van Breda A, Katzen BT, Deutsch AS: Urokinase versus streptokinase in local thrombolysis. Radiology 1987;165:109.

18. Bell WR: Update on urokinase and streptokinase: A comparison of their efficacy and safety. Hosp Formul 1988;23:230.

19. Graor R, Cleveland Clinic, Internal Medicine, Peripheral Vascular Disease Section, personal communication, 1994.

20. McNamara TO, Mednik G, Gardner KR, Curran J: Emission characteristics for multisidehole and endhole-only infusion systems currently available for thrombolysis. Presented at the 2nd International Congress and Comprehensive Course: Vascular and Nonvascular Intervention in the Nineties, Zermatt, Switzerland, April 3, 1995.

21. Bookstein JJ, Fellmeth B, Roberts A: Pulsed-spray pharmacomechanical thrombolysis: Preliminary clinical results. AJR 1989;152:1097.

22. McNamara TO: Thrombolytic therapy for iliac artery occlusions. In Kadir S, ed: Current Practice of Interventional Radiology. Philadelphia, B C Decker, 1991, pp 301–306.

23. McNamara TO, Gardner KR: Results of thrombolytic infusions with single catheter versus coaxial catheter systems. Presented at the 76th Scientific Assembly and Annual Meeting of the Radiological Society of North America, Chicago, Ill. November 26, 1990.

21

Thrombolytic Therapy in the Management of Peripheral Arterial Occlusion

KENNETH OURIEL
ANTHONY J. COMEROTA

Thrombotic and thromboembolic occlusion of the peripheral arterial tree is responsible for over 100,000 major and minor amputations yearly in the United States.[1] Traditionally, operative revascularization has been the mainstay of therapy in the setting of lower extremity ischemia.[2] Operative bypass, endarterectomy, and thromboembolectomy have all been used quite successfully to restore arterial circulation and salvage the threatened limb.

Thrombolytic therapy is gaining increasing acceptance as a treatment modality performed as an adjuvant or alternative to operation in patients with peripheral arterial occlusion. Administration of these clot-dissolving agents provides a potentially less invasive means of restoring arterial continuity both in the angiographic suite and as an adjunct to operative revascularization. The purpose of this chapter is to summarize the important concepts relating to the use of thrombolytic agents in peripheral arterial occlusion, focusing on the rationale, procedural methodology, and ultimate clinical outcome.

HISTORY OF THROMBOLYSIS

Thrombolytic agents have been used clinically since the late 1940s.[3] The early pharmacologic preparations were obtained from impure isolates of the *Streptococcus* bacterium and contained streptodornase and other foreign-protein contaminants in addition to the active agent streptokinase.[4] These contaminants were responsible for a variety of untoward systemic effects and forced investigators to limit the use of thrombolytic agents to extravascular disease processes, specifically, to dissolve the fibrinous septa of loculated hemothorces. It was not until the mid-1950s that Tillet and his group at New York University felt confident enough in the purity of their streptokinase preparation to use it through an intravascular route. In 1955, these investigators reported the results of a clinical trial of intravenous streptokinase in 11 patients, designed to define the safety of the intravascular administration of the agent.[5] Unfortunately, systemic reactions were common, with low-grade fever developing in all the patients and profound hypotension in 4.

In 1956, Cliffton and Grossi[6] reported successful preliminary results with what was assumed to be the direct thrombolytic agent plasmin. Cliffton's agent comprised a mixture of plasminogen and streptokinase designed to generate free plasmin. Despite the theoretical advantages of using the direct fibrinolytic agent plasmin, subsequent work suggested that the effects Cliffton and Grossi observed more likely occurred as a result of the streptokinase in the preparation rather than the plasmin.[7] Nevertheless, 1 year later Cliffton[8] reported his experience with streptokinase-plasmin and documented beneficial effects of direct intra-arterial infusions in two patients with peripheral arterial occlusions. These historical insights confirm that although Dotter et al.[9] are frequently credited with pioneering catheter-directed peripheral arterial thrombolysis in 1974, Cliffton actually documented the use of this technique 17 years earlier.

PATHOPHYSIOLOGY OF ACUTE ARTERIAL OCCLUSION

Acute arterial occlusion frequently occurs suddenly and without warning. A complex of six signs and symptoms are characteristically observed, each beginning with the letter *p:* pain, pallor, poikilothermy, pulselessness, paresthesia, and paralysis. Symptoms are usually of sufficient magnitude that the patient presents early, at a time when the thrombus is relatively susceptible to lytic dissolution. A useful classification of the severity of lower extremity ischemia is provided within a Society for Vascular Surgery/International Society for Cardiovascular Surgery report that places patients into one of three classes; viable and nonthreatened, viable but threatened, and nonviable.[10] In this schema, class II patients are generally the most appropriate candidates for thrombolysis; class I patients do not usually manifest sufficient symptoms to warrant the risks attendant to thrombolytic therapy, and class III patients are, by definition, irretrievable with any treatment modality.

The etiology of acute arterial occlusion can be divided into two categories: thrombosis and embolism. Thrombotic etiologies are observed more frequently by a ratio of 4:1 in most series of acutely compromised lower extremities.[11,12] Irrespective of etiology, the initial occlusive process is rapidly followed by prograde and retrograde propagation of thrombus to the next large collateral channel. The development of propagated thrombus attains significance in the setting of pharmacologic thrombolysis; the red cell-rich, platelet-poor secondary thrombus is easy to lyse, but the occluding head of platelet-rich thrombus or older embolus is relatively resistant[13] (Fig. 21-1).

Thrombotic arterial occlusion may be observed in native arteries or bypass conduits.[14,15] Thrombosis of native arteries usually develops in the setting of a preexisting stenosis, although acute thrombotic occlusion of near normal arterial segments may develop with such entities as the antiphospholipid syndrome or the hypercoagulable state associated with malignancy.[16] Thrombosis of a bypass conduit may occur with or without an anatomic lesion; closure of autogenous conduits is unlikely without a stenotic process, but prosthetic conduits frequently fail in the absence of an identifiable lesion.[17] This observation may relate to the relative nonthrombogenic luminal surface of autogenous grafts, which allows continued patency despite markedly reduced flow rates.

Arterial emboli characteristically originate in the heart on injured ventricular endocardium after an acute myocardial infarction or within the left atrium in the setting of atrial fibrillation. Arterioarterial emboli also account for some cases of acute limb ischemia and consist of cholesterol or fibrin-platelet debris originating in a proximal aneurysm or ulcerated atherosclerotic plaque. Cardiac emboli are typically large and associated with obstruction of the femoral or popliteal vessels, whereas arterioarterial emboli are smaller and usually associated with tibial or digital artery obstruction and such clinical entities as the "blue toe" syndrome.

OPERATION AS THE STANDARD THERAPY IN ACUTE ARTERIAL OCCLUSION

Operative therapy became the standard mode of intervention in acute arterial occlusion with the advent of surgical revascularization in the late 1940s.[18,19] The subsequent four decades witnessed an impressive improvement in technical advances, with the ability to operatively salvage the vast majority of acutely threatened limbs. The introduction of the balloon embolectomy catheter by Fogarty in 1963 offered an effective means of removing emboli and propagated thrombus through a single arteriotomy.[20]

Operative interventions fall into two major categories in acute limb ischemia: thromboembolectomy and bypass. Thromboembolectomy

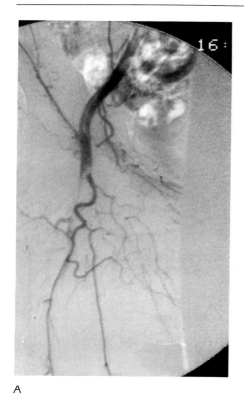

A

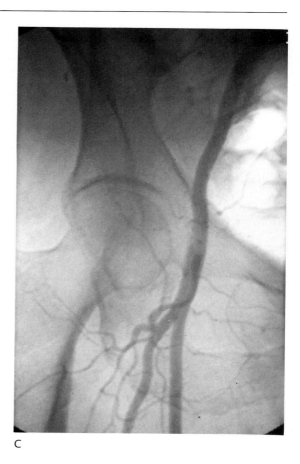

C

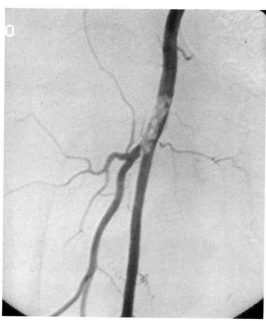

B

Figure 21-1. (**A**) A patient with an embolus, originating in the heart, lodging at the right common femoral bifurcation with prograde and antegrade propagation of clot. (**B**) The propagated clot lyses relatively quickly after 6 hours of urokinase infusion, leaving the more resistant embolic material from the heart. (**C**) However, after 15 hours of lytic infusion, even the resistant embolic material dissolves, leaving a widely patent femoral system.

is reserved for processes not associated with pre-existing anatomic defects, e.g., in patients with common femoral emboli or thrombosis of a prosthetic graft free of fixed narrowing. Alternatively, thrombectomy may be performed in conjunction with a patch angioplasty of an occluded native artery or bypass graft. Bypass is appropriate in all other circumstances, and it has been argued that all graft occlusions should be treated with the insertion of a new conduit, since the secondary patency rates of failed infrainguinal bypass conduits have been disappointing.[21]

Despite these technical advances and the resulting decreased amputation rate, limb salvage has been achieved at the cost of an alarmingly high perioperative mortality rate, approaching 25 percent in the review of Blaisdell et al.[22] and approximately 20 percent in a later series by Jivegård et al.[23] More recently, Edwards and colleagues[21] replaced 111 occluded lower extremity bypass grafts with new autogenous vein conduits and documented a limb salvage rate of 90 percent at 5 years. However, these results were associated with a mortality rate of 26 percent at 6 months, and only 12 percent of patients were alive at 5 years. The observations of these studies suggest that acute limb ischemia develops in a medically compromised subpopulation, a group that may be further jeopardized by invasive reconstructive procedures. It is on this background that the advent of effective thrombolytic agents provided some hope for a treatment modality that would maintain the excellent limb-salvage rates associated with immediate operation concurrent with a decreased periprocedural mortality rate.

PHARMACOLOGY OF THROMBOLYTIC AGENTS

Thrombolytic agents are *plasminogen activators,* converting fibrin-bound plasminogen to fibrin-bound plasmin, which subsequently degrades the fibrin thrombus[24] (Table 21-1). The administration of exogenous plasmin has very little, if any, thrombolytic activity.[25] In vitro studies confirmed that free plasmin was relatively ineffective in degrading fibrin but did result in significant degradation of fibrinogen and factors V and VIII.[26] These studies led to the formulation of a scheme of thrombolysis whereby plasminogen exists in two phases: a gel (thrombus) phase, where it is bound to fibrin, and a soluble (plasma) phase, where it is free.[27] Activation of soluble-phase plasminogen to free plasmin leads to degradation of fibrinogen and other plasma proteins but is ineffective in dissolving fibrin within a thrombus. Free plasmin is also rapidly inactivated by antiplasmins. Gel-phase plasminogen, however, when activated to fibrin-bound plasmin, results in selective fibrinolysis in an environment relatively protected from antiplasmins. This mechanism explains why the degradation of fibrin thrombus is dependent on the concentration of plasminogen activators but independent of the concentration of exogenously administered plasmin.[28]

Table 21-1. Properties of Components of the Thrombolytic System

Component	Molecular Weight	Structure	Plasma Half-life
Streptokinase	46,000	Single chain	11 minutes
Urokinase	54,000	Two chains	10 minutes
rt-PA	70,000	One or two chains	5 minutes
APSAC	131,000	Lys-plasminogen-SK	70 minutes
Pro-urokinase	53,000	Single chain	6 minutes
Plasminogen	88,000	Single chain	2.2 days
Plasmin	88,000	Two chains	0.1 second
α_2-Antiplasmin	70,000	Single-chain	2.6 days
PAI*	40,000	Single chain	

*Plasminogen activator inhibitor.
Source: Reprinted with permission from Marder VJ: The use of thrombolytic agents: Choice of patient, drug administration, laboratory monitoring. Ann Intern Med 1979;90:802.

There exist four thrombolytic agents currently approved by the U.S. Food and Drug Administration (FDA): streptokinase, urokinase, recombinant tissue plasminogen activator (rt-PA), and acylated plasminogen streptokinase activator complex (APSAC). Each agent produces fibrinolysis through an activation of fibrin-bound plasminogen to fibrin-bound plasmin. The plasmin then hydrolyses fibrin, leading to the dissolution of the thrombus and the restoration of blood flow. Streptokinase is a purified isolate from the *Streptococcus* bacterium and is an inactive single-chain 46,000-dalton protein. It forms a complex with plasminogen or plasmin, and this complex requires an additional streptokinase molecule to convert plasminogen to plasmin. Urokinase, clinically employed in both high-molecular-weight (54,000-dalton) and low-molecular-weight (31,000-dalton) forms, is a two-chain compound present in urine. Unlike streptokinase, urokinase directly activates plasminogen without the need for initial binding to an additional plasminogen molecule. rt-PA is a single- or two-chain 70,000-dalton molecule containing two kringle structures, one of which is important in the binding of rt-PA to fibrin.[29] Thus rt-PA has been promoted as an agent with "fibrin specificity" and a low potential for systemic fibrinogen degradation. This contention has not been substantiated in the clinical setting, with similar decreases in plasma fibrinogen concentration following systemic administration of urokinase and rt-PA.[30] APSAC consists of an equimolar complex of streptokinase and plasminogen, originally developed to hasten fibrinolysis by eliminating the initial step of plasminogen binding. In practice, the benefits of APSAC may be related to its increased half-life rather than plasminogen supplementation.

The plasminogen activators differ in their relative rate of fibrin dissolution and in their fibrin specificity.[31] An ideal agent would manifest a high degree of fibrinolytic activity with a low potential for systemic fibrinogen degradation. Reputedly, streptokinase has the lowest activity and is not fibrin-specific. Urokinase is intermediate, but rt-PA has been reported to be associated with the highest rate of fibrinolysis and the greatest degree of fibrin specificity.

Our laboratory studies have corroborated these clinical impressions. In an in vitro model of thrombolysis, human blood was recirculated through a system containing a segment of polytetrafluoroethylene graft material filled with retracted human clot. Using doses similar to those employed clinically, streptokinase was the least efficient agent and rt-PA was the most efficient agent. Urokinase was associated with an intermediate rate of lysis, but the amount of systemic fibrinogen breakdown was substantially less than for either of streptokinase or rt-PA. This observation refutes the widespread belief that rt-PA is a fibrin-specific agent unassociated with significant fibrinogenolysis. The findings of Meyerovitz et al.[32] corroborate our in vitro data; these investigators observed more rapid clot lysis in patients treated with rt-PA, but systemic fibrinogen levels were significantly lower than those in patients treated with urokinase. A retrospective analysis of 465 patients with peripheral arterial occlusion reported by Graor et al.[33] documented successful clot lysis in 94 percent of patients treated with rt-PA and 89 percent of patients treated with urokinase. By contrast, successful lysis was achieved in only 72 percent of patients treated with streptokinase. Systemic fibrinogenolysis was observed in all groups; even the rt-PA–treated patients experienced a decrease in fibrinogen levels to 66 percent of baseline.

TRANSPORT PHENOMENA AS A DETERMINANT OF THROMBOLYTIC RATE

Thrombi can be envisioned as "fibrin gels" consisting of a fluid phase (serum) and a polymer phase (fibrin strands). Red blood cells, platelets, and leukocytes are enmeshed within the gel; the ratio of one specific blood element to another is determined by hemodynamic and chemotactic conditions present at the time the clot forms.[34] Thrombi that form in a high-shear-rate environment are typically rich in platelets (arterial thrombi), while thrombi forming under conditions of low shear rate contain fewer platelets and more red blood cells (venous thrombi).[35,36]

Recent experimental work has suggested that transport of fibrinolytic agents into the clot may be the most important variable determining the rate of recanalization.[37] No matter how effective a specific plasminogen activator is, thrombolysis does not occur if the activator does not reach its substrate. Transport into gels is mediated by two mechanisms: (1) simple diffusion at the fluid-gel interface and (2) bulk flow through tiny channels in the gel. Diffusion is a less efficient process than bulk transport, being dependent on a high concentration of molecules at the fluid-gel interface. Diffusion results in a concentration profile that decreases exponentially and becomes extraordinarily inefficient over distances greater than 10 to 50 μm.[37] It has been estimated that it would take 50 days for streptokinase to reach one-hundredth of its outside concentration at a depth of just 10 cm by diffusion mechanisms alone.

Bulk flow is a transport mechanism of substantially greater efficiency than simple diffusion. Molecules are driven through a porous medium by an energy gradient. In the case of thrombolysis, plasminogen activator agent is transported through microscopic pores in the clot by a pressure differential between the head and tail of the thrombus. Kinetic modeling predicts that bulk flow mechanisms must be at play in the setting of in vivo thrombolysis, and the greater the pressure gradient, the more rapid is the process. In this regard, forceful injection of lytic agent into the substance of the thrombus is much more effective than systemic administration. Valji et al.[38] injected identical doses of plasminogen activator either directly into femoral venous thrombi or adjacent to the thrombus into the blood proximally. Whereas intrathrombic administration resulted in complete clot lysis within 1 hour, parathrombic injection failed to achieve any degree of lysis after periods of up to 2 hours. It is apparent that transport of both plasminogen activator and plasminogen is crucial for effective clot lysis. Experimental evidence suggests that unbound plasminogen entrapped inside the clot is important in the lysis of nonretracted thrombi, while retracted thrombi lyse via activation of preexisting fibrin-bound plasminogen.[39,40] The concentration of fibrin-bound plasminogen is too low in retracted clots to allow effective thrombolysis. Thus transport of additional plasminogen from the bloodstream is necessary, and this process proceeds most efficiently when a pressure differential provides the energy gradient for bulk flow mechanisms to occur.

The dependence of thrombolysis on bulk transport mechanisms also explains the clinical observation that clot dissolution slows markedly once initial recanalization has occurred and the pressure gradient dissipates. Thrombolysis is almost always associated with residual mural thrombus that is exceedingly difficult to dissolve, presumably as a result of the loss of efficient bulk flow transport of activator into the material. Bulk flow mechanisms also explain the observed difference between the rapidity of lysis in retracted and nonretracted thrombi. Clots composed of tightly compacted, thin fibrin strands offer more resistance to flow than clots with loosely interspersed, thick fibrils, decreasing the contact between plasminogen activator molecules and fibrin polymer.[41]

TECHNIQUE OF ARTERIAL THROMBOLYSIS

At the outset, the most important caveat of arterial thrombolysis relates to the goal of therapy. Thrombolysis is designed to rid the arterial tree of occluding thrombus, uncovering the anatomic lesion responsible for the occlusive event in the majority of cases. Operation or endovascular interventions are subsequently employed to correct the unmasked lesion.[14,15,42,43] It is only in the minority of cases without demonstrable anatomic defects that successful thrombolytic therapy can be employed without subsequent operative revascularization or balloon angioplasty. Thus studies designed to document the effectiveness of thrombolysis are flawed when the primary outcome measure is avoidance of operation, since the goal of arterial thrombolysis is to uncover and clearly define the etiologic mechanism and lessen the magnitude of a subsequent remedial intervention.[44]

Irrespective of the agent employed, arterial thrombolysis is best accomplished via a catheter-directed approach, with the delivery of activator agent directly into the substance of the thrombus.[45] In contrast to the setting of acute coronary artery occlusion, intravenous routes of administration have been entirely unsatisfactory in the periphery. Intravenous streptokinase attained popularity in the 1960s but was associated with successful

Table 21-2. Results of Intravenous Streptokinase Thrombolysis in Peripheral Arterial Occlusion

Authors	Fiessinger et al.[46]	Amery et al.[47]	Hess[48]
Year:	1978	1970	1967
Patients:	194	68	438
Success:	29%	31%	46%
Hemorrhage:	9%	24%	15%
Thromboembolism:	11%	9%	10%
Death:	3%	9%	4%

lysis in a minority of patients. Relatively large series reported by Fiessinger et al.,[46] Amery et al.,[47] and Hess[48] employed streptokinase in doses of many millions of units, but demonstrated successful lysis in less than 50 percent of cases (Table 21-2). These marginal rates of success were achieved at the cost of a high rate of hemorrhage, stroke, and distal embolization.

The difference in the success rate of intravenous thrombolysis in the coronary and peripheral arterial setting is presumably a result of the larger size of peripheral thrombi, with an inability of thrombolytic agent to diffuse into the substance of the larger clots. The numerous side branches of coronary arteries also may aid in the efficiency of intravenous thrombolytic therapy. The short length of thrombus between the head of the thrombus and the next side branch is easily lysed, followed by washout of the byproducts of the process through the side branch (Fig. 21-2). Fresh blood containing lytic agent and plasminogen then comes in contact with the new thrombus head just beyond the side branch. Thus short segments of thrombus are dissolved in a sequential fashion from side branch to side branch until the coronary artery is completely open. By contrast, thrombolysis of a long length of thrombus within a branchless peripheral artery or bypass graft is impeded by the absence of washout between branches. Clot dissolution can proceed only through diffusion of new lytic agent through the meniscus of byproducts at the head of the clot, explaining the poor success rates with intravenous (systemic) thrombolysis of peripheral arterial thrombi.

Direct intraarterial infusion of thrombolytics provides a method to achieve high local doses of

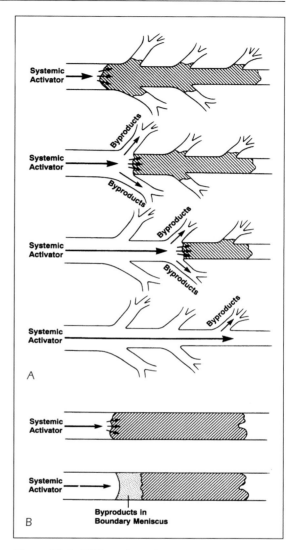

Figure 21-2. (A) Thrombus within arterial segments containing frequent side branches are more susceptible to lysis through an intravenous route of administration, since the side branches allow washout of the byproducts of thrombolysis. The coronary arterial tree is an example of such a system; systemic therapy is associated with a high rate of success. **(B)** By contrast, long, branchless conduits require a catheter-directed approach to achieve adequate contact between the lytic agent, plasminogen, and the fibrin clot.

activator agent. Dotter[9] reintroduced catheter-directed thrombolysis, using a low-dose streptokinase regimen in 1974. Hess et al.[49] reported the results of catheter-directed thrombolysis, with successful clot dissolution in 69 percent of the cases. Subsequently, McNamara and Bomberger[50] employed a high-dose urokinase regimen and observed complete clot lysis in 77 percent of infusions. Our studies have corroborated McNamara and Bomberger's findings; we observed a successful lytic result (greater than 80 percent clot lysis) in 70 percent of 57 patients randomized to urokinase therapy for acute limb ischemia.[12] These data, however, must be analyzed in the context of patient selection and the definition of successful lysis, both of which vary from study to study. For example, if investigators include only those patients in whom successful catheter placement was achieved, a higher lytic success rate will be realized when compared with the data from investigators who included all patients. Similarly, successful lysis may be defined in terms of percentage of clot remaining, avoidance of operative intervention, improvement in hemodynamic noninvasive laboratory parameters, or limb salvage. Different results will be reported depending on the criteria used in defining success.

Both antegrade and contralateral catheter insertion techniques have been employed successfully in catheter-directed peripheral arterial thrombolysis. The ipsilateral femoral artery is the insertion site in the antegrade approach, angling the needle in a distal direction. It is frequently difficult to pass the guidewire into an occluded bypass graft using an antegrade approach; the wire preferentially enters the profunda femoris artery, and the close proximity of the graft orifice to the needle insertion site renders catheter manipulation arduous. The contralateral route is safest, especially in inexperienced hands, since failure to accomplish antegrade access may leave the patient with multiple needle-stick holes in the ipsilateral femoral artery that may bleed during subsequent thrombolytic infusion through a contralateral approach. There is a tendency for thrombus to form on the wall of the catheter during any protracted intraarterial procedure, and embolization of this "pericatheter thrombus" may occur as the thrombus is sheared off the catheter at the time of removal. The frequency of complications can be minimized through the use of small-bore catheters and concurrent heparin or aspirin therapy. An increase in the risk of hemorrhagic complications with systemic anticoagulation or antiplatelet agents, however, has forced some to avoid these adjuvants and rely on low dose heparin flushes through the infusion sheath alone.

The procedure of intraarterial thrombolysis is begun with an adequate diagnostic arteriogram, generally through the contralateral femoral artery, with suitable views of the abdominal aorta and both lower extremities to the foot level. Ample information can usually be obtained from two aortic injections: one with the diagnostic flush catheter at the supraceliac level for visualization of the aorta, and the second with the catheter at the level below the renal orifices to visualize the distal aorta, iliac arteries, and infrainguinal vessels. Once adequate diagnostic information has been obtained, the diagnostic catheter may be replaced with an infusion catheter, and this catheter is threaded around the aortic bifurcation and into the occluded bypass graft or native artery. Alternatively, an antegrade approach through the ipsilateral common femoral artery may be attempted when the diagnostic arteriogram reveals an appropriate anatomic situation. Specifically, an antegrade approach is applicable when a sufficient length of proximal superficial femoral artery is patent to allow an adequate distance between the site of common femoral cannulation and the exit of lytic agent from the catheter.

The choice of infusion catheter is important to ensure accurate and thorough distribution of the lytic agent. A catheter diameter of no. 5 French is usually best. Multisidehole catheters with a series of ports spaced along the distal portion of the catheter are commonly employed, choosing an appropriate length such that the first and last holes are positioned within the proximal and distal portions of the thrombus, respectively (Fig. 21-3). A tip-occluding wire is helpful when using multisidehole catheters, since the bulk of the thrombolytic agent tends to flow out the endhole rather than the smaller sideholes. The lack of a means of occluding the endhole of multihole diagnostic flush catheters makes these catheters inappropriate substitutions for the specialized multisidehole infusion catheters. Coaxial systems with infusion through an outer catheter and inner infusion wire may be useful to split the dose of lytic agent when infusion into two anatomically separate sites is

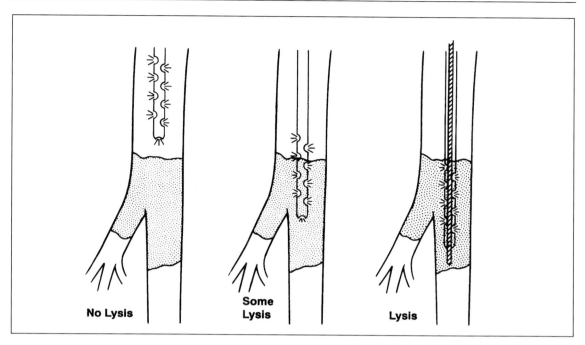

Figure 21-3. It is most important to place all catheter infusion holes into the substance of the thrombus, since the infused agent tends to flow through the path of least resistance.

advantageous. A single-endhole catheter may be required when small thrombi are encountered, especially in cases of emboli without proximal or distal clot propagation. Introducing sheaths are usually employed in sizes approximating the outer diameter of the infusion catheter. Replacement of the initial sheath with a larger sheath may be required during the course of thrombolysis, since catheter manipulation may cause enlargement of the arterial puncture site and produce seepage of blood around the sheath.

Several methods of infusion of thrombolytic agents are in routine use. A pulse-spray technique has been used, bolusing the thrombolytic agent through a multiholed catheter along the length of the occlusive thrombus, potentially increasing the rate of dissolution. *Lacing* refers to the infusion of large amounts of agent along the length of the thrombus as the catheter is withdrawn in an effort to attain even and complete distribution of lytic agent throughout the thrombus. *Burst therapy* refers to the intermittent infusion of thrombolytics, discontinuing therapy for a period of hours to allow hepatic repletion of total-body plasminogen.

Despite theoretical advantages, no consistent benefits have been documented with the use of one technique over another.[51] Presently, the method of thrombolytic administration should be based on the experience of the patient care team and the needs of the specific clinical situation. Continuous infusions of thrombolytic agent are employed most commonly, usually beginning with a larger (e.g., 4000 IU urokinase per minute for 4 hours) dose and tapering thereafter (Table 21-3). A maximum duration of lytic administration of 48 hours is recommended, since a prime correlate of complications appears to be the duration of infusion. Moreover, if no degree of reperfusion has been achieved after 12 to 18 hours of intrathrombus infusion of lytic agent, further attempts are unlikely to be successful.[12]

It is important to follow the progress of thrombolysis with serial arteriographic studies. Catheter manipulation is necessary in the majority of instances, with repositioning of the infusion holes to keep them within the substance of the unlysed thrombus. The use of smaller catheters and sheaths may minimize the chance of clot

Table 21-3. Protocol for Intraarterial Thrombolytic (Urokinase) Infusion

1. 325 mg aspirin on presentation
2. Catheter positioned into substance of thrombus
3. Urokinase infusion, 4000 IU/min for 2 hours (5000 IU/ml, in 5% dextrose)
4. Decrease to 2000 IU/min, continue for 2 hours
5. Decrease to 1000 IU/min, continue to a maximum of 48 hours total therapy

Source: Reprinted with permission from Ouriel K, Shortell CK, De-Weese JA, et al: A comparison of thrombolytic therapy with operative revascularization in the treatment of acute peripheral arterial ischemia. J Vasc Surg 1994;19:1021.

deposition on the catheter, lessening the need for heparin or aspirin.

Distal embolization is a well-known complication of thrombolysis and is heralded by acute deterioration in the status of the foot. We have coined the phrase *secondary embolization* to describe this event. The process occurs as the trailing portion of a thrombus is lysed and the remaining bits of undissolved clot travel distally with the resumption of normal arterial flow. Large prosthetic grafts appear to be prone to secondary embolization, and the techniques of bolusing and lacing may increase this risk. Patients developing secondary embolization of thrombotic debris should not be taken immediately to the angiographic suite or the operating room. Rather, a period of observation is warranted because the process is fortunately treatable with continuation of infusion, sometimes with an increase in the thrombolytic dose. Repositioning of the catheter into the distal emboli is not always immediately necessary, since small particles of embolized material are usually sensitive to upstream administration of lytic agent. Thus secondary embolization represents one of the few exceptions to the caveat of infusing agent directly into the substance of the thrombus, possibly because the embolized material has been presaturated with lytic agent. However, if clinical improvement does not occur within 1 to 2 hours, arteriography and catheter repositioning into the tibial vessels may be necessary.

Monitoring of coagulation parameters during thrombolytic therapy remains controversial. Fibrinogen concentration, thrombin time, and other laboratory tests have been advocated as measures with which to gauge the risk of distant bleeding complications, but conclusive evidence does not exist in this regard.[24,52] Bleeding complications almost always result from defects in vascular integrity, usually at the site of arterial cannulation (Fig. 21-4). These events bear little or no correlation with abnormalities in the coagulation tests, but accumulating evidence indicates that the duration of thrombolytic infusion may be an important predictor of hemorrhage.

Intracranial hemorrhage is one of the most dreaded complications of thrombolytic therapy. Other devastating bleeding complications include retroperitoneal hemorrhage and massive gastrointestinal blood loss. These life-threatening bleeding complications are treated with immediate termination of lytic infusion and replacement of fibrinogen and other clotting proteins with fresh frozen plasma or cryoprecipitate when they are depleted. Epsilon amino caproic acid can be infused intravenously to arrest ongoing fibrinolysis in cases of severe bleeding.

RESULTS OF THROMBOLYSIS IN ACUTE PERIPHERAL ARTERIAL OCCLUSION

Large, retrospective series of patients treated with intraarterial thrombolytic therapy began to appear in the early 1980s.[11,53–55] Success was reported in over 90 percent of cases over a mean duration of infusion of 6 to 12 hours. Amputation rates averaged less than 10 percent, with early mortality rates of less than 5 percent and bleeding complications in 5 to 10 percent of patients. Urokinase and rt-PA were argued to be safer and more efficacious than streptokinase. There were, however, severe limitations with these studies, and their conclusions are not entirely justified by the data. Streptokinase, for example, was utilized early in the course of each series, usually at a time when the medical team had little experience in thrombolytic treatment. Patients with acute and chronic limb ischemia were included in many of the studies, precluding meaningful comparison with data on truly threatened extremities. Moreover, outcome measures were frequently subjective, bearing little clinical relevance to limb salvage or mortality.

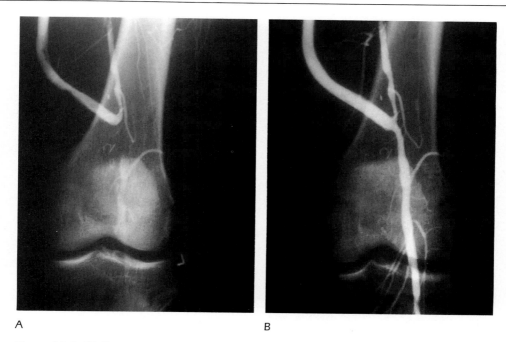

A   B

Figure 21-4. (**A**) The goal of thrombolysis is to uncover the anatomic defect responsible for the occlusive process. A critical stenosis was uncovered after 11 hours of urokinase influsion into this prosthetic graft. (**B**) The patient underwent balloon dilation of the lesion, with an acceptable angiographic result. The graft remained patent for 36 months following this procedure.

These early series triggered several contradictory reports, all retrospective and somewhat anecdotal.[44,56–58] The data generated by these studies argued against the use of thrombolytic agents in acute arterial occlusion, principally on the basis of poor patency rates associated with sole therapy and the frequent need for concurrent operative intervention to achieve an acceptable result. The goal of thrombolysis, however, is not to replace or eliminate surgery. Rather, thrombolytic therapy should be employed in an effort to diminish the magnitude of required interventions and thereby decrease the frequency of morbid and mortal events (Fig. 21-5). Studies that failed to tabulate long-term survival and limb salvage as primary endpoints predictably indicted thrombolysis as a useless therapeutic endeavor.

More recent trials have avoided these limitations by employing a randomized, prospective design and objective, clinically relevant endpoints.[42] In peripheral arterial occlusion, two major issues have been addressed by clinical trials: (1) a comparison of the efficacy of different thrombolytic agents and (2) a comparison of thrombolytic and operative treatment modalities.

Berridge et al.[59] randomized 60 patients to intraarterial rt-PA, intravenous rt-PA, or intraarterial streptokinase in the setting of peripheral arterial thrombosis. Complete lysis was observed in 85 percent of the intraarterial rt-PA group and in 80 percent of the streptokinase group. Intravenous rt-PA, however, was associated with complete lysis in only 30 percent of the patients. The study of Meyerovitz et al.[32] compared rt-PA and urokinase in 32 patients with peripheral arterial or bypass graft occlusions. Near-complete lysis was achieved more rapidly in the rt-PA group. Greater than 95 percent lysis was documented in 44 percent of the rt-PA group at 8 hours following the institution of therapy versus only 6 percent of the urokinase group. Systemic fibrinogen degradation, however, was greater in the rt-PA patients 24 hours after the start of infusion. Thus rt-PA appears to be the agent associated with the most rapid fibrinolysis. This advantage, however, must be weighed

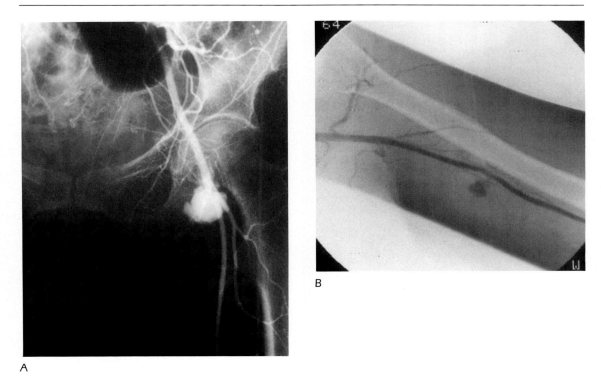

Figure 21-5. (**A**) A femoral false aneurysm that occurred following the removal of a no. 5 French catheter and infusion sheath from the left common femoral artery. Compression for 40 minutes was successful in thrombosing the aneurysm. (**B**) A brachial false aneurysm that developed following an antegrade puncture of the brachial artery for urokinase thrombolysis of an embolus to the brachial bifurcation. Operative intervention was necessary after symptoms of median nerve compression were noted.

against an increased degree of systemic fibrinogen breakdown with rt-PA as well an increased economic cost when compared with either urokinase or streptokinase.

To date, there exist three completed prospective comparisons of thrombolysis and operative management of peripheral arterial occlusion. The first published trial was a small series from Sweden. Thrombolysis with intraarterial rt-PA was contrasted with surgical treatment in 20 ischemic limbs. The small number of patients in this series precluded any meaningful conclusions.

The STILE trial (surgery versus thrombolysis for ischemia of the lower extremity) randomized 393 patients with acute and subacute peripheral arterial occlusion to one of three treatment groups: operation, intraarterial rt-PA, or intraarterial urokinase. Improvement in the rate of limb salvage

was observed in the surgical arm. The results, however, were confounded by an inability to place the catheter into the thrombus in a large percentage of patients randomized to thrombolysis. The third completed trial of operation versus thrombolysis was conducted at the University of Rochester and comprised 114 patients with ischemia of 7 days' duration or less.[12] Intraarterial urokinase was compared with operation in the *initial* management of the patients, realizing that thrombolysis would need to be followed by operative intervention in many of the thrombolytic patients with underlying anatomic lesions responsible for the thrombotic process. A 62 percent reduction in the 1-year mortality rate was seen in the thrombolytic group. This difference was attributed to a lower requirement for surgery concurrent with a decrease in the frequency of cardiopulmonary

Table 21-4. Factors Predictive of Success in a Multivariate Analysis (Stepwise Linear Regression) of 103 Peripheral Arterial and Bypass Graft Occlusions Treated with Thrombolytic Therapy

Parameter	Percent of Patients	Success Rate
Catheter into thrombus		
Yes	86%	88%
No	14%	0
Guidewire traversed thrombus		
Possible	82%	89%
Impossible	18%	16%
Conduit Involved		
Vein graft	18%	55%
Prosthetic graft	34%	80%
Native artery	48%	78%
Arterial segments involved		
One	51%	88%
Two	33%	71%
Three	16%	40%
Diabetes Mellitus		
Present	29%	49%
Absent	71%	80%

complications in the patients randomized to thrombolysis. No increment in the requirement for amputation was observed, with 1-year limb salvage rates of approximately 80 percent in each treatment arm. The conclusion of the study was that thrombolysis with or without subsequent operation was superior to operation alone in the treatment of the acutely ischemic limb, presumably as a result of a reduction in the incidence of in-hospital cardiopulmonary complications in the operative group.

It is likely that different patient categories will benefit from one form of therapy over another. Anecdotal experience suggested that certain patients will be best served with thrombolysis, while others will benefit most from immediate operative intervention. In a multivariate analysis of patients treated with intraarterial thrombolysis, five variables were found to be predictive of successful arteriographic dissolution[60] (Table 21-4). Technical factors appeared most important. Successful lysis was seldom achieved if the infusion catheter could not be threaded into the thrombus or if a

guidewire could not be passed through the occlusive process. Several clinical factors also attained significance as independent predictors of arteriographic success. Vein grafts were less likely to undergo successful lysis than prosthetic grafts or native arteries. Lysis was more frequently achieved in nondiabetics than in diabetics and in patients with fewer arterial segments involved.

The economics of thrombolysis have attained increased significance with the recent emphasis on the cost of health care. Thrombolysis appears to be associated with a similar length of hospital stay when compared with operative intervention.[61] The cost of hospitalization may be somewhat greater when thrombolytic therapy is employed, principally as a result of the cost of the lytic agent (Table 21-5). When professional fees are considered, however, these differences vanish. Clear advantages to the use of thrombolysis are realized when the cost data are expressed in relation to the dollars expended per life saved.

INTRAOPERATIVE THROMBOLYTIC THERAPY

Intraarterial delivery of thrombolytic agents via catheter-directed techniques has become well established in the treatment of arterial and graft occlusion. Activation of fibrin-bound plasminogen is the basis for thrombolytic therapy; therefore, the intraarterial delivery of high concentrations of plasminogen activators should accelerate lysis of pathologic thrombi.

Table 21-5. Economic Costs of Thrombolytic versus Operative Intervention in the Initial Management of Acute Peripheral Arterial Occlusion

	Thrombolysis (n = 57)	Operation (n = 57)
Hospital cost	$22,171	$19,775
Professional fees	$2,445	$3,517
Total costs	$24,616	$23,292
One-year survival rate	84%	58%
Cost per life saved	$29,305	$40,158

Source: From Ouriel K, Shortell CK: Results of thrombolytic therapy in acute limb ischemia, unpublished data.

A recent operation is considered a contraindication to intravenously delivered fibrinolytic therapy due to the risk of bleeding. This principle was extended to the intraoperative use of lytic agents. However, the appreciation that the half-life of most plasminogen activators is short and the observation that thrombus dissolution can occur rapidly with the regional delivery of high concentrations of lytic agents led to their use intraoperatively.[62,63]

These clinical observations were welcome, anticipating that an effective treatment might be developed for the intraarterial thrombi persisting after balloon catheter thromboembolectomy for acute arterial occlusion. Greep et al.[64] showed that almost all patients treated with the standard balloon catheter technique had additional thrombus removed with a modified wire basket catheter retrieval system. Plecha and Pories[65] performed an angiographic study that showed that 36 percent of patients had residual thrombus following their best attempts at balloon catheter thromboembolectomy for acute arterial occlusion. These data were corroborated by Quinones-Baldrich et al.[66] in an experimental study where they demonstrated that 85 percent of dogs had angiographically demonstrable residual thrombi following balloon catheter thromboembolectomy. The existence of residual thrombi provides a strong rationale to administer thrombolytic agents. Moreover, appropriate intraoperative use of lytic agents will minimize or avoid a systemic lytic effect after wound closure.

Dunnant and Edwards[67] demonstrated that experimental hindlimb ischemia produced arteriolar thrombosis following 6 hours of inflow occlusion. The extensive degree of thrombosis indicated that simple mechanical thrombectomy would not restore perfusion to the nutrient vessels from the main arteries.

Quinones-Baldrich et al.,[66] in their controlled canine hindlimb perfusion study, showed that thrombolysis following the best attempts at balloon catheter thromboembolectomy produced significantly improved angiographic results and a marked trend (though not statistically significant) toward improved flow compared with control limbs. Belkin et al.,[68] in an isolated limb ischemic muscle preparation, demonstrated that urokinase infusion salvaged more ischemic muscle compared with the control group. Additionally, significantly less injury (as shown by reperfusion edema) was noted in the lytic group compared with control muscles. In this study, there was also a trend toward improved blood flow. Therefore, experimental animal models confirm the clinical observations that balloon catheter thromboembolectomy frequently leaves residual thrombus. The data also demonstrate that arteriolar perfusion can be restored, tissue salvaged, and reperfusion injury reduced with the judicious use of intraarterial infusion of lytic agents.

CLINICAL APPLICATION OF INTRAOPERATIVE THROMBOLYSIS

An early report on the use of intraoperative streptokinase dampened the enthusiasm of many surgeons for intraoperative thrombolysis. Cohen et al.[69] treated 12 patients with streptokinase in doses ranging from 25,000 to 250,000 IU using a repeated-bolus technique over 30 to 150 minutes of inflow occlusion. There was a high mortality (42 percent), and an equally high rate of bleeding complications. It is likely that patient selection, choice of lytic agent, and a method of infusion that included prolonged repeated-bolus infusions contributed to the high complication rate.

Norem et al.[70] demonstrated that intraoperative thrombolysis promoted additional clot retrieval with thromboembolectomy. In 19 patients having thromboembolectomy for acute arterial ischemia, intraarterial streptokinase was infused in the operating room. After a short waiting period, repeat balloon catheter thrombectomy retrieved additional thrombus, and all patients demonstrated angiographic improvement. Similar findings were demonstrated with the use of intraoperative urokinase infusion.[68]

Parent and colleagues[71] treated 28 patients with acute ischemia and residual thrombus following balloon catheter thrombectomy. Seventeen patients had operative angiograms demonstrating thrombi. Of these 17, 15 had successful lysis when treated with intraoperative thrombolytic therapy. Both streptokinase and urokinase were used and were shown to be equally effective.

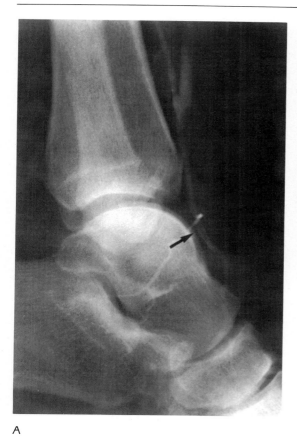

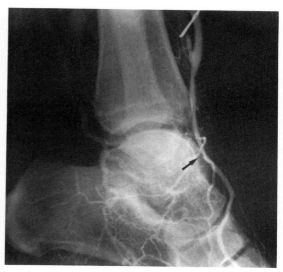

Figure 21-6. Operative arteriogram (**A**) following a femoral–distal anterior tibial bypass for multisegment occlusive disease and gangrene of the great toe. Angiogram demonstrated thrombus in dorsalis pedis artery (*arrow*) which was not present preoperatively. The patient was given additional heparin, the graft occluded, and 250,000 IU urokinase was infused over the next 30 minutes. Upon reperfusion, the Doppler signal improved considerably with triphasic and diastolic signals. A repeat arteriogram (**B**) demonstrated that the thrombus dissolved and the dorsalis pedis was patent. The patient's ischemia resolved and his foot healed.

However, hypofibrinogenemia and bleeding complications were significantly more frequent in those treated with streptokinase compared with those treated with urokinase.

At Temple University Hospital, 53 patients who had impending limb loss and occlusions of their "runoff" vessels have been treated with intraoperative, intraarterial lytic therapy over the past 13 years (Fig. 21-6). Included are patients with extensive distal thrombosis in whom complete thrombectomy was difficult or impossible and in whom it was believed that tissue loss was imminent. Streptokinase, urokinase, or recombinant tissue plasminogen activator (rt-PA) was infused into the most distal artery containing the thrombus with a short duration of infusion (either single- or double-bolus technique). Up to 50,000 IU of streptokinase, 250,000 IU of urokinase, and up to 10 mg of rt-PA were used for routine intraoperative use (excluding those having the isolated limb perfusion technique). Inflow was restored to the site of infusion in each instance by thrombectomy or bypass, whichever was necessary. Limb salvage was achieved in 70 percent. In 47 percent, limb salvage was directly attributable to lysis. Since thrombectomy or bypass procedures also were performed in these patients, in some it was difficult to determine the intervention contributing to the limb salvage. Therefore, 23 percent were identified as indeterminant outcomes. Thirty percent ultimately had a major amputation. Although there was a 9 percent mortality rate, none of the deaths were thought due to the lytic agent. One major bleeding complication occurred on the third postoperative day in a patient who was on heparin, and this was attributed to anticoagulation.

A promising new approach is known as *high-dose isolated limb perfusion.*[72] This procedure is indicated in patients with multivessel occlusion in whom it is judged that a single- or double-bolus infusion would not be effective and in patients in whom any degree of systemic fibrinolysis would pose significant risk. This technique includes full anticoagulation, exsanguination of venous blood from the limb with a rubber bandage, application of a tourniquet to achieve complete arterial and venous occlusion, direct arterial infusion into the affected vessels with a high dose (1 million IU or more) of urokinase or rt-PA (40 mg or more), and drainage of the venous effluent (Fig. 21-7). Infusion of a lytic agent in the limb for 45 to 60 minutes has yielded impressive results in a small number of patients suffering from acute multivessel distal thrombi or emboli. Seven patients have been treated for severe ischemia with the isolated limb perfusion method. Four had a good response with limb salvage, and three patients failed to improve. If distal vessel occlusion is due to atheromatous emboli or well-formed thrombus, treatment has not been successful. This novel approach deserves further evaluation.

PROSPECTIVE, RANDOMIZED STUDY OF INTRAOPERATIVE UROKINASE

The preceding discussion summarized the role to date of intraoperative intraarterial thrombolytic therapy. It has been shown to be effective in dissolving distal thrombi in occluded arteries and grafts, clearing the distal circulation before or after lower extremity operative reconstruction, and assisting in more effective mechanical removal of the thrombus.[73] However, high rates of bleeding complications have been reported.[69] During the evolution of intraarterial catheter directed lytic therapy for arterial and vascular graft occlusion, urokinase has become the preferred agent because of its safety and efficacy profile. rt-PA has been used less frequently.

The goal of intraoperative intraarterial thrombolytic therapy is to deliver a plasminogen activator at a high concentration to the thrombus, thereby promoting regional thrombolysis with minimal effects on plasma fibrinogen or clotting factors and with a low risk of bleeding complications. However, there is little information available on the regional effects compared with the systemic effects of intraoperatively administered plasminogen activators. Moreover, the dose-response relationship to the infused plasminogen activators has not been evaluated. A prospective, multicenter randomized, blinded, and placebo-controlled study was performed to address a number of basic issues regarding intraoperative delivery of urokinase.[74] Several issues were addressed by this investigation, including characterization of the regional and systemic effects of intraoperative intraarterial lytic infusion on plasma fibrinogen and the fibrinolytic system, the determination of dose-response relationships, quantification of the breakdown of cross-linked fibrin in a limb undergoing elective revascularization following a bolus dose of urokinase, and documentation of the risk of excessive bleeding during intraoperative thrombolysis.

One-hundred and thirty-four patients were prospectively randomized to receive one of three doses of urokinase or a saline placebo infusion in a blinded fashion into the distal arterial circulation during routine infrainguinal lower extremity revascularization for chronic limb ischemia. Endpoints analyzed were the degree of plasminogen activation, the regional and systemic breakdown of fibrinogen and fibrin, the degree to which a dose-response relationship could be established, and the clinical safety of intraoperative intraarterially infused urokinase. One of three doses of study drug or placebo was infused in a 30-cc volume as a bolus through the distal arteriotomy at the time of vascular reconstruction. Patient groups included (1) placebo (saline), (2) UK125 (urokinase, 125,000 IU), (3) UK250 (urokinase, 250,000 IU), and (4) UK500 (urokinase, 500,000 IU).

Blood samples (20 cc) were drawn simultaneously from the ipsilateral femoral vein to evaluate regional effects and the arm to evaluate the systemic effects at four time points: (1) preinfusion (pre), i.e., following heparinization but prior to vascular clamping; (2) pre-reperfusion (pre-re), i.e., after vascular reconstruction was completed but before vascular clamps were removed; (3)

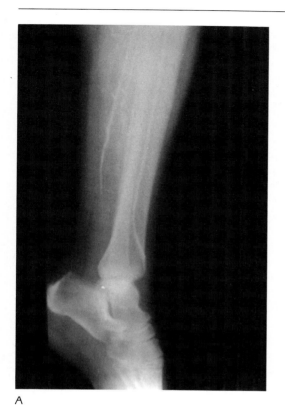

A

Figure 21-7. The technique of high-dose isolated limb perfusion of a thrombolytic agent in a patient who could not have any degree of systemic fibrinolysis (having had a coronary artery bypass 2 days earlier) and who had acute multivessel distal occlusion that was unlikely to resolve with a single bolus of a fibrinolytic agent. The patient had an acute embolic/thrombotic arterial occlusion after percutaneous removal of an intraaortic balloon, which was required following her emergency coronary artery bypass. Shown is the intraoperative arteriogram after balloon catheter thrombectomy of her popliteal and tibial vessels. Additional thrombus could not be removed mechanically. Catheters were placed into the origin of the posterior tibial and anterior tibial arteries, and the arteriogram (**A**) was performed with this selective injection technique. There was no evidence of contrast material entering the foot. Since additional thrombus could not be retrieved with balloon catheters, we believed the patient would suffer a major amputation. The patient's limb was elevated and the venous blood exsanguinated with a rubber bandage. A sterile blood pressure cuff (tourniquet) was placed on the distal thigh and inflated to 350 mmHg. The popliteal vein was cannulated with a red rubber catheter and drained into a basin. (**B**) One million units of UK was infused into the lower leg in a volume of 1 liter of saline (500,000 IU in each of the anterior tibial and posterior tibial arteries) over 20 minutes. Following completion of the UK infusion, the limb was flushed with a heparin-saline solution. The venotomy was closed primarily and the arteriotomy closed with a patch.

Illustration continued on following page

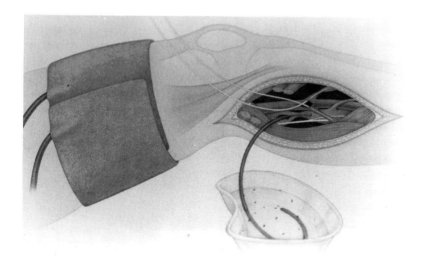

B

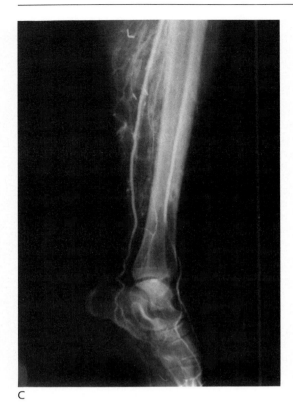

C

Figure 21-7 *continued.* A postinfusion arteriogram **(C)** documented significant improvement of perfusion to the foot. The patient had a palpable dorsalis pedis pulse and a pink foot following wound closure.

post-reperfusion (post-re), i.e., approximately 1 minute after vascular clamps were removed and reperfusion restored; and (4) 2 hours (2 hrs) after the study drug was infused. The 2-hour sample was a systemic sample only because by this time most patients were in the recovery room. A standardized dose of heparin was given intravenously (75 IU/kg) before vascular clamping, and subsequent anticoagulation or dextran was withheld until after the 2-hour blood sample was drawn.

Blood samples were analyzed for (1) plasminogen activity, (2) fibrinogen, (3) fibrin(ogen) degradation products (FDPs), (4) D-dimer, and (5) fibrinopeptide B-β 15-42 breakdown products. When thrombin interacts with fibrinogen, fibrin I and fibrin II are formed by the sequential release of fibrinopeptides A and B. Fibrin II is subsequently cross-linked by activated factor XIII

(Fig. 21-8). Activation of plasminogen results in the formation of plasmin, which has proteolytic effects on fibrinogen, fibrin, and cross-linked fibrin. The assays used to measure degradation products (FDPs) do not distinguish between those from fibrinogen or fibrin. However, specific markers are available to detect plasmin-induced breakdown of fibrin and cross-linked fibrin. Action of plasmin on fibrin results in the formation of fragment B-β 15-42 and on cross-linked fibrin with the production of D-dimer.

For the laboratory data, the change from baseline (pre) values was calculated for each time point of pre-reperfusion, post-reperfusion, and 2-hour post-reperfusion. Changes from baseline were compared between each dosage level and placebo using the maximum change from baseline in the expected direction, assuming a treatment effect.

Patient characteristics were similar between treatment groups, with the exception that those in the placebo group were younger than patients receiving urokinase ($p = 0.042$). There were no significant differences across treatment groups with respect to the distribution of associated risk factors, degree of ischemia at presentation, the type of operative procedure or anesthesia administered.

Figures 21-9 through 21-13 show the plasma levels of the measured proteins by treatment group for each time point. Plasma plasminogen activity (Fig. 21-9) was measured in the systemic circulation only. Compared with the placebo group, there was a dose-dependant decline in plasminogen activity that was significant ($p < 0.001$) only at the highest dose. Even at UK500, however, the mean values were still within the normal range. There was no significant decline in either the regional or systemic plasma fibrinogen levels following bolus urokinase infusion (Fig. 21-10). The plasma FDP levels (Fig. 21-11) were elevated in the treatment group in a dose-related fashion, with increases becoming significant ($p < 0.001$) relative to the placebo group at UK250 and UK500 in the regional circulation and at UK500 systemically ($p = 0.01$). There were significant elevations of D-dimer (Fig. 21-12) regionally at each urokinase dose ($p < 0.001$), which increased in a dose-response fashion. Systemic levels of D-dimer became significantly elevated at UK250

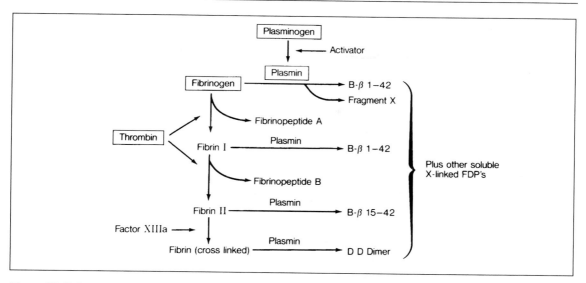

Figure 21-8. Schematic diagram of the markers of thrombin and plasmin-mediated proteolysis of fibrinogen and fibrin.

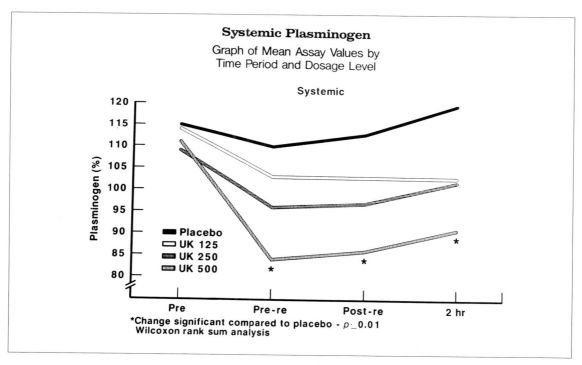

Figure 21-9. Mean plasma plasminogen levels in the systemic circulation by time period and dosage level. There appears to be dose-related decline in plasminogen which is significantly different from the placebo group in the UK 500 group ($p < 0.001$) (normal = 112 ± 22 percent).* $p < 0.001$.

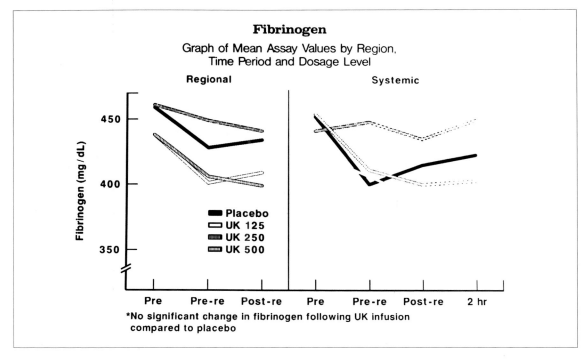

Figure 21-10. Mean plasma fibrinogen levels in the regional and systemic circulations by time period and dosage level. There was no significant change in any of the UK treatment groups compared to placebo (normal = 294 ± 64 mg/dl).

and UK500 ($p < 0.001$). Lastly, fragment B-β 15-42 levels (Fig. 21-13) showed a trend toward elevation at the higher doses of urokinase but achieved significance only at UK500 ($p = 0.009$), at the pre-reperfusion time point in the systemic circulation.

There was no difference in blood loss, blood replaced, excessive operative bleeding, or wound hematomas comparing those receiving urokinase with those receiving placebo. There is a trend toward a shorter length of stay in the placebo group (10.8 days) compared with the treatment groups (15.6–22.7 days, $p = 0.06$). An unexpected finding was the increased mortality in the placebo group (12.1 percent in placebo compared with 2.0 percent in patients receiving urokinase; $p = 0.033$). There were no significant differences between the maximal changes noted in the systemic and regional circulations for any of the plasma measurements.

An important observation of this multicenter, randomized study was the safety of intraopera-

tivelyinfused urokinase in bolus doses up to 500,000 IU. No bleeding complications were identified. The increased mortality (12 percent) in the placebo group was an unexpected finding and cannot be easily explained. Interestingly, in another recent prospective, randomized study comparing catheter-directed thrombolysis with surgery in patients with acute limb ischemia, patients in the thrombolytic group had significantly better survival than patients randomized to surgery.[12] In our study, the postoperative length of stay appeared to be longer in the urokinase groups, although this was not statistically significant. Since two deaths occurred by the second postoperative day and two deaths occurred 1 month postoperatively, the mortality in the placebo group was not a factor influencing length of stay. The longer mean length of stay in the urokinase-treated patients may be due to several outliers, some remaining hospitalized more than 3 months. The facts that patients in the placebo group were significantly younger and more were treated for

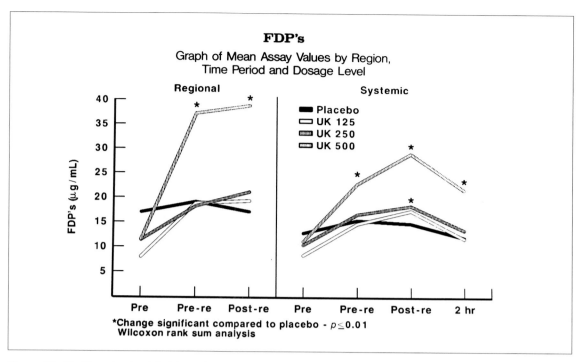

Figure 21-11. Mean levels of fibrin(ogen) degradation products (FDPs) in the regional and systemic circulations by time period and dosage level. The FDPs were significantly elevated regionally and systemically at all time periods in the UK500 group (*p* < 0.001). There was a significant systemic elevation post-reperfusion in the UK250 group (*p* < 0.001).

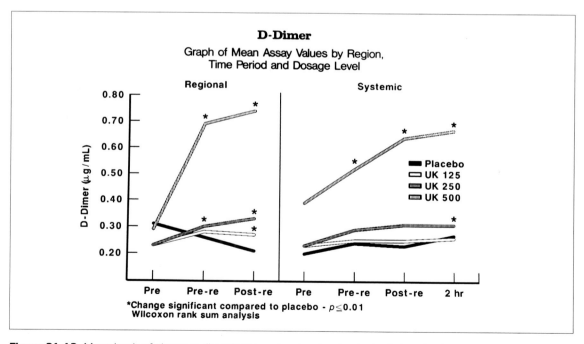

Figure 21-12. Mean levels of plasma D-dimer in the regional and systemic circulations by time period and dosage level (normal = 0.083 ± 0.014 µg/ml). Note significant and dose-related elevations at all doses of UK regionally and at UK250 and UK500 systemically.

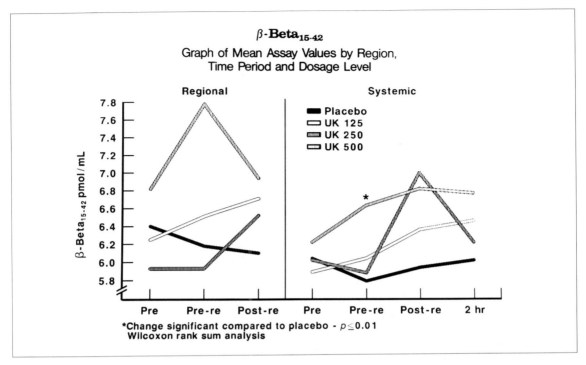

Figure 21-13. Mean levels of B-β 15-42 in the regional and systemic circulations by time period and dosage level (normal = 6.9 ± 1.1 pmol/ml). There appear to be dose-related increases in B-β 15-42; however, the only significant elevation occurred in the UK500-treated patients at the pre-reperfusion times.

intermittent claudication also may have influenced postoperative length of stay. The median values for length of stay, however, are relatively consistent for all treatment groups and placebo.

The goal of regionally delivered plasminogen activators is to achieve fibrinolysis with minimal breakdown of fibrinogen, clotting factors, and other plasma proteins. A major purpose of our study was to assess the impact of the intraoperative use of urokinase on plasminogen activation and lysis of fibrinogen and fibrin in the regional and systemic circulation. There was a dose-dependent decline in plasma plasminogen levels indicating plasminogen activation, particularly at the highest dose. Although regional levels were not measured, it is reasonable to assume the same dose-response occurred locally also, where the urokinase levels would be higher than peripherally. Activation of plasminogen results in the generation of plasmin, which induces lysis of fibrin clots, as well as circulating fibrinogen, with

formation of degradation products. Of particular importance is the finding that even at the highest concentration of urokinase administered, there was no significant decline in plasma fibrinogen levels over those noted in the placebo group. The plasma levels of FDPs, which reflect the breakdown of both fibrin and fibrinogen, were significantly elevated. Overall, the changes in fibrinogen, plasminogen, and FDPs noted in our study are substantially lower than those noted in studies where thrombolytic agents have been administered to patients with acute myocardial infarction,[75,76] where much higher doses of thrombolytic agents are infused systemically over a longer duration. Our patients had relatively small doses of urokinase given intraarterially as a bolus into a relatively stagnant distal circulation.

Of particular interest was whether urokinase would lyse cross-linked fibrin in the distal arterial bed, which might be a potential beneficial effect. Because the FDP assay measures the sum of the breakdown products of fibrin and fibrinogen, additional markers of plasmin-mediated proteolysis were used to differentiate between the breakdown of fibrin and cross-linked fibrin. The action of plasmin on fibrin results in the release of fibrinopeptide B-β 15-42. Fragment D-dimer is derived from the action of plasmin on cross-linked fibrin. There was significant elevation in D-dimer levels regionally at all doses of urokinase and systemically at UK250 and UK500. Levels of fragment B-β 15-42 demonstrated increasing levels with increasing doses of urokinase but were significantly elevated in the systemic circulation at UK500. These findings suggest that there is degradation of fibrin by urokinase. The absence of such a rise in either B-β 15-42 or D-dimer levels in the placebo group indicates that the observed elevations in the urokinase groups are not merely due to lysis by endogenous plasminogen activators of the clot formed during surgery to provide hemostasis. The elevated D-dimer levels suggest lysis of cross-linked fibrin in the regional circulation. It needs to be considered whether the observed high D-dimer levels are influenced by detection of other non-cross-linked fibrin degradation products in the assay as reported Lawler et al.[77] in subjects with extensive fibrinogen breakdown (>80 percent of baseline values) following administration of thrombolytic therapy. This is unlikely to be the case because in our patients the changes in plasma levels of plasminogen, FDPs, and D-dimer were substantially less than the levels observed by these authors, and more important, there was no significant decline in plasma fibrinogen levels. Moreover, no appreciable cross-reactivity with FDPs has been reported with the ELISA assay.[78] Therefore, the elevated D-dimer levels suggest that urokinase-induced dissolution of cross-linked fibrin occurs in the extremity circulation. Whether such lysis of clinically silent fibrin deposits in the ischemic extremity translates into clinical benefit needs to be established.

Although the acutely ischemic limb with suspected distal thrombi is the most frequent indication for intraoperative fibrinolytic therapy, this study was designed to evaluate the effects of urokinase infusion in patients with chronic lower extremity ischemia with respect to its effects on activation of the fibrinolytic system and plasma fibrinogen. The significant dose-related elevation of D-dimer suggests that there is lysis of fibrin in the distal arterial circulation. If this is indeed the case, small distal vessel thrombosis may be part of the pathophysiology of chronic limb ischemia. Since no bleeding complications were observed, it seems reasonable to consider distal infusion of urokinase in patients undergoing operations for chronic severe limb ischemia. Although these results suggest that intraoperative urokinase infusion may be of value for patients undergoing revascularization for chronic limb ischemia, additional randomized studies are indicated to delineate clinical benefits.

SUMMARY

It is likely that some patient subgroups will be most appropriately treated with thrombolytic interventions and other subgroups will be best treated with immediate operation. The definition of these distinct categories awaits the findings of large randomized studies. Intraoperative thrombolytic therapy may be useful in dissolving thrombus in poorly accessible anatomic locations. Initial experience suggests that the modality does not increase perioperative hemorrhagic complications; rather, its use may be associated with a reduction in morbidity and mortality. Pending the availability of data on the results of thrombolysis in distinct subcategories of clinical presentation, appropriate therapy must be planned on the basis of reasonable clinical judgment and the experience of the angiographic and surgical teams.

REFERENCES

1. Rutkow IM, Ernst CB: An analysis of vascular surgical manpower requirements and vascular surgical rates in the United States. J Vasc Surg 1986;3:74.
2. Green RM, DeWeese JA, Rob CG: Arterial embolectomy before and after the Fogarty catheter. Surgery 1975;77:24.
3. Tillett WS, Sherry S: The effect in patients of streptococcal fibrinolysin (streptokinase) and streptococcal desoxyribonuclease on fibrinous, purulent, and sanguinous pleural exudations. J Clin Invest 1949; 28:173.

4. Tillett WS, Sherry S, Christensen LR: Streptococcal desoxyribonuclease: Significance in lysis of purulent exudates and production by strains of hemolytic streptococci. Proc Soc Exp Biol Med 1948;68:184.

5. Tillett WS, Johnson AJ, McCarty WR: The intravenous infusion of the streptococcal fibrinolytic principle (streptokinase) into patients. J Clin Invest 1955;34:169.

6. Cliffton EE, Grossi CE: Investigations of intravenous plasmin (fibrinolysin) in humans; physiologic and clinical effects. Circulation 1956;14:919.

7. Sherry S, Fletcher AP, Alkjaersig N: Developments in fibrinolytic therapy for thromboembolic disease. Ann Intern Med 1959;50:560.

8. Cliffton EE: The use of plasmin in humans. Ann NY Acad Sci 1957;68:209.

9. Dotter CT, Rosch J, Seaman AJ: Selective clot lysis with low-dose streptokinase. Radiology 1974;111:31.

10. Rutherford RB, Flanigan DP, Gupta SK, et al: Suggested standards for reports dealing with lower extremity ischemia. J Vasc Surg 1986;4:80.

11. McNamara TO, Fischer JR: Thrombolysis of peripheral arterial and graft occlusions: Improved results using high-dose urokinase. AJR 1985;144:769.

12. Ouriel K, Shortell CK, DeWeese JA, et al: A comparison of thrombolytic therapy with operative revascularization in the treatment of acute peripheral arterial ischemia. J Vasc Surg 1994;19:1021.

13. Jang IK, Gold HK, Ziskind AA, et al: Differential sensitivity of erythrocyte-rich and platelet-rich arterial thrombi to lysis with recombinant tissue-type plasminogen activator: A possible explanation for resistance to coronary thrombolysis. Circulation 1989;79:920.

14. Gardiner GA Jr, Sullivan KL: Catheter-directed thrombolysis for the failed lower extremity bypass graft. Semin Vasc Surg 1992;5:99.

15. McNamara TO: Thrombolysis as an alternative initial therapy for the acutely ischemic lower limb. Semin Vasc Surg 1992;5:89.

16. Shortell CK, Ouriel K, Green RM, et al: Vascular disease in the antiphospholipid syndrome: A comparison with the patient population with atherosclerosis (discussion). J Vasc Surg 1992; 15:158.

17. Schoenbaum S, Goldman MA, Siegelman SS: Renal arterial embolization. Angiology 1971;22:332.

18. Kunlin J: Le traitement de l'arterite obliterante par la greffe veineuse. Arch Malad Coeur Vaiss 1949; 42:371.

19. Dos Santos JC: Sur la desobstruction des thrombus arterielles anciennes. Mem Acad Chir 1947;73:409.

20. Fogarty TJ, Cranley JJ, Drause RJ, et al: A method for extraction of arterial emboli and thrombi. Surg Gynecol Obstet 1963;116:241.

21. Edwards JE, Taylor LM Jr, Porter JM: Treatment of failed lower extremity bypass grafts with new autogenous vein bypass grafting. J Vasc Surg 1990;11:136.

22. Blaisdell FW, Steele M, Allen RE: Management of acute lower extremity arterial ischemia due to embolism and thrombosis. Surgery 1978;84:822.

23. Jivegard L, Holm J, Schersten T: Acute limb ischemia due to arterial embolism or thrombosis: Influence of limb ischemia versus pre-existing cardiac disease on postoperative mortality rate. J Cardiovasc Surg 1988;29:32.

24. Marder VJ: The use of thrombolytic agents: choice of patient, drug administration, laboratory monitoring. Ann Intern Med 1979;90:802.

25. Alkjaersig N, Fletcher AP, Sherry S: The mechanism of clot dissolution by plasmin. J Clin Invest 1959;38:1086.

26. Marder VJ, Sherry S: Thrombolytic therapy: Current status, part I. N Engl J Med 1988;318:1512.

27. Sherry S, Fletcher AP, Alkjaersig N: Fibrinolysis and fibrinolytic activity in man. Physiol Rev 1959;39:343.

28. Sherry S, Lindemeyer RI, Fletcher AP: Studies on enhanced fibrinolytic activity in man. J Clin Invest 1959;38:810.

29. Agnelli G, Buchanan MR, Fernandez F, Hirsh J: The thrombolytic and hemorrhagic effects of tissue type plasminogen activator: Influence of dosage regimens in rabbits. Thromb Res 1985;40:769.

30. Goldhaber SZ, Heit J, Sharma GVRK, et al: Randomized, controlled trial of recombinant tissue plasminogen activator versus urokinase in the treatment of acute pulmonary embolism. Lancet 1988; 2:293.

31. Kane KK: Fibrinolysis—A review. Ann Clin Lab Sci 1984;14:443.

32. Meyerovitz MF, Goldhaber SZ, Regan K, et al: Recombinant tissue-type plasminogen activator versus urokinase in peripheral arterial and graft occlusions: A randominzed trial. Radiology 1990; 175:75.

33. Graor RA, Olin J, Bartholomew JR, et al: Efficacy and safety of intraarterial local infusion of streptokinasae, urokinase, or tissue plasminogen activator for peripheral arterial occlusion: A retrospective review. J Vasc Med Biol 1990;2:310.

34. Turitto VT, Weiss HJ, Baumgartner HR, et al: Cells and aggregates at surfaces. Ann NY Acad Sci 1987;516:453.

35. Ouriel K, Donayre C, Shortell CK, et al: The hemodynamics of thrombus formation in arteries (discussion). J Vasc Surg 1991;14:757.

36. Blebea J, Ouriel K, Zollo RA, Marder VJ: Deposition of platelets and fibrinogen on ex vivo vascular segments: Dependence on shear rate. Surg Forum 1990;41:357.

37. Blinc A, Planinsic G, Keber D, et al: Dependence of blood clot lysis on the mode of transport of urokinase into the clot. A magnetic resonance imaging study in vitro. Thromb Haemost 1991;65:549.

38. Valji K, Roberts AC, Davis GB, Bookstein JJ: Pulsed-spray thrombolysis of arterial and bypass graft occlusions. AJR 1991;156:617.

39. Sabovic M, Lijnen HR, Deber D, Collen D: Correlation between progressive adsorption of plasminogen to blood clots and their sensitivity to lysis. Thromb Haemost 1990;64:450.

40. Sabovic M, Lijnen HR, Keber D, Collen D: Effect of retraction on the lysis of human clots with fibrin-specific and non-fibrin specific plasminogen activators. Thromb Haemost 1989;62:1083.

41. Okada M, Blomback B: Factors influencing fibrin gel structure studied by flow measurement. Ann NY Acad Sci 1983;408:233.

42. Nilsson L, Albrechtsson U, Jonung T, et al: Surgical treatment versus thrombolysis in acute arterial occlusion: A randomised controlled study. Eur J Vasc Surg 1992;6:189.

43. Allen DR, Smallwood J, Johnson CD. Intra-arterial thrombolysis should be the initial treatment of the acutely ischaemic lower limb. Ann R Coll Surg Engl 1992;74:106.

44. Faggioli GL, Peer RM, Pedrini L, et al: Failure of thrombolytic therapy to improve long-term vascular patency. J Vasc Surg 1994;19:289.

45. McNamara TO, Bomberger RA, Merchant RF: Intra-arterial urokinase as the initial therapy for acutely ischemic lower limbs. Circulation 1991;83 (suppl I):I-106.

46. Fiessinger JN, Aiach M, Vayssairat M, et al: Traitment thrombolytique des arteriopathies. Ann Anesthesiol Fr 1978;19:739.

47. Amery A, Deloof W, Vermylen J, Verstraete M: Outcome of recent thromboembolic occlusions of limb arteries treated with streptokinase. Br Med J 1970;4:639.

48. Hess H: Thrombolytische therapie. *In* Symposion der Deutschen Gesellschaft fur angiologie. Stuttgart, Springer-Verlag, 1967, pp 91–108.

49. Hess H, Ingrisch H, Mietaschk A, Rath H: Local low-dose thrombolytic therapy of peripheral arterial occlusions. N Engl J Med 1982;307:1627.

50. McNamara TO, Bomberger RA: Factors affecting initial and 6 month patency rates after intraarterial thrombolysis with high dose urokinase. Am J Surg 1986;152:709.

51. Kandarpa K, Chopra PS, Aruny JE, et al: Prospective, randomized comparison of forced periodic infusion and conventional slow continuous infusion. Radiology 1993;188:1.

52. Marder VJ, Sherry S: Thrombolytic therapy: Current status, part II. N Engl J Med 1988;318:1585.

53. Graor RA, Risius B, Young JR, et al: Low-dose streptokinase for selective thrombolysis: Systemic effects and complications. Radiology 1984;152:35.

54. Krings W, Roth FJ, Cappius G, Schmidtke I: Catheter-lysis: Indications and primary results. Int Angiol 1985;4:117.

55. Graor RA, Risius B, Lucas FV, et al: Thrombolysis with recombinant human tissue-type plasminogen activator in patients with peripheral artery and bypass graft occlusions. Circulation 1986;74:I-15.

56. Sicard GA, Schier JJ, Totty WG, et al: Thrombolytic therapy for acute arterial occlusion. J Vasc Surg 1985;2:65.

57. Ricotta J: Intra-arterial thrombolysis. A surgical view (comment). Circulation 1991;83:I-120.

58. Lacombe M: Surgical versus medical treatment of renal artery embolism. J Cardiovasc Surg 1977; 18:281.

59. Berridge DC, Gregson RHS, Hopkinson BR, Makin GS: Randomized trial of intra-arterial recombinant tissue plasminogen activator, intravenous recombinant tissue plasminogen activator and intra-arterial streptokinase in peripheral arterial thrombolysis. Br J Surg 1991;78:988.

60. Ouriel K, Andrus CH, Ricotta JJ, et al: Acute renal artery occlusion: When is revascularization justified? J Vasc Surg 1987;5:348.

61. Ouriel K, Shortell CK: Results of thrombolytic therapy in acute limb ischemia. Unpublished data.

62. Comerota AJ, Rubin R, Tyson R, et al: Intra-arterial thrombolytic therapy in peripheral vascular disease. Surg Gynecol Obstet 1987;165:1.

63. Chaise LS, Comerota AJ, Soulen RL, et al: Selective intra-arterial streptokinase therapy in the immediate postoperative period. JAMA 1982;247: 2397.

64. Greep JM, Allman PJ, Janet F, et al: A combined technique for peripheral arterial embolectomy. Arch Surg 1972;105:869.

65. Plecha FR, Pories WJ: Intraoperative angiography in the immediate assessment of arterial reconstruction. Arch Surg 1972;105:902.

66. Quinones-Baldrich WJ, Ziomek S, Henderson TC, et al: Intraoperative fibrinolytic therapy: Experimental evaluation. J Vasc Surg 1986;4:229.

67. Dunnant JR, Edwards WS: Small vessel occlusion in the extremity after periods of arterial obstruction: An experimental study. Surgery 1973;75:240.

68. Belkin M, Valeri R, Hobson RW: Intra-arterial urokinase increases skeletal muscle viability after acute ischemia. J Vasc Surg 1989;9:161.

69. Cohen LJ, Kaplan M, Bernhard VM: Intraoperative fibrinolytic therapy: An adjunct to catheter thromboembolectomy. J Vasc Surg 1985;2:319.

70. Norem RF, Short DH, Kerstein MD: Role of intraoperative fibrinolytic therapy in acute arterial occlusion. Surg Gynecol Obstet 1988;167:87.

71. Parent NE, Bernhard VM, Pabst TS, et al: Fibrinolytic treatment of residual thrombus after catheter embolectomy for severe lower limb ischemia. J Vasc Surg 1989;9:153.

72. Comerota AJ, White JV, Grosh JD: Intraoperative, intra-arterial thrombolytic therapy for salvage of

limbs in patients with distal arterial thrombosis. Surg Gynecol Obstet 1989;169:283.

73. Comerota AJ, White JV: Intraoperative, intraarterial thrombolytic therapy as an adjunct to revascularization in patients with residual distal arterial thrombus. Semin Vasc Surg 1992;5:110.

74. Comerota AJ, Rao AK, Throm RC, et al: A prospective, randomized, blinded, and plcebo-controlled trial of intraoperative intraarterial urokinase infusion during lower extremity revascularization: Regional and systemic effects. Ann Surg 1993;218:534.

75. Rao AK, Pratt C, Berke A, et al: Thrombolysis in myocardial infarction (TIMI) trial: Phase I. Hemorrhagic manifestations and changes in plasma plasminogen activator and streptokinase. J Am Coll Cardiol 1988;11:1.

76. Mueller HS, Rao AK, Forman SA, TIMI Investigators: Thrombolysis in myocardial infarction (TIMI): Comparative studies of coronary reperfusion and systemic fibrinogenolysis with two forms of reconbinant tissue-type plasminogen activator. J Am Coll Cardiol 1987;10:479.

77. Lawler CM, Bovill EG, Stump DC, et al: Fibrin fragment D-dimer and fibrinogen B-beta peptides in plasma as markers of clot lysis during thrombolytic therapy in acute myocardial infarction. Blood 1990;76:1341.

78. Whitaker AN, Elms MJ, Masci PP, et al: Measurements of cross-linked fibrin derivatives in plasma: An immunoassay using monoclonal antibodies. J Clin Pathol 1984;37:882.

Venous Thrombolysis

CHARLES P. SEMBA
MICHAEL D. DAKE

Management of iliofemoral deep venous thrombosis (DVT) remains relatively unchanged over the past two decades. Despite advances in diagnosing DVT with duplex Doppler imaging, treatment is still centered on systemic anticoagulation with heparin followed by warfarin.[1–3] The rationale for anticoagulation is essentially threefold: (1) to minimize the associated complication of pulmonary emboli, (2) to prevent further thrombus formation, and (3) to minimize the risk of postphlebitic syndrome related to deep venous valvular insufficiency. The purpose of this chapter is to review an alternative strategy to anticoagulation using thrombolytic agents and endoluminal techniques in treating symptomatic iliofemoral deep venous thrombosis.

ANTICOAGULATION THERAPY

Anticoagulation theoretically prevents further thrombus formation but does not treat the offending thrombus. With time, the thrombus will retract and eventually resolve if it is present in small quantities. Many treating physicians work under the incorrect notion that heparin therapy directly activates and facilitates clot lysis. Serial ultrasound studies of patients with DVT show that less than 10 percent will spontaneously lyse within 10 days of full anticoagulation therapy and that 40 percent of patients will continue to propagate thrombus despite therapeutic doses of heparin.[4,5] In the patient with massive iliofemoral DVT, dissolution of the thrombus depends on the patient's own ability to fibrinolyse. While the body can dissolve small quantities of thrombus, it is our experience that patients with large segment iliofemoral venous thrombosis (> 5 to 7 cm) usually never recanalize despite adequate anticoagulation.

Valvular function rarely returns to normal even when there is partial return of blood flow through the vein during anticoagulation therapy.[6] Long-term studies in patients with iliofemoral deep venous thrombosis treated with anticoagulation alone have demonstrated that muscle pump function and valvular competency are severely compromised in approximately 95 percent of patients at 5 years of follow-up despite improvement in venous outflow.[7] While anticoagulation is the standard of care in treating DVT, critical evaluation of the data shows that heparin and warfarin alone are not sufficient in reducing long-term lower extremity morbidity.[8]

SURGICAL THERAPY

Surgical venous thrombectomy of the iliofemoral vein was proposed in the early 1960s and has been used at several centers with good results.[9–11] Despite these favorable reports, venous thrombectomy has not gained wide acceptance in the United States because of the high rate of recurrent thrombosis and postphlebitic syndrome.[12–14] This may be related to large quantities of adherent residual mural thrombus following thrombectomy, which then serves as the focal point for rethrombosis and occlusion. Thrombolytic therapy for the reoccluded vein has not been very successful in restoring and maintaining patency.[15] To improve the patency rates, temporary creation of an arteriovenous fistula for 3 to 6 months has been proposed to maintain high-velocity blood flow through the treated venous segment.[16–18] However, the vein tends to thrombose once the fistula is removed. Currently, there is no generally accepted standard surgical therapy for iliofemoral thrombosis.[19,20]

THROMBOLYTIC THERAPY

Thrombolytic agents have been available for the last 10 years but have not been widely used for treating iliofemoral DVT. Several studies have shown significant lysis and better long-term clinical benefits when using thrombolytic agents compared with anticoagulation therapy when treating DVT.[21–26] The main drawback to thrombolytic therapy has been the risk of bleeding, immunologic complications, and the risk of pulmonary emboli arising from partially thrombosed clot. The major studies that demonstrate the benefit of thrombolytic agents over heparin therapy have used systemic infusions. From our experience, we felt that systemic infusion, though effective, would be less efficient than infusing the clot directly using a catheter. Systemic infusion of the thrombolytic agent may not treat the clot, since most of the flow is directed around the occluding thrombus via numerous collateral veins. For the past several years, investigators have been successful at treating thrombosed arterial bypass grafts and upper extremity veins using catheter-directed, locally infused thrombolytic agents.[27–29] Initial reports using catheter-directed techniques for treating iliofemoral venous thrombosis have shown the feasibility of this method.[30–33]

PATIENT SELECTION FOR CATHETER-DIRECTED THROMBOLYSIS

Patients undergoing treatment have symptomatic iliofemoral DVT. Clinical symptoms range from lower extremity pain and swelling to frank phlegmasia. The thrombosis is documented with color-flow Doppler ultrasound and/or ascending venography. Patients are excluded from treatment if they have any contraindications to anticoagulation, bleeding disorders, pregnancy or recent delivery, isolated infrainguinal DVT, metastatic cancer with brain or spinal cord involvement, or a history of a hemorrhagic stroke. Recent major surgery is a relative contraindication. We generally do not treat patients within 14 days of a major operation. The optimal candidates for this procedure have thrombus isolated to the infrarenal inferior vena cava and iliac veins with duration of clinical symptoms of less than 4 weeks. We do not treat patients with isolated infrainguinal DVT.

PROCEDURE

Thrombolysis catheters are placed directly into the thrombosed vein using fluoroscopic guidance in the angiography suite. With the patient in a supine position, the right side of the neck is prepped and draped in sterile fashion, and the skin is anesthetized with 5 cc 1% lidocaine. Using a 20-gauge needle and a no. 5 Fr micropuncture set (Cook, Inc., Bloomington, Ind.), a 0.035-in-diameter guidewire is introduced into the inferior vena cava following placement of a no. 5 Fr sidearm sheath. The clotted inferior vena cava and/or iliac vein is then probed using an hydrophilic guidewire (Terumo Glidewire, Medi-Tech, Waterston, Mass.). The wire is then advanced into the thrombosed vein, and a no. 5 Fr endhole catheter is placed into the midportion of the thrombosed vein. The guidewire is removed, and a 0.035-in endhole thrombolysis wire (Sos wire, USCI, Billerica, Mass.) is then advanced through the catheter and placed near the leading edge of the thrombus. An alternative thrombolysis system consists of a single no. 4.8 Fr dual-lumen catheter (EDM catheter, Peripheral Systems Group, Mountain View, Calif.) that uses a 0.018-in-diameter guidewire instead of a 0.035-in guidewire. Whether using a coaxial system or a single dual-lumen catheter, each type of setup requires the use of two intravenous pumps for urokinase infusion.

Urokinase (Abbokinase, Abbott Laboratories, Abbott Park, Ill.) is reconstituted using 500,000 IU in 250 cc of 0.9% NaCl solution and delivered in split doses of 75,000 to 100,000 IU/h into each thrombolysis catheter or guidewire (total of

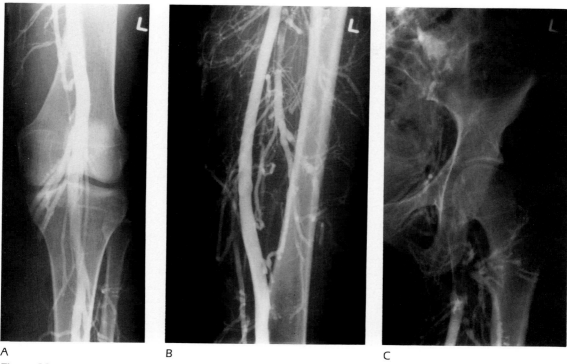

A   B   C

Figure 22-1. Complete thrombolysis using catheter-directed techniques. A 24-year-old woman with acute-onset leg edema and pain. (**A,B**) Ascending venogram shows (**A**) normal popliteal vein and (**B**) normal superficial femoral vein with and acute thrombus in the deep femoral vein (*arrow*). (**C**) There is abrupt occlusion of the common femoral and iliac veins secondary to an acute thrombus.

Illustration continued on the following page

150,000 to 200,000 IU/h). The patient is also heparinized, and the partial thromboplastin time (PTT) is maintained between 50 and 90 seconds and the fibrinogen levels are kept above 100 mg/dl.

Occasionally, the transjugular approach may fail secondary to the inability to pass a guidewire into the clotted iliac vein. An alternative approach is to puncture the thrombosed common femoral vein under ultrasound guidance using micropuncture technique and passing a 0.018-in guidewire into the inferior vena cava. The wire is then snared and pulled out the jugular access site. A no. 5 Fr endhole catheter can then be advanced over the wire into the clotted iliac vein, and the percutaneously placed wire is then removed. A thrombolytic endhole wire is then advanced further into the clotted vein. If this technique is unsuccessful, then the patient is placed prone, and the popliteal vein

is punctured using ultrasound guidance, and the wires and catheters are advanced antegrade into the thrombosed iliac vein.

Follow-up venography is performed within 24 hours from the start of lytic therapy. If there is partial thrombolysis after 24 hours, the catheters are repositioned, and thrombolytic therapy will be continued for another 24 to 48 hours. Lysis is considered to be complete if there is less than 5 percent residual thrombus (Fig. 22-1). Following thrombolysis, further intervention is performed if there is an underlying venous stenosis of greater than 50 percent. Interventions consist of either balloon angioplasty alone or angioplasty and stent placement. Stent placement is performed using either the balloon-expandable, rigid stainless steel Palmaz stent (Johnson and Johnson Interventional Systems, Warren, N.J.) or the self-expanding

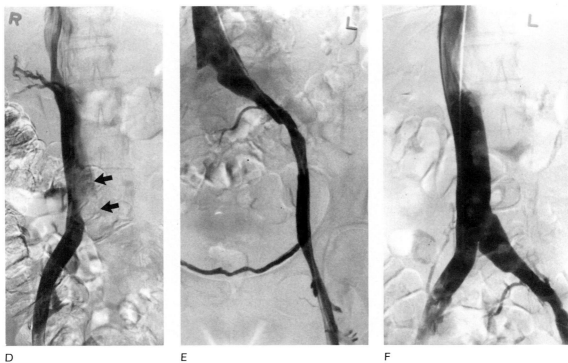

D   E   F

Figure 22-1 *continued.* (**D**) A mural thrombus extends into the IVC (*arrows*). (**E,F**) After 24 hours of thrombolytic therapy with urokinase, patency of the iliac and femoral veins was restored (**E**) with no residual thrombus in the IVC (**F**).

stainless steel Wallstent (Schneider, Inc., Plymouth, Minn.). All stents are placed above the inguinal ligament whenever possible. If the common femoral vein requires stenting, the longitudinally flexible Wallstent is used to avoid crushing the stent during normal hip flexion. Transjugular placement of the Palmaz stent into the iliac veins requires a no. 10 Fr 80-cm-long sidearm sheath (Cook, Inc., Bloomington, Ind.), which serves as a guiding catheter.

Following the procedure, the patients are anticoagulated initially with intravenous heparin and later oral warfarin, which is adjusted to maintain INR value of 2.0–3.0.* In patients with underlying malignancies, warfarin therapy is continued as long as clinically feasible. In all other patients, warfarin is discontinued after 8 to 12 weeks of therapy. Patients are also placed on aspirin (325 mg) daily, and the aspirin is continued indefinitely.

*International normalized ratio[54]

Clinical follow-up consists of a baseline venous Doppler study immediately after completion of the procedure and subsequent examinations at 2 weeks, and 3, 6, and 12 months and annually thereafter.

RESULTS

We have treated 21 patients (10 males and 11 females, mean age 52.8 years, range 24 to 74 years) with symptomatic iliofemoral DVT.[33] In total, 27 limbs were treated using catheter-directed thrombolysis techniques. Initial clinical symptoms and distribution of the thrombi are summarized in Table 22-1. Most of our patients (67 percent) had been on anticoagulation therapy with heparin for approximately 1 week without improvement in symptoms. Treatment outcomes and complications are summarized in Table 22-2.

Table 22-1. Presenting Symptoms and Location and Etiology of DVT in 27 Limbs (21 Patients)

	No. of Limbs	Percent
Initial symptoms		
Lower extremity edema	26	96
Lower extremity pain	27	100
Phlegmasia	2	7
Type of symptoms		
Acute*	20	74
Chronic†	7	26
Location of thrombus		
Left lower extremity	19	70
Right lower extremity	8	30
IVC, iliac vein	1	4
IVC, iliac and femoral veins	9	33
Iliac vein	5	19
Iliac and femoral veins	12	44
Etiology		
Recurrent DVT	2	7
Retroperitoneal fibrosis	2	7
Iliac compression syndrome	2	7
Radiation injury to vein	6	22
Postoperative DVT	7	26
Unknown	8	30

*Average duration of acute symptoms was 10.5 days (range 7 to 28 days).
†Average duration of chronic symptoms was 367.7 days (range 35 to 1095 days).

ROLE OF CATHETER-DIRECTED THROMBOLYSIS

The two main advantages of transcatheter infusion of thrombolytic agents is, first, the ability to deliver high concentrations directly into the thrombus while minimizing the potential for a systemic fibrinolytic effect and second, the ability to identify venous stenoses or obstructions with venography. Our study shows a complete lysis rate of 72 percent and a partial lysis rate of 20 percent using urokinase alone. Following intervention, 85 percent of treated limbs had complete resolution of leg edema and pain. One patient (one limb) had significant symptomatic improvement with only partial recanalization and no further interventions.

Venography is extremely useful in identifying outflow obstructions in the vein, which can be treated using endoluminal stents. In over half our cases, a venous injury or stenosis could be located following thrombolytic therapy. Angioplasty is initially performed on the iliac vein stenoses.[30,34] Owing to the elastic nature of the vein, often angioplasty alone is not sufficient. Stents provide the appropriate support to allow the large diameter vein to remain patent[31] (Fig. 22-2).

The role of thrombolytic agents in treating chronic clots is less certain. Historically, it has been well established that chronic clots are far more difficult to lyse than soft, fresh, acute clot. In a study by Theiss et al., complete or partial thrombolysis was achieved in 94 percent of cases when the occlusion was less than 3 days old. If thrombolysis was performed 5 to 8 weeks after onset of symptoms, success rates dropped to 14 percent when using systemic infusions of thrombolytic agents. In our experience, the best results are achieved when the thrombus is less than 7 days old. Even if the symptoms are of several months' duration, we will still initiate thrombolytic therapy to attempt to lyse any soft thrombus that may be

Table 22-2. Treatment Outcomes in 27 Limbs (21 Patients) Treated for Iliofemoral DVT

	No. of Limbs	Percent
Lysis of thrombus		
Complete	18	72
No further intervention	7	
Angioplasty	2	
Angioplasty and stent	9	
Partial	5	20
No further intervention	1	
Angioplasty and stent	4	
None	2	8
No further intervention	1	
Angioplasty and stent	1	
Technical failure		
Occluded vein unable to cross with wire	2	7
No lysis achieved, no further intervention	1	4
Partial lysis, no further intervention	1	4
Resolution of leg edema and pain		
Complete	21	81
Partial	1	4
None	4	15
Technical success	23	85
Clinical success	23	85

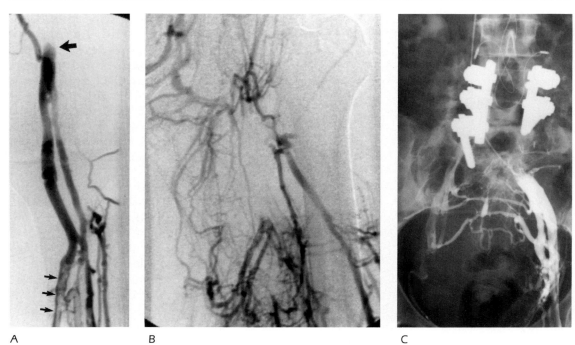

A   B   C

Figure 22-2. Complete thrombolysis with underlying focal stenosis requiring an endoluminal Palmaz stent. A 45-year-old woman with acute left leg swelling and pain 3 weeks after a lumbar fusion was performed. (**A**) Ascending subtraction venogram demonstrates a patent popliteal vein with multiple filling defects in the calf veins (*small arrows*) and abrupt occlusion of the superficial femoral vein (*large arrow*). (**B**) In the region of the femoral head, numerous small collateral vessels were present secondary to complete occlusion of the superficial femoral, common femoral, and iliac veins. The deep veins are thrombosed to the level of the IVC. (**C**) After 24 hours of catheter-directed thrombolysis, brisk flow was restored in the left femoral and external iliac veins; however, the common iliac vein remained occluded, with collateral filling of the presacral veins. The common iliac vein was excessively stretched with a surgical retractor during placement of the lumbar fusion rods by means of an anterior abdominal approach.

present. We feel that a trial of thrombolytic therapy helps to soften the thrombus, which facilitates recanalization procedures with angioplasty and stents. In our series, five of seven patients (71 percent) with chronic venous occlusions (mean 1.0 years) diagnosed by onset of symptoms and/or venography partially responded to thrombolysis.

THROMBOLYTIC AGENTS

Currently approved thrombolytic agents are streptokinase (Streptase, Hoechst-Roussel, Somerville, N.J.), recombinant tissue plasminogen activator (Activase, Genentech, San Francisco, Calif.), and urokinase. We prefer to use urokinase because of its reliability, high degree of safety, and proven efficacy in the arterial system and with upper extremity DVT.[27–29,36] Streptokinase can cause immunogenic side effects such as serum sickness and drug fever, and its efficacy can diminish because of activation of an antibody response. Hemorrhagic complications tend to be much higher with streptokinase and recombinant tissue plasminogen activator than with urokinase.[37,38] Though streptokinase is the least expensive agent, it is less cost-effective than urokinase because the hemorrhagic complications tend to lead to longer hospitalizations and higher overall costs.[39,40]

A handful of patients have experienced a urokinase-induced anaphylactoid reaction.[41,42] This typically occurs immediately following large bolus infusions of urokinase (>250,000 IU) and consists of shaking chills and tachycardia. The general

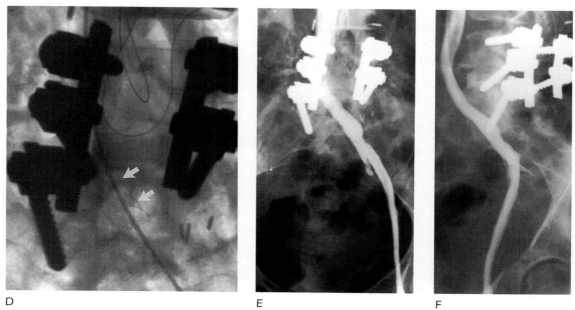

D   E   F

Figure 22-2 *continued.* *(arrows in* **D**) in the common iliac vein (**D**), as seen in the anteroposterior (**E**) and 35-degree left anterior oblique (**F**) projections. Patient is asymptomatic and the vein is patent at 12 months of follow-up.

treatment has been intravenous administration of meperidine hydrochloride (50 mg Demerol, Sanofi Winthrop Pharmaceuticals, New York, N.Y.) and histamine blockers (300 mg Tagamet, Smith, Kline & French Laboratories, Philadelphia, Pa.).[43] The reaction lasts about 5 minutes, and there are no further sequelae.

TECHNICAL CONSIDERATIONS FOR CATHETER-DIRECTED THERAPY

Several possible access routes are available for catheter-directed therapy. These include (1) arterial infusion into the affected lower extremity, (2) infusion into a foot vein with Ace wraps or cuffs employed to direct the drug into the ipsilateral deep veins, (3) ipsilateral popliteal vein puncture for transcatheter treatment of iliofemoral thrombus, (4) ipsilateral femoral vein puncture for catheter-directed lysis of iliac vein clot, (5) contralateral femoral vein puncture with passage of an infusion catheter over the caval bifurcation, and (6) transjugular placement of an infusion catheter directly into the thrombus. Techniques 1 and 2 are

minimally effective in our experience, and an indwelling catheter in the femoral artery or foot vein for up to 3 days is difficult to maintain both for the nursing staff and patient. Technique 3 is most useful for thrombus that has extended from the IVC into the superficial femoral vein, in which the transjugular approach is difficult because of the venous valves or the resistance in passing the guidewire through organized chronic thrombus. Techniques 4 and 5 are the easiest approaches, but we favor a transjugular rather than a femoral approach for three reasons: patient comfort, easier access into the occluded common iliac vein (as opposed to the contralateral approach), and prevention of further DVT by catheter placement in the affected limb. The right internal jugular approach spares the femoral vein from catheter-related trauma, a known risk factor in DVT,[44] especially when balloon-expandable stents are delivered through no. 9 or no. 10 Fr sheaths. Thrombosis in the jugular vein is less likely to lead to significant symptoms or long-term disability. Thrombolysis may require 24 to 48 hours of continuous infusion through the catheter. For patient comfort, a transjugular approach allows the patient to ambulate and sit up in bed with a lesser risk of dislodging the catheter or causing a venous hematoma during ambulation. In addition, the neck usually offers a cleaner site for an indwelling catheter than the groin.

THE ROLE OF ENDOLUMINAL STENTS

Maintaining patency of the successfully treated iliofemoral vein requires establishment of brisk blood flow. Endoluminal stents can treat underlying venous stenoses and restore the normal lumen geometry, thus allowing for brisk blood flow through the treated segment. We advocate stent placement only in the inferior vena cava and the iliac veins. Our experience in placing stents in the smaller infrainguinal veins has been disappointing because of extremely poor patency rates. The ideal candidates for stents are those patients with (1) isolated IVC or iliac vein occlusions or stenoses and (2) normal inflow from the popliteal and femoral veins. Stents placed in the iliac veins or IVC with good inflow tend to develop far less intimal hyperplasia than upper extremity venous stents. The reasons for less hyperplasia are unknown, but based on our studies, the large lumens (10 to 16 mm) created by stents combined with minimal hyperplasia tend to increase long-term durability.[45]

There are two general categories of stents for venous reconstruction currently being studied at our institution; the balloon-expandable, rigid Palmaz stent and the self-expanding, longitudinally flexible Wallstent. The Palmaz stent offers excellent hoop strength and resistance to radial forces but may be difficult to utilize in long segment disease or in tortuous vessels.[46] The Wallstent has less hoop strength but can cover longer segments of vein (up to 90 mm in length) and offers flexibility, which is desirable if a stent needs to extend from the iliac vein below the inguinal ligament.[47] In patients with chronic venous disease or in patients who have received pelvic radiation therapy, stents provide an attractive alternative to lesions that have failed conventional angioplasty alone because of elastic recoil, fibrosis, and intimal thickening.[48,49] Following implantation of the stents, the stainless steel surface develops a fine layer of neointima that will eventually incorporate the stent within the vessel wall in 4 to 6 weeks.[50] The long-term durability of stents is unknown at this time; however, based on our series, there is a 90 percent primary patency rate at 1 year when there is normal inflow from a patent superficial femoral vein.[45]

COMPLICATIONS

We have not encountered any major complications related to urokinase, including hemorrhage, immune reactions, or pulmonary emboli. Initially, we performed ventilation-perfusion lung scans before and after the procedure, but no perfusion defects following thrombolysis were ever detected. There have been no clinically significant cases of pulmonary emboli resulting in increasing dyspnea or arterial oxygen desaturation, and we no longer advocate routine placement of inferior vena cava filters prior to catheter-directed intervention. Other investigators have reported fresh thrombus trapped in temporary IVC filters following thrombolytic therapy for iliofemoral DVT.[32,51,52] While death from pulmonary emboli is extremely rare during thrombolytic therapy, it is likely that microemboli travel to the lung during infusion therapy and eventually dissolve and are of no clinical significance.[53] Minor complications include small venous hematomas at the venous access site or balloon rupture during stent deployment. The stents can be repositioned and deployed with a new balloon catheter. We have not had any cases of stent embolization after implantation.

CONCLUSIONS

Using catheter-directed techniques to deliver thrombolytic agents into acute and chronic DVTs, we have achieved a clinical and technical success rate of 85 percent. Urokinase is the agent of choice because of its margin of safety and low complication rate. The ideal candidates for therapy are patients with fresh, soft thrombus that is less than 1 week old. Using percutaneous techniques has allowed for endoluminal reconstruction of chronically diseased iliac veins using angioplasty and stents. Long-term durability is directly related to establishment of good inflow into the treated segment from a normal and widely patent femoral vein. These techniques provide an attractive alternative to standard anticoagulation and surgical venous interventions.

REFERENCES

1. Hirsh J: Antithrombotic therapy in deep vein thrombosis and pulmonary embolism. Amer Heart J 1992;123(4 pt 2):1115.
2. Hyers TM, Hull RD, Weg JG: Antithrombotic therapy for venous thromboembolic disease. Chest 1989;95:37S.
3. Bounameaux H: Low molecular-weight heparins: A decade with the new class of antithrombotic agents. Vasa 1994;23:3.
4. Sherry S: Thrombolytic therapy for deep vein thrombosis. Semin Intervent Radiol 1985;4:331.
5. Krupski WC, Bass A, Dilley RB, et al: Propagation of deep venous thrombosis identified by duplex ultrasonography. J Vasc Surg 1990;12:467.
6. van Bemmelen PS, Bedford G, Beach K, Strandness DE Jr: Functional status of the deep venous system after an episode of deep venous thrombosis. Ann Vasc Surg 1990;4:455.
7. Akesson H, Brudin L, Dahlstrom JA, et al: Venous function assessed during a five-year period after acute iliofemoral venous thrombosis treated with anticoagulation. Eur J Vasc Surg 1990;4:43.
8. Strandness DE, Langlois YE, Cramer M, et al: Long-term sequelae of acute venous thrombosis. JAMA 1983;250:1289.
9. Mahorner H, Castleberry JW, Coleman WO: Attempts to restore function in major veins which are the sites of massive thrombosis. Ann Surg 1957;146:510.
10. Haller JA, Abrams BL: Use of thrombectomy in the treatment of acute iliofemoral venous thrombosis in forty-five patients. Am Surg 1963;158:561.
11. Fontaine R, Tuchmann L: The role of thrombectomy in deep venous thrombosis. J Cardiovasc Surg 1964;5:298.
12. Karp RB, Wylie EJ: Recurrent thrombosis after iliofemoral venous thrombectomy. Surg Forum 1966;17:147.
13. Lansing AM, Davis WM: Five-year follow-up study of iliofemoral venous thrombectomy. Ann Surg 1968;168:620.
14. Edwards WH, Sawyers JL, Foster JH: Iliofemoral venous thrombosis: Reappraisal of thrombectomy. Ann Surg 1970;171:961.
15. Mavor GE, Ogston D, Galloway JMD, et al: Urokinase in iliofemoral venous thrombosis. Br J Surg 1969;56:571.
16. Delin A, Swedenborg J, Hellgren M, et al: Thrombectomy and temporary arteriovenous fistula for iliofemoral venous thrombosis in fertile women. Surg Gynecol Obstet 1982;154:69.
17. Plate G, Einarsson E, Ohlin P, et al: Thrombectomy with temporary arteriovenous fistula: The treatment of choice in acute iliofemoral venous thrombosis. J Vasc Surg 1984;1:867.
18. Rasmussen A, Mogensen K, Nissen FH, et al: [Acute iliofemoral venous thrombosis: 26 cases treated with thrombectomy, temporary arterio-venous fistula, and anticoagulants]. Ugeskrift for Laeger (Danish) 1990;152:2928.
19. Norgren L: Does thrombectomy still have a place in the treatment of acute deep venous thrombosis? Acta Chir Scand suppl 1990;555:193.
20. Comerota AJ: Venous thrombectomy and arteriovenous fistula versus anticoagulation in the treatment of iliofemoral venous thrombosis. J Vasc Surg 1992;15:887.
21. Comerota AJ, Aldridge SC: Thrombolytic therapy for deep vein thrombosis: A clinical review. Can J Surg 1993;36:359.
22. Robertson BR, Nilsson IM, Nylander GL: Value of streptokinase and heparin in treatment of deep vein thrombosis. Acta Chir Scand 1969;134:203.
23. Kakkar V, Flanc C, Howe CT, et al: Treatment of deep vein thrombosis: A trial of heparin, streptokinase, and arvin. Br Med J 1969;1:806.
24. Elliott MS, Immelman EJ, Jeffrey L, et al: A comparative randomized trial of heparin versus streptokinase in the treatment of acute proximal venous thrombosis: An interim report of prospective trial. Br J Surg 1979;66:838.
25. Arneson H, Hoiseth A, Ly B: Streptokinase or heparin in the treatment of deep vein thrombosis. Acta Med Scand 1982;211:65.
26. Rogers LP, Lutcher CL: Streptokinase therapy for deep vein thrombosis. A comprehensive review of the English literature. Am J Med 1990;88:389.
27. McNamara TO, Fischer JR: Thrombolysis of arterial and graft occlusions: Improved results using high-dose urokinase. AJR 1985;144:769.
28. Becker GJ, Holden RW, Rabe EF, et al: Local thrombolytic therapy for subclavian and axillary vein thrombosis. Radiology 1983;149:663.
29. Druy EM, Trout HH, Giordano JM, Hix WR: Lytic therapy in the treatment of axillary and subclavian vein thrombosis. J Vasc Surg 1985;2:821.
30. Okrent D, Messersmith R, Buckman J: Transcatheter fibrinolytic therapy and angioplasty for left iliofemoral venous thrombosis. JVIR 1991;2:195.
31. Molina JE, Hunter DW, Yedlicka JW: Thrombolytic therapy for iliofemoral venous thrombosis. J Vasc Surg 1992;26:630.

32. Palombo D, Porta C, Brustia P, et al: [Loco-regional thrombolysis in deep venous thrombosis]. Phlebologie (French) 1993;46:293.

33. Semba CP, Dake MD: Iliofemoral deep venous thrombosis: Aggressive therapy using catheter-directed thrombolysis. Radiology 1994;191:487.

34. Marache P, Asseman P, Jabinet JL, et al: Percutaneous transluminal venous angioplasty in occlusive iliac vein thrombosis resistant to thrombolysis. Amer Heart J 1993;125(2 pt 1):362.

35. Theiss W, Worttzfeld A, Fink U, Maubach P: The success rate of fibrinolytic therapy of fresh and old thrombosis of the iliac and femoral veins. Angiology 1983;34:61.

36. Goldhaber SZ, Polak JF, Feldstein ML, et al: Efficacy and safety of repeated boluses of urokinase in the treatment of deep venous thrombosis. Amer J Cardiol 1994;73:75.

37. Califf RM, Stump D, Thorton D, et al: Hemorrhagic complications after tissue plasminogen activator therapy for acute myocardial infarction. Circulation 1987;76:IV-1.

38. Simoons ML, Maggioni AP, Knatterud G, et al: Individual risk assessment for intracranial hemorrhage during thrombolytic therapy. Lancet 1993; 342:1523.

39. Graor RA, Young JR, Risius B, Ruschaupt WF: Comparison of cost-effectiveness of streptokinase and urokinase in treating deep venous thrombosis. Ann Vasc Surg 1987;1:524.

40. van Breda A, Graor RA, Katzen BT, et al: Relative cost-effectiveness of urokinase versus streptokinase in the treatment of peripheral vascular disease. JVIR 1991;2:77.

41. Bell WR: Update on urokinase and streptokinase: A comparison of their efficacy and safety. Hosp Formul 1988;23:230.

42. Matsumoto AH, Selby JB, Tegtmeyer CJ, et al: Recent development of rigors during infusion of urokinase: is it related to endotoxins? JVIR 1994;5:433.

43. Vidovich RR, Heiselman DE, Hudock D: Treatment of urokinase-related anaphylactoid reaction with intravenous famotidine. Ann Pharmacother 1992;26:782.

44. Mewissen MW, Erickson SJ, Foley WD, et al: Thrombosis at venous insertion sites after inferior vena cava filter placement. Radiology 1989; 173:155.

45. Semba CP, Dake MD, Chang H: Endovascular stents for the treatment of lower extremity venous occlusions: Mid-term results. Radiology 1994;193:192.

46. Trerotola SO, Lund GB, Samphilipo MA, et al: Palmaz stent in the treatment of central venous stenosis: safety and efficacy of redilation. Radiology 1994;190:379.

47. Dyet JF, Nicholson AA, Cook AM: The use of the Wallstent endovascular prosthesis in the treatment of malignant obstruction of the superior vena cava. Clin Radiol 1993;48:381.

48. Antonucci F, Salomonowitz E, Stuckmann G, et al: Hemodialysis-related venous stenoses: treatment with self-expanding endovascular stents. Eur J Radiol 1992;14:195.

49. Zollikofer CL, Antonucci F, Stuckmann G, et al: Use of the Wallstent in the venous system including hemodialysis-related stenoses. Cardiovasc Intervent Radiol 1992;15:334.

50. Palmaz JC: Intravascular stenting: tissue-stent interactions and design considerations. AJR 1993; 160:613.

51. Thery C, Asseman P, Amrouni N, et al: Use of a new removable vena cava filter in order to prevent pulmonary embolism in patients submitted to thrombolysis. Eur Heart J 1990;11:334.

52. Pieri A, Santoro G, Duranti A, Mori F, et al: [Temporary caval filters: Our experience. Preliminary analysis of 24 cases]. Phlebologie (French) 1993;46:457.

53. Grimm W, Schwieder G, Wagner T: [Fatal pulmonary embolism in venous thrombosis in the leg and pelvis during lysis therapy]. Dtsch Med Wochenschr 1990;115:1183.

54. WHO Expert Committee on Biological Standardization, 33rd report. World Health Organization Tech Rep Ser 1983;687:24.

CHAPTER

23

Comparison of Thrombolytic Agents

CHRISTOPHER J. WHITE

The three clinically available thrombolytic agents, streptokinase (SK), urokinase (UK), and recombinant tissue plasminogen activator (rt-PA), share the common ability to either directly or indirectly lyse intravascular thrombi. Historically, streptokinase was the first of these agents, discovered in 1933 by Tillet and coworkers,[1] and was the first to be used clinically.[2,3] MacFarland and Pilling[4] in 1946 reported on urokinase isolated from human urine, and Collen and associates[5] described the purification of human tissue-type plasminogen activator in 1982, followed in 1983 by the cloning and expression of recombinant tissue-type plasminogen activator (rt-PA) by Pennica and colleagues.[6]

Indications and dosage regimens for delivering these agents have evolved over several decades since the initial reports of the systemic intravenous administration of streptokinase.[7–11] Further advances have included trials of "local," intraarterial, administration of streptokinase,[12–17] urokinase,[18–23] and recombinant tissue-type plasminogen activator.[24–29] Clinical applications for selective intraarterial thrombolytic therapy include native artery occlusions,[12–29] peripheral bypass graft occlusions,[30–35] and as an adjunct to surgical thrombectomy.[36–43] Intraarterial thrombolytic therapy has emerged as an attractive alternative to surgical embolectomy[44] for acute peripheral vascular thrombotic events.[45–50] Nonrandomized comparisons of surgical therapy and percutaneous thrombolytic therapy appear to favor thrombolysis.[51–55]

Several "lesion-specific" variables significantly affect the outcome of thrombolytic therapy. These variables include (1) the etiology of the obstruction (embolic versus thrombotic), (2) the volume of thrombus to be lysed (clot burden), (3) the age of the thrombus, (4) whether a native vessel or bypass graft occlusion is treated, and (5) the adequacy of runoff vessels.[56–62] Not controlling for these variables is a major source of confusion when attempting to compare the results of nonrandomized trials.

Other factors that make the comparison of nonrandomized studies of thrombolytic agents difficult include the variable drug doses and delivery techniques employed. The method of administration of the thrombolytic agent appears to affect success rates. Mechanical acceleration of thrombolysis with techniques such clot maceration,[63] multilevel catheter infusions,[64] aspiration thrombectomy,[65,66] transthrombus bolus delivery (lacing),[67,68] pulsatile intrathrombic infusions (pulsed-spray technique),[69–72] rotational catheter systems,[73] the use of adjunctive ultrasound energy,[74] and the duration and rate of the infusion may be significant uncontrolled variables in nonrandomized comparisons of lytic agents.

An example of the potential confounding effects of differing delivery techniques is apparent when reviewing the results of the pulse-spray technique using a pulsatile intrathrombic infusion of urokinase.[70] In this study, urokinase was administered at a dose of 5000 IU given two to four times per minute for 10 to 20 minutes through a multiple-sidehole catheter positioned within the thrombus. The dose of urokinase was then reduced to 2000 IU boluses given one to two times per minute until completion. The authors were able to achieve clot resolution in 46 of 47 (98 percent) cases, with lysis complete in 63 ± 35 minutes. The total dose of urokinase needed for lysis averaged 368,000 ± 132,000 IU (range 100,000 to 600,000 IU).

However, in a prospective trial comparing the pulse-spray technique versus a slow continuous infusion of urokinase, Kandarpa and coworkers[75] demonstrated the clinical equivalency of the two methods. Both groups, in this study, received a pretreatment transthrombus bolus (lacing of the thrombus) of urokinase. There was no statistical difference in the time to initial patency or complete lysis between the two treatment groups. The time to completion (complete clot lysis) was 28 ± 26 hours in the continuous-infusion group versus 20 ± 14 hours in the pulse-spray group ($p = $ NS). The authors concluded that the pretreatment transthrombus bolus of urokinase was the most important step in shortening therapy, even though the completion time in this study was almost 20 times greater than that reported by others[70,72] investigating the pulse-spray technique. The authors of this study attributed the difference in treatment time from prior studies of the pulse-spray technique to the incomparability of clinical variables such as limb ischemia status, thrombus burden, age of the thrombus, and different study endpoints. Attempting to draw conclusions from these pulse-spray studies demonstrates the pitfalls of comparing uncontrolled trials.

The mechanism of action of these agents has been presented in detail in prior chapters. There are significant differences in the mechanisms of action of streptokinase, urokinase, and recombinant tissue-type plasminogen activator. Streptokinase is a single-chain polypeptide produced by hemolytic streptococci that must bind with plasminogen to form an activator to convert plasminogen to plasmin. As a foreign protein, it is potentially antigenic, and if a patient has significant levels of streptococcal antibodies present, allergic reactions may result, and the streptokinase may be inactivated.[76–79] Martin and Fiebach[80] used high-dose intravenous streptokinase (1.5 million IU per hour for 6 hours) to treat patients with chronic arterial occlusions or acute deep vein thromboses and found that one-third of patients complained of facial flushing, dyspnea, and back pain. Chills and fever occurred in 6.3 percent, and a skin rash appeared in 4.5 percent of their patients.

Urokinase, a human protein, has no antigenic properties. It differs from streptokinase by acting directly on plasminogen to form plasmin. Tissue plasminogen activator, also a human protein produced by normal vascular endothelium, is clinically available as a recombinant product (rt-PA). It differs from both urokinase and streptokinase in that it is bound by fibrin and therefore potentially acts selectively on clot-bound plasminogen. In reality, however, it is apparent from clinical trials that excess drug is released into the circulation and may cause systemic lysis.

These agents share common indications and contraindications, with the exception that streptokinase should not be readministered within 6 months due to its antigenic nature. Streptokinase has the advantage of being approximately one-tenth the cost of urokinase and recombinant tissue-type plasminogen activator, but cost also must take into account the required duration of infusion, the incidence and severity of side effects, and the overall success rates.

NONRANDOMIZED TRIALS

With the above-mentioned caveats regarding nonrandomized trials in mind, several themes have emerged when comparing thrombolytic agents for peripheral arterial occlusion. The first is that although streptokinase is less expensive than either urokinase or recombinant tissue-type plasminogen activator, the duration of infusion is generally longer, the success rate is lower, and the incidence of major complications is higher. Olin and Graor[58] compared pooled data from 17 studies using intraarterial streptokinase (474 infusions) and 4 studies using intraarterial urokinase (162 infusions) for peripheral arterial occlusion. The average duration of infusion for streptokinase was 40 hours versus 30 hours for urokinase. The reported success rate for streptokinase was 67 percent versus 81 percent for urokinase. Finally, the major complication rate reported in the streptokinase groups was 19 percent versus 12 percent for urokinase.

Lonsdale and coworkers have reported on the immediate[81] and intermediate[82] results of a nonrandomized study comparing recombinant tissue-type plasminogen and streptokinase for local intraarterial thrombolysis. They found that the immediate success rate was significantly higher in the tissue-type plasminogen group (58 versus 41 percent; $p < 0.05$). The infusion duration was shorter in the tissue-type plasminogen group (22 hours) compared with 40 hours for the streptokinase-treated patients. Of interest, there was no difference in major bleeding complications between the groups. The authors concluded that tissue-type plasminogen activator was superior to streptokinase owing to its higher success rate and shorter infusion time.

A large, nonrandomized single-center experience comparing infusions of streptokinase ($n = 200$), urokinase ($n = 200$), and recombinant tissue-type plasminogen activator ($n = 65$) for peripheral arterial occlusion has been reported by Graor et al.[83] This retrospective review of 465 patients compared clinical success, defined as complete thrombus lysis and improvement in clinical status, and complication rates. Clinical success occurred in 60 percent of streptokinase-treated patients versus 95 percent of urokinase-treated patients and 91 percent of recombinant tissue-type plasminogen activator–treated patients. Statistically, both urokinase and tissue-type plasminogen activator were more successful than streptokinase ($p < 0.001$). Successful lysis of thrombus also occurred more frequently with urokinase (89 percent) and tissue-type plasminogen activator (94 percent) than with streptokinase (72 percent) ($p < 0.001$).

Complications were more frequent with streptokinase than with the other two agents, with major bleeding complications occurring in 28 percent of the streptokinase-treated patients compared with 12 percent of the tissue-type plasminogen activator–treated patients and only 6 percent of urokinase-treated patients ($p < 0.001$ for SK versus UK, $p = 0.01$ for SK versus rt-PA, and $p = 0.09$ for UK versus rt-PA).[81] Intracranial bleeding occurred in 2 percent of streptokinase- and tissue-type plasminogen activator–treated patients versus none of the urokinase-treated patients. The authors concluded that although tissue-type plasminogen activator had success rates equal to uroki-

nase, the lower complication rates seen in patients treated with urokinase made it the agent of choice for selective infusion therapy of peripheral arterial occlusions.

The explanation for the relative safety of urokinase and the similarity of bleeding complications with "clot-selective" tissue-type plasminogen activator and streptokinase is uncertain. Although it has not been established that overall bleeding complications are directly related to serum fibrinogen levels, Graor and coworkers[83] suggest that the magnitude of any bleeding complication may be logically related to the fibrinogen available for hemostasis. In a trial comparing intracoronary infusions of streptokinase and urokinase, Tennant and associates[84] demonstrated that streptokinase depleted fibrinogen more severely than urokinase, which was associated with a higher incidence of bleeding complications. The additional antiplatelet effects of streptokinase and tissue-type plasminogen activator[85] also may contribute to a higher incidence of bleeding complications than occurs with urokinase.

RANDOMIZED TRIAL OF rt-PA VERSUS UROKINASE

A single randomized, controlled trial comparing a local infusion of urokinase versus recombinant tissue-type plasminogen activator for peripheral arterial and graft occlusions has been reported by Meyerovitz and coworkers.[86] In both groups, a transthrombus (lacing) bolus was administered prior to beginning a constant infusion. Of the 32 patients randomized in this trial, 29 had bypass graft occlusions (17 saphenous vein grafts) and 3 had native artery occlusions less than 90 days old. The mean length of the occlusions was 44 cm in the rt-PA group and 42 cm in urokinase group, suggesting that a very large clot burden was present.

At 8 hours, 7 of 16 (44 percent) of the tissue-type plasminogen activator–treated patients had achieved 95 percent or greater lysis versus only 1 of 16 (6 percent) of the urokinase-treated patients ($p = 0.04$). Note that a potential bias in favor of rt-PA was introduced into this trial because 4 urokinase patients and 1 rt-PA patient were studied at 16 hours and not at 8 hours, which may have affected the early patency results. At 24 hours, 8 of 16 (50 percent) of rt-PA–treated patients versus 6 of 16 (38 percent) of urokinase-treated patients had achieved success ($p = 0.72$). There was a trend toward more bleeding complications in the rt-PA group ($p = NS$), and the fibrinogen levels at 24 hours were significantly lower in the rt-PA group ($p = 0.01$). At 30 days, there was no difference in the clinical outcomes of the two groups.

CONCLUSIONS

In reviewing the published data comparing the results of thrombolytic therapy for peripheral vascular occlusions, several tentative conclusions can be drawn. First, the paucity of randomized, controlled studies severely limits the accuracy of any comparison. Second, advances in the delivery technique of all the thrombolytic agents has resulted in significant improvements in both safety and success rates. Finally, it appears that both urokinase and recombinant tissue-type plasminogen activator are superior to streptokinase for regional thrombolysis. Urokinase and recombinant tissue-type plasminogen activator would appear to have similar clinical success rates from the published data. Tissue-type plasminogen activator may achieve lysis more rapidly than urokinase, but this may be associated with more frequent bleeding complications.

The preceding evidence suggests that the current treatment of choice for local intraarterial thrombolytic therapy of peripheral vascular occlusion is urokinase. Based on the principle of "doing no harm," urokinase appears to offer a clinical success rate equal to that of tissue-type plasminogen activator and superior to that of streptokinase while being associated with fewer complications than either of those agents.

As newer dosage regimens, infusion techniques, and thrombolytic agents are devised, large randomized trials will be necessary to determine the optimal method of treating patients with peripheral vascular occlusive disease.

REFERENCES

1. Tillet WS, Garner RL: The fibrinolytic activity of hemolytic streptococci. J Exp Med 1933;58:485.
2. Tillet WS, Johnson AJ, McCarthy WF: The intravenous infusion of streptococcal fibrinolytic principle (streptokinase) into patients. J Clin Invest 1955;34:169.
3. Fletcher AP, Aljaersig N, Sherry S: The maintenance of a sustained lytic state in man: I. Induction and effects. J Clin Invest 1959;38:1096.
4. MacFarlane RG, Pilling J: Observations on fibrinolysis: Plasminogen, plasmin and antiplasmin content of human blood. Lancet 1946;2:562.
5. Collen D, Rijken DC, vanDamme T, et al: Purification of human tissue-type plasminogen activator. Thromb Haemost 1982;48:294.
6. Pennica D, Holmes WE, Kohr WJ, et al: Cloning and expression of human tissue-type plasminogen activator cDNA in E. coli. Nature 1983;301:214.
7. Amery A, Deloof W, Vermylen J, et al: Outcome of recent thromboembolic occlusions of limb arteries treated with streptokinase. Br Med J 1970;4:639.
8. Hume M, Gurewich V, Thomas DP, et al: Streptokinase for chronic arterial occlusive disease. Arch Surg 1970;101:653.
9. Martin M, Schoop W, Weitler E: Streptokinase in chronic arterial occlusive disease. JAMA 1970;211:1169.
10. Poliwoda H, Alexander K, Buhl V, et al: Treatment of chronic arterial occlusions with streptokinase. N Engl J Med 1969;280:689.
11. Johnson AJ, McCarty WR: The lysis of artificially induced intravascular clots in man by intravenous infusions of streptokinase. J Clin Invest 1959;38:810.
12. McNicol GP, Reid W, Bain WH, et al: Treatment of peripheral arterial occlusion by streptokinase perfusion. Br Med J 1963;1:1508.
13. Dotter CT, Rosch J, Seamen AJ: Selective clot lysis with low dose streptokinase. Radiology 1974;111:31.
14. Verstraete M, Amery A, Vermylen J: Feasibility of adequate thrombolytic therapy with streptokinase in peripheral arterial occlusions: I. Clinical and arteriographic results. Br Med J 1963;2:1499.
15. Cotten LT, Flute PT, Tsapogas MJC: Popliteal artery thrombosis treated with streptokinase. Lancet 1962;2:1081.
16. Earnshaw JJ: Thrombolytic therapy in the management of acute limb ischaemia. Br J Surg 1991;78:261.
17. Katzen BT, vanBreda A: Low dose streptokinase in the treatment of arterial occlusions. AJR 1981;136:1171.
18. Cragg AH, smith TP, Corson JD, et al: Two urokinase dose regimens in native arterial and graft occlusions: Initial results of a prospective randomized clinical trial. Radiology 1991;178:681.
19. Fiessinger JN, Vayssairat M, Juillet Y, et al: Local urokinase in arterial thromboembolism. Angiology 1974;31:715.

20. McNamara TO, Fischer JR: Thrombolysis of peripheral arterial and graft occlusions: Improved results using high dose urokinase. AJR 1985;144:769.

21. McNamara TO, Bomberger RA: Factors affecting initial and 6 month patency rates after intraarterial thrombolysis with high dose urokinase. Am J Surg 1986;152:709.

22. Pernes JM, Vitous JF, Brenoit P, et al: Acute peripheral and graft occlusion: Treatment with selective infusion of urokinase and lysyl plasminogen. Radiology 1986;158:481.

23. Parent FN, Piotrowski JJ, Bernhard V, et al: Outcome of intraarterial urokinase for acute vascular occlusion. J Cardiovasc Surg 1991;32:680.

24. Berridge DC, Gregson RHS, Makin GS, et al: Tissue plasminogen activator in peripheral arterial thrombolysis. Br J Surg 1990;77:179.

25. Dawson K, Hamilton G: Recombinant tissue-type plasminogen activator versus urokinase in peripheral arterial occlusions. Radiology 1991;178:283.

26. Graor RA, Risius B, Lucas FV, et al: Thrombolysis with recombinant human tissue type plasminogen activators in patients with peripheral artery and bypass graft thrombosis. Circulation 1986;74(suppl I):I-15.

27. Krupski WC, Feldman RK, Rapp JH: Recombinant human tissue-type plasminogen activator is an effective agent for thrombolysis of peripheral arteries and bypass grafts: Preliminary report. J Vasc Surg 1989;10:491.

28. Risius B, Graor RA, Geisinger MA, et al: Recombinant human tissue-type plasminogen activator for thrombolysis in peripheral arteries and bypass grafts. Radiology 1986;160:183.

29. Weimar W, Stibbe J, vanSeyen AJ, et al: Specific lysis of an iliofemoral thrombus by administration of extrinsic (tissue-type) plasminogen activator. Lancet 1981;2:1018.

30. Bandyk D: Thrombolysis in peripheral arterial graft occlusion. Can J Surg 1993;36:372.

31. Browse DJ, Torrie EPH, Galland RB: Low-dose intra-arterial thrombolysis in the treatment of occluded vascular grafts. Br J Surg 1992;79:86.

32. Durham JD, Geller SC, Abbot WM, et al: Regional infusion of urokinase into occluded lower-extremity bypass grafts: Long-term clinical results. Radiology 1989;172:83.

33. Gardiner GA Jr, Koltun W, Kandarpa K, et al: Thrombolysis of occluded femoropopliteal grafts. AJR 1986;147:621.

34. Gardiner GA Jr, Harrington DP, Koltun W, et al: Salvage of occluded arterial bypass grafts by means of thrombolysis. J Vasc Surg 1989;9:426.

35. McNamara TO: The use of lytic therapy with endovascular "repair" for the failed infrainguinal graft. Semin Vasc Surg 1990;3:59.

36. Cohen LH, Kaplan M, Bernhard VM: Intraoperative streptokinase. Arch Surg 1986;121:708.

37. Comerota AJ, White JV, Grosh JD: Intraoperative intra-arterial thrombolytic therapy for salvage of limbs in patients with distal arterial thrombosis. Surg Gynecol Obstet 1989;169:283.

38. Garcia R, Saroyan RM, Senkowsky J, et al: Intraoperative intra-arterial urokinase infusion as an adjunct to Fogarty catheter embolectomy in acute arterial occlusion. Surg Gynecol Obstet 1990;171:201.

39. Norem RF, Short DH, Kernstein MD: Role of intraoperative fibrinolytic therapy in acute arterial occlusion. Surg Gynecol Obstet 1988;167:87.

40. Parent FN, Bernhard VM, Pabstill T, et al: Fibrinolytic treatment of residual thrombus after catheter embolectomy for severe lower limb ischemia. J Vasc Surg 1989;9:153.

41. Quinones-Baldrich WJ, Baker JD, Busuttil RW, et al: Intraoperative infusion of lytic drugs for thrombotic complications of revascularization. J Vasc Surg 1989;10:408.

42. Quinones-Baldrich WJ, Zierler RE, Hiatt JC: Intraoperative fibrinolytic therapy: An adjunct to catheter thromboembolectomy. J Vasc Surg 1985;2:319.

43. Wasselle JA, Bandyk DF: Intraoperative thrombolysis in peripheral arterial occlusion. Can J Surg 1993;36:354.

44. Fogarty TJ, Cranley JJ, Krause RJ, et al: A method for extraction of arterial emboli and thrombi. Surg Gynecol Obstet 1963;116:241.

45. Whittemore A, Clowes A, Couch N, et al: Secondary femoropopliteal reconstruction. Ann Surg 1981;193:35.

46. O'Donnell TFJ: Arterial diagnosis and management of acute thrombosis of the lower extremity. Can J Surg 1993;36:349.

47. Plecha FR, Pories WJ: Intraoperative angiography in the immediate assessment of arterial reconstruction. Arch Surg 1972;105:902.

48. Foster JH, Carter JH, GrahamJr CP, et al: Arterial injuries secondary to the Fogarty catheter. Ann Surg 1970;171:971.

49. Blaisdell FW, Steele M, Allen RE: Management of acute lower extremity ischemia due to embolism and thrombosis. Surgery 1978;84:822.

50. Abbott WM, Maloney RD, McCabe CC, et al: Arterial embolism: A 44-year perspective. Am J Surg 1982;143:460.

51. Dunnant JH, Edwards WW: Small vessel occlusion in the extremity after various periods of arterial obstruction. Surgery 1973;73:240.

52. Earnshaw JJ, Gregson RHS, Makin GS, et al: Acute peripheral arterial ischaemia: A prospective evaluation of differential management with surgery or thrombolysis. Ann Vasc Surg 1989;3:374.

53. Hess H, Mietaschk A, Bruckl R: Peripheral arterial occlusions: A 6-year experience with local low-dose thrombolytic therapy. Radiology 1987;74:753.

54. McNamara TO, Bomberger RA, Merchant RF: Intra-arterial urokinase as the initial therapy for acutely ischaemic lower limbs. Circulation 1991;83(suppl I):I-106.

55. Graor RA, Risius B, Young JR, et al: Thrombolysis of peripheral arterial bypass grafts: Surgical thrombectomy compared with thrombolysis. J Vasc Surg 1988;7:347.

56. Scott DJA, Wyatt MG, Murphy YG, et al: Intraarterial streptokinase infusion in acute lower limb ischaemia. Br J Surg 1991;78:732.

57. Motarjame A: Thrombolytic therapy in arterial occlusion and graft thrombosis. Semin Vasc Surg 1989; 2:155.

58. Olin JW, Graor RA: Thrombolytic therapy in the treatment of peripheral arterial occlusions. Ann Emerg Med 1988;17:1210.

59. Hess H: Thrombolytic therapy in peripheral vascular disease. Br J Surg 1990;77:1083.

60. Ljungman C, Adami HO, Gergqvist D, et al: Time trends in incidence rates of acute, non-traumatic extremity ischaemia: A population-based study during a 19-year period. Br J Surg 1991;78:857.

61. Lawrence PF, Goodman GR: Thrombolytic therapy. Surg Clin North Am 1992;72:899.

62. DeMaioribus CA, Mills JL, Fujitani RM, et al: A reevaluation of intraarterial thrombolytic therapy for acute lower extremity ischemia. J Vasc Surg 1993;17:888.

63. Davis GB, Dowd CF, Bookstein JJ, et al: Thrombosed dialysis grafts: Efficacy of intrathrombic deposition of concentrated urokinase, clot maceration, and angioplasty. AJR 1987;149:177.

64. Shewchun J, Sniderman K: Fibrinolytic therapy in peripheral arterial grafts utilizing the "crossed two catheter" technique. Cardiovasc Intervent Radiol 1989;12:110.

65. Roth F-J, Rieser R, Scheffler A, et al: Intraarterial fibrinolytic therapy of chronic arterial occlusions. Semin Throm Hem 1991;17:39.

66. Starck EE, McDermott JC, Crummy AB, et al: Percutaneous aspiriation thromboembolectomy. Radiology 1985;156:61.

67. Sullivan KL, Gardiner GA, Shapiro MJ, et al: Acceleration of thrombolysis with a high-dose transthrombus bolus technique. Radiology 1989;173:805.

68. Koltun WA, Gardiner GA, Harrington DP, et al: Thrombolysis in the treatment of peripheral arterial vascular occlusions. Arch Surg 1987;122:901.

69. Kandarpa K, Drinker PA, Singer SJ, et al: Forceful pulsatile local infusion of enzyme accelerates thrombolysis: In vivo evaluation of a new delivery system. Radiology 1988;168:739.

70. Bookstein JJ, Fellmet B, Roberts A, et al: Pulsed-spray pharmacomechanical thrombolysis: Preliminary clinical results. AJR 1989;152:1097.

71. Bookstein JJ, Saldinger E: Accelerated thrombolysis: In vitro evaluation of agents and methods of administration. Invest Radiol 1985;20:731.

72. Valji K, Bookstein JJ: Fibrinolysis with intrathrombic injection of urokinase and tissue-type plasminogen activator. Invest Radiol 1987;22:23.

73. Schmitz-Rode T, Gunther RW: Percutaneous mechanical thrombolysis: A comparative study of various rotational catheter systems. Invest Radiol 1991;26:557.

74. Tachibana K: Enhancement of fibrinolysis with ultrasound energy. JVIR 1992;3:299.

75. Kandarpa K, Chopra PS, Aruny JE, et al: Intraarterial thrombolysis of lower extremity occlusions: Prospective, randomized comparison of forced periodic infusion and conventional slow continuous infusion. Radiology 1993;188:861.

76. Baumgartner TG, Davis RG: Streptokinase induced anaphylactic reaction. Clin Pharmacol 1982;1:470.

77. Totty WG, Romano T, Benian GM, et al: Serum sickness following streptokinase therapy. AJR 1982;138:143.

78. van Breda A, Katzen BT: Thrombolytic therapy of peripheral vascular disease. Semin Intervent Radiol 1985;2:354.

79. Weatherbee TC, Esterbrooks DJ, Katz DA, et al: Serum sickness following selective intracoronary streptokinase. Curr Ther Res 1984;35:433.

80. Martin M, Fiebach BJO: Short-term ultrahigh dose streptokinase treatment of chronic arterial occlusions and acute deep vein thromboses. Semin Thromb Hemost 1991;17:21.

81. Lonsdale RG, Berrridge DC, Earnshaw JJ, et al: Recombinant tissue-type plaminogen activator is superior to streptokinase for local intra-arterial thrombolysis. Br J Surg 1992;79:272.

82. Lonsdale RJ, Whitaker SC, Berridge DC, et al: Peripheral arterial thrombolysis: Intermediate-term results. Br J Surg 1993;80:592.

83. Graor RA, Olin J, Bartholomew JR, et al: Efficacy and safety of intraarterial local infusion of streptokinase, urokinase or tissue plasminogen activator for peripheral arterial occlusion: A retrospective review. J Vasc Med Biol 1990;2:310.

84. Tennant SN, Dixon J, Benable TC, et al: Intracoronary thrombolysis in patients with acute myocardial infarction: Comparison of efficacy of urokinase with streptokinase. Circulation 1984;69:756.

85. Vaughan DE, Loscalzo J: Comparative effects of plasminogen activators on platelet disaggregation. J Vasc Med Biol 1989;1:27.

86. Meyerovitz MF, Goldhaber SZ, Reagan K, et al: Recombinant tissue-type plasminogen activator versus urokinase in peripheral arterial and bypass graft occlusions: a randomized study. Radiology 1990;175:75.

C H A P T E R

24

Innovative Approaches to Fibrinolytic Therapy

CHARLES W. FRANCIS

The recent rapid advances in fibrinolytic therapy have resulted from an improved understanding of the biochemistry and physiology of the fibrinolytic system as well as from clinical studies that have demonstrated improved outcomes with appropriate application. Advances in both basic science and clinical application have been driven particularly by the increasing importance of fibrinolytic therapy in managing acute myocardial infarction. Advances in biochemistry and molecular biology have led to elucidation of the primary structures of the principal enzymes and inhibitors of the fibrinolytic system and to an understanding of their functional roles. Interrelations between the coagulation and fibrinolytic systems are better understood, and recent evidence has underscored the importance of interactions of the fibrinolytic system with vascular cells. As a result of these scientific advances, new plasminogen activators are under investigation for potential clinical use. Equally important, new adjunctive therapies to modify the balance between fibrinolysis and coagulation are available, including potent and specific new anticoagulants and platelet inhibitors that are entering clinical trial.

The rapid advances in fibrinolytic therapy also have been spurred by incisive clinical investigations. The seminal studies of DeWood et al.[1] demonstrating thrombotic occlusion of coronary arteries during myocardial infarction and of Rentrop et al.[2,3] in documenting reperfusion with intracoronary administration of streptokinase provided incontrovertible evidence of the importance of thrombosis and the potential role of fibrinolytic

therapy in treating myocardial infarction. A series of increasingly large clinical trials has refined and improved this approach and modified standard therapy, resulting in a substantial decline in acute mortality from this common illness. This intense interest has spurred additional investigations into applications of fibrinolytic therapy in other thrombotic diseases, in minimizing hemorrhagic side effects, and in understanding the biochemical and physiologic changes attendant on administration of plasminogen activators. Fibrinolytic therapy continues to evolve rapidly, and a review of promising new innovations will be the subject of this chapter.

PROBLEMS WITH CURRENT FIBRINOLYTIC THERAPY

Innovative approaches in fibrinolytic therapy must be viewed in the context of limitations of currently available treatment (Table 24-1). In treating arterial thrombosis, the overriding concern is to establish reperfusion as quickly as possible because of the rapid loss of tissue viability with ischemia. The largest experience and data are available for treatment of acute myocardial infarction, and the magnitude of this clinical problem continues to provide the impetus for aggressive new approaches. Much of the information learned in treating myocardial infarction also may be applicable to other arterial thrombotic diseases with modifications. Initial approaches were quite successful, with coronary reperfusion established in over 50

Table 24-1. Current Problems and New Approaches to Fibrinolytic Therapy

Problem	Approaches
Arterial thrombosis	
Speed and frequency of reperfusion	New regimens of activators Combinations of activators New fibrinolytic agents Adjunctive antithrombotic therapies Prehospital treatment Improved delivery of activators
Reocclusion	Improved anticoagulant and antiplatelet therapy Angioplasty, atherectomy, surgery
Venous thromboembolism	
Resistance of deep vein thrombi to lysis	Improved patient selection New activators and regimens
Speed of lysis of pulmonary emboli	New administration regimens New activators
Bleeding complications	Application of "fibrin-specific" agents

percent of patients using either intracoronary administration of streptokinase or high-intensity, brief-duration intravenous therapy. New regimens of administration including accelerated or "front-loaded" recombinant tissue-type plasminogen activator (rt-PA) have improved results. The differing fibrin-binding properties and pharmacokinetic profiles of available plasminogen activators have provided the basis for investigating combinations of agents, but the results have not been clearly better. Tremendous effort has gone into the development of new plasminogen activators with improved properties. One approach has been based on an understanding of the biochemistry and structure of physiologic activators and has used molecular biologic methods to produce "designer" molecules with potentially improved properties. To date, none of these has made a clinical impact. A second approach has been to identify naturally occurring plasminogen activators and anticoagulants in bloodsucking animals, and this has been fruitful in identification and characterization of activators with unique and potentially useful properties. The recognition that thrombus formation and dissolution proceed concurrently and that

fibrinolytic therapy can either generate thrombin or expose thrombin associated with thrombus has led to investigation of the role of concurrent anticoagulant and antiplatelet therapy to block new clot formation during administration of plasminogen activators. Clear evidence is available that this approach is useful and results in increased reperfusion and improved clinical outcomes. Combination therapy including the use of fibrinolytic agents, anticoagulants, and antiplatelet agents is now the standard approach to aggressive management of arterial thrombosis (Fig. 24-1). Optimizing the delivery system to achieve a maximum concentration of activator at the site of thrombosis also may accelerate clot dissolution. Intracoronary delivery of fibrinolytic agents and local or intrathrombotic administration in the treatment of peripheral arterial thrombosis are being actively pursued. Finally, the critical importance of early treatment has moved medical care into mobile units in some communities to provide fibrinolytic therapy prior to delivery of the patient to a hospital, thereby reducing time from onset of symptoms to initiation of thrombolysis.

Another major problem in the treatment of arterial thrombosis is reocclusion. After establishing initial reperfusion, two problems may again lead to acute compromise of arterial flow. The first is residual thrombus, which has procoagulant properties related in part to fibrin-bound thrombin that can generate new fibrin and activate platelets. Since fibrin-bound thrombin is relatively resistant to heparin, the role of new specific antithrombins with activity against clot-associated thrombin is being actively investigated, as are more potent antiplatelet agents that can prevent platelet accumulation. The second problem remaining after establishing reperfusion is the underlying atheromatous lesion, which remains partly occluding and often fissured with procoagulant potential. This problem has provided the impetus for investigation of the use of angioplasty, atherectomy, and surgery in conjunction with fibrinolytic therapy.

The problems with fibrinolytic therapy of venous thromboembolic disease are different. A major impediment is the lack of response of many thrombi, possibly based on age-related changes, since patients may present many days after the

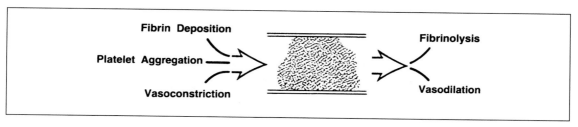

Figure 24-1. The balance of processes determining vessel patency. Fibrin deposition, platelet aggregation, and vasoconstriction promote thrombus growth and vascular occlusion, while fibrinolysis and vasodilation lead to patency. Pharmacologic treatment to promote reperfusion can focus on inhibiting fibrin deposition, platelet aggregation, or vasoconstriction or accelerating fibrinolysis and stimulating vasodilation.

onset of symptoms. Efforts to predict responsiveness based on imaging using venography or magnetic resonance characteristics have shown promise in the ability to select patients most likely to respond. Other initiatives include the use of new plasminogen activators and exploration of the potential for intrathrombic administration to accelerate clot dissolution in some cases. Increased interest in fibrinolytic therapy of pulmonary emboli has resulted from demonstration of rapid improvement in pulmonary hemodynamics with the use of fibrinolytic regimens of shorter duration and higher intensity.

Another major problem with fibrinolytic therapy is the occurrence of bleeding complications, which are frequent at sites of vascular instrumentation and may be fatal if they involve the central nervous system. It is generally recognized that bleeding is most often due to dissolution of needed hemostatic plugs and that this accounts for bleeding at sites of vascular invasion and pathologic lesions such as ulcers in the gastrointestinal tract. As long as there are hemostatic plugs with properties similar to those of occlusive vascular thrombi, the potential for bleeding complications cannot be eliminated during thrombolytic therapy. However, the hypocoagulable state resulting from the systemic action of plasminogen activators, the "lytic state" may exacerbate the bleeding tendency. This has provided the impetus for finding "fibrin-specific" agents that will be effective only at sites of fibrin deposition, such as "designer" recombinant plasminogen activators or the exquisitely fibrin-specific bat plasminogen activator.

NEW PLASMINOGEN ACTIVATORS

Progress in developing new plasminogen activators has followed from understanding the properties and limitations of currently available agents. The first fibrinolytic drugs available included streptokinase (SK), which is purified from cultures of streptococci, and urokinase (UK), derived from urinary sources or cell culture and more recently by recombinant DNA technology. Streptokinase is inexpensive to produce, but its bacterial origin makes it immunogenic and also increases undesirable allergic responses. Its administration results in systemic activation of fibrinolysis with development of the lytic state and hypocoagulability. Urokinase (two-chain urokinase-like plasminogen activator) is a physiologic activator present in the blood in its single-chain form[4] and in relatively high concentrations in the urinary system in the two-chain proteolytic derivative. It has the advantage of being nonimmunogenic, but it also induces a lytic state when administered in high dosage. Tissue plasminogen activator (t-PA) has been introduced more recently, and is a naturally occurring activator secreted from endothelial cells.[5] It has the property of binding to fibrin and also demonstrates increased enzymatic activity in the presence of fibrin,[6-8] properties that serve to localize t-PA physiologically at sites of fibrin deposition. Because of these properties, it is more fibrin-specific than UK or SK, resulting in a less intense lytic state when used pharmacologically. Anistreplase (Eminase) is a complex of SK and plasminogen with an acyl blocking group at the active site.[9] Anistreplase has a longer duration of

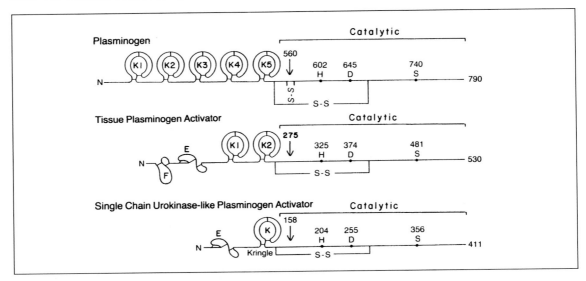

Figure 24-2. Domainal structures of plasminogen, tissue-type plasminogen activator, and single-chain urokinase-like plasminogen activator. All three proteins are similar in the structure of their light chains following activation, which contain the catalytically active site containing the histidine (*H*), aspartic acid (*D*), and serine (*S*). All contain similar kringle structures (*K*) but different numbers of these domains. Tissue-type plasminogen activator contains a single finger domain (*F*) which is similar to those present in fibronectin. Tissue-type plasminogen activator and single-chain urokinase-like plasminogen activator contain an epidermal growth factor–like domain (*E*). The arrows indicate the cleavage sites that activate plasminogen and convert the single-chain forms of tissue plasminogen activator and single-chain urokinase-like plasminogen activator to their two-chain forms.

action after administration, so it can be given by bolus injection, but it induces a lytic state comparable to streptokinase when used therapeutically. Single-chain urokinase-like plasminogen activator (scu-PA) is the single-chain precursor of UK, and it has minimal enzymatic activity until cleaved to the two-chain form. Despite this, scu-PA has potent thrombolytic properties after pharmacologic administration, and it is relatively fibrin-specific, activating fibrin-bound plasminogen more avidly than plasma plasminogen.[10,11]

The available plasminogen activators are effective agents, but impetus for development of new drugs has resulted from clinical experience revealing their limitations. The goal is to develop a highly potent agent with its activity limited to the pathologic thrombus that could be easily administered, nonimmunogenic, and free of bleeding complications. One approach to developing such an agent has resulted from understanding the structures and functional properties of plasminogen and plasminogen activators coupled with the

development of molecular biologic approaches to designing and producing molecules with specific modifications. Studies relating molecular structure and function have associated specific biochemical properties with particular structural motifs that are homologous among different molecules (Fig. 24-2). This commonality of structure and function is supported by characterization of the genetic origin of these molecules demonstrating that different functional domains are encoded by one or more consecutive exons and suggesting a "gene shuffling" concept of molecular evolution. For example, plasminogen, t-PA, and scu-PA all contain "kringle" domains, and scu-PA and t-PA share an epidermal growth factor–like domain, while t-PA also contains a "finger" domain similar to those in fibronectin. Each molecule contains a catalytic domain homologous to that in other serine proteases. As specific functional properties such as fibrin affinity, binding to receptors involved in clearance, and binding to inhibitors were localized to specific domains, the concept was evolved that molecules

Table 24-2. Development of New Plasminogen Activators

Goal	Examples
Prolong clearance of t-PA	Deletion of F and E domains
	Addition of glycosylation sites
	Addition of kringle domains from plasminogen
Create resistance to PAI-1	Alter recognition site for PAI-1
Increase fibrin specificity	Combine domains from t-PA and scu-PA that bind fibrin
	Addition of kringle domains of plasminogen
	Conjugate u-PA or t-PA with fibrin-specific MoAb
	Bifunctional antibodies with fibrin and activator binding
	Bat plasminiogen activator
Increase activity toward platelet-rich thrombin	Conjugate t-PA with platelet-specific MoAb

with desired properties could be generated by combining specific domains from different naturally occurring molecules into a recombinant variant. A full discussion of the production and biochemistry of the large variety of recombinant activators that has been created is beyond the scope of this chapter but has been recently reviewed.[12,13] Only examples will be cited.

The rapid plasma clearance of t-PA necessitates administration of large doses given by a constant infusion in the treatment of myocardial infarction, and this has led to efforts to produce a modified t-PA molecule with a longer plasma half-life. The pharmacokinetic properties of t-PA were studied by Larsen et al.,[14,15] who expressed mutants lacking specific domains and tested their properties in a rat model. Deletion mutants lacking the F and E domains (see Fig. 24-2) had reduced plasma clearances, and modifying glycosylation sites further increased the plasma $t^{1/2}$ by as much as 20-fold. While thrombolytic activity was retained, the overall thrombolytic potency was not substantially increased in the mutants compared with wild-type t-PA. t-PA variants with slower plasma clearance also have been produced by altering glycosylation of the kringle domains.[16–18]

A second property of t-PA that influences its activity is inhibition by plasminogen activator inhibitor type 1 (PAI-1). This property has been altered by using site-directed mutagenesis to change the amino acid sequence involved in interaction with PAI-1 without altering the ability of t-PA to convert plasminogen to plasmin.[19] The resulting molecules were remarkably resistant to PAI-1 inhibition. A mutant also has been expressed that combined altered glycosylation to decrease plasma clearance with decreased PAI-1 binding to prevent inhibition.[17] Despite the power of the recombinant methods and imaginative bioengineering, there are, however, potential problems with using PAI-1–resistant t-PA mutants therapeutically. First, t-PA is usually administered in great excess over the inhibitory capacity of PAI-1, so the advantage of the resistant mutants is small, and a similar result could be achieved by increasing the dose or rate of administration. Also, there is a potential concern over administering an activator resistant to its naturally occurring inhibitor because bleeding complications could be increased.

scu-PA (see Fig. 24-1) is a single-chain molecule with very little enzymatic activity that can cause fibrin-specific thrombolysis, possibly by conversion to the more active two-chain form at the site of thrombosis through a plasmin-mediated feedback mechanism. In an attempt to modify its properties, a molecule has been expressed with an altered cleavage site so that conversion of the single- to the two-chain form is prevented.[20] This molecule had the expected resistance to proteolytic cleavages but also had reduced fibrinolytic activity. Another variant of interest is low-molecular-weight scu-PA that lacks both the F and K domains but retains fibrinolytic activity and resistance to PAI-1.[21,22] This is a potentially useful molecule that shows increased fibrin specificity in an animal model.

Another concept in designing improved fibrinolytic agents is the combination of functional domains from different molecules into "designer" plasminogen activators. This approach relies on the hypothesis that the function associated with a domain in the native molecule will be retained in the new construct. Combining structures from t-PA and scu-PA is an example. The fibrin binding and specificity of t-PA reside in the F and K2 domains of the A chain, whereas the carboxyl-terminal portion of scu-PA has both the fibrin affinity and protease domains (see Fig. 24-2). Several chimeric molecules have been expressed and evaluated consisting of portions of amino-terminal domains of t-PA and carboxyl-terminal regions of scu-PA.[23–28] These molecules have interesting biochemical properties, and some demonstrate increased fibrin binding. However, none has dramatically improved properties as a thrombolytic agent over the native molecules. Chimeras of plasminogen and plasminogen activators also have been constructed to increase fibrin binding activity. The five kringle structures of plasminogen have been combined with the protease domain of scu-PA[29] or of t-PA,[30] resulting in constructs with increased fibrin specificity. The five kringle structures of plasminogen also have been linked to the t-PA K2 and protease domain, resulting in a six-kringle structure that has dramatically decreased plasma clearance with a $t^{1/2}$ of up to 100-fold greater than native t-PA and potential as a useful therapeutic agent.[31]

Antibodies have very high binding affinities, and this property has been exploited to produce hybrid antibody-targeted plasminogen activators. Conversion of fibrinogen to fibrin changes the molecular structure and generates fibrin-specific epitopes to which monoclonal antibodies have been raised with high specificity toward fibrin as compared with fibrinogen. One specific monoclonal antibody directed toward the new amino terminus of the fibrin beta chain has been conjugated to either t-PA or scu-PA[32–34] and demonstrates increased thrombolytic activity. Another antibody directed to the factor XIII cross-linked D domains of fibrin also has been used to create antibody-activator molecules with high fibrin affinity.[35] Greater sophistication using recombinant approaches has allowed synthesis of single molecules combining only the antigen-binding variable region of the antibody molecule with the protease domain of plasminogen activator. Such molecules also can be potentially "humanized" to reduce or eliminate the antigenicity of mouse-derived protein. These approaches have been used to combine fibrin-specific antibodies with protease domains from either t-PA or scu-PA.[36,37] Bispecific antibodies, containing regions binding both fibrin and plasminogen activator, also have been produced chemically or through recombinant methods to increase fibrin specificity of activators.[38] Finally, plasminogen activators have

been coupled with monoclonal antibodies specific for platelets to target plasminogen activators to platelet-rich zones and thrombi that are relatively resistant to thrombolysis.[38]

An enormous effort has gone into these approaches to engineer and synthetically produce better plasminogen activators for clinical application. Insight into structure/function relations, combined with imagination and advanced recombinant technology, has resulted in the production of molecules with unique function. Their study in vitro and in vivo has contributed greatly to improved understanding of the physiology and biochemistry of fibrinolysis. To date, however, none has been sufficiently better than SK, UK, or t-PA in vitro or in animal studies to warrant large-scale production and clinical trials, although this effort continues. It illustrates the formidable problems in engineering proteins with properties improved over those resulting from evolution.

Natural sources have been another productive area for identification of new anticoagulants and fibrinolytic agents. The ability of staphylococci to secrete a protein capable of dissolving blood clots has been known for over 40 years. Recently, the active enzyme staphylokinase has been purified, and subsequently, the gene was cloned and expressed in *Escherichia coli*,[40] providing large amounts of recombinant protein for investigation. Like SK, staphylokinase is an indirect plasminogen activator, first combining stoichiometrically with plasminogen to form a complex which then activates other plasminogen molecules.[41,42] Unlike streptokinase, staphylokinase has high fibrin affinity and activates plasminogen preferentially at the fibrin surface, making it a relatively "fibrin-specific" agent. Studies in animals suggest that it may be a promising fibrinolytic agent for eventual clinical testing.[43]

An even more fibrin-specific plasminogen activator is bat plasminogen activator, derived from the salivary glands of the vampire bat and now produced using recombinant DNA technology.[44] The unique property of bat plasminogen activator is its extreme fibrin specificity, which results in essentially no consumption of plasminogen, α_2-plasmin inhibitor, or fibrinogen at fibrinolytically active concentrations.[44,45] Also, bat plasminogen activator is relatively stable in plasma, possibly the result of decreased susceptibility to inhibition by plasminogen activator inhibitor type 1. These properties make it promising for eventual clinical application, and animal studies are underway.

NEW REGIMENS OF PLASMINOGEN ACTIVATORS

Several recent investigations have examined new dosing regimens to improve the response for both acute myocardial infarction and pulmonary embolism. The regimen of t-PA initially recommended for myocardial infarction was based on several early trials, including that by the TIMI study group, and was 100 mg over 3 hours given as 60 mg in the first hour and then 20 mg/h for the next 2 hours. Subsequent smaller studies[46-48] suggested that accelerating t-PA administration could increase patency of the infarct-related artery, and this formed the basis for the large multicenter GUSTO trial[49] in which patients randomized to the t-PA group received "accelerated t-PA" administered as a 15-mg bolus followed by 0.75 mg/kg over 30 minutes and 0.5 mg/kg over the next 60 minutes. Intravenous heparin was administered concurrently. The group receiving "accelerated t-PA" had a slightly but significantly lower mortality compared with the SK-treated groups. Since there was only one t-PA regimen used in this study, no direct comparison can be made with other t-PA regimens.

Studies evaluating the effects of combinations of fibrinolytic agents have been stimulated by the slightly different biochemical properties and clinical results with these agents. Thus the large GUSTO trial[49] included a group that received a combination of t-PA plus SK but found that this combination was no better than SK alone and slightly less effective than the t-PA regimen. In other studies, a combination of low-dose t-PA and scu-PA did not give improved results in the treatment of myocardial infarction,[50,51] but a combination of low-dose UK followed by scu-PA may provide a synergistic benefit.[52,53]

Accelerated administration may offer some advantages for the treatment of pulmonary embolism. The Food and Drug Administration (FDA)-approved regimens for SK and UK extend treatment for 12 to 24 hours and are based on the USPET and UPET trials.[54,55] The consideration that maximum benefit in acutely ill patients with pulmonary embolism would result from the most rapid lysis provided the stimulus for evaluating shorter and more intensive thrombolytic regimens. Also, longer durations of treatment may increase bleeding complications, and results of small trials showed that pulmonary embolism could be treated effectively with shorter infusions of plasminogen activators.[56,57] These smaller studies were followed by several randomized trials comparing treatment regimens. Levine et al.[58] randomized 58 patients to receive either rt-PA 0.6 mg/kg as a bolus compared with heparin alone and showed significantly better lung scan perfusion in the thrombolytic group at 24 hours. A dose of 100 mg of rt-PA delivered over 2 hours was compared with the standard 24-hour UK regimen in a randomized trial that demonstrated more rapid lysis with the short t-PA regimen.[59] A subsequent trial[60] compared the 2-hour t-PA regimen with an accelerated UK regimen of 3 million units over 2 hours. Both regimens were comparable, with angiographic improvement in 79 and 67 percent of the t-PA- and UK-treated patients, respectively, and no significant difference in bleeding complications. A study reported by Meyer et al.[61] also found that a 2-hour rt-PA infusion was equally effective as a 12-hour UK infusion. High-dose bolus SK also has been used successfully in a small number of patients.[62] Together these findings provide convincing evidence that a short, intensive treatment regimen provides more rapid clot lysis and hemodynamic improvement with no increase in bleeding complications compared with regimens extending up to 24 hours.

PLASMINOGEN

Fibrinolysis depends on the activator-mediated conversion of the zymogen plasminogen to the active enzyme plasmin, which proteolytically solubilizes the fibrin matrix of a thrombus. The rate of plasmin generation is determined in part by the concentration of plasminogen at the site of fibrin deposition. During clot formation, a small amount of plasma plasminogen binds to fibrin and becomes incorporated into the clot.[63,64] Activation of fibrinolysis facilitates additional binding of plasminogen to fibrin as native glu-plasminogen is proteolytically converted to lys-plasminogen, which has a 10-fold higher affinity for fibrin.[65,66] Also, initial plasmic degradation of the fibrin substrate exposes new plasminogen binding sites.[67,68] The binding and activation of plasminogen on fibrin are important in both accelerating and localizing thrombolysis.

Although the plasminogen incorporated into the clot is a determinant of lysis rate, the concentration of soluble plasminogen is also important. This is supported by indirect evidence demonstrating increased clot lysis after preincubation of clots in plasma.[69,70] Studies in vitro also have demonstrated that plasminogen supplementation increases clot lysis with SK.[71] Also, plasminogen depletion of plasma reduces lysis of whole-blood thrombi with UK in an in vitro perfusion system, but enrichment of the perfusate with lys-plasminogen accelerates fibrinolysis.[72,73]

These observations are relevant to fibrinolytic therapy when physiologic regulatory mechanisms are overwhelmed as large amounts of plasminogen activator are infused to accelerate degradation of pathologic thrombi. Circulating activator in excess of the capacity of plasma inhibitors leads to the conversion of plasminogen to plasmin in the blood, with a decrease in plasma plasminogen and degradation of plasma proteins termed the *lytic state*. These effects are less marked with rt-PA and with scu-PA activator than with UK, SK, or Anistreplase, which often decrease plasminogen concentration to less than 25 percent of normal. Since effective fibrinolysis depends on the availability of plasminogen, and since thrombolytic therapy frequently induces a lytic state associated with a decrease in plasma plasminogen concentration, plasminogen supplementation could augment thrombolysis. Önundarson et al.[74] investigated the influence of soluble plasminogen concentration on in vitro lysis of whole-blood clots. Clot lysis was shown to be dependent on soluble plasminogen concentration, with maximum lysis using rt-PA between 0.5 and 1 unit/ml of plasminogen, while lysis increased progressively at higher concentrations of plasminogen with UK. The effect of in vivo activator-induced plasminogen depletion on in vitro clot lysis rates was tested with plasma obtained from patients after they received Anistreplase for treatment of myocardial infarction. Posttreatment plasma showed depletion of plasminogen to 14 ± 2 percent of normal, and these plasma samples produced only 4 ± 1 percent in vitro clot lysis during 4 hours. However, lysis increased progressively after repletion with plasminogen (see Fig. 24-3), suggesting that the reduction in plasminogen associated with the lytic state attenuated thrombolysis.

Purified plasminogen has been administered in small clinical trials to patients in conjunction with activators to increase therapeutic effectiveness. Kakkar et al.[75] found greater thrombolysis with a combination of intermittent plasminogen and low-dose SK than with intermittent low-dose SK alone in patients with deep vein thrombosis. The absence of therapeutic benefit obtained in control patients treated with this regimen of streptokinase alone, however, precludes any definite conclusions about the contribution of supplemental plasminogen in this study. Lys-plasminogen in combination with UK has been used in controlled studies of arterial occlusions,[76,77] myocardial infarction,[78] and pulmonary embolism,[79] but conclusions regarding the clinical benefit of plasminogen supplementation are premature in the absence of a well-designed clinical trial. The report of Tilsner and Whitte,[77] however, suggests that plasminogen supplementation contributed to successful treatment of thrombi with UK previously refractory with lysis. They treated 123 patients with peripheral arterial occlusions with UK and had a 60 percent rate of recanalization. Lys-plasminoge in combination with UK was then administered to 40 patients who had failed initial therapy, with a 78 percent incidence of reperfusion.

ULTRASOUND

The use of ultrasound in the treatment of vascular thrombosis has been investigated using two qualitatively different approaches. In the first, wires vibrating ultrasonic frequency (20 to 25 KHz) and power levels up to 20 W can disrupt clots[80–82] or

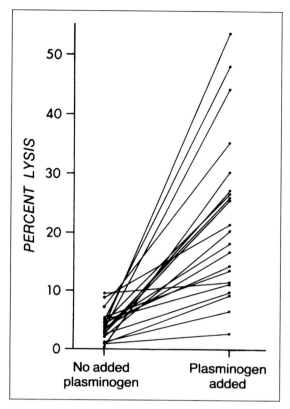

Figure 24-3. Lysis in vitro of whole-blood clots in plasma obtained from patients 90 to 120 minutes after anistreplase administration with or without added plasminogen. Whole-blood clots labeled with ^{125}I-fibrinogen were incubated for 4 hours in citrated plasma obtained from 21 patients with acute myocardial infarction at 90 to 120 minutes after bolus injection of 30 mg of anistreplase. Without added plasminogen, the mean clot lysis was 4.0 ± 0.5 percent, significantly lower than the 22.4 ± 3.0 percent measured in samples to which 1 unit/ml plasminogen had been added ($p < .001$). (Reproduced with permission from Önundarson PT, Francis CW, Marder VJ: Depletion of plasminogen in vitro or during thrombolytic therapy limits fibrinolytic potential. J Lab Clin Med 1992;120:120.)

atherosclerotic plaque[83,84] in vitro, producing fragments with diameters up to 800 μm. A similar approach has been used to ablate thrombi in dog models of femoral artery thrombosis, and the particles that result are either aspirated or embolize distally.[81,82,85,86] A similar device has been used to recanalize obstructed peripheral arteries in several

patients.[87,88] Reported complications with this technique include heating of the catheter, perforation of the vessel wall,[81] and histologic evidence of intimal disruption or medial dissection,[82] and there is concern over potential adverse effects of the embolized clot or plaque fragments.

A completely different approach is the noninvasive use of high-frequency ultrasound to accelerate enzymatic fibrinolysis. Kudo[89] has reported ultrasonic enhancement of rt-PA–mediated fibrinolysis in a dog model of femoral artery thrombosis. The mean time to reperfusion with rt-PA alone was 71 ± 30 minutes, and this was significantly shortened to 17 ± 9 minutes by percutaneous application of 200-KHz ultrasound directed to the thrombus. Hamano[90] also showed accelerated thrombolysis in a dog arterial thrombolysis model with transcutaneous ultrasound. Recently, Kornowski et al.[91] observed faster arterial recanalization during fibrinolytic therapy when using ultrasound in a rabbit femoral artery thrombosis model. However, they found that reocclusion also was increased by ultrasound, an effect they attributed to platelet activation, since the reocclusion was mitigated by concurrent aspirin administration. Francis et al.[92] investigated the effects of ultrasound on fibrinolysis in vitro and demonstrated that 1-MHz ultrasound significantly accelerated enzymatic fibrinolysis (Fig. 24-4). This occurred with SK, UK, or rt-PA.[93] The effect was dependent on ultrasound intensity, with significant increases at 1 W/cm^2 and above. Ultrasound did not cause mechanical fragmentation of the clot but accelerated enzymatic fibrinolysis. High-frequency, low-intensity ultrasound also accelerates fibrinolysis and speeds reperfusion in an in vitro circulating flow system with obstructive thrombus.[94] Acceleration of fibrinolysis with ultrasound in vitro also has been observed by several other investigators.[95–97]

In these experiments, ultrasound caused no mechanical fragmentation of the thrombus but accelerated enzymatic fibrinolysis. The effect was not thermally mediated but may be related to ultrasound-induced cavitation, which refers to the formation and action of microbubbles. These can have the effect of increasing transport of reactants from solution to the fibrin network where fibrinolysis occurs. The noninvasive, percutaneous

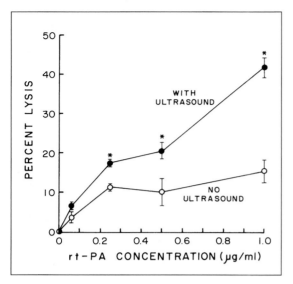

Figure 24-4. Effect of ultrasound on clot lysis with varying concentrations of rt-PA. Radiolabeled plasma clots were incubated for 1 hour at 37°C in normal plasma containing rt-PA at concentrations up to 1 μg/ml. Clots were exposed to ultrasound at 4 W/cm². Individual points represent the mean ± SEM of six experiments. Lysis was significantly greater in the presence of ultrasound at 0.25 μg/ml, 0.5 μg/ml, and 1 μg/ml ($p < 0.0005$ for each). (Reproduced with permission from Francis CW, Önundarson PT, Carstensen EL, et al: Enhancement of fibrinolysis in vitro by ultrasound. J Clin Invest 1992;90:2063.)

application of ultrasound could have significant potential as a fibrinolytic adjunct by augmenting fibrinolysis locally at the site of thrombosis without inducing systemic effects.

INHIBITION OF PLASMIN INHIBITOR

The principal inhibitor of plasmin is α_2-antiplasmin, which is found in both plasma and platelets.[98] During fibrinolytic therapy, the plasma concentration of α_2-plasmin inhibitor falls as it reacts with plasmin, and the inhibitor-enzyme complex is cleared. Factor XIIIa also rapidly crosslinks α_2-plasmin inhibitor to fibrin during clot formation.[99,100] This fibrin-bound inhibitor inhibits locally formed plasmin and contributes to the increased resistance of cross-linked fibrin clots to fibrinolysis. Therefore, inhibition of fibrin-

bound α_2-plasmin inhibitor could potentially accelerate fibrinolysis by preventing inhibition of locally formed plasmin.

Studies in vitro[101,102] have demonstrated that monoclonal antibodies to α_2-plasmin inhibitor bind and inactivate plasmin inhibitor that is crosslinked to fibrin and that this results in acceleration of fibrinolysis. This approach has been extended to studies in a rabbit model in which a clot of human blood was formed in a rabbit jugular vein.[103] In this model, administration of a monoclonal antibody to α_2-plasmin inhibitor significantly accelerated clot lysis in the absence of t-PA administration, indicating that inhibition of α_2-plasmin inhibitor accelerates endogenous fibrinolysis. Administration of both t-PA and the monoclonal antibody significantly accelerated pharmacologic thrombolysis compared with that with t-PA alone without increasing the systemic effects of plasmin. These findings suggest that clot-bound α_2-plasmin inhibitor plays an important regulatory role in fibrinolysis and that inhibition could be a useful approach in augmenting fibrinolytic therapy.

IMPORTANCE OF TRANSPORT

Successful fibrinolytic therapy depends on the delivery of pharmacologic concentrations of plasminogen activator to the site of thrombosis to accelerate the local conversion of plasminogen to plasmin and solubilize the fibrin matrix. The success of this approach depends in part on the adequacy of delivery of plasminogen activator to the thrombus and also on the supply of plasminogen. An acute thrombus is a nonvascularlized structure with only a small fraction of its surface exposed to therapeutically administered plasminogen activator. Since active fibrinolysis will occur only at sites where plasminogen activator is delivered, the progress of fibrinolysis will be slow unless activator is transported into the thrombus. Thus transport of fibrinolytic agents into the clot is an important determinant of the overall rate of thrombolysis.

Mathematical models of fibrinolysis predict that clot lysis occurs along a front where the concentration of plasminogen and activator generate sufficiently high plasmin concentrations.[104–106] These models predict that enzyme transport into the clot is the major determinant of lysis rate, which will be very slow if limited to diffusion alone, since it is very inefficient in transport over distances greater than a few tens of micrometers. Bulk flow or permeation refers to directional movement of a fluid by a pressure gradient. It is a much more effective mode of transport than diffusion, and mathematical models predict that activator transport by permeation will greatly accelerate clot lysis.[105]

Experimental models support the importance of transport in fibrinolysis. Blinc et al.[107] compared the rate of lysis using a simple in vitro model and found that lysis was increased 59-fold at a flow rate of approximately 50 μl/min driven by a pressure gradient of 37 cm of H_2O through an occlusive clot as compared with that with diffusion alone. Studies using high-resolution magnetic resonance imaging to monitor simultaneously the course of fluid permeation and clot lysis in vitro found a close correlation between the flow pattern and the initial channels of thrombolysis.[108] Other evidence demonstrates that clot lysis is faster if plasminogen activator is incorporated throughout the clot than if it diffuses from the surrounding fluid[109] and that fibrinolysis can be accelerated in vitro[110] and in animal models[111,112] by directly injecting activator into a clot. Accelerated transport may explain in part the increased rate of fibrinolysis observed in an ultrasound field.

Clinical experience also suggests that enzyme transport into a clot is an important determinant of therapeutic success. In acute myocardial infarction, higher rates of reperfusion have been observed with intracoronary administration of plasminogen activator that result in a higher concentration at the site of thrombosis.[113] Treatment of peripheral arterial occlusion is more successful if the catheter can be advanced into the clot for direct intrathrombic infusion rather than administration into the blood (see Chap. 21). Also, lysis of upper extremity venous clots was found to be more successful with direct intraclot infusion of activator than with local administration into the blood.[114] Optimizing delivery of both plasminogen and activator, both to the site of thrombosis and into the clot itself, has significant potential to optimize the rate of thrombolysis.

ANTICOAGULANTS

Acute hemostatic activation occurs with myocardial infarction, as evidenced by the fresh thrombotic coronary occlusion and by elevation of markers such as fibrinopeptide A on presentation. Fibrinolytic therapy can result in further activation of the coagulation system, reflected in further elevation of markers of thrombin activation in the plasma.[115–118] Also, arterial thrombi contain enzymatically active thrombin bound to fibrin,[119] and exposure of this clot-associated thrombin during fibrinolytic therapy could lead to additional local fibrin formation and platelet activation concurrent with fibrin lysis. Administration of heparin is routine during thrombolytic therapy with rt-PA and may reduce the otherwise high incidence of reocclusion following treatment. There has been intense recent interest in the development of new anticoagulants and their application during thrombolytic therapy for several reasons. First, there is substantial evidence of thrombin activation during thrombolytic therapy. Second, fibrin-bound thrombin is resistant to inhibition through the heparin–antithrombin III system but remains sensitive to lower-molecular-weight direct thrombin inhibitors.[120] Third, several new direct-acting thrombin inhibitors have become available for clinical evaluation (Table 24-3).

The largest experience has been with hirudin and its derivatives. Hirudin is a highly potent natural direct thrombin inhibitor present in the salivary glands of the European medicinal leech consisting of a 65-amino-acid peptide[121] whose crystallographic structure has been determined.[122] It has been produced in a recombinant form for clinical trials. Variants include a smaller peptide derived from the carboxyl-terminal portion of hirudin that binds to a noncatalytic site of thrombin (Hirugen), thereby reducing its affinity for natural substrates.[123] Also available is Hirulog, a synthetic hirudin analogue composed of the carboxyl-terminal portion that binds to the noncatalytic thrombin site, and a synthetic active site inhibitor linked by glycine residues.[124]

In a dog coronary thrombosis model, hirudin both accelerated thrombolysis and prevented reocclusion better than heparin.[125] Hirudin and its variants inhibit fibrin-bound thrombin[126] and can

Table 24-3. Adjunctive Anticoagulant Agents with Potential to Improve Fibrinolytic Efficacy

Mechanism	Examples
Antithrombin III–dependent inhibition	Unfractionated heparin Low-molecular-weight heparin
Direct thrombin inhibition	Hirudin Hirugen Hirulog Argatroban PPACK
Direct factor Xa inhibition	Tick anticoagulant peptide Antistasin
Inactivation of factors VIIIa and Va	Activated protein C
Inhibition of factor VIIIa–tissue factor and factor Xa	Tissue factor pathway inhibitor

inhibit clot formation after vessel injury in an animal model.[127] A recent clinical study demonstrated that hirudin was as effective as heparin in maintaining coronary patency after PTCA with no increase in bleeding.[128] Other direct thrombin inhibitors include the active site blocker PPACK[129] and the competitive thrombin inhibitor argatroban,[130] both of which have antithrombotic potency in animal models.

Specific inhibitors of factor Xa are other new anticoagulants that may have potential in the setting of thrombolytic therapy. These include the tick anticoagulant peptide (TAP)[131,132] and antistasin, which is derived from the Mexican leech.[133,134] Both are now available in recombinant form. They selectively inhibit factor Xa, including that surface- or platelet-bound, but do not inactivate thrombin. Both have been tested in animal models and show antithrombotic effects, including acceleration of thrombolysis.

Activated protein C is a central element in a natural anticoagulant pathway and is also under investigation as an adjunct to thrombolytic therapy. Thrombin binds to thrombomodulin on endothelial cells, and cell binding changes its properties, converting it from a procoagulant, which is capable of cleaving fibrinogen and activating platelets, to a form that cleaves protein C to activated protein C. Activated protein C functions as an anticoagulant by proteolytically inac-

tivating factors VIIIa and Va.[135] Both natural and recombinant forms of activated protein C have been produced and evaluated in animal models. In a baboon model of thrombolysis with a Dacron graft incorporated into an AV shunt, activated protein C increased the thrombolytic effectiveness of UK, suggesting that it may have value as a thrombolytic adjunct.[136,137] A potential advantage of activated protein C in this setting is that it has less effect on primary hemostasis, with normal bleeding times maintained during infusion. Tissue factor pathway inhibitor (TFPI) inhibits factor Xa and factor VIIa–tissue factor and is an important natural anticoagulant. It has been evaluated as an adjunct to thrombolysis in animal models with rt-PA and shows potential in preventing reocclusion.[138]

ANTIPLATELET AGENTS

Arterial thrombi are rich in platelets, and further platelet activation may occur at a site of thrombosis. Thrombosis is a dynamic process, with clot formation and dissolution occurring simultaneously, and thrombolytic resistance or reocclusion may occur if platelet activation is accelerated during thrombolytic therapy. Evidence supporting the importance of platelet activation during thrombolysis derives from several sources. A particularly compelling clinical trial was ISIS-2.[139] In this prospective, double-blind, and randomized trial, over 17,000 patients with acute myocardial infarction received SK, aspirin, both drugs, or neither. The results showed that either SK or aspirin alone produced a highly statistically significant 25 percent reduction in the 5-week vascular mortality compared with placebo therapy. Aspirin plus SK combined produced an additive benefit (Fig. 24-5). These and other findings strongly support the importance of platelet inhibition in maximizing benefits of thrombolytic therapy so that aspirin has become a standard component of thrombolytic therapy for myocardial infarction.

The evidence for platelet activation and the effectiveness of aspirin has spurred intense interest in the development of more potent antiplatelet agents (Table 24-4). The greatest effort has been in developing inhibitors of glycoprotein IIb/IIIa

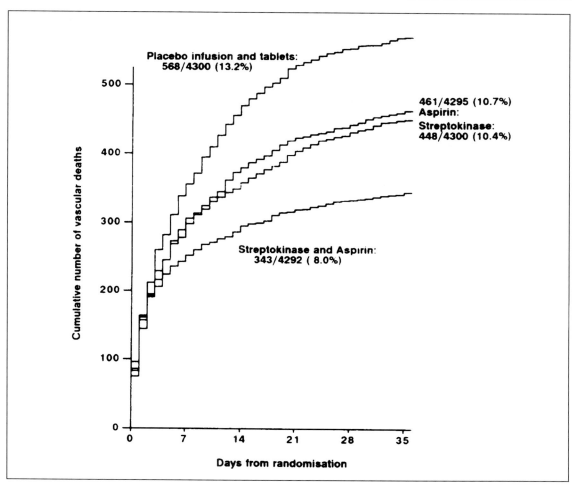

Figure 24-5. Cumulative vascular mortality in days 0 to 35 in the ISIS-2 study. (Reproduced with permission from ISIS-2, Second International Study of Infarct Survival, Collaborative Group: Randomized trial of intravenous streptokinase, oral aspirin, both, or neither among 17,187 cases of suspected acute myocardial infarction: ISIS-2. Lancet 1988;2:349.)

(GPIIb/IIIa), a platelet membrane integrin receptor that plays a critical role in platelet aggregation. GPIIb/IIIa is normally present on platelets in an inactive form, but following platelet activation, it changes conformation and acquires the capacity to bind fibrinogen.[140] Since fibrinogen is bivalent, it combines two activated platelets and results in aggregation. Both fibrinogen and GPIIb/IIIa are required for aggregation, and aggregation does not occur without both components. Detailed studies have identified specific sites on GPIIb/IIIa that interact with an RGD-containing peptide sequence on the A-alpha chain of fibrinogen and

also on the carboxyl terminal of the gamma chain.[141,142] Understanding the biochemistry of this system and the importance of platelet aggregation has led to two new approaches in antiplatelet therapy—blocking the receptor with antibodies or using molecules that mimic the binding site on fibrinogen (Fig. 24-6).

Antibodies that bind to GPIIb/IIIa can effectively block fibrinogen binding and platelet aggregation. An example is monoclonal antibody 7E3 that is currently undergoing clinical testing as an adjunct to fibrinolytic therapy. In vitro, 7E3 blocks fibrinogen binding to platelets and prevents platelet

Table 24-4. Adjunctive Antiplatelet Agents with Potential to Improve Fibrinolytic Efficacy

Mechanism	Examples
Inhibition of activation	
Cyclooxygenase inhibition	Aspirin
Thromboxane synthase inhibition	Dazoxiben
	CGS 13080
	Ridrogel
Thromboxane A$_2$ receptor blockade	Sulatroban
	SQ 30741
Inhibition of platelet-fibrinogen interaction	
Antibody to GPIIb/IIIa	MoAb 7E3 and variants
Competitive inhibition of fibrinogen binding	Echistatin
	Bitistatin
	Kistrin
	DMP728

aggregation.[143] Fab'2 and Fab fragments of 7E3 accelerate thrombolysis in animal models and reduce reocclusion.[144–148] In a recent small clinical trial, Kleiman et al.[149] administered 7E3 in increasing doses to patients being treated with rt-PA, aspirin, and heparin for acute myocardial infarction. The antibody effectively inhibited platelet aggregation, and receptor blockade was demonstrated. The reperfusion rates were high, and bleeding complications were not increased with antibody administration, indicating that the agent was promising for larger clinical trials. Potential problems with 7E3 include immunogenicity due to its murine origin and the occasional occurrence of thrombocytopenia. The side effects may be reduced by the development of a chimeric recombinant 7E3 fragment consisting of the mouse variable region linked to human constant domains.[150]

An alternative approach to blocking the GPIIb/IIIa-fibrinogen interaction is through the

Figure 24-6. Mechanism of action of inhibitors of GPIIb/IIIa-fibrinogen interaction. Platelets normally circulate in a quiescent form but after activation express an activated form of glycoprotein IIb/IIIa (GPIIb/IIIa) on the membrane. This receptor can interact with specific sites on fibrinogen, leading to platelet aggregation. Aggregation can be pharmacologically inhibited with an antibody to GPIIb/IIIa (anti-GPIIb/IIIa), which directly blocks the receptor, or by the use of competitive inhibitors of similar structure to the binding site on fibrinogen (RGD mimetic) that will bind to the receptor and prevent fibrinogen interaction and aggregation.

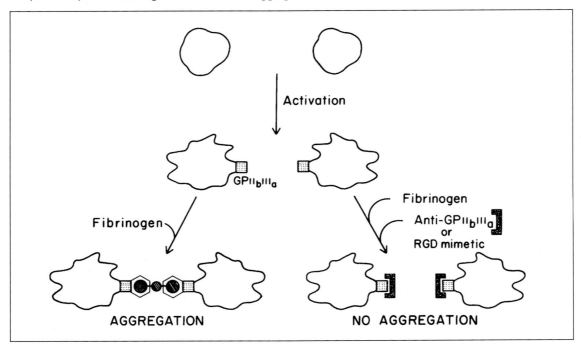

use of molecules that mimic the fibrinogen binding site, and a variety of synthetic and natural agents have been evaluated. The amino acid sequence RGD is involved in the interaction of fibrinogen with its receptor, and acetyl-RGDS has been shown to have some antithrombotic efficacy.[151] Analogues of RGD have been developed to improve pharmacologic properties. A cyclic analogue, DMP728, has been synthesized which is metabolically stable and highly effective in inhibiting platelet function at low concentration. In a dog femoral artery thrombosis model, DMP728 accelerated reperfusion and reduced reocclusion following thrombolysis using rt-PA or SK.[152] Naturally occurring inhibitors of GPIIb/IIIa occur in snake venoms, and purified agents have an RGD sequence that binds tightly to the receptor. Examples are bitistatin,[153,154] kistrin,[155] and echistatin.[156]

Although aspirin is clearly effective in improving fibrinolytic therapy, it is not a specific inhibitor of platelet function because it inhibits cyclooxygenase, an enzyme that is needed to synthesize pro-aggregatory and vasoconstrictor endoperoxides in platelets but also platelet inhibitory and vasodilatory endoperoxides in endothelial cells. The effects on endothelial cells are unwanted. A more specific inhibitor of platelet function would be an agent capable of blocking synthesis or action of thromboxane A_2. Examples are the thromboxane A_2 receptor antagonists SQ 30741[157] and sulatroban,[158] which have been tested in animal models of thrombolysis and demonstrate effectiveness in accelerating reperfusion and decreasing reocclusion. Similar results have been obtained with the selective thromboxane synthase inhibitors dazoxiben[159] and CGS 13080.[160] A novel agent is Ridgrogel, a synthetic agent that is a potent inhibitor of thromboxane A_2 synthase as well as a weak competitive inhibitor of the thromboxane A_2 receptor. In a canine model, this agent enhanced the thrombolytic activity of rt-PA and SK, decreasing the time to reperfusion, decreasing reocclusion, and decreasing infarct size.[161,162] Ridgrogel was evaluated clinically in a randomized, double-blind study in 907 patients with acute myocardial infarction who received SK and either aspirin or Ridgrogel.[163] The primary endpoint,

angiographic patency of the infarct-related artery prior to hospital discharge, was similar in the aspirin and Ridgrogel groups, 75.5 and 72.2 percent, respectively. The drug was well tolerated. Although there was some benefit in secondary endpoints, the results show that the combined inhibitor approach was not substantially better than aspirin alone. Other antiplatelet agents that have been evaluated include the prostacycline analogue, iloprost,[164,165] prostaglandin E1,[166,167] and organic nitrates, which have antiplatelet properties as well as vasodilation-inducing properties.

REFERENCES

1. DeWood MA, Spores J, Notske R, et al: Prevalence of total coronary occlusion during the early hours of transmural myocardial infarction. N Engl J Med 1980;303:897.
2. Rentrop KP, Blanke H, Karsch KR, et al: Acute myocardial infarction: Intracoronary application of nitroglycerin and streptokinase. Clin Cardiol 1979;2:254.
3. Rentrop P, Blanke H, Karsch KR, et al: Selective intracoronary thrombolysis in acute myocardial infarction and unstable angina pectoris. Circulation 1981;63:307.
4. Wun TC, Schleuning D, Reich E: Isolation and characterization of urokinase from human plasma. J Biol Chem 1982;257:3276.
5. Loscalzo J, Braunwald E. Tissue plasminogen activator. N Engl J Med 1988;319:925.
6. Rijken DC, Hoylaerts M, Collen D: Fibrinolytic properties of one-chain human extrinsic (tissue-type) plasminogen activator. J Biol Chem 1982;257:2920.
7. Ranby M: Studies on the kinetics of plasminogen activation by tissue plasminogen activator. Biochem Biophys Acta 1982;704:461.
8. Hoylaerts M, Rijken DC, Lijnen HR, Collen D: Kinetics of the activation of plasminogen by human tissue plasminogen activator: Role of fibrin. J Biol Chem 1982;257:2912.
9. Smith RAG, Dupe RJ, English PD, et al: Fibrinolysis with acylenzymes: A new approach to thrombolytic therapy. Nature 1981;290:505.
10. Lijnen HR, Zamarron C, Blaber M, et al: Activation of plasminogen by pro-urokinase: I. Mechanism. J Biol Chem 1986;261:1253.
11. Pannell R, Gurewich V: Pro-urokinase: A study of its stability in plasma and of a mechanism for its selective fibrinolytic effect. Blood 1986;67:1215.
12. Haber E, Quertermous T, Matsueda GR, Runge MS: Innovative approaches to plasminogen activator therapy. Science 1989;243:51.

13. Lijnen HR, Collen D: Annotation: Towards the development of improved thrombolytic agents. Br J Haematol 1991;77:261.

14. Larsen GR, Henson K, Blue Y: Variants of human tissue-type plasminogen activator: Fibrin binding, fibrinolytic, and fibrinogenolytic characterization of genetic variants lacking the fibronectin finger-like and/or the epidermal growth factor domains. J Biol Chem 1988;263:1023.

15. Larsen GR, Hensen K, Blue Y, Horgan P: The finger domain: A primary determinant in the clearance of t-PA in rat. Fibrinolysis 1988;2:29.

16. Gething MJ, Sambrook J, McGookey D: Addition of an oligosaccharide side-chain at an ectopic site on the EGF-like domain of t-PA prevents binding to specific receptors on hepatic cells. Thromb Haemost 1989;62:338.

17. Paoni NF, Keyt BA, Refino CJ, et al: A slow clearing, fibrin-specific, PAI-1 resistant variant of t-PA (T103N, KHRR 296–299 AAAA). Thromb Haemost 1993;70:307.

18. Berg DT, Bruck PJ, Berg DH, Grinnell BW: Kringle glycosylation in a modified human tissue plasminogen activator improves functional properties. Blood 1993;81:1312.

19. Madison EL, Goldsmith EJ, Gerard RD, et al: Serpin-resistant mutants of human tissue-type plasminogen activator. Nature 1989;339:721.

20. Collen D, Mao J, Stassen JM, et al: Thrombolytic properties of lys-158 mutants of recombinant single chain urokinase-type plasminogen activator (scu-PA) in rabbits with jugular vein thrombosis. J Vasc Med Biol 1989;1:46.

21. Stump DC, Lijnen HR, Collen D: Purification and characterization of a novel low molecular weight form of single-chain urokinase-type plasminogen activator. J Biol Chem 1986;261:17120.

22. Lijnen HR, Nelles L, Holmes WE, Collen D: Biochemical and thrombolytic properties of a low molecular weight form (comprising Leu144 through Leu411) of recombinant single-chain urokinase-type plasminogen activator. J Biol Chem 1988;263:5594.

23. Nelles L, Lijnen HR, Collen D, Holmes WE: Characterization of a fusion protein consisting of amino acids 1 to 263 of tissue-type plasminogen activator and amino acids 144 to 411 of urokinase-type plasminogen activator. J Biol Chem 1987;262:10855.

24. Lijnen HR, Nelles L, Van Hoef B, et al: Characterization of a chimeric plasminogen activator consisting of amino acids 1 to 274 of tissue-type plasminogen activator and amino acids 138 to 411 of single-chain urokinase-type plasminogen activator. J Biol Chem 1988;263:19083.

25. Nelles L, Lijnen HR, Van Nuffelen A, et al: Characterization of domain deletion and/or duplication mutants of a recombinant chimera of tissue-type plasminogen activator (rt-PA/u-PA). Thromb Haemost 1990;64:53.

26. Collen D, Lu HR, Lijnen HR, et al: Thrombolytic and pharmacokinetic properties of chimeric tissue-type and urokinase-type plasminogen activators. Circulation 1991;81:1216.

27. Agnelli G, Pascucci C, Nenci GG, et al: Thrombolytic and haemorrhagic effects of bolus doses of tissue-type plasminogen activator and a hybrid plasminogen activator with prolonged plasma half-life (K_2tu-PA: CGP 42935). Thromb Haemost 1993; 70:294.

28. Colucci M, Cavallo LG, Agnelli G, et al: Properties of chimeric (tissue-type/urokinase-type) plasminogen activators obtained by fusion at the plasmin cleavage site. Thromb Haemost 1993; 69:466.

29. Robbins KC, Boreisha: A covalent molecular weight ~92,000 hybrid plasminogen activator derived from human plasmin-binding and tissue plasminogen activator catalytic domains. Biochemistry 1987;26:4661.

30. Robbins KC, Tanaka Y, Gulba DL, et al: Covalent molecular weight ~92,000 hybrid plasminogen activator derived from human plasmin amino-terminal and urokinase carboxy-terminal domains. Biochemistry 1986;25:3603.

31. Browne MJ, Carey JE, Chapman CG, et al: Protein engineering and comparative pharmacokinetic analysis of a family of novel recombinant hybrid and mutant plasminogen activators. Fibrinolysis 1993; 7:357.

32. Bode C, Matsueda GR, Hui KY, Haber E: Antibody-directed urokinase: A specific fibrinolytic agent. Science 1985;229:765.

33. Runge MS, Bode C, Matsueda GR, et al: Conjugation to an antifibrin monoclonal antibody enhanced the fibrinolytic potency of tissue plasminogen activator in vitro. Biochemistry 1988; 27:1153.

34. Runge MS, Bode C, Matsueda GR, et al: Antibody-enhanced thrombolysis: Targeting of tissue plasminogen activator in vivo. Proc Natl Acad Sci USA 1987;84:7659.

35. Dewerchin M, Lijnen HR, Van Hoef B, et al: Biochemical properties of conjugates of urokinase-type plasminogen activator with a monoclonal antibody specific for cross-linked fibrin. Eur J Biochem 1989;185:141.

36. Schnee JM, Runge MS, Matsueda GR, et al: Construction and expression of a recombinant antibody-targeted plasminogen activator. Proc Natl Acad Sci USA 1987;84:6904.

37. Holvoet P, Laroche Y, Stassen JM, et al: Pharmacokinetic and thrombolytic properties of chimeric plasminogen activators consisting of a single-chain Fv fragment of a fibrin-specific antibody fused to single-chain urokinase. Blood 1993;81:696.

38. Bode C, Runge MS, Branscomb EE, et al: Antibody-directed fibrinolysis. An antibody specific for both fibrin and tissue plasminogen activator. J Biol Chem 1989;264:944.

39. Dewerchin M, Lijnen HR, Stassen JM, et al: Effect of chemical conjugation of recombinant single-chain urokinase-type plasminogen activator with monoclonal antiplatelet antibodies on platelet aggregation and on plasma clot lysis in vitro and in vivo. Blood 1991;78:1005.

40. Sako T, Sawaki S, Sakurai T, et al: Cloning and expression of the staphylokinase gene of *Staphylococcus aureus* in *Escherichia coli*. Mol Gen Genet 1983;190:271.

41. Kowalska-Loth B, Zakrzewski K: The activation by staphylokinase of human plasminogen. Acta Biochim Pol 1975;22:327.

42. Lijnen HR, Van Hoef B, DeCock F, et al: On the mechanism of fibrin-specific plasminogen activation by staphylokinase. J Biol Chem 1991;266:11826.

43. Matsuo O, OkadaK, Fukao H, et al: Thrombolytic properties of staphylokinase. Blood 1990; 76:925.

44. Gardell SJ, Duong LT, Diehl RE, et al: Isolation, characterization, and cDNA cloning of a vampire bat salivary plasminogen activator. J Biol Chem 1989;264:17947.

45. Gardell SJ, Hare TR, Bergum PW, et al: Vampire bat salivary plasminogen activator is quiescent in human plasma in the absence of fibrin unlike human tissue plasminogen activator. Blood 1990;76:2560.

46. Neuhaus KL, Feurer W, Jeep-Tebbe S, et al: Improved thrombolysis with a modified dose regimen of recombinant tissue-type plasminogen activator. J Am Coll Cardiol 1989;14:1566.

47. Neuhaus KL, Von Essen R, Tebbe U, et al: Improved thrombolysis in acute myocardial infarction with front-loaded administration of alteplase: Results of the rt-PA-APSAC patency study (TAPS). J Am Coll Cardiol 1992;19:885.

48. Carney RJ, Murphy GA, Brandt TR, et al: Randomized angiographic trial of recombinant tissue-type plasminogen activator (alteplase) in myocardial infarction. J Am Coll Cardiol 1992;20:17.

49. The GUSTO Investigators: An international randomized trial comparing four thrombolytic strategies for acute myocardial infarction. N Engl J Med 1993;329:673.

50. Tranchesi B Jr, Belloitti G, Chamone DF, Verstraete M: Effect of combined administration of saruplase and single-chain alteplase on coronary recanalization in acute myocardial infarction. Am J Cardiol 1989;64:229.

51. Kirshenbaum JM, Bahr RD, Flaherty JT, et al: Clot-selective coronary thrombolysis with low-dose synergistic combinations of single chain urokinase-type plasminogen activator and recombinant tissue-type plasminogen activator. Am J Cardiol 1991; 1991;68:1564.

52. Gulba DCL, Fischer K, Barthels M, et al: Low-dose urokinase preactivated natural prourokinase for thrombolysis in acute myocardial infarction. Am J Cardiol 1989;63:1025.

53. Kasper W, Hohnloser H, Engler H, et al: Coronary reperfusion studies with pro-urokinase in acute myocardial infarction: Evidence for synergism of low-dose urokinase. J Am Coll Cardiol 1990;16:733.

54. The Urokinase Pulmonary Embolism Trial: A national cooperative study. Circulation 1993;47(suppl II):108.

55. Urokinase-Streptokinase Embolism Trial: Phase 2 results: A cooperative study. JAMA 1974; 229:1606.

56. Dickie KJ, deGroot WJ, Cooley RN, et al: Hemodynamic effects of bolus infusion of urokinase in pulmonary thromboembolism. Am Rev Respir Dis 1974;109:48.

57. Petitpretz P, Simmoneau G, Cerrina J, et al: Effects of a single bolus of urokinase in patients with life-threatening pulmonary emboli: A descriptive trial. Circulation 1984;70:861.

58. Levine MN, Hirsh J, Weitz J, et al: A randomized trial of a single bolus dosage regimen of recombinant tissue plasminogen activator in patients with acute pulmonary embolism. Chest 1990; 98:1473.

59. Goldhaber SZ, Kessler CM, Heit J, et al: A randomized controlled trial of recombinant tissue plasminogen activator versus urokinase in the treatment of acute pulmonary embolism. Lancet 1988;2:293.

60. Goldhaber SZ, Kessler CM, Heit JA, et al: Recombinant tissue-type plasminogen activator versus a novel dosing regimen of urokinase in acute pulmonary embolism: A randomized controlled multicenter trial. J Am Coll Cardiol 1992;20:24.

61. Meyer G, Sors H, Charbonnier B, et al: Effects of intravenous urokinase versus alteplase on total pulmonary resistance in acute massive pulmonary embolism: A European multicenter double-blind trial. J Am Coll Cardiol 1992; 19:239.

62. Ozbeck C, Sen S, Frank S, et al: Rapid high dose streptokinase in severe pulmonary embolism. Lancet 1989;1:229.

63. Rakoczi I, Wiman B, Collen D: On the biologic significance of the specific interaction between fibrin, plasminogen and antiplasmin. Biochim Biophys Acta 1978;540:295.

64. Sakata Y, Mimuro J, Aoki N: Differential binding of plasminogen to crosslinked and non-crosslinked fibrins: Its significance in hemostatic defect in factor XIII deficiency. Blood 1984;63:1393.

65. Thorsen S: Differences in the binding to fibrin of native plasminogen and plasminogen modified by

proteolytic degradation influence of ε-aminocarboxylic acids. Biochim Biophys Acta 1975; 393:55.

66. Lucas MA, Fretto LJ, McKee PA: The binding of human plasminogen to fibrin and fibrinogen. J Biol Chem 1983;258:4249.

67. Suenson E, Lutzen O, Thorsen S: Initial plasmin-degradation of fibrins the basis of a positive feedback mechanism in fibrinolysis. Eur J Biochem 1984;140:513.

68. Harpel PC, Change T-S, Verderber E: Tissue plasminogen activator and urokinase mediate the binding of glu-plasminogen to plasma fibrin I. J Biol Chem 1985;260:4432.

69. Ogston D, Ogston CM, Fullerton HW. The plasminogen content of thrombi. Thromb Diath Haemorrh 1966;15:220.

70. Whitaker AN, Rowe EA, Masci PP, et al: The binding of glu- and lys-plasminogen to fibrin and their subsequent effects on fibrinolysis. Thromb Res 1980;19:381.

71. Gottlob R, Blümel G Studies on thrombolysis with streptokinase: I. On the penetration of streptokinase into thrombi. Thromb Diath Haemorrh 1968; 19:94.

72. Iga Y, Stella SR, Chandler AB: Kinetics of urokinase-induced thrombolysis in a biphasic in vitro system. Haemostasis 1985;15:189.

73. Watahiki Y, Scully MR, Ellis V, Kakkar VV: Potentiation by lys-plasminogen of clot lysis by single or two chain urokinase-type plasminogen activator or tissue-type plasminogen activator. Thromb Haemost 1989;61:502.

74. Onundarson PT, Francis CW, Marder VJ: Depletion of plasminogen in vitro or during thrombolytic therapy limits fibrinolytic potential. J Lab Clin Med 1991;120:120.

75. Kakkar VV, Sagar S, Lewis M: Treatment of deep vein thrombosis with intermittent streptokinase and plasminogen infusion. Lancet 1975;2:674.

76. Pernes JM, Vitoux JF, Brenoit P, et al: Acute peripheral arterial and graft occlusion: Treatment with selective infusion of urokinase and lysyl plasminogen. Radiology 1986;158:481.

77. Tilsner V, Witte G: Effectiveness of intraarterial plasminogen application in combination with percutaneous transluminal angioplasty (PTA) or catheter assisted lysis (CL) in patients with chronic peripheral occlusive disease of the lower limbs (POL). Haemostasis 1988;18:139.

78. deProst D, Guerot C, Laffay N, et al: Intra-coronary thrombolysis with streptokinase or lys-plasminogen/urokinase in acute myocardial infarction: Effects on recanalization and blood fibrinolysis. Thromb Haemost 1983;50:792.

79. Ellis DA, Neville E, Hall RJC: Subacute massive pulmonary embolism treated with plasminogen and streptokinase. Thorax 1983;38:903.

80. Hong AS, Chae JS, Dubin SB, et al: Ultrasonic clot disruption: An in vitro study. Am Heart J 1990; 120:418.

81. Rosenschein U, Bernstein JJ, DiSegni E: Experimental ultrasonic angioplasty: Disruption of atherosclerotic plaque and thrombi in vitro and arterial recanalization in vivo. J Am Coll Cardiol 1990; 15:711.

82. Ariani M, Fishbein MC, Chae JS, et al: Dissolution of peripheral arterial thrombi by ultrasound. Circulation 1988;84:1680.

83. Siegel RJ, Fishbein MC, Forrester J: Ultrasonic plaque ablation. A new method for recanalization of partially or totally occluded arteries. Circulation 1988;78:1443.

84. Ernst A, Schenk EA, Gracewski SM, et al: Ability of high-intensity ultrasound to ablate human arthrosclerotic plaques and minimize debris size. Am J Cardiol 1991;68:242.

85. Trübestein G, Engel C, Etzel F, et al: Thrombolysis by ultrasound. Clin Sci Mol Med 1976; 51:697s.

86. Stumpff U. Ultrasonic thrombolysis. J Acoust Soc Am 1979;65:541.

87. Siegel RJ, Cumberland DC, Myler RK, Don-Michael AT: Percutaneous ultrasonic angioplasty: Initial clinical experience. Lancet 1989;2:772.

88. Rosenschein U, Rozenszajn LA, Kraus L, et al: Ultrasonic angioplasty in totally occluded peripheral arteries: Initial clinical, histological and angiographic results. Circulation 1991;83:1976.

89. Kudo S: Thrombolysis with ultrasound effect. Tokyo Jukeikai Med J 1989;104:1005.

90. Hamano K: Thrombolysis enhanced by transcutaneous ultrasonic irradiation. Tokyo Jikeikai Med J 1991;106:533.

91. Kornowski R, Meltzer RS, Chernine A, et al: Does external ultrasound accelerate thrombolysis? Results from a rabbit model. Circulation 1994; 89:339.

92. Francis CW, Önundarson PT, Carstensen EL, et al: Enhancement of fibrinolysis in vitro by ultrasound. J Clin Invest 1992;90:2063.

93. Blinc A, Francis CW, Trudnowski JL, Carstensen EL: Characterization of ultrasound-potentiated fibrinolysis in vitro. Blood 1993;81:2636.

94. Harpaz D, Chen X, Francis CW, et al: Ultrasound enhancement of thrombolysis and reperfusion in vitro. J Am Coll Cardiol 1993;21:1507.

95. Lauer CG, Burge R, Tang DB, et al: Effect of ultrasound on tissue-type plasminogen activator-induced thrombolysis. Circulation 1992;86:1257.

96. Luo H, Steffen W, Cercek B, et al: Enhancement of thrombolysis by external ultrasound. Am Heart J 1993;125:1564.

97. Shlansky-Goldberg R, LeVeen RF, Sehgal CM: The use of ultrasound to enhance thrombolysis. Circulation 1991;84:422.

98. Plow EF, Collen D: The presence and release of α2-plasmin from human platelets. Blood 1981; 58:1069.

99. Sakata Y, Aoki N: Cross-linking of α2-plasmin inhibitor to fibrin by fibrin-stabilizing factor. J Clin Invest 1980;65:290.

100. Sakata Y, Aoki N: Significance of cross-linking of α2-plasmin inhibitor to fibrin in inhibition of fibrinolysis and in hemostasis. J Clin Invest 1982; 69:536.

101. Sakata Y, Eguchi Y, Mimuro J, et al: Clot lysis induced by a monoclonal antibody against α2-plasmin inhibitor. Blood 1989;74:2692.

102. Reed GL III, Matsuedo GR, Haber E: Synergistic fibrinolysis: The combined effects of plasminogen activators and an antibody that inhibits α2-antiplasmin. Proc Natl Acad Sci USA 1990; 87:1114.

103. Reed GL III, Matsueda GR, Haber E: Inhibition of clot-bound α2-antiplasmin enhanced in vivo thrombolysis. Circulation 1990;82:164.

104. Zidansek A, Blinc A: The influence of transport parameters and enzyme kinetics of the fibrinolytic system on thrombolysis: Mathematical modelling of two idealised cases. Thromb Haemost 1991; 65:553.

105. Diamond SL, Anand S: Inner clot diffusion and permeation during fibrinolysis. Biophys J 1993; 65:2622.

106. Zidansek A, Blinc A, Lahainar G, et al: Lysing patterns of blood clots: A nuclear magnetic resonance imaging study in vitro and mathematical modelling of the lysing pattern kinetics. J Mol Struct 1993;294:283.

107. Blinc A, Planinsic G, Keber D, et al: Dependence of blood clot lysis on the mode of transport of urokinase into the clot—A magnetic resonance study in vitro. Thromb Haemost 1991;65:549.

108. Blinc A, Kennedy SD, Bryant RG, et al: Flow through clots determines the rate and pattern of fibrinolysis. Thromb Haemost 1994;71:230.

109. Matsuo O, Rijken DC, Collen D: Comparison of the relative fibrinogenolytic, fibrinolytic and thrombolytic properties of tissue plasminogen activtora and urokinase in vitro. Thromb Haemost 1982;45:225.

110. Brookstein JJ, Saldinger E: Accelerated thrombolysis: In vitro evaluation of agents and methods of administration. Invest Radiol 1985;20:731.

111. Valji K, Bookstein JJ: Fibrinolysis with intrathrombic injection of urokinase and tissue-type plasminogen activator results in a new model of subacute venous thrombosis. Invest Radiol 1987; 22:23.

112. Kandarpa K, Drinker PA, Singer SJ, Caramore D: Forceful pulsatile local infusion of enzyme accelerates thrombolysis: In vivo evaluation of a new delivery system. Radiology 1988;168:739.

113. Marder VJ, Sherry S: Thrombolytic therapy: Current status. N Engl J Med 1988;318:1512, 1585.

114. Fraschini G, Jadeja K, Lawson M, et al: Local infusion of urokinase for the lysis of thrombosis associated with permanent central venous catheters in cancer patients. J Clin Oncol 1987;5:672.

115. Eisenberg PR, Sherman LA, JAffe AS: Paradoxic elevation of fibrinopeptide A after streptokinase: Evidence for continued thrombosis despite intense fibrinolysis. J Am Coll Cardiol 1987;10:527.

116. Owen J, Friedman KD, Grossman BA, et al: Thrombolytic therapy with tissue plasminogen activator or streptokinase induces transient thrombin activity. Blood 1988;72:616.

117. Rapold HJ, Kuemmerli H, Eiss M, et al: Monitoring of fibrin generation during thrombolytic therapy of acute myocardial infarction with recombinant tissue-type plasminogen activator. Circulation 1989;79:980.

118. Rapold HJ, Grimaudo V, Declerck PJ, et al: Plasma levels of plasminogen activator inhibitor type 1, β-thromboglobulin, and fibrinopeptide A before, during and after treatment with acute myocardial infarction with alteplase. Blood 1991;78:1490.

119. Francis CW, Markham RE Jr, Barlow GH, et al: Thrombin activity of fibrin thrombi and soluble plasmic derivatives. J Lab Clin Med 1983;102:220.

120. Weitz JI, Hudoba M, Massel D, et al: Clot-bound thrombin is protected from inhibition by heparin-antithrombin III but is susceptible to inactivation by antithrombin III-independent inhibitors. J Clin Invest 1990;86:385.

121. Harvey RP, Degryse E, Stefani L, et al: Cloning and expression of a cDNA coding for the anticoagulant hirudin from the blood-sucking leech, *Hirudo medicinalis*. Proc Natl Acad Sci USA 1986;83:1084.

122. Rydel TJ, Ravichandran KG, Tulinsky A, et al: The structure of a complex of recombinant hirudin and human α-thrombin. Science 1990;249:277.

123. Naski MC, Fenton JW 2d, Maraganore JM, et al: The COOH-terminal domain of hirudin. An exosite-directed competitive inhibitor of the action of alpha-thrombin on fibrinogen. J Biol Chem 1990;265:13484.

124. Maraganore JM, Bourdon P, Jablonsi J, et al: Design and characterization of hirulogs: A novel class of bivalent peptide inhibitors of thrombin. Biochemistry 1990;29:7095.

125. Haskel EJ, Prager NA, Sobel BE, Abendschein DR: Relative efficacy of antithrombin compared with antiplatelet agents in accelerating coronary thrombolysis and preventing early reocclusion. Circulation 1991;83:1048.

126. Mirshashi M, Soria J, Soria C, et al: Evaluation of the inhibition of heparin and hirudin of coagulation activation during rt-PA induced thrombolysis. Blood 1989;74:1025.

127. Kelly AB, Marzec UM, Krupsi W, et al: Hirudin interruption of heparin-resistant arterial thrombus formation in baboons. Blood 1991;77:1006.

128. van den Bos AA, Deckers JW, Heyndrickx GR, et al: Safety and efficacy of recombinant hirudin (CGP 39 393) versus heparin in patients with stable angina undergoing coronary angioplasty. Circulation 1993;88:2058

129. Hansen SR, Harker LA: Interruption of acute platelet-dependent thrombosis by the synthetic antithrombin D-phenylalanyl-L-prolyl-L-arginyl chloromethyl ketone. Proc Natl Acad Sci USA 1988;85:3184.

130. Kikumoto T, Tamao Y, Tezuka T, et al: Selective inhibition of thrombin by (2R,4R)-4-methyl-1-[N2] [3-methyl-1,2,3,4-tetrahydro-8-quinolinyl) sulfonyl]-2-pepeiridine-carboxylic acid. Biochemistry 1984;23:85.

131. Wasman L, Smith D, Arcuri K, Vlasuk G: Tick anticoagulant peptide (TAP) is a novel inhibitor of coagulation factor Xa. Science 1990;248:593.

132. Neeper MP, Waxman L, Smith DE: Characterization of recombinant tick anticoagulant peptide. J Biol Chem 1990;265:17746.

133. Nutt E, Gasil T, Rodkey J: The amino acid sequence of antistasin. J Biol Chem 1988;263:10162.

134. Dunwiddie C, Thornberry NA, Bull HG, et al: Antistasin, a leech-derived inhibitor of factor Xa. Kinetic analysis of enzyme inhibition and identification of the reactive site. J Biol Chem 1989;264:16694.

135. Esmon CT: Brief review. Protein C: Biochemistry, physiology, and clinical implications. Blood 1983;62:1155.

136. Gruber A, Griffin JH, Harker LA, Hanson SR: Inhibition of platelet-dependent thrombus formation by human activated protein C in a primate model. Blood 1989;73:639.

137. Gruber A, Hanson SR, Kelly AB: Inhibition of thrombus formation by activated recombinant protein C in a primate model of arterial thrombosis. Circulation 1989;82:578.

138. Haskel EJ, Torr SR, Day KC, et al: Prevention of arterial reocclusion after thrombolysis with recombinant lipoprotein-associated coagulation inhibitor. Circulation 1991;84:821.

139. ISIS-2 (Second International Study of Infarct Survival) Collaborative Group: Randomised trial of intravenous streptokinase, oral aspirin, both, or neither among 17,187 cases of suspected acute myocardial infarctions: ISIS-2. Lancet 1988;2:349.

140. Phillips DR, Charo IF, Scarborough RM: GPIIb-IIIa: The responsive integrin. Cell 1991;65:359.

141. Kloczewiak M, Timmons S, Lukas TJ, Hawiger J: Platelet receptor recognition site on human fibrinogen. Synthesis and structure-function relationship of peptides corresponding to the carboxy-terminal segment of the γ chain. Biochemistry 1984;23:1767.

142. Andrieux A, Hudry-Clergeon G, Ryckewaert J-J, et al: Amino acid sequences in fibrinogen mediating its interaction with its platelet receptor, GPI-IbIIIa. J Biol Chem 1989;264:9258.

143. Coller BS, Scudder LE, Beer J, et al: Monoclonal antibodies to platelet glycoprotein IIb/IIIa as antithrombotic agents. Ann NY Acad Sci 1991;614:193.

144. Mickelson JK, Simpson PJ, Cronin M, et al: Antiplatelet antibody [7E3 F(AB')2] prevents rethrombosis after recombinant tissue-type plasminogen activator-induced coronary artery thrombolysis in a canine model. Circulation 1990;81:617.

145. Gold HK, Coller BS, Yasuda T, et al: Rapid and sustained coronary artery recanalization with combined bolus injection of recombinant tissue-type plasminogen activator and monoclonal antiplatelet GP IIb/IIIa antibody in a canine preparation. Circulation 1988;77:670.

146. Yasuda T, Gold HK, Leinbach RC, et al: Lysis of plasminogen activator–resistant platelet-rich coronary bypass thrombus with combined bolus injection of recombinant tissue-type plasminogen activator and antiplatelet GP IIB/IIIa antibody. J Am Coll Cardiol 1990;16:1728

147. Yasuda T, Gold HK, Yaoita H, et al: Comparative effects of aspirin, a synthetic thrombin inhibitor, and a monoclonal antiplatelet glycoprotein IIb/IIIa antibody on coronary artery reperfusion, reocclusion, and bleeding with recombinant tissue-type plasminogen activator in a canine preparation. J Am Coll Cardiol 1990; 16:714.

148. Yasuda T, Gold, HK, Fallon JT, et al: Monoclonal antibody against the platelet glycoprotein (GP)IIb/IIIa receptor prevents coronary artery reocclusion after reperfusion with recombinant tissue-type plasminogen activator in dogs. J Clin Invest 1988;81:1284.

149. Kleiman NS, Ohman EM, Califf RM, et al: Profound inhibition of platelet aggregation with monoclonal antibody 7E3 Fab after thrombolytic therapy. Results of the thrombolysis and angioplasty in myocardial infarction (TAMI) 8 pilot study. J Am Coll Cardiol 1993;22:381.

150. Simoons ML, de Boer J, Marcel JBM, et al: Randomized trial of a GPIIb/IIIa platelet receptor blocker in refractory unstable angina. Circulation 1994;89:596.

151. Shebuski RJ, Berry DE, Bennett DB, et al: Demonstration of Ac-Arg-Gly-Asp-Ser-NH2 as an antiaggregatory agent in the dog by intracoronary administration. Thromb Haemost 1989;61:183.

152. Mousa SA, Bozarth JM, Forsythe MS, et al: Antiplatelet and antithrombotic efficacy of DMP728,

a novel platelet GPIIb/IIIa receptor antagonist. Circulation 1994;89:3.

153. Shebuski RJ, Ramjit DR, Benson GH, Polokoff MH: Characterization and platelet inhibitory activity of a potent RGD containing peptide from the venom of the viper *Bitis arietans*. J Biol Chem 1989;264:21550.

154. Shebuski RJ, Stabilito IJ, Sitko GR, Polokoff MH: Acceleration of recombinant tissue-type plasminogen activator induced thrombolysis and prevention of reocclusion by the combination of heparin and the Arg-Gly-Asp containing peptide bitistatin in a canine model of coronary thrombosis. Circulation 1990;82:169.

155. Yasuda T, Gold HK, Leinbach RC, et al: Kistrin, a polypeptide platelet GP IIb/IIIa receptor antagonist enhances and sustains coronary arterial thrombolysis with recombinant tissue-type plasminogen activator in a canine preparation. Circulation 1991;83:1038.

156. Holahan MA, Mellot MJ, Garsky VM, Shubuski RJ: Prevention of reocclusion following tissue-type plasminogen activator-induced thrombolysis by the RGD-containing peptide, echistatin, in a canine model of coronary thrombosis. Pharmacology 1991;42:340.

157. Schumacher WA, Grover GJ: The thromboxane receptor antagonist SQ 30741 reduces myocardial infarct size in monkeys when given during reperfusion at a threshold dose for improving reflow during thrombolysis. J Am Coll Cardiol 1990; 15:883.

158. Shebuski RJ, Smith JR Jr, Storer BL, et al: Influence of selective endoperoxide/thromboxane A_2 receptor antagonism with sulatroban on lysis time and reocclusion rate after tissue plasminogen activator-induced coronary thrombolysis in the dog. J Pharmacol Exp Ther 1988;246:760.

159. Golino, P. Rosolowsky M, Yao SK, et al: Endogenous prostaglandin endoperoxides and prostacylin modulate the thrombolytic activity of tissue plasminogen activator. Effect of simultaneous inhibition of thromboxane A_2 synthase and block-ade of thromboxane A_2/prostaglandin H_2 receptors in a canine model of coronary thrombolysis. J Clin Invest 1990;86:1095.

160. Shebuski RJ, Storer BL, Fujita T: Effect of thromboxane synthase inhibition on the thrombolytic action of tissue-type plasminogen activator in a rabbit model of peripheral arterial thrombosis. Thromb Res 1988;52:381.

161. Collen D, Masuda M, Rong Lu H, et al: Effect of ridogrel, a combined thromboxane A_2 synthase inhibitor/prostaglandin endoperoxide receptor antagonist, on the lysis of platelet-rich coronary arterial thrombi with recombinant tissue-type plasminogen activator in a canine model. Fibrinolysis 1992;6:7.

162. Yao S-K, Ober JC, Ferguson JJ, et al: Combination of inhibition of thrombin and blockage of thromboxane A_2 synthetase and receptors enhances thrombolysis and delays reocclusion in canine coronary arteries. Circulation 1992;86:1993.

163. The RAPT Investigators: Randomized trial of Ridogrel, a combined thromboxane A_2 synthase inhibitor and thromboxane A_2/prostaglandin endoperoxide receptor antagonist, versus aspirin as adjunct to thrombolysis in patients with acute myocardial infarction The Ridogrel versus aspirin patency trial (RAPT). Circulation 1994;89:588.

164. Topol EJ, Ellis SG, Califf RM, et al: Combined tissue-type plasminogen activator and prostacyclin therapy for acute myocardial infarction. J Am Coll Cardiol 1989;14:877.

165. Nicolini FA, Mehta JL, Nichols WW, et al: Prostacycline analogue iloprost decreases thrombolytic potential of tissue-type plasminogen activator in canine coronary thrombosis. Circulation 1989; 81:1115.

166. Sharma B, Wyeth RP, Giminez HJ, Franciosa JA: Intracoronary prostaglandin E_1 plus streptokinase in acute myocardial infarction. Am J Cardiol 1986;58:1161.

167. Vaughan DE, Plavin SR, Schfer AI, Loscalzo AI: PGE_1 accelerates thrombolysis by tissue plasminogen activator. Blood 1989;73:1213.

Complications of Local Intraarterial Thrombolysis for Lower Extremity Occlusions

KRISHNA KANDARPA

Local or regional thrombolytic therapy for peripheral arterial occlusions has gained favor as the limitations of balloon thromboembolectomy have become recognized.[1] Thromboembolectomy has been associated with a high incidence of residual thrombus, the inability to clear thrombus in smaller peripheral branches, and disruption of the endothelium, which results in diffuse luminal narrowing over the long term.[2] Local infusion of plasminogen activators for arterial and graft occlusions, guided by high-quality fluoroscopy and arteriography, has the primary goal of restoring blood flow to the ischemic limb by dissolving a substantial amount of the occlusive thrombus.[3,4] Initially successful lysis can be achieved in over 90 percent of cases.[3–7] An angiogram at the termination of a successful infusion almost always identifies the underlying lesions that caused the thrombotic occlusion and defines which are amenable to repair by percutaneous and/or surgical means. Following such intervention, a 30-day successful therapeutic outcome can be achieved in about 80–85 percent of patients.[3,8] Surgery is seldom compromised by an initial trial of thrombolytic therapy,[3] and the extent of required surgery may be decreased while the outcome is improved in the majority of successfully lysed patients.[3,9] However, as discussed below, regional (local) thrombolytic therapy does pose some risks to the patient. The reported overall *total* complication rate associated with this treatment may range as high as 50 percent.[10,11] For-tunately, the vast majority of these complications do not have significant clinical consequences.

The overall rate for a *major* complication such as stroke, acute myocardial infarction, amputation as result of distal embolization during treatment, and death is under 1 percent.[10,11] This rate varies only slightly between different plasminogen activators and dosage regimens.[7,12–14] Serious complications may be the result of judgment errors such as inappropriate patient selection, failure to recognize bleeding or mismanagement of it, and failure to adhere to a fixed, well-tested infusion protocol.[15] In addition, the probability of a major complication associated with lower extremity thrombolysis increases with the duration of infusion from 4 percent at 8 hours to 34 percent at 40 hours.[5] Therefore, the risks of regional thrombolytic therapy can be minimized by selecting patients who meet the clinical and angiographic criteria associated with successful and safe outcome, by understanding the safety profiles of the available plasminogen activators, and by using techniques and protocols that expedite treatment.

PATIENT SELECTION

The key to minimizing the risk of complication from local thrombolysis is proper patient selection. Table 25-1 lists the usual indications and contraindications to thrombolytic therapy. As can be noted, the list of contraindications is based on the

Table 25-1. Indications and Contraindications for Local Thrombolytic Therapy[4,37,40–42]

Indication

Thrombotic or embolic occlusion of a native artery or bypass graft causing new-onset claudication or limb-threatening ischemia.

Contraindications

Absolute
1. Active internal bleeding
2. Irreversible limb ischemia (severe sensory deficits, muscle rigor)
3. Recent stroke (arbitrary guideline: TIA within 2 months or CVA within 6 months; some prefer to wait up to 12 months)
4. Intracranial neoplasm or recent (2 months) craniotomy

*Relative**
1. History of gastrointestinal bleeding
2. Recent (10 to 14 days) major surgery, including biopsy
3. Recent trauma
4. Recent cardiopulmonary resuscitation
5. Severe uncontrolled high blood pressure (diastolic bp > 125 mmHg)
6. Subacute bacterial endocarditis
7. Coagulopathy
8. Pregnancy and postpartum period (< 10 days)
9. Severe cerebrovascular disease
10. Diabetic hemorrhagic retinopathy

---

*Thrombolysis should be considered infrequently in this group of patients, and the need should far outweigh the risk of treatment. Careful clinical evaluation and sound judgment in patient selection are essential. Prophylactic measures should be taken to minimize risk.

---

potential hazards of reperfusing a severely ischemic limb, internal bleeding, or thrombus embolization as a result of treatment.

Limb Ischemia Status

The risks of rapidly reperfusing a severely ischemic limb have long been recognized.[16–18] Restoration of blood flow may result in (1) compartment syndrome, which is clinically manifested by excruciating pain, a tenseness over the muscle compartment, and progressive loss of muscle (loss of ability to dorsiflex the foot) and nerve function as a consequence of the elevated intracompartmental pressure from fluid retention and muscle edema, and (2) the more serious, and potentially fatal, consequences of reperfusion syndrome, such as *cardiac dysfunction* from systemic acidemia and hyperkalemia, resulting from washout of the metabolites of necrotic mus-

cle such as lactate and potassium, and *renal failure* from entrapment of myoglobin released from necrotic muscle. Compartment syndrome has been noted in about 2 percent of patients undergoing regional thrombolysis for acute lower extremity ischemia,[11] and reperfusion syndrome has been seen in under 1 percent.[10] When indicated, fasciotomy successfully relieves the high pressure causing compartment syndrome. However, when serious systemic metabolic disturbances occur from reperfusion, they are far more difficult to treat.

In consideration of the preceding, when selecting patients, thrombolytic therapy is best avoided in those with irreversibly ischemic limbs (SVS/ISCVS category III), especially when a large amount of muscle mass is jeopardized. On examination, these limbs are characterized by the absence of distal pulses and capillary return (marbling of the skin), muscle paralysis (rigor), and severe sensory deficits (anesthesia). Noninvasive examination demonstrates an absence of both arterial and venous Doppler signals. Arteriographically, all major branches and their collaterals are typically thrombosed, and there is no reconstitution of the calf runoff vessels.[3] In their patients who fell into this category, McNamara et al.[3] reported a high rate of amputation (25 percent) and their only death (from the systemic consequences of reperfusion syndrome). An earlier study utilizing streptokinase also reported on the unacceptably high risk of attempting to treat irreversibly ischemic limbs with signs of massive muscle necrosis.[19] It should be emphasized that the larger the amount of jeopardized muscle mass (i.e., more proximal occlusion) and the more profound the ischemia, the greater is the risk of complications from reperfusion of necrotic tissue. Even then, the overall incidence of complications, including death, from the systemic consequences of "reperfusion syndrome" is well below 1 percent.[10]

In the previously cited study by McNamara et al.,[3] no patients with viable (SVS/ISCVS category I) or threatened (SVS/ISCVS category II) limbs died, and the amputation rates were 0 and 8 percent, respectively. Therefore, patients in these two acute limb ischemia categories are ideal candidates for regional thrombolytic therapy, barring other contraindications.

Propensity for Bleeding

Absolute contraindications to thrombolytic therapy such as active internal bleeding, recent intracranial or other neurosurgery, and recent stroke or intracranial neoplasm are based on avoiding the disastrous consequences of the increased propensity for bleeding during infusion of plasminogen activators.[7,10,12–14,20,21] There are clinical settings where the increased risk for bleeding may constitute a relative contraindication to local thrombolytic therapy (see Table 25-1), such as *recent* major (abdominal or intrathoracic) surgery, organ biopsy, trauma, gastrointestinal bleeding, postpartum status, and uncontrolled hypertension or diabetic hemorrhagic retinopathy. Sound clinical judgment should be exercised before initiating thrombolytic therapy in these latter patients. The reported rates for bleeding complications depend on the specific plasminogen activator's ability to produce a systemic lytic state, the route and duration of infusion, dosage, and whether or not anticoagulants are administered concomitantly.[7,13,14]

Major bleeding is generally defined by episodes requiring discontinuation of infusion, blood transfusion, or surgical intervention, with minor bleeding being primarily clinically insignificant puncture-site hematomas. In a review of 1767 published cases of peripheral intraarterial thrombolysis, Gardiner and Sullivan[10] found a major bleeding complication rate of about 7 percent, and a minor bleeding complication rate of about 6 percent. However, overall bleeding complication rates can range anywhere from 3 to 30 percent, depending on the series and the influencing factors cited above.[7,14] Hemorrhagic complications are higher with streptokinase (SK) and recombinant tissue-type plasminogen activator (rt-PA) than with urokinase (UK).[7,12,14] The results of one small dose-ranging study using tissue-type plasminogen activator for peripheral arterial thrombolysis suggest that major hemorrhagic complications are more frequent at higher doses.[22]

Among the most devastating of the major hemorrhagic complications are stroke and remote internal bleeding. In the above-mentioned review,[10] the overall incidence of intracranial hemorrhage was 0.5 percent. Comparable overall rates are reported by McNamara et al.,[11] who reviewed their experience with 1000 patients. Higher rates of intracranial bleeding have been associated with streptokinase and recombinant tissue-type plasminogen activator than with urokinase for peripheral arterial thrombolysis,[7,14,20] but the numbers of patients in these series are small. Notably, intracranial hemorrhage is more frequent in patients undergoing systemic thrombolytic infusions (with much larger doses) for acute myocardial infarction (AMI).[11] Specifically, elderly patients (age greater than 70 years) with hypertension (blood pressure greater than 150/95 mmHg) being treated with *intravenous* thrombolytic infusion for AMI are reported to have a greater risk for intracerebral hemorrhage.[23] In as much as direct extrapolation of the AMI experience to the peripheral system should be made with caution, it would appear to be prudent to screen and monitor such patients carefully when they are being considered for regional thrombolysis, especially if prolonged infusion is anticipated.

A limb that has recently undergone vascular surgery bears special consideration. The traditional and somewhat arbitrary waiting period before initiating thrombolytic therapy has been a week to 10 days to allow for wound healing. Occasionally, an operative complication or a technical problem may force the surgeon to request thrombolytic therapy much earlier. I have on rare occasion initiated infusions as early as 2 days after peripheral arterial surgery limited to the limb. However, this requires a careful analysis of the extent of the problem and potential risks and sound clinical judgment on the part of all involved. The decision to proceed with a brief trial of infusion should be based on a clear therapeutic goal and an agreement on the part of the surgeon and interventional radiologist to stop infusion or intervene surgically if problems arise.

Unfortunately, routine laboratory assessment of systemic lytic and coagulation parameters (e.g., fibrinogen, fibrin degradation products, plasminogen levels, etc.) has proved of little use in the prediction and prevention of hemorrhagic complications.[10,11,13,14] However, baseline assessment of hematocrit, aPTT or ACT, and fibrinogen levels and periodic reassessment of these parameters may be useful for early detection and/or management of bleeding.

Risk of Embolization

Some patients undergo thrombolytic therapy for embolic occlusions in the lower extremity from a remote site such the heart or aorta. Patients with intracardiac thrombi have a greater risk of repeat embolization during lytic therapy,[24] and if the heart is the suspected source of the embolus, some would suggest that an echocardiogram is indicated prior to the initiation of thrombolytic therapy. In general, patients with left ventricular thrombi (LVT) are six times more likely to experience an embolic event on follow-up (mean of 22 months) than matched controls without LVT.[25] Protrusion and mobility of the thrombus on echocardiography are predictive of a higher risk for embolization[25]; patients with such findings should be excluded from consideration for thrombolysis. Notably, in one small study of 16 post-AMI patients, no peripheral embolization occurred following intravenous urokinase administration for dissolving adherent left ventricular mural thrombi.[26] On the other hand, a case of death from recurrent massive embolization from the left ventricle during regional thrombolysis also has been reported.[24] Fortunately, the risk of embolic stroke from regional thrombolysis, in the absence of the preceding echocardiographic findings, appears to be extremely low to negligible based on both experience and theoretical considerations.[11]

Other potential sources for peripheral embolization, such as free-floating thrombi in the aorta, also should be evaluated carefully prior to initiating thrombolytic therapy. Thrombosed popliteal aneurysms carry a potentially high risk of distal embolization, but thrombolysis may be considered if all runoff vessels are occluded and there is a need to open a distal vessel prior to surgical bypass.[27,28]

PROCEDURE-RELATED COMPLICATIONS

Undetected remote internal bleeding can have disastrous consequences. For example, a retroperitoneal hematoma, reported to occur in under 0.5 percent of patients,[11] if massive, will result in hypotension and may cause myocardial infarction and possibly death, since most patients with peripheral atherosclerosis have coronary artery disease as well. Nonetheless, the overall risk of myocardial infarction associated with regional thrombolysis is low, about 0.2 percent.[10] Most retroperitoneal hematomas are attributable to high arterial punctures (above the inguinal ligament), from which blood can dissect into the pelvic and retroperitoneal spaces without manifesting superficial signs of bleeding. Careful attention to complaints such as unexplained persistent nausea and back pain and frequent monitoring of vital signs and hematocrit should provide early clues to the possibility of retroperitoneal bleeding, which, if suspected, can be definitively diagnosed by computed tomography of the abdomen. Unless the bleeding stops spontaneously with the cessation of lytic and anticoagulant therapy or with measures to reverse the hemorrhagic state, surgical intervention may be needed.

Distal migration (embolization) of thrombus fragments into the limb during treatment is not uncommon and is noted overall in about 5 percent of cases.[10] Clinically, such embolization is manifested as a sudden onset of pain or loss of a distal Doppler pulse during infusion. Patients should be warned of this possibility. Fortunately, most of these emboli resolve without significant clinical consequences with continued lytic therapy. Occasionally, a small (no. 3 Fr) coaxial catheter might have to be placed distally for infusion of concentrated lytic agent directly into the embolized vessel or thrombus. Less than 1 percent of cases may need limited amputation as a direct result of such clot migration.[10] The risk of distal embolization can be minimized by avoiding excessive clot fragmentation and premature balloon angioplasty. In general, amputation is more likely to be needed because of the preexisting ischemic status of the limb rather than as a result of a complication of lytic therapy.[3,11]

Concurrent rethrombosis is noted in about 3 percent of patients undergoing regional thrombolytic therapy,[10] and may be more likely to occur if concomitant intravenous heparin is not administered. Rethrombosis following successful recanalization can result from a low blood flow rate within the conduit and the presence of the infusion catheter, which can both be occlusive to flow and serve as a thrombogenic surface.[29] The high thrombogenicity of residual thrombus itself has been recognized and is attributed to the presence of fibrin-bound thrombin.[30] The administration of systemic heparin has resulted in a significant decrease in the incidence of this setback during thrombolytic therapy.[29] Careful maintenance of therapeutic aPTT or ACT levels during lytic therapy serves to avoid rethrombosis and unnecessary prolongation of the infusion.

Puncture-site hematomas constitute the majority of the 6 percent of minor bleeding complications associated with regional thrombolysis[10] and are easily managed by local arterial compression. Occasionally, the size of the catheter or sheath in the artery may need to be increased in order to tamponade the puncture site, and the heparin intravenous infusion rate may need adjustment. Catheter-related trauma resulting in arterial dissection or a puncture site pseudoaneurysm occurs in under 1 percent of cases and may on rare occasion necessitate surgical intervention.[10,11,21]

Extravasation of contrast-mixed blood through prosthetic graft materials (e.g., knitted Dacron) can occur from a graft of any age.[31] Frequently, the site of extravasation is at the anastomosis, but seepage through the body of the graft also can occur. Often, infusion may simply be discontinued with no further consequence. If the extravasation is superficial and within the limb, it is usually more easily detected and corrected than when it is within the abdomen, when greater diligence in monitoring the patient is indicated in order to avoid the consequences of massive retroperitoneal or intrapelvic hemorrhage.

Other rare ($\leqslant 0.5$ percent) complications include (1) acute renal failure related to the use of iodinated radiographic contrast agents (proper hydration and use of digital subtraction angiography with diluted contrast media can minimize this risk[32]), (2) allergic reactions to the lytic agents, primarily to streptokinase (see section on plasminogen activators), and (3) sepsis.[10,11,21] Extremely rare occurrences of spontaneous splenic rupture and hemorrhage have been reported.[33]

Death from local thrombolytic therapy is rare, under 1 percent, and is usually the result of remote bleeding (e.g., intracranial, retroperitoneal) or systemic complications from reperfusion of an irreversibly ischemic limb.[7,10,11,14] In one small series, all deaths associated with regional thrombolysis occurred during infusion of streptokinase or rt-PA, and no deaths were associated with urokinase.[7]

PLASMINOGEN ACTIVATOR–SPECIFIC COMPLICATIONS

Few prospective studies have compared lytic agents specifically for regional thrombolysis. A small study ($n = 16$ in each group) comparing urokinase with rt-PA found that although rt-PA caused rapid early lysis in a greater number of patients, by 24 hours, the success rates were similar, and at 30 days, there was no significant difference in clinical outcome.[12] Additionally, rt-PA caused more frequent complications and a significantly greater decrement in fibrinogen levels. A retrospective review by Graor et al.[7] compared the efficacy and safety of urokinase ($n = 200$), streptokinase ($n = 200$), and rt-PA ($n = 65$) for regional thrombolysis and found the highest clinical success rates (defined as complete lysis of thrombus and improvement in clinical status) with urokinase (95 percent) and rt-PA (91 percent) and the lowest rates with streptokinase (60 percent). In addition, urokinase had the lowest rates for major bleeding (6 percent) and streptokinase the highest (28 percent), with rt-PA in between (12 percent). Intracranial hemorrhage occured in 2 percent of patients treated with streptokinase or rt-PA and no patients treated with urokinase. Death occurred in 4 percent of patients treated with streptokinase, 2 percent with rt-PA, and none treated with urokinase. Also, as noted in prior studies, fibrinogen depletion was more profound with SK and rt-PA than with UK infusions. The conclusion from this study that urokinase has higher efficacy and safety compared with the other two agents is generally supported in the literature.[34–37]

The incidence of a major true allergic reaction with SK or rt-PA is under 0.5 percent, and it is 0 percent with UK.[14] Allergic reactions to streptokinase are attributed to the presence of streptococcal antibodies in a significant proportion of the population.[13,14,20,21] Antigen-antibody interaction also decreases the bioavailibility of streptokinase in vivo, thereby reducing its efficacy and prolonging infusion times. For similar reasons, once a patient is exposed to streptokinase, a delay of about 6 months may be required before repeat treatment can be given with this agent. Occasional episodes of mild bronchospasm, skin rash, and transient fever have been reported with UK. Recently, however, there have been reports of chills and rigors following large (> 250,000 units), rapid-bolus infusions of urokinase (e.g., given for thrombolysis of dialysis fistulas). These symptoms may be treated prophylactically with hydrocortisone 100 mg IV, acetaminophen 1 g PO, and benadryl 50 mg IV given 30 to 60 minutes prior to UK infusion.

CONCLUSIONS

The key factors in avoiding and minimizing complications during local intraarterial thrombolytic therapy are proper patient selection, expeditious infusions, diligent monitoring of the patient in an intensive care setting, and selection of a plasminogen activator and protocol with which one is familiar and comfortable. All efforts should be made to complete the infusion therapy expeditiously and to avoid unnecessarily prolonged infusions, which increase the probability of a complication. Initial intrathrombic bolusing of the lytic agent with either endhole or pulse-spray catheters may decrease infusion times.[5,38] The most important factor in preventing complications during thrombolysis is to pursue the underlying cause of seemingly innocuous and nonspecific signs and symptoms (e.g., nausea, which could occur with a retroperitoneal hemorrhage or with ongoing myocardial ischemia). Persistent and inexplicable complaints of back pain or discomfort (retroperitoneal hemorrhage) or headache (intracranial hemorrhage) should be assessed expeditiously and investigated with computed tomography if necessary. Attention to details such as placing a Foley catheter to monitor urine output and avoid bladder overdistension (causing vasovagal hypotension) and avoiding intramuscular injections, aspirin, and concomitant dextran infusion improve the safety of this therapy. Frequent vital sign assessment, physical examination, and appropriate laboratory evaluation should be used to monitor for indications of bleeding or deterioration in the status of the patient or limb. A high index of suspicion and prompt corrective action can prevent most of the potentially disastrous consequences to the patient.

REFERENCES

1. Graor Ra, Risius B, Young Jr, et al: Thrombolysis of peripheral arterial bypass grafts: Surgical thrombectomy compared with thrombolysis. J Vasc Surg 1988;7:347.
2. Bowles CR, Olcott C, Pakter RL, et al: Diffuse arterial narrowing as a result of intimal proliferation: A delayed complication of embolectomy with the Fogarty balloon catheter. J Vasc Surg 1988;7:487.
3. McNamara TO, Bomberger RA, Merchant RF: Intraarterial urokinase as the initial therapy for acutely ischemic limbs. Circulation 1991;83[suppl I]:106.
4. Sullivan KL, Gardiner GA, Kandarpa K, et al: Efficacy of thrombolysis in infrainguinal bypass grafts. Circulation 1991;83 [suppl I]:99.
5. Sullivan KL, Gardiner GA, Shapiro MJ, et al: Acceleration of thrombolysis with a high-dose transthrombus bolus technique. Radiology 1989; 173:805.
6. LeBlang SD, Becker GJ, Benenati JF, et al: Low-dose urokinase regimen for the treatment of lower extremity arterial and graft occlusions: Experience in 132 cases. JVIR 1992;3:475.
7. Graor RA, Olin J, Bartholomew JR, et al: Efficacy and safety of intraarterial local infusion of streptokinase, urokinase, or tissue plasminogen activator for peripheral arterial occlusion: A retrospective review. J Vasc Med Biol 1990;2:310.
8. Clouse ME, Stokes KR, Perry LJ, Wheeler HG: Percutaneous intraarterial thrombolysis: analysis of factors affecting outcome. JVIR 1994;5:93.
9. Ouriel K: Thrombolysis Versus Operation in Acute Peripheral Arterial Occlusion. Presented at the Twentieth Annual Symposium on Current Critical Problems and New Techniques in Vascular Surgery, New York, N.Y., November 1993.
10. Gardiner GA, Sullivan KL: Complications of regional thrombolytic therapy. In Kadir S (ed): Current Practice of Interventional Radiology. Philadelphia, B C Decker, 1991, pp 87–91.
11. McNamara TO, Goodwin SC, Kandarpa K: Complications associated with thrombolysis. Semin Intervent Radiol 1994;2:134.
12. Meyerovitz MF, Goldhaber SZ, Reagan K, et al: Recombinant tissue-type plasminogen activator versus urokinase in peripheral arterial and graft occlusions: A randomized trial. Radiology 1990; 175:75.
13. Holden RW: Plasminogen activators: Pharmacology and therapy. Radiology 1990;174:993.

14. Woo KS, White HD: Comparative tolerability profiles of thrombolytic agents: A review. Drug Safety 1993;8:19.

15. Hirshberg A, Schneiderman J, Garniek A, et al: Errors and pitfalls in intraarterial thrombolytic therapy. J Vasc Surg 1989;10:612.

16. Haimovici H: Arterial embolism with acute massive ischemic myopathy and myoglobinuria. Surgery 1960;47:739.

17. Fisher DR, Fogarty TJ, Morrow AG: Clinical and biochemical observations of the effect of transient femoral occlusion in man. Surgery 1970;68:323.

18. Beyersdorf F, Matheis G, Kruger S, et al: Avoiding reperfusion injury after revascularization: Experimental observations and recommendations for clinical application. J Vasc Surg 1989;9:757.

19. Lang EK: Streptokinase therapy: Complications of intra-arterial use. Radiology 1985;154:75.

20. Graor RA, Risius B, Young JR, et al: Low-dose streptokinase for selective thrombolysis: Systemic effects and complications. Radiology 1984;152:35.

21. Palaskas C, Totty WG, Gilula LA: Complications of local intraarterial fibrinolytic therapy. Semin Intervent Radiol 1985;2:396.

22. Earnshaw JJ, Westby JC, Gregson RHS, et al: Local thrombolytic therapy of acute peripheral arterial ischemia with tissue plasminogen activator: A dose-ranging study. Br J Surg 1988;75:1196.

23. Anderson JL, Karagounis L, Allen A, et al: Older age and elevated blood pressure are risk factors for intracerebral hemorrhage after thrombolysis. Am J Cardiol 1991;68:166.

24. Paulson EK, Miller FJ: Embolization of cardiac mural thrombosis: Complication of intraarterial fibrinolysis. Radiology 1988;168:95.

25. Stratton JR: Embolic risk due to left ventricular thrombi. Cardiol Board Rev 1988;5:81.

26. Kremer P, Fiebig R, Tilsner V, et al: Lysis of left ventricular thrombi with urokinase. Circulation 1985;72:112.

27. Carpenter JP, Barker CF, Roberts B, et al: Popliteal Artery Aneurysms: Improved Results with Thrombolytic Therapy. Presented at the North American Chapter ISCVS and SVS Annual Meeting, Washington, D.C., June 1993.

28. Leen VH, Shlansky-Goldberg RD, Carpenter JP, et al: Thrombolysis of thrombosed popliteal aneurysms. JVIR 1994;5:46.

29. Eskridge JM, Becker GJ, Rabe FE, et al: Catheter-related thrombosis and fibrinolytic therapy. Radiology 1983;149:429.

30. Fuster V, Stein B, Ambrose JA, et al: Atherosclerotic plaque rupture and thrombosis: evolving concepts. Circulation 1990;82(suppl II):II-47.

31. Becker GJ, Holden RW, Rabe FE: Contrast extravasation from a Gore-Tex graft: A complication of thrombolytic therapy. AJR 1984;142:573.

32. Eisenberg, RL Bank WO, Hedgkock MW: Renal failure after major angiography can be avoided with hydration. AJR 1981;136:855.

33. Lambert GW, Cook PS, Gardiner GA, Regan JR: Spontaneous splenic rupture associated with thrombolytic therapy and/or concomitant heparin anticoagulation. Cardiovasc Intervent Radiol 1992;15:177.

34. Van Breda A, Groar RA, Katzen BT, et al: Relative cost-effectiveness of urokinase versus streptokinase in the treatment of peripheral vascular disease. JVIR 1991;2:77.

35. Janosik JE, Bettmann MA, Kaul AF, Souney PF: Therapeutic alternatives for subacute peripheral arterial occlusion: Comparison by outcome, length of stay, and hospital charges. Invest Radiol 1991; 26:921.

36. Traughber PD, Cook PS, Micklos TJ, Miller FJ: Intraarterial fibrinolytic therapy for popliteal and tibial artery obstruction: Comparison of streptokinase to urokinase. AJR 1987;149:543.

37. Belkin M, Belkin B, Buckman CA, et al: Intraarterial fibrinolytic therapy: efficacy of streptokinase vs urokinase. Arch Surg 1986;121:769.

38. Kandarpa K, Chopra PS, Aruny JE, et al: Intraarterial thrombolysis of lower extremity occlusions: A prospective, randomized comparison of forced periodic infusion and conventional slow continuous infusion. Radiology 1993;188:861.

39. McNamara TO, Fischer JR: Thrombolysis in peripheral arterial and graft occlusions: Improved results using high dose urokinase. AJR 1985; 144:764.

40. Gardiner GA, Koltun W, Kandarpa K, et al: Thrombolysis of occluded femoropopliteal grafts. AJR 1986;147:621.

41. McNamara TO: Thrombolysis as an alternative initial therapy for the acutely ischemic limb. Semin Vasc Surg 1992;5:89.

42. Physicians' Desk Reference, 41st ed. Oradell, NJ: Medical Economics Company, 1987.

26

Cost-Effectiveness of Thrombolytic Agents in Peripheral Arterial Occlusion

KENNETH OURIEL
MICK KOLASSA

The use of thrombolytic therapy has been criticized on the basis of increased costs associated with the lytic agent.[1] The cost of the agent, however, is only one of the many parameters determining the economic impact of thrombolysis. Devices necessary to deliver the agent, professional fees, and technical charges must all be in the equation. Similarly, the effectiveness of thrombolytic intervention must be compared with that of standard intervention. A logical and thorough analysis of cost-effectiveness must weigh the economic impact with clinical benefit. Decisions regarding the appropriate use of thrombolytic intervention await the demonstration of substantial advantages in the cost-benefit ratio.

CONCEPT OF COSTS VERSUS CHARGES

An important factor in the determination of the economic impact of a pharmaceutical agent is the cost of that agent to the consumer. A major problem thwarting the estimation of these costs is their dependence on who is paying for the patient's care. For example, the government is paying the hospital when the patient has Medicare insurance coverage. The amount of the payment is determined under the schedule of diagnosis-related groups (DRGs) and is relatively independent of the resources used by the hospital. In the setting of Medicare reimbursement, it is the cost of the pharmaceutical agent to the patient that determines economic impact. By contrast, the DRG system is not usually invoked when a patient does not have third-party coverage for hospital care. In these cases of "self-pay" reimbursement, it is the patient who must bear the cost of any intervention. Hospitals may mark up the charge of a particular pharmaceutical agent as much as 100 percent. The economic impact of the agent is best estimated by "hospital cost" in the setting of Medicare reimbursement but is estimated by "hospital charges" when care is rendered outside the DRG system. This irregularity makes the estimation of economic impact imprecise unless the reimbursement distribution of the patient population is taken into consideration. Fortunately, the care of the vast majority of patients requiring thrombolysis for arterial ischemia is rendered under a DRG-based system. Economic impact is best estimated by tabulating hospital cost data rather than charges.

ECONOMICS OF VARIOUS THROMBOLYTIC AGENTS

Scant information exists in the literature with regard to comparisons of different thrombolytic agents in the peripheral vascular setting. Most studies have focused on coronary thrombolysis, comparing streptokinase with recombinant tissue plasminogen activator (rt-PA), urokinase, or acylated

Table 26-1. Comparative Costs of Thrombolytic Agents, Data from In Vitro Perfusion Studies.

	Streptokinase	Urokinase	rt-PA
Percent lysis at 30 min.	10%	31%	54%
Relative cost of agent	100	280	490
Cost-effectiveness	10	9	9

Note: Cost-effectiveness was calculated as the relative cost required to lyse 1 percent of the thrombus after 30 minutes.

plasminogen-streptokinase complex (APSAC).[2,3] The lack of a standardized method of determining the in vivo activity of the different agents makes any attempt at cost comparison difficult, since there are no accurate means to compare the cost of similar doses of each agent.

We have used in vitro activity data to provide an approximation of cost comparisons between streptokinase, urokinase, and rt-PA. Retracted human whole-blood clots were packed into polytetrafluoroethylene graft segments 5 cm in length. Perfusion with heparinized blood was instituted, concurrent with infusion of lytic agents through a microcatheter placed directly into the clot. Cost comparisons could be calculated as the cost of lytic agent required to lyse a given volume of thrombus (Table 26-1). Although rt-PA was associated with the most rapid lytic rate, its cost was also the greatest. Urokinase and rt-PA were the most cost-effective agents in our laboratory evaluation; streptokinase was the least.

Van Breda et al.[4] examined the costs and benefits associated with urokinase and streptokinase therapy in the setting of peripheral arterial occlusion. The experience of two institutions were compared: Alexandria Hospital and the Cleveland Clinic. The cost of therapy was greater at the Cleveland Clinic for all modalities studied. Despite the greater costs of urokinase compared with streptokinase, the total cost of care was less with the more expensive agent. When expressed as the cost per therapeutic success, urokinase was less expensive than streptokinase by a factor of 0.73 and 0.32 at the two hospitals.

A study by Janosik and colleagues[5] compared the resources used when patients with peripheral arterial occlusions of less than 30 days' duration were treated with surgery, urokinase, or streptokinase. The length of stay was identical for surgery and streptokinase, averaging 21 days. Urokinase, however, was associated with a significant reduction in hospitalization, averaging 11.5 days ($p < 0.001$). Although the cost of the thrombolytic agent used in the urokinase patients was almost 10 times that in the streptokinase patients, the total hospital charges were similar (Table 26-2). Of note, patients treated with surgery had a mean cost of hospitalization not different from the two thrombolytic groups. A subgroup analysis was then tabulated, subcategorizing the data on the basis of therapeutic outcome. The total hospital charges were equal in the streptokinase patients, irrespective of whether the agent was successful in restoring arterial patency. By contrast, the charges associated with a urokinase therapeutic failure were over twice the charges associated with a urokinase success ($16,818 versus $40,295).

LIMITATIONS OF THE ECONOMIC STUDIES

The results of these studies must be evaluated in the context of marked differences in the cost of the agents within geographic areas, as well as differences in the cost of individual agents over time. For example, the cost of streptokinase may vary by a factor of 1.5 between two institutions just miles apart. Similarly, the cost may vary substantially from one year to the next, especially when major shifts in distribution occur. This phenomenon was observed when a new company began distributing streptokinase in the early 1990s and the cost to some hospitals rose over 300 percent. A third factor that confounds cost-comparison studies relates to inflationary trends in currency. Adjustments for inflation should be made in any economic analysis, and the data should be specified in terms of dollars of a given calendar year (e.g., "1990 U.S. dollars"). Even with these concerns accounted for, a remaining issue of contention is the choice of the most appropriate economic index with which to standardize inflationary trends. Some of the indices include the consumer price index, the producer price index, the rate of inflation, and

Table 26-2. Retrospective Comparison Data—Surgery Versus Thrombolysis

	Length of Stay	Cost of Agent	Total Hospital Charges
Surgery	21.1	—	$25,336
Streptokinase	21.3	$690	$25,978
Urokinase	11.5	$6,429	$22,203

Reprinted with permission from Janosik JE, Bettmann MA, Kaul AF, Sonney PF: Therapeutic alternatives for subacute peripheral arterial occlusion: Comparison by outcome, length of stay, and hospital charges. Invest Radiol 1991;26:921.

various indices specific to the health care industry. The value of each index is unique and may differ considerably from the other indices over time.

RANDOMIZED COMPARISONS OF THROMBOLYSIS WITH SURGERY

At the present time, surgical intervention must be considered to be the standard with which to compare the results of thrombolytic therapy. The results of different treatment modalities are best achieved through a randomized trial. As such, four randomized comparisons of surgery and thrombolysis have been completed. A small trial comparing surgical thrombectomy and thrombolysis appeared in the British literature in 1992.[6] The size of this series, and its size precluded any meaningful conclusions relating to the two treatment modalities. The Rochester trial was a larger study that compared the results of urokinase thrombolysis and surgery in the initial management of acute arterial occlusion.[7] The STILE trial (surgery versus thrombolysis for ischemia of the lower extremity) was a multicenter study that randomized patients to urokinase, rt-PA, or surgery.[8] The STILE trial appeared in the literature just 3 months after the Rochester trial. A final study, the TOPAS trial (thrombolysis or peripheral arterial surgery), compared recombinant urokinase with surgery in a protocol analogous to that of the Rochester trial and was conducted on a multicenter, international level. The results of the TOPAS trial are not available at the time of this writing.

The Rochester trial randomized 114 patients to urokinase (57 patients) or surgery (57 patients) in the initial treatment of limb-threatening ischemia of less than 7 days' duration. Thrombolysis was followed by an operative procedure in two-thirds of the thrombolytic group, directed at repair of an unmasked anatomic lesion responsible for the occlusive event. There were no differences observed in the rate of amputation, averaging approximately 20 percent at 1 year of follow-up. The 1-year survival rate was greater in the thrombolytic treatment group (84 versus 58 percent; $p = 0.01$). The mortality difference appeared to be associated with a higher incidence of in-hospital cardiopulmonary complications in the surgical group.

The STILE trial comprised 393 patients with peripheral arterial occlusive disease randomized to urokinase, rt-PA, or surgery. The primary inclusion criterion was a change in symptomatology over the previous 6 months. As such, the length of time between worsening symptoms and randomization averaged almost 2 months. Several conclusions were drawn from an analysis of the STILE data. First, there was no clinical difference in the results of rt-PA or urokinase thrombolysis. Second, patients with acute ischemia of less than 14 days' duration had a lower rate of amputation with thrombolysis than with surgery (11.1 versus 30.0 percent at 6 months; $p = 0.01$). By contrast, patients with more chronic symptoms had a greater risk of amputation with thrombolytic intervention (12.1 versus 3.0 percent at 6 months; $p = 0.01$). Mortality rates were not significantly different in the two treatment groups, irrespective of whether the patient presented before or after 14 days of worsening symptoms.

ECONOMIC ANALYSIS OF RANDOMIZED GROUPS

Many of the limitations of economic data obtained from retrospective series are avoided when cost

Table 26-3. Comparison of Hospital Costs

	Thrombolytic Group (n = 57)	Operative Group (n = 57)
Nonpharmaceutical costs	$17,176 ± $4328	$16,365 ± $4408
Medication, including urokinase	$ 4995 ± $630	$ 3410 ± $764
Medication, urokinase only	$ 2653 ± $243	0
Total costs	$22,171 ± $4959	$19,775 ± $5253

Table 26-4. Comparison of Charges

	Thrombolytic Group	Operative Group
Total hospital charges	$38,377 ± $8583	$45,447 ± $9622
Medication with urokinase	$ 7259 ± $916	$ 4790 ± $1073
Urokinase alone	$ 3854 ± $353	0
No. of primary consultations	1.3	1.8
No. of secondary consultations	3.0	1.4
Total consultation fees	$ 186 ± $76	$ 314 ± $100
Surgeon fees	$ 863 ± $173	$ 1417 ± $127
Anesthesiologist fees	$ 787 ± $165	$ 1356 ± $227
Radiologist fees	$ 609 ± $21	$ 428 ± $7
Total fees	$ 2445 ± $315	$ 3517 ± $318
Total charges	$40,823 ± $8764	$41,930 ± $10,398

Table 26-5. Cost-effectiveness of Thrombolytic and Operative Therapy

	Thrombolysis	Operation
Life expectancy (years)	12.4 ± 1.3	9.4 ± 1.3
Cost per life saved	$49,508	$70,295
Cost per life-year saved	$ 3980	$ 7489

and charge information is available from a randomized trial. The ability to cull hospital cost and physician charge data from the Rochester trial provided the opportunity to compare the resource utilization of urokinase and surgery in similar groups of patients. Hospital costs and professional fees were summed to provide an index of the total economic impact of one therapy over another. These data are tabulated in Table 26-3 and document a slight, statistically insignificant increase in the hospital expenditures associated with urokinase therapy, concurrent with a significant decrease in the professional fees. Although the economic data were generated for the first hospital admission only, the lack of differences in the rate of subsequent admission, the frequency of subsequent operative interventions, and the long-term amputation rate would suggest that differences in the use of economic resources is unlikely through at least 1 year of follow-up (Tables 26-4 and 26-5).

CONCLUSIONS

The available data would suggest that, at present, urokinase is the most cost-efficient agent in the armamentarium of the vascular specialist. The lower cost of streptokinase is overshadowed by a lower rate of success, while the higher cost of rt-PA is not sufficiently compensated by greater effectiveness. A direct comparison of the economic impact of surgery versus thrombolysis suggests that the costs of the two treatment modalities are approximately equal in the setting of acute peripheral arterial occlusion. The results of the STILE trial would suggest that surgery may be more efficient in the setting of more chronic occlusions, specifically, those of greater than 2 weeks' duration.

REFERENCES

1. Faggioli GL, Peer RM, Pedrini L, et al: Failure of thrombolytic therapy to improve long-term vascular patency. J Vasc Surg 1994;19:289.
2. Gruppo Italiano per lo Studio della Streptochinasi nell'Infarto Miocardico (GISSI): Long-term effects of intravenous thrombolysis in acute myocardial infarction: Final report of the GISSI study. Lancet 1987;2:871.
3. Mueller HS, Rao AK, Forman SA, TIMI Investigators: Thrombolysis in myocardial infarction (TIMI): Comparative studies of coronary reperfusion and systemic fibrinogenolysis with two forms of recombinant tissue-type plasminogen activator. J Am Coll Cardiol 1987;10:479.
4. van Breda A, Graor RA, Katzen BT, et al: Relative cost-effectiveness of urokinase versus streptokinase in the treatment of peripheral vascular disease. JVIR 1991;2:77.
5. Janosik JE, Bettmann MA, Kaul AF, Souney PF: Therapeutic alternatives for subacute peripheral arterial occlusion: Comparison by outcome, length of stay, and hospital charges. Invest Radiol 1991;26:921.
6. Nilsson L, Albrechtsson U, Jonung T, et al: Surgical treatment versus thrombolysis in acute arterial occlusion: a randomized controlled study. Eur J Vasc Surg 1992;6:189.
7. Ouriel K, Shortell CK, DeWeese JA, et al: A comparison of thrombolytic therapy with operative revascularization in the treatment of acute peripheral arterial ischemia. J Vasc Surg 1994;19:1021.
8. The STILE Investigators: Results of a prospective randomized trial evaluating surgery versus thrombolysis for ischemia of the lowest extremity: The STILE trial. Ann Surg 1994;220:251.

Lower Extremity Venous Disease

Venous Stasis Disease

JOHN J. BERGAN

Varicose veins, telangiectatic blemishes, and dilated, tortuous, flat, blue-green reticular veins are not normal physical findings. They are evidence of venous dysfunction. This, in the lower extremities, may manifest itself in a number of different ways. These include the visible findings mentioned above as well as the production of disabling pain, eczematoid dermatitis, brawny ankle induration, and intractable cutaneous ulceration. It is the visible presence of varicose veins that is subtle evidence for the manifestations of venous stasis which may precede severe complications of venous insufficiency.

Venous dysfunction has occupied the attention of many great minds. These include Ambrose Paré, John Hunter, Frederich Trendelenburg, and John Homans. Homans is of particular importance because it was he who tied development of severe sequelae of venous dysfunction to prior deep venous thrombosis,[1] hence the condition of brawny induration, lipodermatosclerosis, and the medial and lateral ankle hyperpigmentation in gaiter areas and characteristic punched-out ulceration that has been referred to as the *postphlebitic* or *postthrombotic state*.

Gradually, it has become known that the disability produced by these conditions and the advanced skin changes are not dependent on a prior episode of deep venous thrombosis.[2] This new knowledge has important therapeutic implications. If the advanced condition of venous stasis is referred to as *chronic venous insufficiency* or, even better, *chronic venous dysfunction*, it is implied that correction can be obtained through surgical or pharmacologic manipulation. If the term *postphlebitic state*

is used, the implication is that there is very little that can be done for the patient or his or her limb.[3] Amplification and elucidation of the details of this distinction are the subject of this chapter.

SIGNS AND SYMPTOMS

Early evidence of venous dysfunction, including varicose veins, is very common and may occur in up to 60 percent of adults. The incidence of these findings increases with advancing age.[4,5] The ultimate target of venous insufficiency is the skin (Fig. 27-1). Changes produced there are entirely predictable. Early darkening of the skin occurs, and it has been found that this is due to hemosiderin deposition. This characteristically occurs in areas of most severe venous hypertension, and these are in the most dependent portions of the leg and ankle, usually on the medial aspect and in the region of perforating veins connected to the posterior arch vein and/or the greater saphenous circulation.[6] Nearly 70 percent of patients are said to have symptoms from such varicosities, but careful evaluation of the population under study will reveal that 98 percent of patients with clinically relevant venous changes have symptoms.[7,8]

Aching pain is the most common symptom, and this is related to pressure on the dense network of somatic nerve fibers present in subcutaneous tissues adjacent to affected veins.[9] Symptoms may be aggravated during periods of limb hyperemia such as warm ambient temperatures combined with high humidity during prolonged standing or

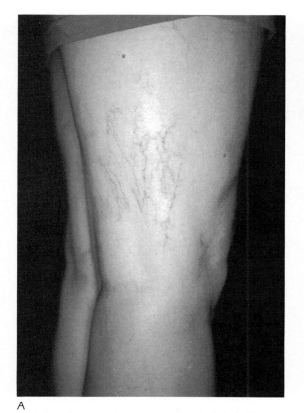

A

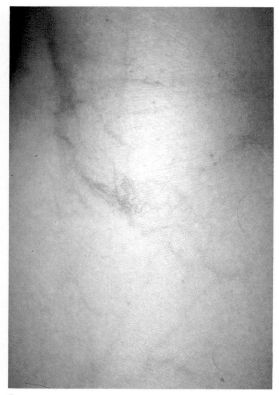

B

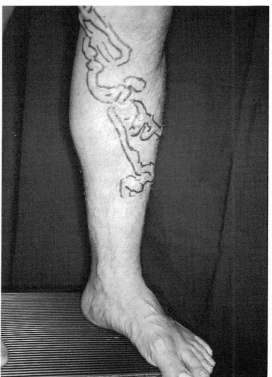

C

Figure 27-1. It is helpful to understand that telangiec-tasias as shown in **A**, reticular varicosities as shown in **B**, and varicose veins as shown in **C** are anatomically and physiologically elongated, dilated veins with incompetent valves that are of hereditary origin and are acted on by hormonal influences and hydrostatic and hydrodynamic forces.

prolonged sitting.[10] Pain also may be due to nociceptor stimulation of the distended vein wall or to an accumulation of tissue metabolites with a subsequent increase in interstitial pressure.[11]

A confusing aspect to venous dysfunction is that some patients, particularly men, have been found to have significant valvular dysfunction and the presence of protuberant, saccular varicosities without any symptoms. This may be attributed to success of the calf muscle pump to compensate for venous reflux and also the absence of female hormonal stimuli to venous distension. Another confusing factor in studying patients with venous dysfunction is the fact that cutaneous pathologic changes produced by chronic venous insufficiency, although related to increases in venous pressure, are not linearly related to it.[12] Identical venous pressure data can be found in limbs with and without the stigmata of chronic venous dysfunction.

Venous pressure measurement is historically important, but because of the observed facts mentioned earlier, its use has given way to more direct imaging techniques in evaluation of dysfunction. Pressure studies did show that there are two sources of venous hypertension. The first is gravitational and is a result of venous blood coursing in a distal direction down linear axial venous segments.[13] This is referred to as *hydrostatic pressure* and is the weight of the blood column from the right atrium. The highest pressure generated by this mechanism is evident at the ankle and foot, where measurements are expressed in centimeters of water or millimeters of mercury.

The second source of venous hypertension is dynamic. It is the force of muscular contraction, usually contained within the compartments of the leg. In the abnormal state, this pressure is transmitted through perforating veins that penetrate the deep crural fascia. Although many of these perforating veins have no valves, their anatomic angulation prevents reflux into the subcutaneous tissues under normal conditions. Valves that are present in some of the perforating veins allow blood flow to be directed from the superficial to the deep tissues. Both the anatomic angulation and the valves may be referred to as *check mechanisms* that protect the venules of the subcutaneous tissue and skin from compartmental hypertension. Failure of this mechanism allows the intercompartmental forces to be transmitted directly to unsupported subcutaneous veins and dermal capillaries.[14] These pressures are expressed in hundreds of millimeters of mercury.[15]

An understanding of the source of venous hypertension and its differentiation into hydrostatic and hydrodynamic is important. The presence of hydrostatic reflux implies surgical correction of this abnormality, and the presence of hydrodynamic reflux implies ablation of the perforating vein mechanism which allows exposure of the subcutaneous circulation to compartmental pressures.

HORMONAL INFLUENCE

Circumstantial evidence and scientific observations confirm the fact that profound hormonal influences affect venous function. In particular, progesterone liberated by the corpus luteum stabilizes the uterus by causing relaxation of smooth muscle fibers. This effect directly influences venous function. The result is passive venous dilation, which, in many instances, causes valvular dysfunction. The multiparous woman with some venous dysfunction will know that she is experiencing a new pregnancy when new varicose veins appear even before the first menstrual period is missed.

Epidemiologic studies show an increased incidence of varicose veins in women who have been pregnant.[16,17] In fact, some studies show that as few as 12 percent of women with varicose veins have never been pregnant.[18] As many as 80 percent of patients develop their varicose veins during the first trimester. This is important because it is at this time that the uterus is only slightly enlarged.[19,20] The obstructive effects of the uterus on the venous circulation do not develop until the second and third trimesters. Venous distensibility increases during pregnancy, and this has been noted both in the forearm and in calf veins.[21] The distensibility observed is greater in the calf veins than in the forearm and returns to normal by the eighth postpartum week. Although progesterone is implicated in the first appearance of varicosities in pregnancy, estrogen also has profound effects. It produces the relaxation of smooth muscle and a softening of collagen fibers.[22,23] Further, the estrogen/progesterone ratio influences venous distensibility. This ratio may explain the predominance of venous insufficiency symptoms on the first day of a menstrual period when there is a profound shift from the progesterone phase of the menstrual cycle to the estrogen phase.[24,25]

INFLUENCE OF HEREDITY

The familial incidence of varicose veins has been identified and described by many, but it has not been uniformly characterized.[26] Most studies are not conclusive but tend toward a demonstration of a simple dominant type of inheritance. Other studies describe a recessive characteristic.[27] Rose and Ahmed[19] postulate an inherited alteration in vein wall collagen and/or elastin. They have observed an increased collagen deposition with separation of smooth muscle cells as a major etiologic precursor to the development of varicose veins.

Although relationships are not clear, the conclusion of multiple studies of population groups documents a significant relationship between heredity and development of varicosities. In addition, there is a significant difference in the incidence of varicose veins among different cultures, with a rarity of varicosities in non-Westernized populations.[28]

CUTANEOUS STIGMATA OF VENOUS DYSFUNCTION

Although elevated distal venous pressure has been linked to venous ulceration, more recent observations relative to lower extremity white blood cell trapping in situations of venous hypertension are more informative.[29] Such white cell trapping is found to be excessive in limbs with lipodermatosclerosis.[30] If leukocytes, when trapped, are then activated, it would be expected that proteolytic enzymes would be released and free radical activity observed. Such a phenomenon would be the fundamental basic common pathophysiologic pathway that explains tissue damage in myocardial ischemia, stroke, shock, and other conditions.[31] Leukocyte trapping and then release also would produce a reperfusion phenomenon, the effects of which in limbs, mesentery, and myocardium have already been shown to be due to white cell trapping and activation.[32]

Studies have shown that the predominant infiltrating cells in limbs with lipodermatosclerosis are T lymphocytes and macrophages.[33] However, it is uncertain whether this accumulation of macrophages and T cells is the cause of chronic venous insufficiency or an effect of it. An inflammatory response to tissue damage from any cause would lead to similar findings.

DIAGNOSTIC EVALUATION IN VENOUS DYSFUNCTION

Physical examination reveals the evidence of venous varicosities and, in many instances, of axial reflux through saphenous trunks. Visual examination can be supplemented by noting a downward-going impulse on coughing. Tapping the venous column of blood also demonstrates pressure transmission through the static column to incompetent distal veins. Also, historically important tests such as the Perthes test for deep venous occlusion[34] and the Brodie-Trendelenburg test of axial reflux are heavily quoted.[35,36] These tests have been replaced by in-office use of the continuous-wave, hand-held Doppler instrument supplemented by duplex evaluation.[37,38] The hand-held Doppler can confirm an impression of saphenous reflux, and this, in turn, dictates the operative procedure to be performed in a given patient. Duplex technology more precisely defines which veins are refluxing by imaging the superficial and deep veins. The duplex examination is commonly done with the patient supine, but this gives an erroneous evaluation of reflux. In the supine position, even when there is no flow, the valves remain open. Valve closure requires a reversal of flow with a pressure gradient that is higher proximally than distally.[39] Thus the duplex examination should be done with the patient standing or in the markedly trunk-elevated position.[40,41]

As the two ultrasound modes of direct evaluation of venous function have emerged, other earlier, indirect tests have been discarded. Though they may have utility in specific situations, their clinical importance has been displaced in the evaluation of venous insufficiency (Table 27-1). These methods include photoplethysmography (PPG), light reflection rheography (LRR), mercury strain gauge plethysmography (MSG), and newer, but still unproven, air plethysmography (APG).

Table 27-1. Methods of Assessing Venous Stasis

Testing Modality	Detects Chronic Obstruction	Detects Reflux	Useful Physiologically	Useful Clinically
Dynamic venous pressure	No	Yes	Yes	No
Photoplethysmography (PPG)	No	Yes	Yes/no	Yes
Light reflection rheography (LLR)	No	Yes	Yes/no	Yes
Air plethysmography	Yes	Yes	Yes	No
Phlebography, ascending	Yes	No	No	Yes
Phlebography, descending	Yes	Yes	No	Yes
MRI phlebography	Yes	No	No	Yes
Continuous-wave Doppler	Yes*	Yes	No	Yes
Duplex, supine	Yes	No	No	No
Duplex, standing	No	Yes	Yes/no	Yes

*Requires experience.

It is important in deciding on therapy in a limb with chronic venous insufficiency to know which pathologic process, obstruction or reflux, is dominant. While reflux is easily detected by physical examination, and hand-held Doppler, and confirmed by duplex techniques, functional obstruction is much more difficult to assess. Further, it is important to know whether one or both of these is present in each major vein segment. The PPG, LRR, MSG, and APG instruments do not provide this information. Only imaging techniques can identify the anatomic location of obstructions. Physiologic venous obstruction is more difficult to ascertain, and no single method emerges that is entirely reliable. At present, imaging techniques include magnetic resonance phlebography, which is totally patient acceptable, radiologic contrast phlebography, which provides anatomic information as well as physiologic venous pressure changes before and after limb exercise, and duplex evaluation, which can identify obstruction. When a surgical decision is made toward reconstruction of major veins by valvuloplasty or bypass, phlebography is mandatory. This must be done in both the ascending and descending modes before surgical therapy.

OPTIONS FOR TREATMENT

Physical examination and history taking supplemented by noninvasive evaluation will determine the need for therapy. Options in therapy include a conservative, nonoperative approach that employs various techniques of compression therapy, a minimally invasive approach to ablation of abnormally functioning vein segments as achieved by sclerotherapy, or detachment with or without removal of malfunctioning veins, venous ligation, and stripping. Improved understanding of cellular mechanisms in venous disease will make a pharmacologic approach to therapy possible in the future.

What is new in treatment of venous stasis is a rearranging of and modifications to older methodology.[42] What has not changed is that conservative treatment of chronic venous insufficiency always precedes consideration of intervention. Such conservative treatment relies on limb compression to counteract the effects of venous hypertension.[43] This is achieved by various forms of gradient elastic support, which does not affect intravascular pressure as much as it compresses interstitial tissue. In order of ascending pressure effects, external compression can be applied as support stockings, gradient elastic supports, long-stretch and short-stretch elastic bandages, gelatin-cast boots (Unna), and a most recent addition, the semirigid Velcro support (CircAid appliance). All the elastic supports should provide a progressively decreasing pressure from distal to proximal.[44]

Patients with class 1* venous insufficiency may derive benefit from simple over-the-counter

*Classification of Joint Councils of the American Vascular Societies, J Vasc Surg 1988;8:172.

support stockings. Those with class 2* venous insufficiency will require ankle pressures in the range of 20 to 30 mmHg, and those with class 3* venous insufficiency with present or healed ulcerations will require 40 mmHg ankle pressure. Treatment of stasis ulceration, complicated sepsis, and cellulitis demands more aggressive therapy. This will include bed rest, leg elevation, antibiotics and special wound care.[43] Organism-specific antibiotics tailored to bacteria cultured from the ulcer bed may be used, but tetracycline is thought to have a nonspecific effect on the cytokine activation phenomenon.

Specific drug therapy for venous insufficiency is not available in the United States. However, methylxanthines have a certain attraction. These improve red cell deformability and also, more important, white cell deformability. They inhibit alterations in the microvasculature induced by interleuken 2 (IL-2). Placebo-controlled trials have suggested a more rapid rate of healing and more complete healing in a shorter time in drug-treated individuals compared with placebo-treated controls.[45,46]

In a multi-institutional cooperative study, oxypentoxifylline, 400 mg three times a day orally, was compared with placebo. Complete healing of the ulcers occurred in 28 of 30 limbs in which the patients received the active agent. This was compared with 12 of 42 limbs in patients treated with placebo ($p < 0.01$).

Following ulcer healing, ulcer recurrence is the rule rather than the exception, although Porter's group[43] has reported an exceptional recurrence rate of only 29 percent at 5 years.

OPERATIVE INTERVENTION

While conservative therapy is being pursued or ulcer healing achieved, appropriate diagnostic studies should reveal patterns of venous reflux or segments of venous occlusion so that specific therapy can be prescribed for the individual limb being examined (Table 27-2). As mentioned earlier, imaging techniques must be used to detect obstruction because maximum venous outflow studies may prove inaccurate as a result of profuse collateralization. Imaging by duplex Doppler will suffice

Table 27-2. Options for Treatment of Venous Stasis

Compression, support
Unna boot, CircAid
Proximal ligation (with sclerotherapy, phlebectomy)
Proximal stripping (with phlebectomy)
Perforator interruption (superficial, subfascial, subfascial endoscopic)
Valveplasty (open, external, external angioscope-assisted)
Bypass of obstruction

for detection of reflux if the examination is carried out in the standing individual. Such noninvasive imaging may prove to be the only testing necessary beyond the hand-held, continuous-wave Doppler instrument if superficial venous ablation is contemplated. If direct venous reconstruction by bypass or valvuloplasty techniques is planned, ascending and descending phlebography will be requisite.

Superficial reflux may be the only abnormality uncovered by diagnostic testing.[42] This is almost always true in simple varicose veins and telangiectasias. It is also a surprising fact that in advanced chronic venous stasis, superficial reflux may be the only abnormality present. Obviously, correction of such pathophysiology will go a long way toward permanent relief of the chronic venous dysfunction and its cutaneous effects. Using duplex technology, Menzoian[48] found that in 95 extremities with current venous ulceration, 16.8 percent had only superficial incompetence, and another 19 percent showed superficial incompetence combined with perforator incompetence. Similarly, the Middlesex group, in a study of 118 limbs, found that "in just over half of the patients with venous ulceration, the disease was confined to the superficial venous system."[49]

In our own study of 58 limbs with class 3 venous insufficiency, 10 (17 percent) exhibited only superficial reflux, and superficial reflux was a major contributor to the chronic venous dysfunction in another 17 limbs. Of some importance is the fact that primary, nonthrombotic deep (superficial femoral vein and popliteal vein) incompetence may accompany superficial reflux. This is explained by reflux proceeding distally down the greater saphenous vein and reentering perforating veins in a proper direction, thus overloading the deep venous system.[50] Presumably, this causes dilatation and elongation of the deep vessels so that their valves become incompetent. Our own study of limbs following greater saphenous vein stripping in which superficial femoral and popliteal venous incompetence was present has revealed correction of the deep reflux by superficial venous stripping in a vast majority of limbs.[51]

Dealing with perforating veins has been of major concern since the early 1940s when Cockett and Linton emphasized their importance.[52] Direct surgical attack, especially using Linton's technique, has fallen into disfavor because of wound healing complications occurring postoperatively. A shearing operation with subcutaneous instrument disruption of perforating veins has been advocated by DePalma.[53,54] However, video techniques of direct visualization through small-diameter scopes has allowed subfascial exploration with minimal invasion to come into current use.[55,56] This operation, done with a vertical proximal incision, accomplishes the objective of perforator vein interruption on an outpatient basis.

VENOUS RECONSTRUCTION

Perforator interruption combined with superficial venous ablation has been effective in controlling venous ulceration in 75 to 85 percent of patients. However, emphasis on failures of this technique has led to a continuing interest in developing techniques of venous reconstruction. A significant breakthrough in direct venous reconstruction was the invention of valvuloplasty by Kistner in 1968 and the general recognition of this procedure after 1975.[57] Late evaluation of direct valve reconstruction indicates good to excellent long-term results in over 80 percent of the patients.[58]

One cannot overestimate the contributions of Kistner. Next, he invented the technique of directing the incompetent venous stream through a competent proximal valve: venous segment transfer. After Kistner's developments, surgeons were provided with an armamentarium of procedures that included the venous bypass of Palma,[59] a modification of that procedure using externally supported prosthetic grafts,[60] direct valvuloplasty (of Kistner), and venous segment transfer (of Kistner). Further, external valve repair as performed by a number of techniques, including monitoring

by endoscopic control, suggests that there will be a renewed interest in this form of treatment of venous insufficiency. These procedures, preceded by direct, noninvasive visualization of reflux and/or obstruction, provide an acceptable therapeutic algorithm for venous stasis disease.

Axillary-to-popliteal autotransplantation of valve-containing venous segments has been interesting since the early observations of Taheri.[61] While excellent results have been reported from some clinics, verification of these by other groups will require time and effort.

CONCLUSIONS

The decade of the 1980s provided a considerable advance in understanding of venous pathophysiology. This is being utilized in the 1990s. Not only have the abnormal venous hemodynamics been uncovered by application of physiologic investigations, but cellular mechanisms involved in chronic venous dysfunction also have been partially elucidated. Future research directions will undoubtedly include investigation of vein wall, venous valve, and perivenous tissue functions. Predictably, in therapy, more direct surgical approaches will be applied with increasing success. Further, wider application of the principle of correcting deep venous incompetence by superficial venous ablation will allow a larger number of patients with severe chronic venous dysfunction to be treated effectively.

REFERENCES

1. Homans J: The late results of femoral thrombophlebitis and their treatment. N Engl J Med 1946;235:249.
2. Browse NL, Burnand KG: The postphlebitic syndrome: A new look. *In* Bergan JJ, Yao JST (eds): Venous Problems. Chicago, Year Book Medical Publishers, 1978, pp 395–404.
3. Dean R, Yao J, Brewster D. (eds): Diagnosis and Treatment of Vascular Disorders. Philadelphia, JB Lippincott, 1995.
4. Widmer LK: Peripheral Venous Disorders: Prevalence and Sociomedical Importance Observations in 4529 Apparently Healthy Persons (Basic Study III). Bern, Hans Huber, 1978.

5. Dodd H, Cockett FB: The Pathology and Surgery of the Veins of the Lower Limbs. London, Churchill-Livingstone, 1976.

6. Bergan JJ: Patterns of venous varicosities. *In* Bergan JJ, Goldman MP (eds): Varicose Veins and Telangiectasias: Diagnosis and Treatment. St. Louis, Quality Medical Publishing, 1993.

7. Wilder CS: Prevalence of selected chronic circulatory conditions. Vital Health Stat 1974;94:1.

8. Fischer H: Socioepidemiological study on distribution of venous disorders among a residental population. Int Angiol 1984;3:89.

9. Goldman MP, Weiss RA, Bergan JJ: Treatment of varicose veins: A review of varicose veins. J Am Acad Derm 1994;31:393.

10. Conrad P: Painful legs: The GP's dilemma. Austral Fam Physician 1980;9:691.

11. Cockett FB, Thomas ML: The iliac compression syndrome. Br J Surg 1965;52:816.

12. Moulton S, Bergan JJ, Beeman S, et al: Gravitational reflux does not correlate with clinical status of venous stasis. Phlebology 1993;8:2.

13. Bjordal RI: Hemodynamic studies of varicose veins and the postthrombotic syndrome. *In* Hobbs JT (ed): The Treatment of Venous Disorders. London, MTP Press, 1977, pp 37–56.

14. Arnoldi CC: Venous pressure in patients with valvular incompetence of the veins of the lower limb. Acta Chir Scand 1966;132:628.

15. Bergan JJ: New developments in the surgical treatment of venous disease. J Cardiovasc Surg 1993; 1:624.

16. Maffei FHA, Magaldi C, Pinho SZ, et al: Varicose veins and chronic venous insufficiency in Brazil: Prevalence among 1755 inhabitants of a country town. Int J Epidemiol 1986;15:210.

17. Brand FN, Dannenberg AL, Abbott RD, Kannel WB: The epidemiology of varicose veins: The Framingham Study. Am J Preventive Med 1988; 4:96.

18. Henry MEF, Corless C: The incidence of varicose veins in Ireland. Phlebology 1989;4:133.

19. Rose SS, Ahmed A: Some thoughts on the aetiology of varicose veins. Int J Cardiovasc Surg 1985;27:584.

20. McCausland AM: Varicose veins in pregnancy. Cal West Med 1939;50:258.

21. Barwin BN, Roddie IC: Venous distensibility during pregnancy determined by graded venous congestion. Am J Obstet Gynecol 1976;125:921.

22. Wahl LM: Hormonal regulation of macrophage collagenase activity. Biochem Biophys Res Commun 1977;74:838.

23. Woolley DE: On the sequential changes in levels of oestradiol and progesterone during pregnancy and parturition and collagenolytic activity. *In* Piez KA, Eddi AH (eds): Extracellular Matrix Biochemistry. New York, Elsevier Science, 1984.

24. McCausland AM, Holmes F, Trotter AD: Venous distensibility during the menstrual cycle. Am J Obstet Gynecol 1963;86:640.

25. Marazita AJD: The action of hormones on varicose veins in pregnancy. Med Rec 1946;159:422.

26. Arnoldi C: The heredity of venous insufficiency. Dan Med Bull 1958;5:169.

27. Troisier J, Le B: Etude genetique des varices. Ann Med Fr 1937;41:30.

28. Alexander CJ: The epidemiology of varicose veins. Med J Aust 1972;1:215.

29. Moyses C, Cederholm-Williams SA, Michel C: Haemoconcentration and the accumulation of white cells in the feet during venous stasis. Int J Microcirc Clin Exp 1987;5:311.

30. Thomas PRS, Nash GP, Dormandy JA: White cell accumulation in the dependent legs of patients with venous hypertension: A possible mechanism for trophic changes in the skin. Br Med J 1988;296:1693.

31. Schmid-Schonbein GW: Granulocyte: Friend or foe? NIPS 1988;3:6.

32. Scurr JH, Coleridge-Smith PD: Pathogenesis of venous ulceration. Phlebology Suppl 1992;13.

33. Scott HJ, Coleridge-Smith PD, Scurr JH: Histological study of white blood cells and their association with lipodermatosclerosis and venous ulceration. Br J Surg 1991;78:210.

34. Perthes G: Uber die operation der untershenkelvaricen nach Trendelenburg. Dtsch Med Wochenschr 1895;21:253.

35. Brodie B: Lectures Illustrative of Various Subjects in Pathology and Surgery, vol 12. London, Longmans, Green, 1840.

36. Trendelenburg J: Uber die unterbinding der vena saphena magna bei unter-schekelvaricen. Beitr Klir Chir 1890–91;7:195.

37. Hoare MC, Royle JP: Doppler ultrasound detection of saphenofemoral and saphenopopliteal incompetence and operative venography to ensure precise saphenopopliteal ligation. Aust NZ J Surg 1984;54:49.

38. Bergan JJ, Moulton SL, Poppiti R, Beeman S: Patient selection for surgery of varicose veins using venous reflux quantitation. *In* Veith FJ (ed): Current Critical Problems in Vascular Surgery 4. St. Louis, Quality Medical Publishers, 1992, pp 138–148.

39. van Bemmelen PS, Beach K, Bedford G, Strandness DE Jr: The mechanisms of venous valve closure. Arch Surg 1990;125:617.

40. van Bemmelen PS, Beach K, Bedford G, Strandness DE Jr: Quantitative segmental evaluation of venous valvular reflux with ultrasound scanning. J Vasc Surg 1989;10:425.

41. Vasdekis SN, Clarke GH, Nicolaides AN: Quantification of venous reflux by means of duplex scanning. J Vasc Surg 1989;10:670.

42. Bergan JJ: New developments in surgery of the venous system. J Cardiovasc Surg 1993;1:624.

43. Mayberry JC, Moneta GL, Taylor LM, Porter JM: Nonoperative treatment of venous ulceration. *In* Bergan JJ, Kistner RL (eds): Atlas of Venous Surgery. Philadelphia, WB Saunders Company, 1992.

44. Bergan JJ: Conrad Jobst and the development of pressure gradient therapy for venous disease. *In* Bergan JJ, Yao JST (eds): Surgery of the Veins. Orlando, Fla, Grune & Stratton, 1985, pp 529–540.

45. Weitgasser H: The use of pentoxifylline (Trental 400) in the treatment of leg ulcers: Results of a double-blind trial. Pharmatherapeutica 1983;3:143.

46. Barbarino C: Pentoxifylline in the treatment of venous ulcers of the leg. Am Med Res Opin 1992; 12:547.

47. Lees TH, Lambert D: Patterns of venous reflux in limbs with skin changes associated with chronic venous insufficiency. Br J Surg 1993;80:725.

48. Hanrahan LM, Araki CT, Rodriguez AA, et al: Distribution of valvular incompetence in patients with venous stasis ulceration. J Vasc Surg 1991; 13:805.

49. Shami SK, Sarin S, Cheatle TR, et al: Venous ulcers and the superficial venous system. J Vasc Surg 1993;17:487.

50. Hach W: Sekundare popliteal und femoralveneninsuffizienz, die Cockettschen Vv. perforantes und die paratibiale fasziotomie. Die Med Welt 1989;32.

51. Walsh JC, Bergan JJ, Beeman S, Comer TP: Femoral venous reflux is abolished by greater saphenous vein stripping. Ann Vasc Surg 1994;8:566.

52. Linton RR: The communicating veins of the lower leg and the operative technique for their ligation. Ann Surg 1938;107:582.

53. DePalma RG: Surgical therapy for venous stasis. Surgery 1975;76:910.

54. DePalma RG: Surgical therapy for venous stasis: Results of a modified Linton operation. Am J Surg 1979;137:810.

55. Jugenheimer M, Junginger TH: Endoscopic subfascial sectioning of incompetent perforating veins in treatment of primary varicosis. World J Surg 1992;16:971.

56. Fischer R: Erfahrungen mit der endoskopischen perforantensanierung. Phlebologie 1992;21:224.

57. Kistner RL: Surgical repair of the incompetent femoral vein valve. Arch Surg 1975;110:1336.

58. Kistner RL: Late results of venous valve repair. *In* Yao JST, Pearce WL (eds): Long-Term Results of Vascular Surgery. Philadelphia, WB Saunders Company, 1993, pp 451–466.

59. Palma EC, Esperon R: Vein transplants and grafts in the surgical treatment of the postphlebitic syndrome. J Cardiovasc Surg 1960;1:94.

60. Gruss JD: Zur modifikation des femoralisbypass nach may. VASA 1975;4:59.

61. Taheri SA, Lazar L, Elias S, et al: Surgical treatment of postphlebitic syndrome with vein valve transplant. Am J Surg 1982;144:221.

Deep Venous Thrombosis and Anticoagulation

RUSSELL D. HULL
GRAHAM F. PINEO

Pulmonary embolism is responsible for approximately 150,000 to 200,000 deaths per year in the United States.[2,3] Despite significant advances in the prevention and treatment of venous thromboembolism (venous thrombosis and pulmonary embolism), pulmonary embolism remains the most common preventable cause of hospital death.[1] Many patients who die from pulmonary embolism succumb suddenly or within 2 hours after the acute event, i.e., before therapy can be initiated or take effect.[4] Venous thromboembolism usually complicates the course of patients who are sick and hospitalized, but it also may affect ambulant and otherwise healthy individuals. It is therefore vital that efforts continue to find more effective and safer means of managing venous thromboembolism. Effective and safe means of prophylaxis against venous thromboembolism are now available in most high-risk patients.[5–7] Prophylaxis is more effective for preventing death and morbidity from venous thromboembolism than is the treatment of established disease.

PATHOGENESIS OF VENOUS THROMBOEMBOLISM

Deep venous thrombosis (DVT) usually arises in the deep veins of the calf muscles or less commonly in the proximal deep veins of the leg. DVT that remains confined to the calf veins is associated with a low risk of clinically important pulmonary embolism.[9–12] However, without treatment approximately 20 percent of calf vein thrombi extend into the proximal venous system,[13,14] where they may pose a serious and potentially life-threatening risk. Untreated proximal venous thrombosis is associated with a 10 percent risk of fatal pulmonary embolism and at least a 50 percent risk of pulmonary embolism or recurrent venous thrombosis.[11,12,15] Furthermore, the postphlebitic syndrome is associated with extensive proximal venous thrombosis and carries its own long-term morbidity.

Pulmonary emboli in most cases (90 percent) originate from thrombi in the deep venous system of the legs. Other less common sources of pulmonary emboli include the deep pelvic veins, renal veins, the inferior vena cava, the right side of the heart, and occasionally, axillary veins. It is now well established that clinically important pulmonary emboli arise from thrombi in the proximal deep veins of the legs.[16–20] The clinical significance of pulmonary embolism depends on the size of the embolus and the cardiorespiratory reserve of the patient.

It is widely accepted that venous thromboembolism is a single disorder.[21–23] Therefore, the diagnostic approach may be to the legs or the lungs, starting with the least invasive testing and proceeding to more invasive tests. The treatment of venous thrombosis or pulmonary embolism is basically the same.

CLINICAL FEATURES

Clinical features of venous thrombosis include leg pain, swelling, tenderness, discoloration, venous distension, prominence of the superficial veins, and the presence of a palpable cord (a palpable thrombosed vessel). The clinical diagnosis of venous thrombosis is very nonspecific because none of the symptoms or signs is unique and each may be caused by nonthrombotic disorders. The diagnosis is not confirmed by objective testing[24] in more than 50 percent of patients with a clinical suspicion of venous thrombosis. Furthermore, patients with relatively minor symptoms and signs (or none at all) may have extensive deep venous thrombosis with or without pulmonary embolism when the appropriate tests are performed. Thus objective testing is mandatory to confirm or exclude a diagnosis of venous thrombosis. The rare exception is the patient with phlegmasia cerulea dolens, in whom the diagnosis of massive iliofemoral thrombosis usually is clinically obvious. This syndrome occurs in less than 1 percent of patients with symptomatic venous thrombosis but is important because treatment is required on an urgent basis.

LABORATORY FEATURES

A number of laboratory abnormalities have been associated with venous thromboembolism. These include increased levels of fibrinopeptide A and fibrinogen degradation products, thrombin-antithrombin complexes, prothrombin fragment 1.2, and D-dimer. Patients with venous thromboembolism frequently have other comorbid conditions, including cancer, recent surgery or trauma, infection, and inflammation, and many of the laboratory changes associated with venous thromboembolism are highly nonspecific.

The search for a simple blood test to detect or eliminate venous thromboembolism continues. The only reasonable contender is measurement of the D-dimer using either an enzyme-linked immunosorbent assay (ELISA) or latex agglutination.[25,26] A cutoff value can be determined below which the sensitivity and negative predictive value of the tests are extremely high.[25,26] The specificity and positive predictive value, however, remain in the 50 percent range. A recent study demonstrated

that a rapid red cell agglutination assay (SIMPLI-RED test), when performed in patients with suspected DVT in whom the diagnosis was confirmed by either compression ultrasonography or venography yielded a sensitivity of 89 percent and a negative predictive value of 95 percent for all DVT.[27] For proximal DVT, the sensitivity was 92 percent and the negative predictive value 96 percent. This assay can be performed in minutes and could therefore be useful in making management decisions.

DIFFERENTIAL DIAGNOSIS

As shown in Table 28-1, a number of clinical conditions can mimic DVT. The alternate diagnosis is frequently not evident at presentation, and it is impossible to exclude venous thromboembolism without the use of objective tests. In a number of patients who do not have DVT, the cause of pain, tenderness, and swelling may remain uncertain even after careful follow-up.

OBJECTIVE TESTS FOR THE DIAGNOSIS OF VENOUS THROMBOEMBOLISM

In the diagnosis of venous thrombosis, objective tests include impedance plethysmography (IPG),

Table 28-1. The Alternative Diagnosis in 87 Consecutive Patients with Clinically Suspected Venous Thrombosis and Negative Venograms*

Diagnosis	Patients (%)
Muscle strain	24
Direct twisting injury to leg	10
Leg swelling in paralyzed limb	9
Lymphangitis, lymphatic obstruction	7
Venous reflux	6
Muscle tear	5
Baker's cyst	3
Cellulitis	2
Internal abnormality of knee	26
Unknown	

*The diagnosis was made once venous thrombosis had been excluded by the finding of a negative venogram.
Reproduced with permission from Hull RD, Hirsh J, Sackett DL, et al. Clinical validity of a negative venogram in patients with clinically suspected venous thrombosis. Circulation 1981;64:622.

B-mode ultrasound, duplex ultrasound, color-flow ultrasonography, and ascending venography.

Impedance Plethysmography

Impedance plethysmography (IPG) is sensitive and specific for proximal vein thrombosis in symptomatic patients but is insensitive to calf vein thrombosis.[28–34] In patients with clinically suspected venous thrombosis, positive IPG results can be used to make therapeutic decisions in the absence of clinical conditions known to produce false-positive results.[31,34] A normal result essentially excludes the diagnosis of proximal vein thrombosis but does not exclude calf vein thrombosis. This potential limitation can be overcome by performing serial IPG. The use of serial IPG is based on the concept now confirmed by clinical observation that calf vein thrombi are only clinically important when extension into the proximal veins occurs, at which point detection with IPG is possible. The effectiveness and safety of IPG have been evaluated by prospective clinical trials in patients with clinically suspected venous thrombosis. Based on the data provided by these studies, the following recommendations can be made: (1) a positive result by IPG is highly predictive of acute proximal vein thrombosis (positive predictive value greater than 90 percent), and (2) it is safe to withhold anticoagulant therapy in symptomatic patients who remain negative by serial IPG for 10 to 14 days.

Although the IPG has a high sensitivity and specificity for symptomatic venous thrombosis, it lacks sensitivity for the detection of asymptomatic venous thrombosis following surgery, such as total hip replacement, or in trauma patients.[25–36] In such circumstances, the only reliable method for detection of DVT is bilateral ascending venography.

Impedance plethysmography has certain limitations. False-positive results may occur with disorders that interfere with arterial inflow or venous outflow. These include severe congestive cardiac failure, constrictive pericarditis, severe arterial insufficiency, hypotension, and external compression of veins. Most of these disorders are readily recognized on clinical grounds. False-positive results also may occur if the test is performed incorrectly or if the patient is not relaxed. The test cannot be performed on some patients, i.e., those who are in plaster casts or who cannot be positioned adequately because of immobilization or pain.

Ultrasonography

Venous imaging using real-time B-mode ultrasound with or without Doppler assessment is becoming the standard technique for evaluating patients with clinically suspected DVT.[37–41] It has been shown in prospective studies that the single criterion of vein compressibility is highly sensitive and specific for proximal vein thrombosis (sensitivity and specificity both greater than 95 percent).[37–41] Other criteria such as echogenicity or change in venous diameter during a Valsalva maneuver are less useful. The visualization of an echogenic band is highly sensitive but nonspecific (specificity 50 percent). The percentage of change in venous diameter during a Valsalva maneuver is both insensitive and nonspecific.

Both real-time B-mode venous ultrasound and duplex ultrasonography are insensitive for isolated calf vein thrombosis, and like IPG, serial testing is required to detect patients who develop proximal extension. B-mode venous ultrasound may fail to detect isolated iliac vein thrombi. This is a practical clinical limitation in patient groups in whom isolated vein thrombosis is not uncommon, such as the pregnant patient with clinically suspected venous thrombosis. Color flow imaging and other technologic advances have improved the ability of B-mode venous imaging to detect isolated iliac vein thrombi and calf vein thrombi.[42–50]

The Doppler ultrasound is highly sensitive and specific in the diagnosis of proximal vein thrombosis in symptomatic patients. Doppler ultrasound is more sensitive than IPG to symptomatic calf vein thrombosis and is more reliable than IPG for detecting proximal vein thrombosis in patients with increased central venous pressure or arterial insufficiency. This technique can be used in patients who have their leg in a plaster cast or external fixation, who are in traction, or who have had leg amputation.

Although the Doppler ultrasound is rapidly replacing venography in verifying the diagnosis of DVT in symptomatic patients, it lacks both sensitivity and specificity for the detection of asymptomatic venous thrombosis in postoperative patients.[51–56] Ultrasonography is now readily available and has replaced IPG as the most popular noninvasive test for the detection of venous thrombosis.

Venography

Venography has been accepted as the standard objective method for the diagnosis of venous thrombosis until recently. Although the diagnosis of proximal venous thrombosis can now be established with noninvasive tests (i.e., ultrasonography and IPG), venography remains the only reliable test for making the diagnosis of DVT in asymptomatic patients, e.g., following orthopedic surgery or trauma.[57–59] Venography is a difficult technique to perform well and requires considerable experience to execute adequately and to interpret accurately. A number of venographic abnormalities have been defined as criteria for the diagnosis of acute DVT.[24] The most reliable of these is the presence of an intraluminal filling defect that is constant in all films and is seen in a number of projections. Other venographic abnormalities such as nonfilling of a segment of the deep venous system or nonfilling of the entire deep venous system above the knee may be caused by technical artifacts, particularly if the dye is injected too far proximally into the dorsal foot vein. These artifacts may then be interpreted as either being caused by thrombus because the vein is not filled or as normal because a filling defect is not seen. The common femoral, external iliac, and common iliac veins may not be adequately filled by ascending venography. This can lead to an incorrect diagnosis based on inadequate venography. In the case of nonfilling of an entire segment of the deep venous system, the diagnosis of acute or recurrent venous thrombosis must depend on the use of other tests such as the IPG or ultrasound.[28]

There are a number of problems related to venography. Even in the best of circumstances, it may be impossible to cannulate a vein on the dorsum of the foot, making ascending venography impossible on one or both legs. If there is inadequate filling of the common femoral or iliac systems, a femoral venogram may be necessary.

Venography is associated with a number of clinically troublesome side effects. Pain may occur in the foot while dye is being injected, or there may be delayed pain in the calf 1 or 2 days after injection. The procedure may be complicated by superficial phlebitis and even DVT in a small percentage of patients with normal venograms (1 to 2 percent).[28] Other less common complications of venography include hypersensitivity to the radiopacque dye and local skin or tissue necrosis due to extravasation of dye at the site of injection. Both nonionic and high-ionic contrast media may cause or aggravate renal insufficiency in patients at high risk for these complications, e.g., patients with established renal disease, hypertension, heart failure, diabetes, or multiple myeloma.[60,61] The risks of venography must be carefully weighed in such circumstances and reviewed with the patient before venography is performed.

DIAGNOSIS AND TREATMENT OF PULMONARY EMBOLISM BASED ON OBJECTIVE TESTING FOR PROXIMAL DVT

At least 80 percent of patients with pulmonary embolism have thrombi originating in the lower leg veins.[9–11,63,64] Because of the diagnostic inaccuracy of noninvasive tests for pulmonary embolism, the concept of using objective tests for the detection of proximal venous thrombosis in the legs was developed in patients suspected of having pulmonary embolism.[12,21–23,65,66] This combined strategy for the diagnosis and treatment of pulmonary embolus or venous thrombosis (i.e., venous thromboembolism) has been applied in prospective clinical trials.[12,65,66]

Noninvasive tests such as IPG or B-mode venous ultrasound have advantages because they are free of morbidity and readily repeatable. Proximal vein thrombosis is revealed by impedance plethysmography in 10 to 25 percent of patients with nondiagnostic ventilation-perfusion scans. This has important implications for management; untreated or inadequately treated proximal-vein thrombosis is associated with a high risk (20 to 50 percent) of recurrent venous thromboembolism.

A positive result by venography or noninvasive testing is an indication for therapy; however, the venogram is negative in approximately 30 percent of patients with angiographically documented pulmonary embolism. There are two possible explanations for this finding. The first is that pulmonary embolism may have originated from a source other than the deep veins of the legs. Alternatively, the emboli may have originated from the deep veins of the legs, but all or most of the thrombus embolized, leaving no residual thrombosis detectable at the time of presentation.

In patients with abnormal but nondiagnostic lung scans and negative objective tests for venous thrombosis, pulmonary angiography is required to confirm or exclude pulmonary embolism. This may be impractical or unavailable, however. In patients who do not have severely limited cardiorespiratory reserve, serial objective testing for proximal vein thrombosis is an alternative approach, based on the concept that clinically important recurrent pulmonary embolism is unlikely (< 1 percent) in the absence of proximal vein thrombosis. This concept is supported by the findings of studies of the natural history of venous thrombosis and by clinical trials of noninvasive testing in patients with symptoms or signs suggesting deep vein thrombosis.[9,10,12] Furthermore, prospective studies indicate that the use of serial objective testing for proximal vein thrombosis is an effective and practical alternative to pulmonary angiography in patients with nondiagnostic lung scans who have adequate cardiorespiratory reserve.[65,66]

PREVENTION OF VENOUS THROMBOEMBOLISM

Without prophylaxis, the frequency of fatal pulmonary embolism ranges from 0.1 to 0.8 percent in patients undergoing elective general surgery,[67–69] 2 to 3 percent in patients undergoing elective hip replacement,[70] and 4 to 7 percent in patients undergoing surgery for fractured hip.[71] It is surprising that physicians and surgeons still do not comply with recommendations for prophylaxis of venous thromboembolism despite the fact that there is convincing evidence for the efficacy and safety of a number of agents.[5–8,71,72] In a recent retrospective audit of hospitals in Massachusetts, it was shown that prophylaxis of venous thromboembolism, even in high-risk patients, was grossly underutilized, particularly in nonteaching hospitals.[73] In orthopedic surgery, as was shown in surveys conducted in England and Sweden, some form of prophylaxis, usually in the form of drugs, is used in the majority of cases.[74,75]

There are two approaches to the prevention of fatal pulmonary embolism. These are (1) secondary prevention by the early detection and treatment of subclinical venous thrombosis by screening postoperative patients with objective tests that are sensitive for venous thrombosis and (2) primary prophylaxis using either drugs or physical methods that are effective for preventing DVT. The latter approach of primary prophylaxis is preferred in most clinical circumstances. Furthermore, prevention of DVT and pulmonary embolism is more cost-effective than treating the complications where they occur.[76–80] Secondary prevention by case-finding studies should never replace primary prophylaxis. It is reserved for patients in whom primary prophylaxis is either contraindicated or relatively ineffective.

The ideal primary prophylactic method is described in Table 28-2. The prophylactic measures most commonly used are low-dose or adjusted-dose unfractionated heparin, low-molecular-weight heparin, oral anticoagulants [international normalized ratio (INR) of 2.0 to 3.0], and intermittent pneumatic leg compression. Other less commonly used measures include aspirin and intravenous dextran.

Ideally, prophylaxis should be started before operation and continued until the patient is fully ambulant. In North America, prophylaxis for high-risk procedures such as total joint replacement has been started postoperatively because of concern for perioperative bleeding. Clinical trials

Table 28-2. Features of an Ideal Prophylactic Method

Effective compared with placebo or active approaches
Safe
Good compliance with patient, nurses, and physicians
Ease of administration
No need for laboratory monitoring
Cost effective

are currently underway to compare the efficacy and safety of preoperative with postoperative commencement of prophylaxis. No data are available to allow specific recommendations for continued prophylaxis in patients discharged from hospital, and this is also being studied in clinical trials.

SPECIFIC PROPHYLACTIC MEASURES

Low-Dose Heparin

The effectiveness of low-dose heparin for preventing DVT has been established by multiple, randomized clinical trials. Low-dose subcutaneous heparin is usually given in a dose of 5000 units 2 hours preoperatively and then postoperatively every 8 or 12 hours. Most of the patients in these trials underwent abdominothoracic surgery, particularly for gastrointestinal disease, but also included were gynecologic and urologic surgery as well as some patients having mastectomy or vascular procedures. Pooled data from meta-analyses confirm that low-dose heparin reduces the incidence of all DVT, proximal DVT, and all pulmonary emboli, including fatal pulmonary emboli.[5–8,69] The International Multicentre Trial also established the effectiveness of low-dose heparin for preventing fatal pulmonary embolism, a clinically striking reduction from 0.7 to 0.1 percent.[69]

Although individual clinical trials reported failure of low-dose heparin to prevent thrombosis following total hip replacement surgery, one meta-analysis demonstrated a 68 percent risk reduction with no increased risk of bleeding.[6] This risk reduction is similar to that seen with low-molecular-weight heparin, although low-molecular-weight heparin has been shown to be superior to low-dose heparin in individual trials. The incidence of major bleeding complications is not increased by low-dose heparin, but there is an increase in minor wound hematomas. The platelet count should be monitored regularly in all patients on low-dose heparin to detect the rare but significant development of heparin-induced thrombocytopenia.

Low-dose heparin has the advantage that it is relatively inexpensive, it is easily administered, and it does not require anticoagulant monitoring.

Adjusted-Dose Heparin

The use of adjusted-dose subcutaneous heparin was shown to be an effective approach for prophylaxis when compared with low-dose heparin in patients undergoing total hip replacement.[81] Adjusted-dose heparin therapy decreased the incidence of DVT significantly (13 versus 39 percent) without any increase in the frequency of bleeding complications. In a more recent study by the same group, adjusted-dose heparin was compared with low-molecular-weight heparin.[82] The decrease in the incidence of DVT was not as striking (16 percent), and there was a surprisingly high incidence of proximal vein thrombosis (13 percent). Adjusted-dose heparin has not become popular because of the time and expense required for laboratory monitoring.

Low-Molecular-Weight Heparin

A number of low-molecular-weight heparin fractions have been evaluated by randomized clinical trials in moderate-risk general surgical patients.[83–90] The low-molecular-weight heparins that have been evaluated include Fragmin, Fraxiparine, Enoxaparin, and Logiparin. In randomized clinical trials comparing low-molecular-weight heparin with unfractionated heparin, the low-molecular-weight heparins given once or twice daily have been shown to be as effective or more effective in preventing thrombosis.[83–90] Most of the trials documented similarly low frequencies of bleeding for low-molecular-weight heparin and low-dose unfractionated heparin, although the incidence of bleeding was somewhat higher with unfractionated heparin when various bleeding endpoints were combined.[83]

There have been several large, randomized clinical trials in patients undergoing total joint replacements (hip ± knees).[91–102] Different low-molecular-weight heparins have been compared with either placebo, unfractionated heparin, adjusted-dose heparin, dextran 40, or warfarin sodium. Compared with placebo, low-molecular-weight heparin significantly decreased the rates of both distal and proximal DVT with no significant increase in bleeding rates.[92,97,99] Low-molecular-weight heparins were at least as effective as or more effective than low-dose unfractionated heparin given two to three times daily.[93,94,102] Bleeding rates were comparable in the unfractionated heparin and low-molecular-weight heparin groups with the exception of one study[93] using unfractionated heparin, 7500 units twice daily. Studies comparing low-molecular-weight heparin with dextran 70 showed a significant improvement in thrombosis rates with low-molecular-weight heparin with no significant differences in bleeding rates.[95]

Two large multicenter studies compared the use of low-molecular-weight heparin once[100] or twice[101] daily with warfarin sodium, both started postoperatively, in the prevention of DVT following total hip or total knee replacement. For patients undergoing hip replacement, both studies showed that low-molecular-weight heparin was as effective as warfarin, but for those undergoing total knee replacements, low-molecular-weight heparin was superior. When the data for patients undergoing hip or knee replacements were pooled, low-molecular-weight heparin was statistically superior to warfarin.[100] The incidence of major and minor bleeding and wound hematomas was higher in the low-molecular-weight heparin group.[100]

The low-molecular-weight heparinoid ORG-10172 (Lomoparin) effectively reduced the rates of DVT following total hip replacement when compared with placebo (15.5 versus 56.6 percent).[103] It was evaluated in two clinical trials involving patients with hip fracture.[104,105] The DVT rates were significantly lower when compared with intravenous dextran[104] (13 versus 35 percent) and with low-intensity warfarin[105] (7 versus 21 percent). More blood transfusions were required in the dextran group.[104]

In recent meta-analyses, low-molecular-weight heparin has been shown to be more effective than unfractionated heparin in the prevention of venous thrombosis, but with a slightly higher risk of bleeding.[106] The low-molecular-weight heparins have the advantage that they can be given once a day at a constant dose without any laboratory monitoring. Studies comparing the cost-effectiveness of low-molecular-weight heparin and either warfarin or unfractionated heparin are currently underway.

Oral Anticoagulants

For prophylaxis, oral anticoagulants can be commenced preoperatively, at the time of operation, or in the early postoperative period. Oral anticoagulants commenced at the time of surgery or early postoperatively may not prevent small venous thrombi that form during surgery or soon after surgery, because the anticoagulant effect is not achieved until the third or fourth postoperative day. However, they are effective in inhibiting the extension of these thrombi and thereby preventing clinically important venous thromboembolism.

The postoperative use of warfarin has been compared with low-molecular-weight heparin[100,101] or intermittent pneumatic compression with little or no difference in the incidence of postoperative venous thrombosis or bleeding.[107–109] Initiation of warfarin in small doses 7 to 10 days preoperatively to prolong the prothrombin time 1.5 to 3.0 seconds followed by less intense warfarin started the night of surgery yielded results similar to warfarin started postoperatively.[107]

In hip fracture patients, warfarin was compared with aspirin and placebo with the following rates of DVT: warfarin 20 percent, aspirin 40.9 percent, and placebo 46 percent.[110]

Very low dose oral anticoagulants (warfarin 1 mg/day), when compared with placebo, were shown to decrease the postoperative thrombosis rate in patients undergoing gynecologic surgery or major general surgery[111] and to decrease the thrombosis rate in patients with indwelling central line catheters.[112] There was no increase in bleeding rates. Very low dose warfarin, however, did not provide protection against DVT following hip or knee replacement.[113]

Intermittent Leg Compression

The use of intermittent pneumatic leg compression prevents venous thrombosis by enhancing blood flow in the deep veins of the legs, thereby preventing venous stasis. It also increases blood fibrinolytic activity, which may contribute to its antithrombotic properties. Intermittent pneumatic leg compression is effective for preventing venous thrombosis in moderate-risk general surgical patients[114] and in patients undergoing neurosurgery.[115–117] In patients undergoing hip surgery, intermittent pneumatic compression of the calf is effective for preventing calf vein thrombosis but is relatively ineffective against proximal vein thrombosis.[118] Sequential compression using calf and thigh cuffs produces greater acceleration of femoral venous blood flow than compression of the calf alone. Recent clinical trials indicate that sequential calf and thigh compression is effective for preventing venous thrombosis in patients undergoing elective total hip replacement, but the incidence of proximal venous thrombosis remains moderately high.[107,118]

Intermittent pneumatic compression of the calf decreased distal venous thrombosis following knee replacement, but proximal thrombosis rates remained high.[119] Studies with calf and thigh compression significantly decreased the incidence of both distal and proximal thrombosis.[120]

Intermittent pneumatic compression is virtually free of clinically important side effects and offers a valuable alternative in patients who have a high risk of bleeding. It may produce discomfort in the occasional patient and should not be used in patients with overt evidence of leg ischemia caused by peripheral vascular disease. A variety of well-accepted, comfortable, and effective intermittent pneumatic devices are currently available that may be applied preoperatively, at the time of operation, or in the early postoperative period. These devices should be used for the entire period until the patient is fully ambulatory.

Graduated Compression Stockings

The use of graduated compression stockings reduces venous stasis in the limb by applying a graded degree of compression to the ankle and the calf, with greater pressure being applied more distally in the limb. Clinical trials have demonstrated graduated compression stockings to be effective for preventing postoperative venous thrombosis in low-risk general surgical patients[121–123] and in selected moderate-risk patients (neurosurgical).[115,117] A recent meta-analysis confirmed the reduction of venous thrombosis following moderate-risk surgery with the use

of graduated compression stockings.[124] However, there was inadequate information to verify whether the use of graduated compression stockings in combination with other forms of prophylaxis resulted in any further risk reduction.[124] Furthermore, the use of graduated compression stockings along with other prophylactic measures in patients undergoing high-risk surgery has not been adequately studied.

Other Agents

Although aspirin decreases the percentage odds reduction of venous thrombosis following general or orthopedic surgery, this reduction is significantly less than seen with other agents, and aspirin therefore cannot be recommended for the prevention of venous thrombosis in high-risk patients.[125] Also, although intravenous dextran has been shown to be effective in the prevention of venous thrombosis following major orthopedic surgery, it is cumbersome, expensive, and associated with significant side effects, and it has been replaced by other agents.

SPECIFIC RECOMMENDATIONS

The recommended primary prophylactic approach depends on the patient's risk category (Table 28-3) and the type of surgery.

Low Risk Patients

Prophylaxis for low-risk patients is recommended in certain circumstances.[8,126] It is clinical custom in some countries to use graduated compression stockings.

Moderate-Risk Patients

GENERAL ABDOMINAL, THORACIC, OR GYNECOLOGIC SURGERY

In moderate-risk patients, the use of subcutaneous low-dose heparin (5000 units every 8 or 12 hours) or subcutaneous low-molecular-weight heparin is recommended.[5,8,126] Subcutaneous low-molecular-weight heparin is as effective as subcutaneous heparin prophylaxis and has the advantage of

Table 28-3. Risk of Venous Thromboembolism (Assessed by Objective Tests)

Risk Category	Calf Vein Thrombosis	Proximal Vein Thrombosis	Fatal Pulmonary Embolism
High Risk Major orthopedic surgery of lower limbs General and urologic surgery in patients over 40 years with recent history of DVT or PE Extensive pelvic or abdominal surgery for malignant disease	40–80%	10–30%	1–5%
Moderate Risk General surgery in patients over 40 years lasting 30 minutes or more and in patients below 40 years on oral contraceptives	10–40%	2–10%	0.1–0.8%
Low Risk Minor surgery (i.e., less than 30 minutes) in patients over 40 years without additional risk factors Uncomplicated surgery in patients under 40 years without additional risk factors	< 10%	< 1%	< 0.01%

Reproduced with permission from Nicolaides AN, Arcelus J, Belcaro G, et al: Prevention of venous thromboembolism. Int Angiol 1992;11(3):151.

once per day injection. An alternative recommendation is the use of intermittent pneumatic compression until the patient is ambulatory. This method is indicated in patients at a high risk of bleeding. Pharmacologic methods may be combined with graduated compression stockings in selected patients.

NEUROSURGERY

These patients should receive intermittent pneumatic compression. This approach may be used in conjunction with graduate compression stockings.[8,126]

High-Risk Patients

The optimal approach remains uncertain because not all approaches have been compared directly in this high-risk patient category. The possible approaches include oral anticoagulants, low-molecular-weight heparin,[8,126] intermittent pneumatic compression, subcutaneous low-dose heparin using the 8-hourly regimen, adjusted-dose subcutaneous heparin, and intravenous dextran. Primary prophylaxis may be supplemented by postoperative screening to detect patients who develop DVT despite prophylaxis.

ELECTIVE HIP REPLACEMENT

Several approaches are effective. Prophylaxis with oral anticoagulants adjusted to maintain an INR of 2.0 to 3.0 is effective and is associated with a low risk of bleeding.[8,126] Subcutaneous low-molecular-weight heparin given once or twice daily is effective and safe. Several such agents are approved for use in Europe, and one is available in North America.[5,8,94] Other effective approaches include adjusted-dose subcutaneous heparin, intravenous dextran, and intravenous dextran combined with intermittent pneumatic leg compression.[8,126]

FRACTURED HIP

Prophylaxis with oral anticoagulants (INR of 2.0 to 3.0) is the preferred approach.[8,126] Where available, low-molecular-weight heparin can be used.[103–105] Intravenous dextran is effective but inconvenient and relatively expensive.

MAJOR KNEE SURGERY

Intermittent pneumatic compression is the preferred approach.[126]

OTHER CONDITIONS

Pregnancy

The use of subcutaneous low-dose heparin is the prophylaxis of choice for pregnant patients who are at high risk of DVT and pulmonary embolism, although data on efficacy from controlled trials are lacking.[8] The benefits of prophylaxis are uncertain in patients undergoing cesarean section, particularly if they have no additional risk factors.[8] Oral anticoagulants are contraindicated throughout pregnancy.

Medical Patients

These patients should be classified as low, moderate, or high risk for suffering from venous thromboembolism. Low-risk patients should be considered for graduated pressure stockings. Moderate-risk patients should receive either subcutaneous low-dose heparin or intermittent pneumatic leg compression (if at high risk of bleeding). High-risk patients should receive adjusted oral anticoagulants (INR of 2.0 to 3.0), subcutaneous low-dose heparin, or subcutaneous low-molecular-weight heparin where these are approved.[8,126]

TREATMENT OF VENOUS THROMBOSIS

The accepted anticoagulant therapy for venous thromboembolism is a combination of continuous intravenous heparin and oral warfarin sodium.[127,128] The use of heparin and warfarin simultaneously has become clinical practice for all patients with venous thromboembolism who are medically stable.[129,130] Exceptions include patients who require immediate medical or surgical intervention such as thrombolysis or insertion of a vena cava filter or patients in the intensive care unit with multiple invasive lines. The length of the initial intravenous heparin therapy has been reduced to 5 days, thus shortening the hospital stay and leading to significant cost saving.[129,130]

HEPARIN THERAPY

The anticoagulant activity of unfractionated heparin depends on a unique pentasaccharide that binds to antithrombin III (ATIII) and potentiates the inhibition of thrombin and activated factor X (Xa) by ATIII.[131–134] In addition, heparin catalyzes the inactivation of thrombin by another plasma cofactor, heparin cofactor II, that acts independently of ATIII.[135] Heparin has a number of other effects, including the release of tissue factor inhibitor, the binding to numerous plasma and platelet proteins, endothelial cells, and leukocytes, and then increased vascular permeability.[136,137] These latter effects may explain some of the nonanticoagulant effects as well as the hemorrhagic effects of heparin and the variability in the action of heparin among individuals. The basic biochemistry, pharmacology, and pharmacokinetics of heparin have recently been reviewed.[136] The anticoagulant response to a standard dose of heparin varies widely among patients, making it necessary to monitor the anticoagulant response of heparin either with activated partial thromboplastin time (aPTT) or heparin levels and to titrate the dose to the individual patient.[136,140]

The laboratory test most commonly used to monitor heparin therapy is the aPTT. The traditional approach has been to adjust the heparin infusion dose to maintain the aPTT within a defined "therapeutic range." Over the years, this therapeutic range evolved, based on clinical custom, to the use of an upper and lower limit (an aPTT ratio of 1.5 to 2.5 times control). The clinical practice of adjusting the heparin dose to maintain the aPTT response within this range is based on two concepts: (1) that maintaining the aPTT ratio above the lower limit of 1.5 will minimize recurrent venous thromboembolic events and (2) that maintaining the aPTT ratio below the upper limit of 2.5 will minimize the risk of bleeding complications.[139,141]

It has been established from experimental studies and clinical trials that the efficacy of heparin therapy depends on achieving a critical therapeutic level of heparin within the first 24 hours of treatment. The critical therapeutic level of heparin as measured by the aPTT is 1.5 times the mean of the control value or the upper limit of the normal aPTT range. This corresponds to a heparin blood level of 0.2 to 0.4 units/ml by the protamine sulfate titration assay.[142] However, there is a wide variability in the aPTT and heparin blood levels with different reagents and even with different batches of the same reagent. It is therefore vital for each laboratory to establish the minimal therapeutic level of heparin as measured by the aPTT that will provide a heparin blood level of at least 0.2 units/ml by the protamine titration assay for each batch of thromboplastin reagent being used, particularly if the reagent is provided by a different manufacturer.[142]

The variability in the aPTT response to different heparin blood levels supports the need for an aggressive approach to heparin therapy to ensure that all patients achieve adequate therapy early in the course of their treatment. The use of low-molecular-weight heparin will eliminate this problem because laboratory monitoring is not required. However, until these agents are approved for use, the problem of aPTT standardization will remain.

Data from three randomized clinical trials[141,143,144] provide firm support for the use of an aPTT ratio of 1.5 as the lower limit of the therapeutic range. The first randomized trial evaluated the clinical outcomes in patients with proximal vein thrombosis who were treated with either continuous intravenous heparin or intermittent subcutaneous heparin adjusted to prolong the aPTT greater than 1.5 times the control.[141] The subcutaneous regimen resulted in an initial anticoagulant response below the lower limit in the majority (63 percent) of patients and a high frequency of recurrent venous thromboembolism (11 of 57 patients, 19.3 percent), which was virtually confined to patients with a subtherapeutic anticoagulant response.[141] In contrast, continuous intravenous heparin resulted in an adequate anticoagulant response in the majority (71 percent) of patients and a low frequency of recurrent thromboembolic events (3 of 58 patients, 5.2 percent); the recurrences in this group also were limited to patients with an initial subtherapeutic anticoagulant response.[141] Thus 13 of 53 patients (24.5 percent) with an aPTT response below the lower limit for 24 hours or more had recurrent venous thromboembolism, compared with only 1 of 62 patients (1.6 percent) in whom an aPTT ratio of 1.5 or more was achieved ($p < 0.001$), a relative risk for recurrent venous thromboembolism of 15:1. Similar results were found when a weight-based heparin dosing nomogram (starting dose 90-units/kg bolus and 18 units/kg per hour infusion) was compared with a standard care nomogram (starting dose 5000-unit bolus and 1000 units/hour infusion).[144] Using the weight-based nomogram, 60 of 62 patients (97 percent) exceeded the therapeutic threshold within 24 hours, compared with 37 of 48 (77 percent) of patients in the standard care group ($p < 0.002$). Recurrent thromboembolism in the 3-month treatment period was more

frequent in the standard care group, relative risk 5.0 (95 percent CI 1.1 to 21.9).[144]

These findings are strongly supported by a randomized trial that compared intravenous heparin plus oral anticoagulants for the initial treatment of patients with proximal vein thrombosis.[143] The latter treatment group, by the nature of their treatment, have an inadequate aPTT response for at least the first 48 hours, since the onset of the anticoagulant effect of oral anticoagulants is delayed. Recurrent venous thromboembolism occurred in 12 of 60 patients (20 percent) treated with oral anticoagulants alone over the subsequent 3 months, compared with 4 of 60 patients (6.7 percent) who received initial intravenous heparin plus oral anticoagulants ($p = 0.058$).[143]

In all these trials, recurrent thromboembolism typically occurred between 3 and 12 weeks. Thus it was not previously recognized that these recurrent clinical events relate to failure of initial therapy.

A recent randomized trial (level I) provides important new information about the upper limit of the therapeutic range for the aPTT.[139] This study evaluated the clinical outcomes in patients with proximal vein thrombosis who were randomized to receive initial treatment with either intravenous heparin alone or intravenous heparin with simultaneous warfarin sodium. Both regimens achieved adequate therapy in almost all patients, but the combined heparin and warfarin group received more intensive anticoagulation, with the majority of patients exceeding the predefined upper limit (aPTT ratio 2.5) for sustained periods of time.[139] Despite this more intense therapy in the combined group, bleeding complications occurred with similar frequency in the two groups: 9 of 99 patients in the combined group (9.1 percent) had bleeding complications, compared with 12 of 100 patients (12.0 percent) in the group given heparin alone.[139] Major bleeding occurred in 3 of 93 patients (3.2 percent) with supratherapeutic aPTT findings, compared with 10 of 106 patients (9.4 percent) without supratherapeutic aPTT findings (relative risk 0.3, $p = 0.09$).[139] The incidence of major bleeding correlated with the clinical risk of bleeding. Patients considered at a low risk for bleeding and who received the higher heparin dose had a low frequency of major bleeding (1 percent), whereas those considered at high risk of bleeding who received a lower dose of heparin had a higher frequency of major bleeding (11 percent) ($p = 0.007$).[139]

These findings refute the findings of retrospective reviews[145] suggesting an association between a supratherapeutic aPTT result (ratio 2.5 or more) and the risk of clinically important bleeding complications.

Numerous audits of heparin therapy indicate that administration of intravenous heparin is fraught with difficulty[146–149] and that the clinical practice of using an ad hoc or intuitive approach to heparin dose titration frequently results in inadequate therapy. For example, an audit of physician practices at three university-affiliated hospitals[148] documented that 60 percent of patients failed to achieve an adequate aPTT response (ratio 1.5) during the initial 24 hours of therapy and, further, that 30 to 40 percent of patients remained subtherapeutic over the next 3 to 4 days. Several practices were identified that led to inadequate therapy. The common theme that explains these practices is an exaggerated fear of bleeding complications on the part of clinicians. Consequently, it has been common practice for many clinicians to start treatment with a low heparin dose and to cautiously increase this dose over several days to achieve the therapeutic range. The data indicate that this practice is inappropriate and indeed dangerous, because it places the patient at an unacceptably high risk for recurrent venous thromboembolism[141] and may induce the development of heparin resistance.[150]

The use of a prescriptive approach or protocol for administering intravenous heparin therapy has been evaluated in two studies in patients with venous thromboembolism.[139,144] In one clinical trial, patients were given either intravenous heparin alone followed subsequently by warfarin sodium or intravenous heparin and simultaneous warfarin in the treatment of proximal venous thrombosis.[139] This heparin nomogram is summarized in Tables 28-4 and 28-5. Only 2 and 1 percent of the patients were subtherapeutic for more than 24 hours in the heparin and warfarin group and the heparin group, respectively.[139] Recurrent venous thromboembolism (objectively documented) occurred infrequently in both groups (7 percent),[139] rates similar to those

Table 28-4. Heparin Protocol

1. Initial intravenous heparin bolus: 5000 units
2. Continuous intravenous heparin infusion: commence at 42 ml/h of 20,000 units (1680 units/h) in 500 ml of two-thirds dextrose and one-third saline (a 24-h heparin dose of 40,320 units), except in the following patients, in whom heparin infusion will be commenced at a rate of 31 ml/h (1240 units/h) (i.e., a 24-h dose of 29,760 units)
   a. Patients who have undergone surgery within the previous 2 weeks.
   b. Patients with a previous history of peptic ulcer disease or gastrointestinal or genitourinary bleeding.
   c. Patients with recent stroke (i.e., thrombotic stroke within 2 weeks previously).
   d. Patients with a platelet count $<150 \times 10^9$ per liter.
   e. Patients with miscellaneous reasons for a high risk of bleeding (e.g., hepatic failure, renal failure or vitamin K deficiency).
3. Heparin dose adjusted using the aPTT. The aPTT is performed in all patients as outlined below:
   a. 4–6 h after commencing heparin; the heparin dose is then adjusted according to the nomogram shown below.
   b. 4–6 h after implementing the first dosage adjustment.
   c. The aPTT is then performed as indicated by the nomogram for the first 24 h of therapy.
   d. Thereafter, the aPTT will be performed once daily, unless the patients is subtherapeutic, in which case the aPTT will be repeated 4–6 h after increasing the heparin dose.

Reproduced with permission from Hull RD, Raskob GE, Rosenbloom D, et al: Optimal therapeutic level of heparin therapy in patients with venous thrombosis. Arch Intern Med 1992;152:1589.

reported previously.[22,32,33] These findings demonstrated that subtherapy was avoided in most patients and that the heparin protocol resulted in effective delivery of heparin therapy in both groups.

This heparin nomogram also was used in a randomized clinical trial comparing the use of fixed-dose subcutaneous low-molecular-weight heparin with continuous intravenous heparin in the initial treatment of proximal venous thrombosis.[151] Warfarin was started on day 2 in all patients. Use of the heparin nomogram in the 15 different treatment centers ensured that the vast majority of patients were within the therapeutic range within 24 hours. A review of the findings from one of the treatment centers indicated that 91 percent of patients were within the therapeutic range (aPTT > 1.5 × control) within 24 hours compared with 60 percent of the patients who were treated without the use of a heparin protocol.[149]

In the other clinical trial, a weight-based heparin dosing nomogram was compared with a

Table 28-5. Intravenous Heparin Dose-Titration Nomogram for aPTT* (IV Infusion)

aPTT	Rate Change, ml/h	Dose Change, U/24 h[†]	Additional Action
≤45	+6	+5760	Repeated aPTT[‡] in 4–6 h
46–54	+3	+2880	Repeated aPTT in 4–6 h
55–85	0	0	None[§]
86–110	−3	−2880	Stop heparin sodium treatment for 1 h; repeated aPTT 4–6 h after restarting heparin treatment
>110	−6	−5760	Stop heparin treatment for 1 h; repeated aPTT 4–6 h after restarting heparin treatment

*aPTT indicates activated partial thromboplastin time; IV, intravenous.
[†]Heparin sodium concentration, 20,000 U in 500 ml = 40 U/ml.
[‡]With the use of Actin-FS thromboplastin reagent (Dade, Mississauga, Ontario).
[§]During the first 24 h, repeated aPTT in 4 to 6 h. Thereafter, the aPTT will be determined once daily, unless subtherapeutic.
Reproduced with permission from Hull RD, Raskob GE, Rosenbloom D, et al: Optimal therapeutic level of heparin therapy in patients with venous thrombosis. Arch Intern Med 1992;152:1589.

standard care nomogram[144] (Table 28-6). Patients on the weight-adjusted heparin nomogram received a starting dose of 80 units/kg as a bolus and 18 units/kg per hour as an infusion. Patients on the standard care nomogram received a bolus of 5000 units followed by 1000 units/hour by infusion. Heparin dose was suggested to maintain an aPTT of 1.5 to 2.3 times control. The primary outcomes were (1) the time to exceed the therapeutic threshold of an aPTT greater than 1.5 times control and (2) the time to achieve the therapeutic range (aPTT 1.5 to 2.3 × control). Ninety-seven percent of patients in the weight-based heparin group exceeded the therapeutic threshold within 24 hours compared with 77 percent in the standard care group. In the weight-adjusted group, 89 per-

cent of patients achieved the therapeutic range within 24 hours compared with 75 percent in the standard care group.[144] The risk of recurrent thromboembolism was more frequent in the standard care group, supporting the previous observation that subtherapeutic heparin during the initial 24 hours is associated with a higher incidence of recurrences.[141] This study included patients with unstable angina and arterial thromboembolism in addition to venous thromboembolism, indicating that the principles applied to a heparin nomogram for the treatment of venous thromboembolism may be generalizable to other clinical conditions.

ORAL ANTICOAGULANT THERAPY

There are two distinct chemical groups of oral anticoagulants: the 4-hydroxy coumarin derivatives (e.g., warfarin sodium) and the indane-1,3-dione derivatives (e.g., phenindione).[152] The coumarin derivatives are the oral anticoagulants of choice because they are associated with fewer nonhemorrhagic side effects than are the indanedione derivatives.

The anticoagulant effect of warfarin occurs by the inhibition of the vitamin K-dependent gamma-carboxylation of coagulation factors II, VII, IX, and X.[152–154] This results in the synthesis of immunologically detectable but biologically inactive forms of these coagulation proteins. Warfarin also inhibits the vitamin K-dependent

Table 28-6. Weight-Based Nomogram

Initial dose	80 U/kg bolus, then 18 U/kg/h
aPTT* <35 s (<1.2 × control)	80 U/kg bolus, then 4 U/kg/h
aPTT, 35–45 s (1.2–1.5 × control)	40 U/kg bolus, then 2 U/kg/h
aPTT, 46–70 s (1.5–2.3 × control)	No change
aPTT, 71–90 s (2.3–3.0 × control)	Decrease infusion rate by 2 U/kg/h
aPTT > 90 s (>3.0 × control)	Hold infusion 1 h, then decrease infusion rate by 3 U/kg/h

*aPTT × activated partial thromboplastin time.
Reproduced with permission from Raschke RA, Reilly BM, Guidry JR, et al: The weight-based heparin dosing nomogram compared with a "standard care" nomogram. Ann Intern Med 1993;119:874.

gamma-carboxylation of proteins C and S.[155] Protein C circulates as a proenzyme that is activated on endothelial cells by the thrombin-thrombomodulin complex to form activated protein C. Activated protein C inhibits activated factor VIII activity directly, and in the presence of protein S, it also inhibits activated factor V.[155] Therefore, vitamin K antagonists such as warfarin create a biochemical paradox by producing an anticoagulant effect due to the inhibition of procoagulants (factors II, VII, IX, X) and a potentially thrombogenic effect by impairing the synthesis of naturally occurring inhibitors of coagulation (proteins C and S).[155] Heparin and warfarin treatment should be overlapped by 4 to 5 days when initiating warfarin treatment in patients with thrombotic disease.[154]

The anticoagulant effect of the vitamin K antagonists is delayed until the normal clotting factors are cleared from the circulation, and the peak effect does not occur until 36 to 72 hours after drug administration.[156] During the first few days of warfarin therapy, the prothrombin time reflects mainly the depression of factor VII, which has a half life of 5 to 7 hours. Equilibrium levels of factors II, IX, and X are not reached until about 1 week after the initiation of therapy. The use of small initial daily doses (e.g., 10 mg) is the preferred approach for initiating warfarin treatment. The dose-response relationship to warfarin therapy varies widely between individuals, and therefore, the dose must be monitored carefully to prevent overdosing or underdosing. There is some evidence that elderly subjects are more sensitive to the effects of warfarin and greater caution is required in establishing maintenance doses in order to prevent overanticoagulation.[157]

A number of drugs interact with warfarin. Critical appraisal of the literature reporting such interactions indicates that the evidence substantiating many of the claims is limited.[158] Nonetheless, patients must be warned against taking any new drugs without the knowledge of their attending physician.

LABORATORY MONITORING AND THERAPEUTIC RANGE

The one-stage prothrombin time is the laboratory test used most commonly to measure the effects of warfarin. The prothrombin time (PT) is sensitive to reduced activity of factors II, VII, and X but is insensitive to reduced activity of factor IX. Confusion about the appropriate therapeutic range has occurred because the different tissue thromboplastins used for measuring the PT vary considerably in sensitivity to the vitamin K–dependent clotting factors and in response to warfarin.[154] Rabbit brain thromboplastin, which is widely used in North America, is less sensitive than is standardized human brain thromboplastin, which has been widely used in the United Kingdom and other parts of Europe. A PT ratio of 1.5 to 2.0 using rabbit brain thromboplastin (i.e., the traditional therapeutic range in North America) is equivalent to a ratio of 4.0 to 6.0 using human brain thromboplastin.[37,46] Conversely, a two- to threefold increase in the PT using standardized human brain thromboplastin is equivalent to a 1.25- to 1.5-fold increase in the PT using a rabbit brain thromboplastin such as Simplastin or Dade-C.[154,159]

The optimal therapeutic range for warfarin therapy in patients with venous thrombosis has recently been established.[154,159] Several randomized trials indicate that venous thrombosis can be treated effectively and more safely with a therapeutic range of 1.25 to 1.5 times control using a rabbit brain thromboplastin such as Simplastin or Dade-C rather than the range of 1.5 to 2.0 times control conventionally recommended in North America.[154,159]

In order to promote standardization of the PT for monitoring oral anticoagulant therapy, the World Health Organization (WHO) has developed an international reference thromboplastin from human brain tissue and has recommended that the PT ratio be expressed as the international normalized ratio (INR).[154] The INR is the PT ratio obtained by testing a given sample using the WHO reference thromboplastin. For practical clinical purposes, the INR for a given plasma sample is equivalent to the PT ratio obtained using a standardized human brain thromboplastin known as the *Manchester comparative reagent,* which has been used widely in the United Kingdom. The currently recommended therapeutic range of 1.25 to 1.5 times control using a rabbit brain thromboplastin such as Simplastin or Dade-C corresponds to an INR of 2.0 to 3.0.[154]

In a survey of 53 hospital laboratories, only 21 percent reported PTs as INR results and 30 percent of hospitals could not provide data on the ISI (international sensitivity index) of the thromboplastin being used.[160] In a survey of 860 laboratories in Canada in 1992, 50.9 percent reported INR alone or with the PT ratio.[161] Only 42 percent of physicians requested INR results for anticoagulant control. Similar results were shown in a survey of laboratories in Utah.[162] These studies indicate that the current recommendations regarding ISI and INR are being disregarded by many laboratories and that anticoagulant monitoring will therefore be substandard.

Warfarin is administered in an initial dose of 10 mg/day for the first 2 days, and the daily dose is then adjusted according to the INR. Heparin therapy is discontinued on the fourth or fifth day following initiation of warfarin therapy, provided the INR is prolonged into the therapeutic range (INR of 2.0 to 3.0).[154] The selection of the correct dosage of warfarin must be individualized because some individuals are either fast or slow metabolizers of the drug. Therefore, frequent INR determinations are required initially to establish therapeutic anticoagulation.

Once the anticoagulant effect and patient's warfarin dose requirements are stable, the INR should be monitored weekly throughout the course of warfarin therapy. However, if there are factors that may produce an unpredictable response to warfarin (e.g., concomitant drug therapy),[158] the INR should be monitored more frequently to minimize the risk of complications due to poor anticoagulant control.

Several attempts have been made to improve the control of warfarin therapy while at the same time decreasing the risk of bleeding complications. These have included the use of warfarin protocols to predict dosing requirements[163] and the use of a prothrombin home monitor device.[164] An alternative to measurement of the INR is the use of an immunoassay to detect native prothrombin antigen.[165]

LONG-TERM TREATMENT OF VENOUS THROMBOEMBOLISM

Patients with established venous thrombosis or pulmonary embolism require long-term anticoagulant therapy to prevent recurrent thromboembolism.[119] Warfarin therapy is highly effective and is preferred in most patients. In patients with proximal vein thrombosis (popliteal, femoral, or iliac vein thrombosis), long-term therapy with warfarin reduces the frequency of objectively documented recurrent venous thromboembolism from 47 to 2 percent.[119] The less intense warfarin regimen (INR of 2.0 to 3.0) markedly reduces the risk of bleeding (from 20 to 4 percent) without loss of effectiveness when compared with more intense warfarin.[159]

Long-term warfarin therapy is continued for 3 months in patients with a first episode of proximal venous thrombosis or pulmonary embolism. In the past, attempts were made to decrease the treatment period with warfarin in an attempt to decrease bleeding risks (approximately 20 percent with higher-intensity warfarin treatment, i.e., INR of 3.0 to 4.5).[166–170] There was limited evidence from either the randomized clinical trials or the retrospective studies to indicate that treatment with warfarin for 12 weeks was superior to treatment for 4 or 6 weeks, but all these studies had significant limitations. In the British Thoracic Society study evaluating the optimal duration of less intense warfarin therapy for venous thromboembolism, patients were randomized to receive either 4 or 12 of weeks treatment.[170] There was a higher recurrence rate of venous thromboembolism in patients treated for 4 weeks (7.8 percent) as opposed to 12 weeks (4.0 percent) during an unspecified follow-up period. A post hoc analysis suggested that patients being treated for postoperative venous thromboembolism had a low rate of recurrence regardless of duration of warfarin therapy, whereas the recurrence rate of venous thromboembolism in "medical patients" was higher, particularly for those receiving only 4 weeks of treatment.[170] For the present, it is recommended that all patients with the first episode of venous thrombosis receive warfarin therapy for 12 weeks. If the finding of the preceding studies are confirmed, it may be possible to shorten the length of therapy for patients with postoperative venous thrombosis to 4 weeks.

The recurrence rate following a 3-month period of treatment with less-intense warfarin for first-episode venous thromboembolism is low (4 to 7 percent).[141,159] However, the long-term prognosis of patients treated for a first episode of venous thrombosis was shown to be poor, with a cumulative 3-year mortality rate of 30 percent in an audit of 16 short-stay hospitals in Massachusetts.[3] Also, in a prospective follow-up study of consecutive patients treated for 3 months with oral anticoagulants for first-episode DVT, the recurrence rate of venous thromboembolism was high (24 percent over 80 weeks) for patients with idiopathic venous thrombosis compared with patients with a known risk factor such as surgery (4.8 percent).[171] Therefore, although treatment with warfarin for 3 months may be adequate for most patients with first-episode DVT, there may be other patients such as those with idiopathic venous thrombosis who would benefit from a longer treatment period, and clinical trials are currently underway to test this hypothesis.

Warfarin treatment for more than 3 months is indicated for patients with recurrent venous thromboembolism or in patients in whom there is a continuing risk factor for venous thromboembolism.[154] Discontinuation of warfarin therapy at 3 months in patients with recurrent venous thrombosis was associated with a 20 percent risk of recurrent venous thromboembolism during the following year and a 5 percent risk of fatal pulmonary embolism.[3] The recent consensus report on antithrombotic therapy of the American College of Chest Physicians recommended an indefinite period of warfarin treatment for patients with recurrent venous thrombosis, although this statement was not based on published data.[171] The optimal duration of therapy in patients with recurrent venous thromboembolism is the subject of clinical trials currently underway.

In those patients with a continuing risk factor that is potentially reversible (e.g., prolonged bed rest), long-term therapy should be continued until the risk factor is reversed. Anticoagulant therapy should probably be continued indefinitely in patients with an irreversible risk factor, such as a deficiency of antithrombin III or protein C.[171]

While there is definitive evidence from clinical trials supporting the use of long-term warfarin therapy for proximal venous thrombosis, the treatment of calf vein thrombosis remains controversial. Without treatment, the likelihood of proximal extension of calf vein thrombosis is approximately 20 percent, and this usually occurs in the first 1 to 2 weeks following diagnosis. Proximal extension of calf vein thrombosis can be detected by noninvasive testing with IPG or Doppler ultrasound.[10,65,66] Where these tests are readily available, it is safe to withhold anticoagulants, providing proximal extension of the thrombosis is not detected.[10,65,66] If facilities to monitor extension of calf vein thrombosis are not available, these patients should be treated with heparin and warfarin in the usual fashion.[14]

OTHER APPROACHES TO THE TREATMENT OF VENOUS THROMBOEMBOLISM

Low-molecular-weight heparin has been shown to be effective in the treatment of proximal venous thrombosis. A number of studies used repeat venography 5 to 7 days after commencing therapy.[173-180] Low-molecular-weight heparin given intravenously or by once- or twice-daily subcutaneous injection was compared with subcutaneous or intravenous unfractionated heparin. These studies showed equal or improved effectiveness of low-molecular-weight heparin over unfractionated heparin with a similar bleeding risk.[173-180]

Two multicenter randomized clinical trials using clinical endpoints compared the use of low-molecular-weight heparin subcutaneously once or twice daily with continuous intravenous heparin with warfarin commenced at the beginning of the study[151] or after 10 days of treatment.[177] In the largest treatment trial to date,[151] fixed-dose subcutaneous low-molecular-weight heparin (Logiparin 175 Xa units/kg) once daily was compared with intravenous heparin by continuous infusion adjusted to maintain an aPTT of 1.5 to 2.5 times the mean normal control value. All patients had venographically proven proximal vein thrombosis. New episodes of venous thromboembolism were seen in 6 of 213 patients receiving low-molecular-weight heparin (2.8 percent) and in 15 of 219 patients receiving intravenous unfractionated heparin (6.9 percent; $p = 0.07$; 95 percent Cl for the difference = 0.02 to 8.1 percent).[151] Major bleeding associated with initial therapy occurred in one patient receiving low-molecular-weight heparin (0.5 percent) and in 11 patients receiving intravenous unfractionated heparin (5.0 percent), a reduction in risk of 95 percent ($p = 0.006$). During long-term warfarin therapy, major hemorrhage was seen in 5 patients who had received low-molecular-weight heparin (2.3 percent) and in none of those receiving intravenous heparin ($p = 0.028$). Ten patients who received low-molecular-weight heparin (4.7 percent) died, as compared with 21 patients who received intravenous unfractionated heparin (9.6 percent), a risk reduction of 51 percent ($p = 0.049$). The most striking difference was in abrupt deaths in patients with metastatic carcinoma, and the majority of these deaths occurred within the first 3 weeks.[151]

Low-molecular-weight heparin (CY216 Fraxiparine) was compared with continuous-intravenous unfractionated heparin in the treatment of patients with proximal venous thrombosis.[176] Either low-molecular-weight heparin or intravenous heparin was continued for 10 days and was then followed by oral warfarin sodium treatment for 3 months. Patients in the low-molecular-weight heparin groups received subcutaneous injections every 12 hours according to body weight (12,500 anti-Xa ICU for patients < 55 kg; 15,000 anti-Xa ICU for patients between 55 and 80 kg; and 17,500 anti-Xa ICU for patients > 80 kg). Patients in the adjusted-dose intravenous heparin group received a continuous infusion to maintain the aPTT within 1.5 to 2.0 times the mean normal control value. In this study, contrast venography was repeated on day 10 or earlier if new symptoms developed. The frequency of objectively diagnosed recurrent venous thromboembolism did not differ significantly between the unfractionated heparin and the low-molecular-weight heparin groups [12 (14 percent) versus 6 (7 percent); 95 percent Cl = − 3 to + 15 percent; $p = 0.13$].[177] There was no significant difference in clinically evident bleeding between the two groups (3.5 percent for unfractionated heparin versus 1.1 percent for low-molecular-weight heparin; $p > 0.2$). In the 6-month follow-up period, there were 12 deaths in the unfractionated heparin group versus 6 in the CY216 group, and this difference was largely due to cancer deaths (8 of 18 in the unfractionated

heparin group versus 1 of 15 in the low-molecular-weight heparin group).[177]

The long-term use of low-molecular-weight heparin has been shown to be safe in the treatment of patients experiencing side effects on oral anti coagulants[181] and in small case series in pregnant patients.[182,183] Randomized clinical trials assessing the effectiveness of long-term use of low-molecular-weight heparin are currently underway. Low-molecular-weight heparin is at least as effective and as safe as unfractionated heparin in the treatment of proximal venous thrombosis, and it is more cost-effective.[184] Furthermore, the drug can be given by a once-daily subcutaneous injection without laboratory monitoring, and this will permit the use of outpatient treatment.

Thrombolysis has a limited role in the treatment of proximal venous thrombosis. Randomized studies comparing the use of streptokinase with intravenous heparin show a higher degree of thrombolysis with streptokinase and a trend toward reduction in postthrombotic sequelae.[185] However, there is an increased risk of major bleeding with streptokinase when compared with heparin, particularly in older subjects.[185] Thrombolysis may be of benefit in younger patients with the recent onset of extensive ileofemoral thrombosis, particularly if there is threatened vascular insufficiency. The hope that the early use of thrombolytic therapy can decrease the incidence of postphlebitic changes has not been substantiated by randomized clinical trials.

REFERENCES

1. Dismuke SE, Wagner EH: Pulmonary embolism as a cause of death. The changing mortality in hospitalized patients. JAMA 1986;255:2039.
2. Dalen JE, Alpert JS: Natural history of pulmonary embolism. Prog Cardiac Dis 1975;17:257.
3. Anderson FA, Wheeler HB, Goldberg RJ, et al: A population-based perspective of the hospital incidence and case-fatality rates of deep vein thrombosis and pulmonary embolism. Arch Intern Med 1991;151:933.
4. Donaldson GA, Williams C, Scanell J, et al: A reappraisal of the application of the Trendelenburg operation to massive fatal embolism. N Engl J Med 1963;268:171.

5. Clagett GP, Reisch JS: Prevention of venous thromboembolism in general surgical patients: Results of meta-analysis. Ann Surg 1988;208:227.

6. Collins R, Scrimgeour A, Yusef S, et al: Reduction in fatal pulmonary embolism and venous thrombosis by perioperative administration of subcutaneous heparin. N Engl J Med 1988;318:1162.

7. Colditz GA, Tuden RL, Oster G: Rates of venous thrombosis after general surgery: Combined results of randomized clinical trials. Lancet 1986; 19:143.

8. Nicolaides AN, Arcelus J, Belcaro G, et al: Prevention of venous thromboembolism. Int Angiol 1992;11(3):151.

9. Hull RD, Hirsh J, Carter CJ, et al: Diagnostic efficacy of impedance plethysmography for clinically suspected deep-vein thrombosis: A randomized trial. Ann Intern Med 1985;102:21.

10. Huisman MV, Buller HE, ten Cate JW, et al: Serial impedance plethysmography for suspected deep venous thrombosis in outpatients. The Amsterdam General Practitioner Study. N Engl J Med 1986;314:823.

11. Moser KM, Le Moine JR: Is embolic risk conditioned by location of deep venous thrombosis? Ann Intern Med 1981;94:439.

12. Huisman MV, Buller HR, ten Cate JW, et al: Management of clinically suspected acute venous thrombosis in outpatients with serial impedanceplethysmography in a community hospital setting. Arch Intern Med 1989;149:511.

13. Kakkar VV, Flanc C, Howe CT, et al: Natural history of post-operative deep-vein thrombosis. Lancet 1969;2:230.

14. Lagerstedt CI, Fagher BO, Olsson CG, et al: Need for long-term anticoagulant treatment in symptomatic calf-vein thrombosis. Lancet 1985;2:515.

15. Hull RD, Delmore T, Genton E, et al: Warfarin sodium versus low-dose heparin in the long-term treatment of venous thrombosis. N Engl J Med 1979;301:855.

16. Huisman MV, Buller HR, ten Cate JW, et al: Unexpected high prevalence of silent pulmonary embolism in patients with deep venous thrombosis. Chest 1989;95:498.

17. Sevitt S, Gallagher N: Venous thrombosis and pulmonary embolism. A clinico-pathological study in injured and burned patients. Br J Surg 1961; 48:475.

18. Mavor GE, Galloway JMD: The iliofemoral venous segment as a source of pulmonary emboli. Lancet 1967;1:871.

19. Hull RD, Hirsh J, Carter CJ, et al: Diagnostic value of ventilation-perfusion lung scanning in patients with suspected pulmonary embolism. Chest 1985; 88:819.

20. A collaborative study by the PIOPED Investigators: Value of the ventilation/perfusion scan in acute pulmonary embolism: Results of the Prospective Investigation of Pulmonary Embolism Diagnosis (PIOPED). JAMA 1990;263:2753.

21. Bone RC: Ventilation/perfusion scan in pulmonary embolism: "The emperor is incompletely attired." JAMA 1990;263:2794.

22. Secker-Walker RH: On purple emperors, pulmonary embolism, and venous thrombosis. Ann Intern Med 1983;98:1006.

23. Stein PD, Hull RD, Saltzman HA, et al: Strategy for diagnosis of patients with suspected acute pulmonary embolism. Chest 1993;103(5):1553.

24. Rabinov K, Paulin S: Roentgen diagnosis of venous thrombosis in the leg. Arch Surg 1972; 104:134.

25. Ginsberg JS, Brill-Edwards PA, Demers C, et al: D-dimer in patients with clinically suspected pulmonary embolism. Chest 1993;104(6):1679.

26. Harrison KA, Haire WD, Pappas AA, et al: Plasma D-dimer: A useful tool for evaluating suspected pulmonary embolus. J Nucl Med 1993;34(6):896.

27. Wells PS, Stevens P, Massicotte P, et al: A rapid D-dimer (DD) assay with high sensitivity and negative predictive value (NPV) in patients with suspected deep vein thrombosis (DVT). Blood 1993; 82(10):407a.

28. Hull RD, Carter C, Jay R, et al: The diagnosis of acute recurrent deep-vein thrombosis: A diagnostic challenge. Circulation 1983;67:901.

29. Richards KL, Armstrong DJ, Tikoff G, et al: Noninvasive diagnosis of deep venous thrombosis. Arch Intern Med 1976;136:1091.

30. Hull RD, van Aken WG, Hirsh J, et al: Impedance plethysmography using the occlusive cuff technique in the diagnosis of venous thrombosis. Circulation 1976;53:696.

31. Hull RD, Hirsh J, Sackett DL, et al: Combined use of leg scanning and impedance plethysmography in suspected venous thrombosis: An alternative to venography. N Engl J Med 1977;296:1497.

32. Hull RD, Hirsh J, Sackett DL, et al: Replacement of venography in suspected venous thrombosis by impedance plethysmography and ^{125}I-fibrinogen leg scanning: A less invasive approach. Ann Intern Med 1981;94:12.

33. Prandoni P, Lensing AWA, Huisman MV, et al: A new computerized impedance plethysmograph: Accuracy in the detection of proximal deep vein thrombosis in symptomatic outpatients. Thromb Haemost 1991;65:229.

34. Heijboer H, Cogo A, Büller HR, et al: Detection of deep vein thrombosis with impedance plethysmography and real-time compression ultrasonography in hospitalized patients. Arch Intern Med 1992; 152:1901.

35. Paiement G, Wessinger SJ, Waltman AC, et al: Surveillance of deep vein thrombosis in asymptomatic total hip replacement patients: Impedance plethysmography and fibrinogen scanning versus

roentgenographic phlebography. Am J Surg 1988; 155:400.

36. Cruickshank MK, Levine MN, Hirsh J, et al: An evaluation of impedance plethysmography and ^{125}I-fibrinogen leg scanning in patients following hip surgery. Thromb Haemost 1989;62:830.

37. Cronan JJ, Dorfman GS, Scola FH, et al: Deep venous thrombosis: US assessment using vein compressibility. Radiology 1987;162:191.

38. Lensing AWA, Prandoni P, Brandjes D, et al: Detection of deep-vein thrombosis by real-time B-mode ultrasonography. N Engl J Med 1989;320:342.

39. Monreal M, Montserrat E, Salvador R, et al: Real-time ultrasound for diagnosis of symptomatic venous thrombosis and for screening of patients at risk. Angiology 1989;40:527.

40. Habscheid W, Hohmann M, Wilhelm T, et al: Real-time ultrasound in the diagnosis of acute deep venous thrombosis of the lower extremity. Angiology 1990;599.

41. Gudmundsen TE, Vinje B, Pedersen T: Deep vein thrombosis of lower extremities. Diagnosis by real-time ultrasonography. Acta Radiol 1990;31:473.

42. Baxter GM, McKechnie S, Duffy P: Colour Doppler ultrasound in deep venous thrombosis: A comparison with venography. Clin Radiol 1990;42:32.

43. Rose ST, Zwiebel WJ, Nelson BD, et al: Symptomatic lower extremity deep venous thrombosis: accuracy, limitations, and role of colour duplex flow imaging in diagnosis. Radiology 1990;175: 639.

44. Mitchell DC, Grasty MS, Stebbings WSL, et al: Comparison of duplex ultrasonography and venography in the diagnosis of deep venous thrombosis. Br J Surg 1991;78:611.

45. Quintavalla R, Larini P, Miselli A, et al: Duplex ultrasound diagnosis of symptomatic proximal deep vein thrombosis of lower limbs. Eur J Radiol 1992;15:32.

46. Schindler JM, Kaiser M, Gerber A, et al: Colour coded duplex sonography in suspected deep vein thrombosis of the leg. Br Med J 1990;301:1369.

47. Mattos MA, Londey GL, Leutz DW, et al: Color-flow duplex scanning for the surveillance and diagnosis of acute deep venous thrombosis. J Vasc Surg 1992;15:366.

48. Vogel P, Laing FC, Jeffrey RB, et al: Deep venous thrombosis of the lower extremity: US evaluation. Radiology 1987;163:747.

49. O'Leary DH, Kane RA, Chase BM: A prospective study of the efficacy of B-scan sonography in the detection of deep venous thrombosis in the lower extremities. J Clin Ultrasound 1988;16:1.

50. Mantoni M: Diagnosis of deep venous thrombosis by duplex sonography. Acta Radiol 1989;30:575.

51. Ginsberg JS, Caco CC, Brill-Edwards P, et al: Venous thrombosis in patients who have undergone major hip or knee surgery: Detection with compression US and impedance plethysmography. Radiology 1991;181:651.

52. Borris LC, Christiansen HM, Lassen MR, et al: Comparison of real-time B-mode ultrasonography and bilateral ascending phlebography for detection of postoperative deep vein thrombosis following elective hip surgery. Thromb Haemost 1989;61:363.

53. Barnes RW, Nix ML, Barnes CL, et al: Perioperative asymptomatic venous thrombosis: Role of duplex scanning versus venography. J Vasc Surg 1989;9:251.

54. Elliott GC, Suchyta M, Rose SC, et al: Duplex ultrasonography for the detection of deep vein thrombi after total hip or knee arthroplasty. Angiology 1993;44:26.

55. Davidson B, Elliott GC, Lensing AWA: Low accuracy of color Doppler ultrasound to detect proximal leg vein thrombosis during screening of asymptomatic high-risk patients. Ann Intern Med 1992;117:735.

56. Rose SC, Zwiebel WJ, Murdock LE, et al: Insensitivity of color Doppler flow imaging for detection of acute calf deep venous thrombosis in asymptomatic postoperative patients. J Vasc Intervent Radiol 1993;4:111.

57. Lensing AWA, Prandoni P, Büller HR, et al: Lower extremity venography with iohexol: Results and complications. Radiology 1990;177:503.

58. Lensing AWA, Büller HR, Prandoni P, et al: Contrast venography, the gold standard for the diagnosis of deep vein thrombosis: Improvement in observer agreement. Thromb Haemost 1992;67:8.

59. McLachlan MSF, Thomson JG, Taylor DW, et al: Observer variation in the interpretation of lower limb venograms. AJR 1979;132:227.

60. Parfrey PS, Griffiths SM, Barrett BJ, et al: Contrast material-induced renal failure in patients with diabetes mellitus, renal insufficiency or both. N Engl J Med 1989;320:143.

61. Schwab SJ, Hlarky MA, Pieper KS, et al: Contrast nephrotoxicity: A randomized, controlled trial of a non-ionic and an ionic radiographic contrast agent. N Engl J Med 1989;320:149.

62. Nicolaides AN, Kakkar VV, Field ES, et al: The origin of deep vein thrombosis: A venographic study. Br J Radiol 1971;44:653.

63. Hull RD, Hirsh J, Sackett DL, et al: Clinical validity of a negative venogram in patients with clinically suspected venous thrombosis. Circulation 1981; 64:622.

64. Hull RD, Taylor DW, Hirsh J, et al: Impedance plethysmography: The relationship between venous filling and sensitivity and specificity for proximal-vein thrombosis. Circulation 1978;58:898.

65. Hull RD, Raskob GE, Coates G, et al: A new non-invasive management strategy for patients with suspected pulmonary embolism. Arch Intern Med 1989;149:2549.

66. Hull RD, Raskob GE, Ginsberg JS, et al: A non-invasive strategy for the treatment of patients with suspected pulmonary embolism. Arch Intern Med 1994;154:289.

67. Skinner DB, Salzman EW: Anticoagulant prophylaxis in surgical patients. Surg Gynecol Obstet 1967; 125:741.

68. Shephard RM, White HA, Shirkey AL: Anticoagulant prophylaxis of thromboembolism in postsurgical patients. Am J Surg 1966;112:498.

69. International Multicentre Trial: Prevention of fatal postoperative pulmonary embolism by low doses of heparin. Lancet 1975;2:45.

70. Coventry MB, Nolan DR, Beckenbaugh RD: "Delayed" prophylactic anticoagulation: A study of results and complications in 2,012 total hip arthroplasties. J Bone Joint Surg 1973;55A:1487.

71. Eskeland G, Solheim K, Skhorten F: Anticoagulant prophylaxis, thromboembolism and morality in elderly patients with hip fracture: A controlled clinical trial. Acta Chir Scand 1986;131:16.

72. Kakkar V, Stamatakis JD, Bentley PG, et al: Prophylaxis for post-operative deep-vein thrombosis. JAMA 1979;241:39.

73. Anderson FA, Wheeler HB, Goldberg RJ, et al: Physician practices in the prevention of venous thromboembolism. Ann Intern Med 1991;115:581.

74. Bergqvist D: Prevention of postoperative deep vein thrombosis in Sweden: Results of a survey. World J Surg 1980;4:489.

75. Laverick MD, Croak SA, Mollan RA: Orthopedic surgeons and thromboprophylaxis. Br Med J 1991;303(6802):549.

76. Salzman EW, Davies GC: Prophylaxis of venous thromboembolism: Analysis of cost-effectiveness. Ann Surg 1980;191:207.

77. Hull R, Hirsh J, Sackett DL, et al: Cost-effectiveness of primary and secondary prevention of fatal pulmonary embolism in high-risk surgical patients. Can Med Assoc J 1982;127:990.

78. Oster G, Tuden RL, Colditz GA: A cost-effectiveness analysis of prophylaxis against deep vein thrombosis in major orthopedic surgery. JAMA 1987;257:203.

79. Bergbqvist D, Matzsch T, Jendteg S, et al: The cost-effectiveness of prevention of postoperative thromboembolism. Acta Chir Scand Suppl 1990; 556:36.

80. Hauch O, Kyattar SC, Jorensen LN: Cost-benefit analysis of prophylaxis against deep vein thrombosis in surgery. Semin Thromb Hemost 1991; 17(suppl 3):280.

81. Leyvrax PF, Richard J, Bachmann F, et al: Adjusted versus fixed dose subcutaneous heparin in the prevention of deep-vein thrombosis after total hip replacement. N Engl J Med 1983;309:954.

82. Leyvraz PF, Bachmann F, Hoek J, et al: Prevention of deep vein thrombosis after hip replacement: Randomised comparison between unfractionated heparin and low molecular weight heparin. Br Med J 1991;303:543.

83. Kakkar VV, Cohen AT, Edmonson RA, et al: Low-molecular-weight versus standard heparin for prevention of venous thromboembolism after major abdominal surgery. Lancet 1993; 341:259.

84. Kakkar VV, Murray WJG: Efficacy and safety of low-molecular-weight heparin (CY216) in preventing postoperative venous thromboembolism: A cooperative study. Br J Surg 1985;72:786.

85. Bergqvist D, Matzsch T, Brumark U, et al: Low-molecular-weight heparin given the evening before surgery compared with conventional low-dose heparin in prevention of thrombosis. Br J Surg 1988;75:888.

86. Fricker JP, Vergnes Y, Schach R, et al: Low-dose heparin versus low-molecular-weight heparin Kabi 2165 in the prophylaxis of thromboembolic complications of abdominal oncological surgery. Eur J Clin Invest 1988;18:561.

87. Samama M, Bernard P, Bonnardot JP, et al: Low-molecular-weight heparin compared with unfractionated heparin in prevention of postoperative thrombosis. Br J Surg 1988;75:128.

88. The European Fraxiparin Study Group: Comparison of a low-molecular-weight heparin and unfractionated heparin for the prevention of deep vein thrombosis in patients undergoing abdominal surgery. Br J Surg 1988;75:1058.

89. Caen JP: A randomized double-blind study between a low-molecular-weight heparin Kabi 2165 and standard heparin in the prevention of deep-vein thrombosis in general surgery: A French multicentre trial. Thromb Haemost 1988;59:216.

90. Leizorovicz A, Picolet H, Peyrieux JC, et al: Prevention of perioperative deep vein thrombosis in general surgery: A multicentre double-blind study comparing two doses of Logiparin and standard heparin. Br J Surg 1991;78:412.

91. Dechavanne M, Ville D, Berruyer M, et al: Randomized trial of a low-molecular-weight heparin (Kabi 2165) versus adjusted-dose subcutaneous standard heparin in the prophylaxis of deep-vein thrombosis after elective hip surgery. Haemostasis 1989;1:5.

92. Turpie AG, Levine MN, Hirsh J, et al: A randomized, controlled trial of a low-molecular-weight heparin (Enoxaparin) to prevent deep-vein thrombosis in patients undergoing elective hip surgery. N Engl J Med 1986;315:925.

93. Levine MN, Hirsh J, Gent M, et al: Prevention of deep vein thrombosis after elective hip surgery: A randomized trial comparing low-molecular-weight heparin with standard unfractionated heparin. Ann Intern Med 1991;114(7):545.

94. Eriksson BI, Kälebo P, Anthmyr BA, et al: Prevention of deep vein thrombosis and pulmonary

embolism after total hip replacement. J Bone Joint Surg 1991;73A(4):484.

95. The Danish Enoxaparin Study Group: Low-molecular weight heparin (Enoxaparin) vs dextran 70. Arch Intern Med 1991;151:1621.

96. Tœrholm C, Broeng L, Jœrgensen PS, et al: Thromboprophylaxis by low-molecular-weight heparin in elective hip surgery: A placebo-controlled study. J Bone Joint Surg 1991;73B:434.

97. Lassen MR, Borris LC, Christiansen HM, et al: Prevention of thromboembolism in 190 hip arthroplasties. Acta Orthop Scand 1991;62(1):33.

98. Planes A, Vochelle N, Fagola M, et al: Prevention of deep vein thrombosis after total hip replacement: The effect of low-molecular-weight heparin with spinal and general anesthesia. J Bone Joint Surg 1991;73B:418.

99. Leclerc JR, Geerts WH, Desjardins L, et al: Prevention of deep vein thrombosis after major knee surgery—A randomized, double-blind trial comparing a low-molecular-weight heparin fragment (Enoxaparin) to placebo. Thromb Haemost 1992;67 (4):417.

100. Hull RD, Raskob GE, Pineo GF, et al: A comparison of subcutaneous low-molecular-weight heparin with warfarin sodium for prophylaxis against deep-vein thrombosis after hip or knee implantation. N Engl J Med 1993;329:1370.

101. Heit J, Kessler C, Mannen E, et al: Efficacy and safety of RD heparin (a LMWH) versus warfarin for prevention of deep-vein thrombosis after hip or knee replacement. Blood 1991;78(10) (suppl):739.

102. Colwell CW, Spiro TE, Trowbridge AA, et al: Use of Enoxaparin, a low-molecular-weight heparin, and unfractionated heparin for the prevention of deep venous thrombosis after elective hip replacement. J Bone Joint Surg 1994;76A (1):3.

103. Hoek J, Nurmohamed MT, ten Cate H, et al: Prevention of deep vein thrombosis following total hip replacement by a low-molecular-weight heparinoid. Thromb Haemost Suppl 1989;62:1637.

104. Bergqvist D, Kettunen K, Fredin H, et al: Thromboprophylaxis in hip fracture patients—A prospective, randomized comparative study between ORG 10172 and dextran. Surgery 1991; 109:617.

105. Gerhart TN, Yett HS, Robertson LK, et al: Low-molecular-weight heparinoid compared with warfarin for prophylaxis of deep vein thrombosis in patients who are operated on for fracture of the hip: A prospective, randomized trial. J Bone Joint Surg 1991;73A(4):494.

106. Nurmohamed MT, Rosendaal FR, Büller HR, et al: Low molecular weight heparin in the prophylaxis of venous thrombosis: A meta-analysis. Lancet 1992;340:152.

107. Francis CW, Pellegrini VD, Marder VJ, et al: Comparison of warfarin and external pneumatic compression in prevention of venous thrombosis after total hip replacement. JAMA 1992;267(21):2911.

108. Paiement F, Wessinger SJ, Waltman WC, et al: Low-dose warfarin versus external pneumatic compression for prophylaxis against venous thromboembolism following total hip replacement. J Arthroplasty 1987;2:23.

109. Kaempffe FA, Lifeso RM, Meinking C: Intermittent pneumatic compression versus Coumadin: Prevention of deep vein thrombosis in lower-extremity total joint arthroplasty. Clin Orthop 1991;269:89.

110. Powers PJ, Gent M, Jay R, et al: A randomized trial of less intense postoperative warfarin or aspirin therapy in the prevention of venous thromboembolism after surgery for fractured hip. Arch Intern Med 1989;149:771.

111. Poller L, McKernan A, Thomson JM, et al: Fixed minidose warfarin: A new approach to prophylaxis against venous thrombosis after major surgery. Br Med J 1987;285:1309.

112. Bern MM, Lokich JJ, Wallach SR, et al: Very low doses of warfarin can prevent thrombosis in central venous catheters. Ann Intern Med 1990;112:423.

113. Dale C, Gallus A, Wycherley A, et al: Prevention of venous thrombosis with minidose warfarin after joint replacement. Br Med J 1991;303: 224.

114. Roberts VC, Sabri S, Beely AH, et al: The effect of intermittently applied external pressure on the hemodynamics of the lower limb in man. Br J Surg 1972;59:233.

115. Turpie AGG, Gallus A, Beattie WS, et al: Prevention of venous thrombosis in patients with intracranial disease by intermittent pneumatic compression of the calf. Neurology 1977;27:435.

116. Turpie AG, Delmore T, Hirsh J, et al: Prevention of venous thrombosis by intermittent sequential calf compression in patients with intracranial disease. Thromb Res 1979;16:611.

117. Skillman JJ, Collins RR, Coe NP, et al: Prevention of deep vein thrombosis in neurosurgical patients: A controlled, randomized trial of external pneumatic compression boots. Surgery 1978;83:354.

118. Hull RD, Raskob G, Gent M, et al: Effectiveness of intermittent pneumatic leg compression for preventing deep vein thrombosis after total hip replacement. JAMA 1990;263:2313.

119. Hull RD, Delmore TJ, Hirsh J, et al: Effectiveness of intermittent pulsatile elastic stockings for the prevention of calf and thigh vein thrombosis in patients undergoing elective knee surgery. Thromb Res 1979;16:37.

120. Mckenna R, Galante J, Bachmann F, et al: Prevention of venous thromboembolism after total knee replacement by high-dose aspirin or intermittent calf and thigh compression. Br Med J 1980;1:514.

121. Turner GM, Cole SE, Brooks JH: The efficacy of graduated compression stockings in the prevention of deep vein thrombosis after major gynaecological surgery. Br J Obstet Gynaecol 1984;91:588.

122. Ishak MA, Moreley KD: Deep venous thrombosis after total hip arthroplasty: A prospective, controlled study to determine the prophylactic effect of graded pressure stockings. Br J Surg 1981;68:429.

123. Allan A, Williams JT, Bolton JP, et al: The use of graduated compression stockings in the prevention of postoperative deep vein thrombosis. Br J Surg 1983;70:172.

124. Wells PS, Lensing AWA, Hirsh J: Graduated compression stockings in the prevention of postoperative venous thromboembolism. Arch Intern Med 1994;154:67.

125. Antiplatelet Trialists' Collaboration: Collaborative overview of randomized trials of antiplatelet therapy: III. Reduction in venous thrombosis and pulmonary embolism by antiplatelet prophylaxis among surgical and medical patients. Br Med J 1994;308:235.

126. Clagett GP, Salzman EW, Brownell Wheeler H, et al: Prevention of venous thromboembolism. Chest 1992;102(4):391S.

127. Moser KM: Venous thromboembolism. Am Rev Respir Dis 1990;141:235.

128. Salzman EW, Deykin D, Shapiro RM, et al: Management of heparin therapy: Controlled prospective trial. N Engl J Med 1976;292:1046.

129. Gallus A, Jackaman J, Tillett J, et al: Safety and efficacy of warfarin started early after submassive venous thrombosis or pulmonary embolism. Lancet 1986;2:1293.

130. Hull RD, Raskob GE, Rosenbloom D, et al: Heparin for 5 days as compared with 10 days in the initial treatment of proximal venous thrombosis. N Engl J Med 1990;322:1260.

131. Bjork I, Lindahl U: Mechanism of the anticoagulant action of heparin. Mol Cell Biochem 1982;48:161.

132. Lindahl U, Backstrom G, Cook M, et al: Structure of the antithrombin-binding site of heparin. Proc Natl Acad Sci USA 1979;76:3198.

133. Rosenberg RD, Damus PS: The purification and mechanism of action of human antithrombin-heparin co-factor. J Biol Chem 1973;248:6490.

134. Rosenberg RD, Lam L: Correlation between structure and function of heparin. Proc Natl Acad Sci USA 1979;76:1218.

135. Tollefsen DM, Majerus DW, Blank MK: Heparin co-factor II: Purification and properties of thrombin in human plasma. J Biol Chem 1982;257:2162.

136. Hirsh J, Dalen JE, Deykin D, et al: Heparin: Mechanism of action, pharmacokinetics, dosing considerations, monitoring, efficacy, and safety. Chest 1992;102(4):337S.

137. Colvin BT, Barrowcliffe TW on behalf of BCSH Haemostasis and Thrombosis Task Force: The British Society for Haematology Guidelines on the use and monitoring of heparin 1992: Second revision. J Clin Pathol 1993;46:97.

138. Hirsh J, van Aken WG, Gallus AS, et al: Heparin kinetics in venous thrombosis and pulmonary embolism. Circulation 1976;53:691.

139. Hull RD, Raskob GE, Rosenbloom DR, et al: Optimal therapeutic level of heparin therapy in patients with venous thrombosis. Arch Intern Med 1992;152:1589.

140. Levine MN, Hirsh J, Gent M, et al: A randomized trial comparing activated thromboplastin time with heparin assay in patients with acute venous thromboembolism requiring large daily doses of heparin. Arch Intern Med 1994;154:49.

141. Hull RD, Raskob GE, Hirsh J, et al: Continuous intravenous heparin compared with intermittent subcutaneous heparin in the initial treatment of proximal-vein thrombosis. N Engl J Med 1986;315:1109.

142. Brill-Edwards P, Ginsberg S, Johnston M, et al: Establishing a therapeutic range for heparin therapy. Ann Intern Med 1993;119:104.

143. Brandjes DPM, Heijboer H, Buller HR, et al: Acenocoumarol and heparin compared with acenocoumarol alone in the initial treatment of proximal-vein thrombosis. N Engl J Med 1992;327:1485.

144. Raschke RA, Reilly BM, Guidry JR, et al: The weight-based heparin dosing nomogram compared with a "standard care" nomogram. Ann Intern Med 1993;119:874.

145. Levine MN, Hirsh J, Kelton JG: Heparin-Induced Bleeding. Boca Raton, Fla, CRC Press, 1989, p 517.

146. Cruickshank MK, Levine MN, Hirsh J, et al: A standard nomogram for the management of heparin therapy. Arch Intern Med 1991;151:333.

147. Fennerty A, Thomas P, Backhouse G, et al: Audit of control of heparin treatment. Br Med J 1985;290:27.

148. Wheeler AP, Jaquiss RD, Newman JH: Physician practices in the treatment of pulmonary embolism and deep-venous thrombosis. Arch Intern Med 1988;148:1321.

149. Elliott GC, Hiltunen SJ, Suchyta M, et al: Physician guided treatment compared with a heparin protocol for deep vein thrombosis. Arch Intern Med 1994;154:999.

150. Hull RD, Brant RF, Pineo GF, et al: Heparin (H) resistance as a predictor of recurrent venous thromboembolism (RVTE). Blood 1993;82(10)(suppl 1):1613.

151. Hull RD, Raskob GE, Pineo GF, et al: Subcutaneous low-molecular weight heparin compared with continuous intravenous heparin in the treatment of proximal-vein thrombosis. N Engl J Med 1992;326:975.

152. Freedman MD: Oral anticoagulants: Pharmacodynamics, clinical indications and adverse effects. J Clin Pharmacol 1992;32:196.

153. Furie B, Furie BC: Molecular basis of vitamin K–dependent gamma-carboxylation. Blood 1990; 75:1753.

154. Hirsh J, Dalen JE, Deykin D, et al: Oral anticoagulants: Mechanism of action, clinical effectiveness, and optimal therapeutic range. Chest 1992;102 (4)(suppl):312S.

155. Clouse LH, Comp PC: The regulation of haemostasis: The protein C system. N Engl J Med 1986; 314:1298.

156. O'Reilly RA, Aggeler PM: Studies on coumarin anticoagulant drugs: Initiation of warfarin therapy without a loading dose. Circulation 1968; 38:169.

157. Gurwitz JH, Avorn J, Ross-Degnan D, et al: Aging and the anticoagulant response to warfarin therapy. Ann Intern Med 1992;116:901.

158. Wells PS, Holbrook AM, Crowther R, et al: Warfarin and its drug/food interactions: A critical appraisal of the literature. Thromb Haemost 1993; 69(6):1133.

159. Hull R, Hirsh J, Jay R, et al: Different intensities of oral anticoagulant therapy in the treatment of proximal-vein thrombosis. N Engl J Med 1982; 307:1676.

160. Bussey HI, Force RW, Bianco TM, et al: Reliance on prothrombin time ratios causes significant errors in anticoagulation therapy. Arch Intern Med 1992;152:278.

161. Turpie AGG (on behalf of Thrombosis Interest Group): Control of anticoagulant therapy: A cross Canada survey. Thromb Haemost 1993;69(6):677.

162. Garr SB, Rodgers GM: Laboratory monitoring of warfarin therapy in Utah. Am J Hematol 1994; 45:85.

163. Ovesen L, Lyduch S, Ott P: A simple technique for predicting maintenance dosage of warfarin—is it better than empirical dosing? Eur J Clin Pharmacol 1989;37:573.

164. White RH, McCurdy SA, von Marensdorff H, et al: Home prothrombin time monitoring after the initiation of warfarin therapy. Ann Intern Med 1989;111:730.

165. Furie B, Liebman HA, Blanchard RA, et al: Comparison of the native prothrombin antigen and the prothrombin time for monitoring oral anticoagulant therapy. Blood 1984;64:445.

166. Holmgren K, Andersson G, Fagrell B, et al: One-month versus six-month therapy with oral anticoagulants after symptomatic deep-vein thrombosis. Acta Med Scand 1985;218:279.

167. O'Sullivan EF: Duration of anticoagulant therapy in venous thromboembolism. Med J Aust 1972; 2:1104.

168. Petitti DB, Strom BL, Melmon KL: Duration of warfarin anticoagulant therapy and the probabilities of recurrent thromboembolism and hemorrhage. Am J Med 1986;81:255.

169. Schulman S, Lockner D, Juhlin-Dannfelt A: The duration of oral anticoagulants after deep-vein thrombosis: A randomized study. Acta Med Scand 1985;217:547.

170. Research Committee of the British Thoracic Society: Optimum duration of anticoagulation for deep-vein thrombosis and pulmonary embolism. Lancet 1992;340:873.

171. Hyers TN, Hull RD, Weg JG: Antithrombotic therapy for venous thromboembolic disease. Chest 1992;102(4):408S.

172. Prandoni P, Lensing AWA, Buller HR, et al: Deep-vein thrombosis and the incidence of subsequent symptomatic cancer. N Engl J Med 1992;327:1128.

173. Bratt G, Tornebohm E, Granqvist S, et al: A comparison between low-molecular-weight heparin (KABI 2165) and standard heparin in the intravenous treatment of deep venous thrombosis. Thromb Haemost 1985;54:813.

174. Bratt G, Aberg W, Johansson M, et al: Two daily subcutaneous injections of Fragmin as compared with intravenous standard heparin in the treatment of deep venous thrombosis (DVT). Thromb Haemost 1990;64:506.

175. Holm HA, Ly B, Handeland GF, et al: Subcutaneous heparin treatment of deep venous thrombosis: A comparison of unfractionated and low molecular weight heparin. Haemostasis 1986; 16:30.

176. Albada J, Nieuwenhuis HK, Sixma JJ: Treatment of acute venous thromboembolism with low-molecular-weight heparin (Fragmin). Results of a double-blind, randomized study. Circulation 1989; 80:935.

177. Prandoni P, Lensing AW, Buller HR, et al: Comparison of subcutaneous low-molecular-weight heparin with intravenous standard heparin in proximal deep-vein thrombosis. Lancet 1992; 339:441.

178. Huet Y, Janvier G, Bendriss PH, et al: Treatment of established venous thromboembolism with Enoxaparin: Preliminary report. Acta Chir Scand Suppl 1990;556:116.

179. Siegbahn A, Y-Hassan S, Boberg J, et al: Subcutaneous treatment of deep venous thrombosis with low molecular weight heparin. A dose finding study with LMWH-Novo. Thromb Res 1989; 55:767.

180. Simonneau G, Charbonnier B, Decousus H, et al: Subcutaneous low-molecular-weight heparin compared with continuous intravenous unfractionated heparin in the treatment of proximal deep vein thrombosis. Arch Intern Med 1993; 153:1541.

181. Harenberg J, Leber G, Dempfle CE, et al: Long-term anticoagulation with low molecular weight heparin in outpatients with side effects on oral anticoagulants. Nouv Rev Fr Hematol 1989; 31:363.
182. Melissari E, Parker CJ, Wilson NV, et al: Use of low-molecular-weight heparin in pregnancy. Thromb Haemost 1992;68(6):652.
183. Forestier F, Sole Y, Aiach M, et al: Absence of transplacental passage of Fragmin (Kabi) during the second and the third trimesters of pregnancy. Thromb Haemost 1992;67(1):180.
184. Hull RD, Rosenbloom D, Pineo GF, et al: A cost-effectiveness analysis of low-molecular-weight heparin compared with continuous intravenous heparin in the treatment of proximal-vein thrombosis. Circulation 1993;88(4)(2):I-516.
185. Goldhaber SZ: Pooled analyses of randomized trials of streptokinase and heparin in phlebographically documented acute deep venous thrombosis. Am J Med 1984;76:393.

Pulmonary Embolism and Vena Caval Interruption

CYNTHIA K. SHORTELL

Pulmonary embolism is responsible for approximately 50,000 deaths annually.[1] The source of embolus is deep venous thrombosis of the lower extremities in the majority of patients.[2] Consequently, the primary focus in the acute management of patients with lower extremity deep venous thrombosis is the prevention of clinically significant pulmonary embolism. Of secondary importance is local control of the thrombotic process and prevention of the postphlebitic syndrome. With regard to both these goals, anticoagulation traditionally has been the mainstay of therapy. Anticoagulation therapy greatly reduces the risk of pulmonary embolism in patients with deep venous thrombosis[3] and reduces long-term venous morbidity.[4–9] In approximately 10 percent of patients, however, anticoagulation is either contraindicated or fails to prevent pulmonary embolism.[10] Under these circumstances, it may be necessary to employ a physical barrier to prevent pulmonary embolism. Over the past two decades, transvenous intraluminal devices have been employed successfully in this regard. In fact, with increasing evidence of the safety and efficacy of many of these devices, it has been suggested that indications for their use be liberalized. Some investigators have advocated vena caval interruption as the primary therapy for acute deep venous thrombosis in subsets of patients in whom anticoagulation is expected to be excessively hazardous, ineffective, or both.[11–14]

BACKGROUND OF VENA CAVAL INTERRUPTION DEVICES

Although anticoagulation with heparin is presently the mainstay of therapy for acute deep venous thrombosis, the use of mechanical means to prevent venous thromboembolism actually predated the discovery of anticoagulants. The earliest of these efforts included simple ligation of the femoral vein[15–18] and later of the inferior vena cava.[19] However, the perioperative mortality associated with vena caval ligation was approximately 20 percent, recurrent pulmonary embolism was seen in up to 36 percent of patients, and long-term venous morbidity was observed in 65 percent of patients.[20] The need to maintain vena caval patency while trapping embolic fragments was thus recognized, and efforts were directed at developing such a device. An additional consideration was the avoidance of an intraabdominal procedure in an already compromised patient.

The earliest attempts at filtration of emboli without vena caval ligation included direct plication using sutures[21,22] or staples.[23] Unfortunately, the channels created by these techniques frequently dilated over time, allowing the passage of embolic debris. This problem was overcome by the development of external plication devices such as the Adams-DeWeese clip.[24] All these modalities, however, have the disadvantage of requiring laparotomy and in addition are associated with a high long-term rate of vena caval occlusion, possibly due to the intimal injury induced.[15]

A number of experimental devices, including the Eichelter sieve,[25] the Hunter[26] and Moser[27] balloons, and the Pate clip,[28] were introduced between 1969 and 1971 but never gained popularity. The first transvenous filtration device to be widely utilized was the Mobin-Uddin umbrella. This device consists of an umbrella-like frame with multiple circular perforations, supported by a series of radial supports providing fixation to the vena caval wall.[29,30] Advantages of this device included insertion via the right internal jugular vein and a reduction in the long-term rate of recurrent pulmonary embolism to 3 to 10 percent. Vena caval occlusion, however, remained high at approximately 60 percent, and a high rate of significant proximal migration resulted in discontinuation of its use.[29,30]

From the experience with these first efforts at transvenous vena caval filtration, criteria have emerged that define the ideal vena caval filtration device, and great strides have been made toward the development of devices that now more closely approximate these criteria. The ideal caval filtration device (1) is readily inserted and precisely positioned using a local anaesthetic only, (2) effectively prevents recurrent pulmonary embolism, (3) is associated with a low rate of long-term caval occlusion, (4) does not migrate significantly from its original position, and (5) is not associated with erosion or perforation of the vena cava.[15]

TRANSVENOUS/INTRALUMINAL DEVICES

General Principles

INDICATIONS AND ALTERNATIVE THERAPIES

Anticoagulation with heparin is the standard of care in patients with acute deep venous thrombosis and is successful in the majority of patients. In some patients, however, anticoagulation therapy may be ineffective or contraindicated, and prevention of pulmonary embolus must be accomplished by mechanical means. Specific indications have been established to delineate those patients in whom vena caval interruption is indicated[15,31]:

1. Clinically significant pulmonary embolism in the presence of adequate anticoagulation
2. Clinically significant pulmonary embolism in a patient with an absolute contraindication to anticoagulation (e.g., gastrointestinal, intracranial, or other life-threatening hemorrhage, severe diastolic hypertension, or development of heparin-induced thrombocytopenia)
3. Clinically significant pulmonary embolism secondary to iliofemoral venous thrombosis
4. Following pulmonary embolectomy (catheter or surgical)

The use of transvenous intraluminal vena caval filtration in the preceding settings is well accepted by most surgeons. Additional indications that remain controversial include the use of vena caval filtration in patients with proximal propagation of iliofemoral thrombi despite adequate anticoagulation,[31,32] a single but massive pulmonary embolism, regardless of anticoagulation status,[31] and patients with a history of pulmonary embolism and a relative contraindication to anticoagulation (e.g., the elderly patient who lives alone).[32]

PRINCIPLES AND GENERAL TECHNIQUES

Insertion of the filtration device is accomplished via the right femoral vein in the majority of patients, with the right internal jugular vein being the second most commonly used delivery site.[32] The left femoral vein may be used for placement of a vena caval filter if the right femoral and internal jugular sites are unavailable, but anatomic considerations make placement from this delivery site technically challenging.

The anatomy of the venous system, including vena caval diameter and clot extension, should be evaluated prior to placement of the filtration device. Both these issues can be addressed using either venacavograhy or ultrasonography. If the thrombotic process involves or extends beyond the right femoral vein, this approach is unsuitable for filter placement, and the right jugular vein should be used. If the vena caval diameter exceeds the maximal expansion capability of the intended device (e.g., 28 mm for the Greenfield filter), filters should be placed in the bilateral iliac veins, or a larger device should be selected.

In most patients, the desired location for a vena caval filtration device is below the renal veins, usually at the level of the second and third lumbar vertebrae (Fig. 29-1). This position should be confirmed by dye injection through the introducer prior to deployment of the filter. In less than 10 percent of patients,[33] suprarenal placement is necessary (Fig 29-2). Indications for suprarenal placement include propagation of thrombus to the level of the renal veins and lower extremity deep venous thrombosis in pregnant patients or patients in whom pregnancy is anticipated or in patients in whom the thromboembolic source is the pelvic or gonadal veins.[33]

Available Devices

GREENFIELD FILTER

The Greenfield filter, introduced in its original stainless steel form in 1972, is the most commonly employed transvenous vena caval interruption device. The conical shape of the filter is ideally suited to allow effective trapping of fragments 3 mm or larger in its apex while maximizing flow through the outer circumference of the filter.[35] When 70 percent of the filter is filled with thrombus, only 49

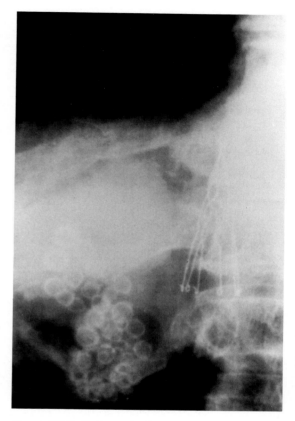

Figure 29-2. Radiograph depicting Greenfield filter in suprarenal position.

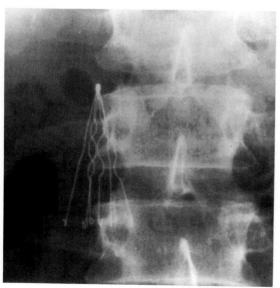

Figure 29-1. Radiograph depicting Greenfield filter in standard infrarenal position.

percent of the cross-sectional area is occluded. When fully expanded, the filter is 28 mm across the base and 4.6 cm long, and it is anchored to the caval wall by six radial spokes.[35] Long-term follow-up in almost 500 patients demonstrated a 4 percent rate of recurrent pulmonary embolism and a 95 percent vena caval patency rate when placed in the infrarenal position.[36] In a series of 71 patients with suprarenal Greenfield filters, the results were similar, with no report of vena caval thrombosis or renal dysfunction[33] Complications of placement include malposition, penetration, and migration, occurring in a small percentage of patients and rarely causing clinically significant sequelae. Penetration is almost invariably localized, and migration usually is minimal. Occasionally, interventional radiologic techniques may be required to retrieve filters that migrate or

Table 29-1. Comparison of Transvenous Vena Caval Filtration Devices

Filter	Author	No. of Patients	Recurrent Pulmonary Embolism	IVC Occlusion	Insertion-Site Occlusion	Migration
Stainless steel Greenfield	Greenfield (1988)[36]	469	4%	5%	40%	10%
Titanium Greenfield	Greenfield (1994)[38]	173	3%	1%	2%	7%
Bird's nest	Roehm (1988)[39]	440	3%	3%	N/A	9%
Venatech	Millward (1994)[42]	63	6%	24%	8%	12%
Nitinol	Simon (1989)[45]	44	4%	20%	28%	2%
Amplatz	Epstein (1989)[46]	42	2%	17%	3%	2%

are accidentally discharged in the heart.[37] A more frequent complication observed with percutaneous placement of the stainless steel Greenfield filter, because of the no. 26 French dilator system required for insertion, is the 30 to 40 percent incidence of insertion-site thrombosis when the right femoral vein is used.[15] The titanium Greenfield filter was developed in order to reduce the incidence of insertion-site thrombosis. The flexibility of titanium enabled a reduction in the size of introducer to no. 12 French. Initial experience with the titanium Greenfield filter was comparable with that of the stainless steel Greenfield filter in most respects. An unacceptably high rate of distal migration (30 percent), however, necessitated revision of the hook design. The modified hook titanium Greenfield filter has been in use since 1989, with rates of recurrent pulmonary embolism, vena caval patency, and distal migration that are comparable with those of the stainless steel Greenfield filter and with a reduction in the incidence of insertion-site thrombosis to 8 percent.[38]

BIRD'S NEST FILTER

The bird's nest filter, introduced in clinical trials in 1982,[39] consists of four stainless steel wires preshaped with multiple, short, nonmatching bends. Each wire ends in a V-shaped strut with a hook attachment for vena caval fixation. The present model is introduced via a no. 12 French sheath, and the first set of hooks is engaged, followed by

extrusion of the wires over a 7-cm length of inferior vena cava, and finally, the remaining hooks are set.[15,39] In 440 patients in whom the bird's nest filter was placed, the incidence of recurrent pulmonary embolism was 3 percent, and the rate of vena caval occlusion was 3 percent. Proximal migration has been a significant problem, even with modification of the strut design.[39,40] The bird's nest filter affords a number of advantages over other vena caval filters: the tight network of wires traps even the smallest emboli, it is suitable for use in vena cavae up to 40 mm in diameter, and its nonsymmetrical configuration eliminates the need for centering the device.[39,41] The major disadvantages of the bird's nest filter are the relatively high rates of vena caval occlusion and the difficulties with proximal migration.

VENATECH FILTER

The Venatech, or LGM, filter is a cone-shaped device formed by six radial struts anchored to the vena cava by hooked stabilizing struts. The filter is usually placed via the right internal jugular approach, using a no. 12 French introducer.[42] The filter must be released abruptly or incomplete opening may occur.[15,32,42] The major experience with the filter reported in the literature is a single series of 100 patients.[43] The authors report a 2 percent incidence of recurrent pulmonary embolism and a vena caval occlusion rate of 8 percent. Incomplete opening, malpositioning, or tilting (usually attributed to failure to effect brisk release of the device) resulted in incorrect placement of the filter in about 15 percent of patients. Caudal migration occurred immediately in 13 percent and was noted later in an additional 13 percent of patients at 1 year. More recent reports showed slightly improved rates of migration (12 to 14 percent)[42,44] and incomplete opening (3 to 6 percent),[42,44] with insertion-site thrombosis in 8 to 23 percent,[42,44] but a 6 percent rate of recurrent pulmonary embolism and a disturbing 24 percent incidence of vena caval occlusion.[42]

SIMON NITINOL FILTER

The unique thermal shape-memory properties of the nickel-titanium alloy nitinol confer the capability of instant configuration transformation on this filter. When cool, the alloy can exist as a soft, straight set of wires, but when exposed to body temperature, it immediately regains its preformed shape. This consists of a conical base, topped by a more spherical and tightly knit crown, designed to trap larger- and smaller-sized fragments, respectively.[45] The filter is inserted through a no. 9 French sheath and adapts to a maximal caval diameter of 28 mm. Because of its thermal dependence, the filter must be introduced using an iced saline infusion system.[45] Short- and long-term follow-up[32,45] demonstrate a 4 percent incidence of recurrent pulmonary embolism, a 2 percent incidence of proximal migration, a 28 percent incidence of insertion-site thrombosis, and a 20 percent incidence of caval occlusion, including 3 patients in whom massive thrombosis was fatal.[32,45]

AMPLATZ RETRIEVABLE FILTER

The Amplatz filter is an inverted cone-shaped device with an apical loop that can be used for filter retrieval. In a series of 52 patients,[46] the incidence of recurrent pulmonary embolism was 2 percent, with a vena caval occlusion rate of 21 percent, and insertion-site thrombosis rate of 2 percent. Migration and tilting were each noted in 2 percent of patients. The most disturbing finding was that of thrombus in the apex on the cardiac side of the filter in 25 percent patients. Filters were retrieved

in 5 patients, with varying difficulty. Technical problems were usually related to hook inaccessibility, and in 2 patients removal of the device resulted in a localized vena caval injury without clinical significance.[46] Potential indications for temporary filter placement include transient contraindications to anticoagulation (e.g., the postoperative state) and protection against pulmonary embolism during thrombolytic therapy for iliofemoral deep venous thrombosis.[15]

Based on the presently available data, the stainless steel Greenfield filter must be considered the "gold standard" by which other transvenous vena caval filtration devices are measured. Initial data on the titanium Greenfield filter appears to demonstrate a similar performance record. In light of the increasing body of evidence documenting the safety and efficacy of the Greenfield filter, many authors have advocated liberalizing the indications for placement of this device, particularly in subsets of patients in whom anticoagulation confers an excessive risk (elderly patients),[11] is likely to be less effective in preventing pulmonary embolism (high-risk patients undergoing total joint replacement),[14] or both (patients with malignancy).[12,13]

PULMONARY CATHETER EMBOLECTOMY

In approximately 10 percent of patients who sustain a pulmonary embolism, the event is considered "massive," resulting in severe hypoxia (PaO_2 < 50 mmHg, $PaCO_2$ < 30 mmHg) and hypotension requiring inotropic support.[15] Under these circumstances, aggressive treatment is needed if survival is to be accomplished, with the three therapeutic options being thrombolytic therapy, operative pulmonary embolectomy, and pulmonary catheter embolectomy. Use of thrombolytic agents was discussed in Chap. 22, but in general, its utility is limited by the presence of contraindications to lytic therapy and the gravity of the patient's condition or both. Operative embolectomy requires mobilization of considerable personnel and resources, including cardiopulmonary bypass, and may not be feasible in all hospital settings. In a meta-analysis of 651 patients undergoing open pulmonary embolectomy for pulmonary embolism,[47] the overall survival rate was 58 percent, with postoperative complications including pulmonary hemorrhage and stroke. Transvenous pulmonary catheter embolectomy was first introduced in 1969[48] in an effort to provide a more rapid, less invasive method with applicability in a wider number of hospital settings. A steerable catheter is introduced using the jugular or femoral approach and advanced into the pulmonary artery. Positioning of the catheter into the clot is guided by use of contrast dye, and suction is then applied on a repeated basis until the clot is cleared, as determined by changes in arteriographic and hemodynamic criteria.[15] Immediate placement of a vena caval interruption device is recommended. In a recent series of 32 patients,[49] the authors reported a 91 percent rate of procedural success, with a 78 percent survival rate. Transvenous pulmonary catheter embolectomy should be considered in patients with massive pulmonary embolism and contraindictions to lytic therapy or in those who have failed to respond to lytic therapy, particularly in institutions or situations in which a cardiothoracic surgical team with cardiopulmonary bypass capabilities is not immediately available.

REFERENCES

1. Consensus Development Panel: Prevention of venous thrombosis and pulmonary embolism. JAMA 1986;256:744.
2. Sevitt S, Gallagher NG: Venous thrombosis and pulmonary embolism: A clinicopathological study in injured and burned patients. Br J Surg 1961; 48:475.
3. Coon WW, Willis PW, Symons MJ: Assessment of anticoagulant treatment of venous thromboembolism. Ann Surg 1969;170:599.
4. Greenfield LJ, Michna BA: Twelve-year clinical experience with the Greenfield vena caval filter. Surg 1988;104:706.
5. Dorfman GS, Cronan JJ, Paolella LP, et al: Iatrogenic changes at the venotomy site after percutaneous placement of the Greenfield filter. Radiology 1989;173:159.
6. Greenfield LJ, Zocco J, Wilk J, et al: Clinical experience with the Kimray Greenfield vena caval filter. Ann Surg 1977;185:692.
7. Wingerd M, Bernhard VM, Maddison F, et al: Comparison of caval filters in the management of venous thrombolism. Arch Surg 1978;113:1264.

8. Cimochowski GE, Evans RH, Zarins CK, et al: Greenfield filter versus Mobin-Uddin umbrella. J Thorac Cardiovasc Surg 1980;79:358.
9. Greenfield LJ, Peyton R, Crute S, et al: Greenfield vena caval filter experience. Arch Surg 1981; 116:1451.
10. Bell WR, Simon TL: Current status of pulmonary thromboembolic disease: Patho-physiology, diagnosis, prevention and treatment. Am Heart J 1982;103:239.
11. Fink J, Jones BT: The greenfield filter as the primary means of therapy in venous thromboembolic disease. Surgery 1991;172:253.
12. Cohen JR, Tenenbaum N, Citron M: Greenfield filter as primary therapy for deep venous thrombosis and/or pulmonary embolism in patients with cancer. Surgery 1991;109:12.
13. Cohen JR, Grella L, Citron M: Greenfield filter instead of heparin as primary treatment for deep venous thrombosis or pulmonary embolism in patients with cancer. Cancer 1992;70:1993.
14. Vaughn BK, Knezevich S, Lombardi AV, et al: Use of the greenfield filter to prevent fatal pulmonary embolism associated with total hip and knee arthroplasty. J Bone Joint Surg 1989;71A:1542.
15. Greenfield LJ, DeLucia A: Endovascular therapy of venous thromboembolic disease. Endovasc Surg 1992;72:969.
16. Greenfield LJ: Evolution of venous interruption for pulmonary thromboembolism. Arch Surg 1992; 127:622.
17. Hunter J: Observation on inflammation of internal coat of veins. Trans Soc Improv Med Chir Knowledge (Lond) 1973;1:18.
18. Homans J: Deep quiet venous thrombosis in the lower limb. Surg Gynecol Obstet 1944;79:70.
19. Bottini. Cited by Dale WA: Ligation of the inferior vena cava for thromboembolism. Surgery 1958; 43:22.
20. Garner AMN: Inferior vena caval interruption in the prevention of fatal pulmonary embolism. Am Heart J 1972;84:537.
21. DeWeese MS, Kraft RO, Nichols WK, et al: Fifteen-year clinical experience with the vena cava filter. Ann Surg 1973;178:247.
22. Spencer FC, Jude J, Rheinhott WF, et al: Plication of the inferior vena cava for pulmonary embolism. Ann Surg 1965;161:788.
23. Ravitch MM, Snodgrass E, McEnany T: Compartmentation of the vena cava with the mechanical stapler. Surg Gynecol Obstet 1966;122:561.
24. Adams JT, Feingold BE, DeWeese JA: Comparative evaluation of ligation and partial interruption of the inferior vena cava. Arch Surg 1971;103:272.
25. Eichelter P, Schenk WG: Prophylaxis of pulmonary embolism: A new experimental approach with initial results. Arch Surg 1968;97:348.

26. Hunter JA, Sessions R, Buenger R: Experimental balloon obstruction of the inferior vena cava. Ann Surg 1970;171:315.
27. Moser KM, Harsnay PG, Harvey-Smith W, et al: Reversible interruption of the inferior vena cava by means of a balloon catheter: Preliminary report. J Thorac Cardiovasc Surg 1971;62:205.
28. Pate JW, Melvin D, Cheek RC: A new form of vena caval interruption. Ann Surg 1969;169:873.
29. Mobin-Uddin K, McLean R, Jude JR: A new catheter technique of interruption of the inferior vena cava for prevention of pulmonary embolism. Am Surg 1969;35:889.
30. McIntyre AB, McCready RA, Hyde GL, et al: A ten year follow-up study of the Mobin-Uddin filter for vena cava interruption. Surg Gynecol Obstet 1984;158:513.
31. Bernstein EF: Caval Interruption Procedures. In Rutherford RB, ed: Vascular Surgery, 3d ed. Philadelphia, WB Saunders, 1989, pp 1575–1582.
32. Dorfman GS: Percutaneous inferior vena caval filters. Radiology 1990;174:987.
33. Greenfield LJ, Cho KJ, Proctor MC, et al: Late results of suprarenal Greenfield vena cava filter placement. Arch Surg 1992;127:969.
34. Greenfield LJ, Proctor MC: Experimental embolic capture by asymmetric Greenfield filters. J Vasc Surg 1992;16:436.
35. Greenfield LJ, McCurdy JR, Brown PP, et al: A new intracaval filter permitting continued flow and resolution of emboli. Surgery 1973;73:599.
36. Greenfield LJ, Michna BA: Twelve-year clinical experience with the Greenfield vena caval filter. Surgery 1988;104:706.
37. Greenfield LJ, Crute SL: Retrieval of the Kim-Ray Greenfield vena caval filter. Surgery 1980;88:719.
38. Greenfield LJ, Proctor MC, Cho KJ, et al: Extended evaluation of the titanium Greenfield vena caval filter. J Vasc Surg 1994;20:458.
39. Roehm JOF Jr, Johnsrude IS, Barth MH, et al: The bird's nest inferior vena cava filter: Progress report. Radiology 1988;168:745.
40. McCowan TC, Ferris EJ, Keifsteck JE, et al: Retrieval of dislodged bird's nest inferior vena caval filter. J Intervent Radiol 1988;3:179.
41. Martin B, Martyak TE, Stoughton TL, et al: Experience with the Gianturco-Roehm bird's nest vena cava filter. Am J Cardiol 1990;66:1275.
42. Millward SF, Peterson RA, Moher D, et al: LGM (Vena Tech) vena caval filter: Experience at a single institution. J Vasc Interven Radiol 1994;5:351.
43. Ricco JB, Crochet D, Sebilotte P, et al: Percutaneous transvenous caval interruption with the "LMG" filter: Early results of a multicenter trial. Ann Vasc Surg 1988;3:242.
44. Murphy TP, Dorfman G, Yedlicka JW, et al: LGM vena cava filter: Objective evaluation of early results. J Vasc Intervent Radiol 1991;12:107.
45. Simon M, Athanasoulis CA, Kim D, et al: Simon Nitinol inferior vena cava filter: Initial clinical experience. Radiology 1989;172:99.
46. Epstein DH, Darcy MD, Hunter DW, et al: Experience with the Amplatz retrievable vena cava filter. Radiology 1989;172:105.
47. Del Campo C: Pulmonary embolectomy: A review. Can J Surg 1985;28:111.
48. Greenfield LJ, Kimmel GO, McCurdy WC: Transvenous removal of pulmonary emboli by vacuum-cup catheter technique. J Surg Res 1969;9:347.
49. Greenfield LJ: Catheter embolectomy for pulmonary thromboembolism. In Current Critical Problems in Vascular Surgery. St. Louis, Quality Medical Publishing, 1991.

30

Valvular Incompetence and Venous Reconstructive Procedures

SESHADRI RAJU

Venous valvular incompetence may be primary or postthrombotic. It is estimated that 20 to 30 percent of cases fall under the first category and the remainder in the postthrombotic group. The hemodynamic abnormality is usually pure reflux with the uncomplicated primary condition. Distal thrombosis, however, can develop in the calf as a complication of reflux stasis.[1] Under these conditions primary valve reflux may develop some of the features of postthrombotic syndrome. Postthrombotic syndrome encompasses a spectrum of hemodynamic pathology ranging from obstruction to reflux. Mixed obstruction/reflux is common.

Important information regarding the evolution of postthrombotic syndrome has recently become available[2] with the advent of duplex scanning technology. Morphologically, there is rapid resolution/recanalization of thrombotic segments in as many as 85 percent of cases by 90 days after initial thrombosis. Since duplex cannot adequately assess the development of collaterals, the functional import of this morphologic observation remains unknown. It appears that a certain significant percentage of patients is left with functionally obstructive lesions in the recanalized venous segment. While the process of recanalization has occurred maximally at 6 months, the process of collateralization proceeds much longer, extending over a period of years. This results in the evolution of an extremity from hemodynamic obstruction to reflux gradually over a period of years. By 3 years after initial onset of thrombosis, one-third of the patients are asymptomatic due to successful recanalization/collateralization, another one-third express mild to moderate symptoms, while the remaining one-third are already suffering from severely symptomatic postphlebitic syndrome.[3] Clinical observations suggest that obstructive lesions predominately result in swelling and pain without ulceration. Hemodynamic reflux also may be accompanied by swelling and pain, but the swelling is typically related to limb dependency. By contrast, swelling is more constant in nature with obstruction. Stasis ulceration with the classic stigmata of discoloration and other stasis changes is invariably an indicator of significant reflux. By the time substantial reflux occurs in postthrombotic syndrome, extensive collateral development has occurred, and the initial hemodynamic obstruction has become well compensated. Occasionally, however, significant obstruction (grade II and higher) may coexist with substantial reflux. Often obstructions are located in the proximal veins (i.e., iliac), with reflux being present in the infrainguinal veins. The proper surgical approach in such mixed lesions remains undetermined.

It is obviously important to identify the underlying hemodynamic abnormality to direct specific treatment. A number of diagnostic methods are currently available to diagnose and assess the extent of reflux.[4] Diagnostic tools to assess obstruction have been limited, cumbersome, or unreliable. Most centers continue to rely on ascending venography. Ascending venography is a morphologic technique that does not provide reliable information on the functional severity of obstruction or the adequacy of collaterals.[5] Impressive-looking collaterals may be poorly functional, and conversely, functional collaterals may not opacify on ascending venography due to technique or flow patterns. For example, when the inferior vena cava is obstructed, one of the lower limbs can present with compensated obstruction (grade I or II), while the opposite limb has high-grade obstruction (grade III or IV), a feature not discernible from venographic appearance (Fig. 30-1). Outflow fractions measured with occlusion plethysmography have been used to quantify obstruction. This technique is hampered by the fact that compliance changes alone independent of any obstructive lesion may influence the result.[4] The arm/foot venous pressure differential technique[4] appears to be the most reliable currently available methodology to diagnose and grade obstruction. An arm/foot differential of more than 4 mmHg in the supine patient indicates the presence of significant obstruction at rest. A differential of less than 4 mmHg in the post-thrombotic patient is indicative of recanalization/collateralization. The functional adequacy of these compensatory mechanisms can be further assessed by inducing reactive hyperemia by ischemic thigh cuff occlusion for 2 minutes and monitoring the resulting elevation of foot venous pressure. A foot venous pressure elevation of greater than 6 mmHg indicates decompensation and inadequate recanalization/collateralization during hyperemia stress; a foot venous pressure elevation of less than 6 mmHg indicates a compensated extremity that provides for adequate outflow even during substantially increased inflow that occurs with hyperemia. A method of grading the severity of venous obstruction by the arm/foot differential and reactive hyperemia methods is shown in Table 30-1. Grade IV obstruction with a resting arm/foot venous pressure differential of greater than 4 mmHg is associated with a paradoxically normal (<6 mmHg) foot venous pressure elevation following ischemic thigh cuff occlusion. It appears that the reactive hyperemia response itself is either muted or altogether absent in the presence of high-grade

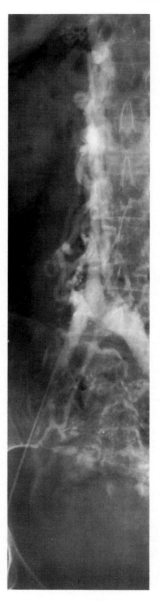

Figure 30-1. Ascending venography is a poor guide to the functional status of venous obstruction. In a patient with inferior vena cava obstruction (*above*), one limb presented with grade II obstruction, while the opposite limb with high grade IV obstruction.

venous obstruction.[6] The basis of this phenomenon is not known.

Duplex examination of the venous system for reflux has supplanted earlier indirect techniques

Table 30-1. A Method of Grading Venous Obstruction

Grade	Arm/Foot Venous Pressure Differential*	Foot Venous Pressure Elevations with Reactive Hyperemia[†]	Comment
I	<4 mmHg	<6 mmHg	Compensated obstruction, adequate collaterals at rest and exercise
II	<4 mmHg	>6 mmHg	Partially compensated obstruction, collaterals adequate at rest only
III	>4 mmHg	>6 mmHg	Partially decompensated obstruction, collaterals inadequate during rest and exercise
IV	>4 mmHg	<6 mmHg	Decompensated high-grade obstruction, no significant pressure increase during reactive hyperemia, paradoxical response

*Normal value < 4 mmHg.
[†]Normal value < 6 mmHg.

such as photoplethysmography that were unreliable due to extremely poor specificity.[7] Van Bemmelen and colleagues[8] have introduced a method of measuring valve closure times utilizing the duplex instrument. Rapid inflation/deflation cuffs are necessary to apply the technique. Valve closure times exceeding 1.2 s for the femoral valve were considered abnormal. Other modifications of the technique to quantify duration of reflux have been described.[9] The practical utility of such methods in chronic venous reflux is yet to be determined. The introduction of air plethysmography allows us to quantify many parameters of reflux and calf muscle function.[10] The usefulness of this technique in selecting patients for valve reconstruction and its role as an aid to postoperative follow-up remain to be evaluated. The ambulatory venous pressure measurement remains the gold standard for assessing venous reflux. Measurement of recovery time is more reliable than postexercise pressure as an index of reflux pathology in my experience.[11] When surgery is contemplated, ascending and descending venography is essential to identify anatomic features of the venous tree in the affected limb and to obtain information regarding the morphology and location of the valve to be operated on.

INDICATIONS FOR SURGERY

Obstruction

A venovenous bypass is indicated in a severe symptomatic limb with documented high-grade obstruction (grade III or IV). Painful swelling sometimes associated with patchy skin necrosis is frequently present in such limbs. Some have argued for early bypass surgery following the onset of deep venous thrombosis to prevent the distal venous valves becoming secondarily incompetent from persistent obstructive venous hypertension.[12] When venous obstruction results in venous *claudication*, venous bypass surgery should be considered. This interesting but rare phenomenon is characterized by increasing pain with ambulation associated with documented elevation of foot venous pressure above resting levels.[6]

Reflux

Conservative measures, i.e., elevation and compression therapy, continue to be the mainstay of treatment for stasis ulceration.[13] However, noncompliance is common, and recurrence is high. Recurrence is frequently associated with repeated hospitalizations (and high cost) for enforced bed rest and elevation to manage the acute phase of recurrence as well as to treat associated cellulitis and suspected recurrent thrombosis. Such patients frequently undergo multiple debridement and skin-graft procedures. Since the disease frequently affects the working-age population, work days lost and the socioeconomic costs of failed conservative therapy can be high. Noncompliance can be attributed to a number of factors: lack of personal discipline to pursue a strict regimen of daily compression, cosmetic considerations in using thick stockings (which some women may consider unattractive), stockings that are poorly fitted and uncomfortable to wear due to binding, sensory intolerance to the degree of compression provided, warm weather-related discomfort from constant stocking use, the relatively high cost of the stockings on a recurring basis, and finally, the inability of some older patients, because of age or other infirmities (arthritis, paresis, etc.), to summon the manual dexterity required to apply the compression device on a daily basis without help. There is general agreement that failure of compression therapy with recurrence of ulcer is a solid indication for applying valve reconstructive surgery. Recurrent complications such as cellulitis, distal thrombosis from reflux, and recurrent painful breakdowns in the stasis area are also appropriate indications for antireflux venous surgery. Centers with established experience in valve reconstruction surgery may selectively include those others for surgery who are unable to employ compression therapy consistently or effectively.

Patients with disabling pain or swelling from documented severe venous reflux constitute a group with a relative indication for surgery. Some patients with chronic pain of long duration have developed a low threshold for pain with central fixation. Correction of the reflux abnormality may not translate into pain relief in such patients. With careful selection, however, the degree of pain relief can be substantial in some. Even though 60 percent of patients report relief of swelling 6 to 12 months after surgery,[14] there is temporary worsening of leg edema following surgical intervention before improvement is discernible. Since pain and swelling often coexist in symptom presentation, pain relief is often immediate after surgery, even though resolution of swelling may take time. Painless swelling is a relative contraindication for surgery.

PATHOLOGY

In primary reflux, the valve apparatus exhibits redundancy of one or more valve cusps. Congenital anomalies,[15] such as tricuspid or monocuspid valve, also may be present; refluxive duplicated conduits and refluxive duplicated valve stations are common anomalies. In postthrombotic syndrome, the valve may be destroyed to a variable extent (Fig. 30-2). In a surprisingly large number of patients, the postthrombotic valve, especially in the proximal superficial femoral vein, may be sufficiently preserved to employ direct repair techniques that were utilized initially in the repair of primary reflux. The preservation of the superficial femoral vein valve in the postthrombotic patient may initially appear surprising. Since most venous thrombosis occurs in the distal portion of the venous tree, the upper valves in the superficial femoral vein may be spared. It appears possible that in some instances the valve structure may survive a thrombotic episode with subsequent speedy clot lysis. Direct proof of this concept, however, is lacking. It is known, however, that rapid clot lysis takes place in a significant proportion of patients.[2] The redundant postthrombotic valve may represent some instances of primary valve reflux complicated by distal thrombosis. In others, valve redundancy may be the result of postthrombotic wall compliance changes around the valve station. Because of vein wall fibrosis affecting valve sinuses, a relative leaflet redundancy may result. Postthrombotic wall changes in association with a redundant valve similar to a primary refluxive valve have been observed by this author during angioscopic repair. Postthrombotic wall changes are known to extend beyond the radiologic limits of venous thrombosis.[16]

SURGICAL TECHNIQUE

Procedures to Correct Reflux

Direct valvuloplasty, as originally described by Ferris and Kistner[17] and later modified by others,[18] remains the mainstay of direct repair of the refluxive valve in primary valve reflux. Since reflux is mostly axial in this pathology, repair of a single valve, usually the most proximal superficial femoral valve, is adequate. When direct valvuloplasty is not feasible, a variety of other techniques can be used (Table 30-2). Internal valvuloplasty is direct and a precise technique, but it remains time-consuming. The indirect techniques such as

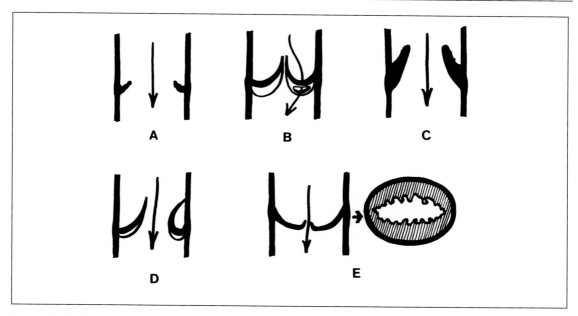

Figure 30-2. *Pathophysiology of venous thrombosis.*

Dacron sleeve in situ and external valvuloplasty are less precise but rapid and are applicable to even small-caliber veins below the knee. The recently introduced technique of angioscopic repair uses an external/internal repair under direct angioscopic vision.[19] A limited venotomy for introduction of the angioscope is necessary. Axillary vein transfer may be the only technique available when the entire valve structure has been destroyed. Because of compliance mismatch between the compliant axillary vein segment and the postthrombotic vein into which the segment is transferred, dilation of the transferred axillary vein segment with recurrence of reflux is common. A restricting prosthetic sleeve to avoid late dilation is recommended.[1] Many of these techniques originally utilized in repairing primary valve reflux have now been adapted for use in the postthrombotic syndrome. The pathology of postthrombotic reflux is more complex than that of primary reflux. Collateral reflux is an important feature of postthrombotic syndrome. In addition, significant axial reflux due to destruction of the axial valve may be present. Because of postthrombotic wall thickening, calf venous pump capacitance may be reduced, and the efficiency of calf pump mechanism may be im-

paired due to compliance changes.[20] While little can be done to correct the calf venous pump abnormality, collateral and axial reflux can be corrected. Collateral reflux may be due to collaterals that arise and end in the axial vein or arise from an adjoining tributary such as the profunda connecting with the popliteal vein (profunda popliteal collateral connection).[21] Direct repair of valves in the collateral vein itself is seldom feasible either because the collateral is small, the valves are absent, or they are oriented in the same direction as reflux flow. To control collateral reflux, multiple valve repair at multiple levels in the axial vein encompassing the origin and end of the axial collateral is necessary.[22] When tributary collaterals are present, valve repair in the specific tributary (i.e., profunda) may be required. Ligation of refluxive collaterals may be inadvisable because outflow obstruction can result when the axial vein is incompletely recanalized. Multiple valve reconstruction is therefore recommended in postthrombotic syndrome. The wide variety of technical options available for valve reconstruction affords the opportunity to choose the optimal technique best suited to a particular patient according to existing valve pathology and other considerations.

Table 30-2. Techniques Currently in Use for Valve Reconstruction

Technique	Comment
Internal valvuloplasty	Precise, direct technique, time-consuming
External valvuloplasty	Indirect technique, rapid, applicable even in small veins, e.g., posterior tibial vein
Dacron sleeve in situ	Indirect technique, rapid, applicable even in small veins, e.g., posterior tibial vein, recommended only when valve becomes competent with surgically induced venoconstriction
Kistner segment transfer	Competent profunda valve required
Angioscopic valvuloplasty	Combined internal/external technique, valve function can be assessed by angioscopy
Axillary vein transfer	Prone to dilatation, may be the only technique available to repair a totally destroyed valve

Procedures to Relieve Obstruction

Patients with postthrombotic obstruction rather than reflux require a bypass to relieve obstruction. High-grade obstruction must be present, and the conduit used should be appropriate for the site of obstruction. The saphenous vein is usually too small to bypass iliac vein obstruction.[23] An externally supported prosthetic polytetrafluoroethylene (PTFE) graft (14 mm) is optimal. External support of the graft is required to avoid compression of the low-pressure venous graft by intraabdominal pressure. The bypass should be performed above the inguinal ligament if at all possible to avoid crossing the hip joint line. The bypass is placed in the space of Retzius behind the rectus muscle,[24] forming a gentle S-shaped curve from side to side. An adjunctive AV fistula between the saphenous vein or tributary and the adjoining superficial femoral artery provides increased flow during the critical early postoperative period. An externally applied prosthetic sleeve should be used to restrict the fistula size to 4 mm. The restricting sleeve helps to avoid distal venous hypertension and aids in later percutaneous closure by coil embolization. A 6-mm or larger coil embolized into the fistula will be trapped by the 4-mm restricting sleeve, leading to fistula occlusion. However, if the adjunctive fistula is well tolerated, it may be left alone without closure, especially in patients in whom flow is judged to be poor at the bypass inflow site. In selected patients with grade II obstruction (significant gradient percentage during exercise only), the fistula will aid in maintaining graft patency during rest when a large gradient is absent. Crural bypasses for venous obstruction (Husni, perforator bypass) may be indicated occasionally in the rare instances when peripheral venous obstruction is high grade and symptomatic. More proximal vena cava bypasses also may be indicated occasionally.

RESULTS

Sufficient experience with valve reconstruction has been accumulated worldwide[25] at the present time to offer some generalizations: (1) Valvuloplasty is superior to axillary vein transfer in long-term results. (2) Healing of stasis ulceration may be expected in about 90 percent of patients in the early postoperative period. There is a 10 to 20 percent decay in these early results over the subsequent 2 to 3 years. Beyond this period, durability of valve reconstruction is sustained in 60 to 80 percent of patients, with healing of the stasis ulceration and without recurrence. Even in those patients in whom ulcer recurs, such recurrence appears to be transitory and less episodic than before. While similar good results are reported by patients who are primarily operated on for pain or swelling,[14] objective assessment of surgical outcome is obviously more difficult than in patients presenting with stasis ulceration.

These clinical results are matched by improvement in venous functional studies[11]; notably ambulatory venous pressure recovery time is significantly prolonged. Improvement in postexercise pressure is less dramatic because of the nonlinear volume-pressure relationship that occurs in collapsible tubes.[26] The absence of improvement in postexercise pressure had been mistakenly interpreted in the past as signifying a failure to abolish reflux.

Prosthetic venous bypasses for iliac or vena caval obstruction[23,27] enjoy excellent short-term patency of about 75 percent. Similar long-term patency has been reported,[24] but experience with these procedures is, however, limited. Crural bypasses are surprisingly durable.[28] The perforator bypass is associated with a curious phenomenon of early postoperative thrombosis with 100 percent recanalization and excellent long-term patency.[28] This may be related to the high incidence of spontaneous thrombolysis that occurs in calf vein thromboses.[29]

REFERENCES

1. Raju S: Venous insufficiency of the lower limb and stasis ulceration: Changing concepts and management. Ann Surg 1983;197:688.
2. Killewich LA, Bedford GR, Beach KW, Strandness DE Jr: Spontaneous lysis of deep venous thrombi: Rate and outcome. J Vasc Surg 1989;9:89.
3. Browse NL, Burnand KG, Thomas ML: Disease of the Veins: Pathology, Diagnosis and Treatment. London, Edward Arnold, 1988.
4. Neglén P, Raju S: Detection of outflow obstruction in chronic venous insufficiency. J Vasc Surg 1993;17:583.
5. Raju S: A pressure-based technique for the detection of acute and chronic venous obstruction. Phlebology 1988;3:207.
6. Raju S, Fredericks R: Venous obstruction: An analysis of 137 cases with hemodynamic, venographic and clinical correlations. J Vasc Surg 1991;14:305.
7. Raju S, Fredericks R: Evaluation of methods for detecting venous reflux: Perspectives in venous insufficiency with descending venography. Arch Surg 1990;125:1463.
8. van Bemmelen PS, Bedford G, Beach KW, Strandness DE Jr: Quantitative segmental evaluation of venous valvular reflux with ultrasonic duplex scanning. J Vasc Surg 1989;10:425.
9. Beckwith TC, Richardson GD, Sheldon M, Clarke GH: A correlation between blood flow volume and ultrasonic Doppler waveforms in the study of valve efficiency. Phlebology 1993;8:12.
10. Christopoulos D, Nicolaides AN, Szendro G: Venous reflux: Quantitation and correlation with the clinical severity of chronic venous disease. Br J Surg 1988;75:352.
11. Raju S, Fredericks RK, Neglén P: Venous function studies after valve reconstruction. J Vasc Surg (submitted).
12. Eklöff B, Neglén P: Venous thrombectomy. In Raju S, Villavicencio L (eds): Surgical Management of Venous Disorders. Baltimore, Williams & Wilkins, 1994.
13. Mayberry JC, Moneta GL, DeFrang RD, Porter JM: The influence of elastic compression stockings on deep venous hemodynamics. J Vasc Surg 1991;13:91.
14. Raju S, Fredericks R: Valve reconstruction procedures for non-obstructive venous insufficiency: Rationale, techniques, and results in 107 procedures with 2–8 year follow-up. J Vasc Surg 1988;7:301.
15. Raju S: In Johnson GJ Jr, Rutherford RB (eds): Operative Management of Chronic Venous Insufficiency. Philadelphia, WB Saunders Company, 1994.
16. Neglén P, Raju S: Occlusion plethysmography is more influenced by compliance changes than venous outflow obstruction in chronic venous insufficiency. (in press).
17. Ferris EB, Kistner RL: Femoral vein reconstruction in the management of chronic venous insufficiency: A 14-year experience. Arch Surg 1982;117:1571.
18. Bergan JJ, Kistner RL: Atlas of Venous Surgery. Philadelphia, WB Saunders Company, 1992.
19. Gloviczki P, Merrell SW, Bower TC: Femoral vein valve repair under direct vision without venotomy: A modified technique with use of angioscopy. J Vasc Surg 1991;14:645.
20. Raju S: Venous reconstruction for treatment of post-phlebitic syndrome. In Haimovici H (ed): Haimovici's Vascular Surgery: Principles and Techniques, 4th ed. Cambridge, Mass, Blackwell Scientific, in press.
21. Raju S: Operative management of chronic venous insufficiency. In Rutherford RB, Johnson G (eds): Review of Vascular Surgery, 4th ed. Philadelphia, WB Saunders Company, 1994.
22. Raju S: Multiple-valve reconstruction for venous insufficiency: Indications, optimal technique, and results. In Veith FJ (ed): Current Critical Problems in Vascular Surgery, vol. 4. St. Louis, Quality Medical Publishing, 1992.
23. Raju S: New approaches to the diagnosis and treatment of venous obstruction. J Vasc Surg 1986;4:42.
24. Gruss J: Bypass procedures for venous obstruction: Palma and Husni bypasses, Raju perforator bypass, prosthetic bypasses, primary and adjunctive AV fistulae. In Raju S, Villavicencio L, (eds): Surgical Management of Venous Disorders. Baltimore, Williams & Wilkins, 1994.
25. O'Donnel T: Angioscopic valvuloplasty. In Raju S, Villavicencio L (eds): Surgical Management of Venous Disorders. Baltimore, Williams & Wilkins, 1994.
26. Raju S, Fredericks R, Lishman P, et al: Observations on the calf venous pump mechanism: Determinants of post-exercise pressure. J Vasc Surg 1993;17:459.

27. Gloutzky P: Vena caval syndromes. *In* Raju S, Villavicencio L (eds): Surgical Management of Venous Disorders. Baltimore, Williams & Wilkins, 1994.

28. Raju S, Fredericks R: Venous obstruction: Diagnosis and treatment. *In* Veith FJ (ed): Current Critical Problems in Vascular Surgery, vol 3. St Louis, Quality Medical Publishing, 1991.

29. Kakkar VV, Lawrence D: Hemodynamic and clinical assessment after therapy for acute deep vein thrombosis. Am J Surg 1985;150:54.

Index

NOTE: Page numbers in *italics* refer to illustrations; page numbers followed by a (t) refer to tables.

Abdominal aortic aneurysm. *See also* Infrarenal aortic aneurysm.
 Dacron graft for, 57
 inflammatory, 81–82
 rupture of, 81
 ultrasound with angiography versus computed tomography in, 234–236, *235, 236*
Abdominal surgery, 392–393
ABI (ankle-brachial pressure index), 4–6
 in ischemia, 41
 in peripheral arterial occlusive disease, 25, 31–32, 32t
Acetaminophen, 364
Acetyl-RGDS, 351
Acquired hypercoagulability, 46t, 46–47
Activated partial thromboplastin time (aPTT), 394–397, 396t, 397t
Activated protein C, 348, 348t
Acute lower limb ischemia (ALLI), 277
Acute myocardial infarction (AMI), 361
Acylated plasminogen streptokinase activator complex (APSAC), economics of, 367–368
 pharmacology of, 299
 properties of, 298t
Adamkiewicz artery, 116–117
Adams-DeWeese clip, 409
AFB. *See* Aortofemoral bypass (AFB).
Air plethysmography (APG), 9
 in venous dysfunction, 378–379, 379t
Allergy, in aortography, 106t
 in thrombolytic therapy, 363
 urokinase-induced, 326–327
ALLI (acute lower limb ischemia), 277
Allopurinol, 117
Alpha$_2$-plasmin inhibitor, 346
Ambulation, in free-tissue transfer, 214
AMI (acute myocardial infarction), 361
Amino acid sequence RGD, 351
Aminocaproic acid, 304
Amplatz filter, 412t, 413
Amputation, in lower extremity ischemia, 215–216
 in peripheral arterial graft infection, 270

Anaphylactoid reaction, urokinase-induced, 326–327
Anastomosis, in aortoenteric fistula, 262, *262*
 in aortofemoral bypass, 162–163
 in axillofemoral bypass, 178
 in femoral artery aneurysm, 137
 in femorofemoral bypass, 172
 in popliteal artery aneurysms, 129, 130
Anastomotic aneurysm, 83
 false, 167
Anastomotic prosthetic enteric fistula, 261, *261*
Ancef. *See* Cephazolin (Ancef).
Anesthesia, in aortic aneurysm repair, 78–79, 108–109
 in aortofemoral bypass, 164
 in femorofemoral bypass, 171
Aneurysm, abdominal aortic. *See* Abdominal aortic aneurysm.
 anastomotic, 83
  false, 167
 brachial false, *306*
 Crawford's type IV (thoracoabdominal), 87, 98
 defined, 71
 dissecting, 71
 endovascular repair of, 141–153. *See also* Endovascular aneurysm repair.
 femoral, 135–138, 136t
  false, *306*
 femoropopliteal, 72
 iliac artery, 72, 143
 juxtarenal. *See* Juxtarenal aneurysm.
 paraanastomotic. *See* Paraanastomotic aneurysm.
 pararenal. *See* Pararenal aneurysm.
 popliteal artery. *See* Popliteal artery aneurysm.
 suprarenal, 87
 thoracoabdominal. *See* Thoracoabdominal aneurysm.
Aneurysm neck, 141–143
Aneurysm thrombus, 143
Aneurysmal dilatation, from aortic dissection, 71
Aneurysmectomy, 127–128, 129
Angina, chronic mesenteric, 8
Angiogenesis, 42
Angiography, iliac, 220–221
 in aortoiliac reconstruction, 160
 in arterial bypass, 196
 in endovascular grafting, 149, *150,* 151
 in endovascular procedures, 223

Angiography, *continued*
  in juxtarenal and pararenal aneurysms, 92, *94, 95*
  interventional, 219–222
  intravascular ultrasound versus, 234–236, *235, 236*
Angioplasty, angioscopy in, 228–229
  balloon, 221, 237
  complications of, 220
  in aortic aneurysms, 78
  percutaneous transluminal coronary, 78
Angioscopy, 223–229
  equipment for, 224
  in angioplasty, 228–229
  in in-situ vein bypass, 227, *228*
  in thrombectomy, 225–227, *226*
  in valve reconstruction, 422t
  intraoperative, 225
  technique of, 224–225, *225*
Anistreplase (Eminase), 339–340
  in fibrinolytic therapy, 344, *345*
Ankle muscle flaps, 213
Ankle-brachial pressure index (ABI), 4–6
  in ischemia, 41
  in peripheral arterial occlusive disease, 25, 31–32, 32t
Antegrade approach, to percutaneous intraarterial
      thrombolysis, 282–283
Antibiotics. *See also specific agent.*
  Dacron grafts and, 57
  in femoropopliteal bypass, 191
  in graft infections, 264, 268
  in graft preservation, 273
  in ischemic ulcers, 41
  in thoracoabdominal aortic aneurysm repair, 109
  polytetrafluoroethylene grafts and, 59
Antibodies, binding to glycoprotein IIb/IIIa, 349–350, 350t
  plasminogen activators and, 342
Anticoagulants, after vascular surgery, 48
  contraindications to, 394
  in deep venous thrombosis, 391, 397–398
  in fibrinolytic therapy, 347–348, 348t
  in fractured hip, 393
  in hypercoagulability, 49t, 50
  in lupus, 46–47
  in venous thromboembolism, 389, 394
  in venous thrombolysis, 321
Antioxidant therapy, 40–41
Antiphospholipid syndrome (APS), 46–47
  management of, 49t, 50
  vascular surgery and, 47–48
α$_2$-Antiplasmin, 298t
Antiplatelet agents, in fibrinolytic therapy, 348–351, *349, 350,* 350t
  in hypercoagulability, 49t, 50
  in peripheral arterial occlusive disease, 38–39
Antistasin, 348t
Antithrombin III (AT III), 49
  deficiency of, 45, 47
Aorta, in aortoiliac reconstruction, 157
Aortic aneurysm, abdominal. *See* Abdominal aortic
      aneurysm.
  infrarenal, 71–85. *See also* Infrarenal aortic aneurysm.
  mycotic, 174
  thoracoabdominal, 103–120. *See also* Thoracoabdominal
      aneurysm.
Aortic dissection, aneurysmal dilatation from, 71
  in thoracoabdominal aortic aneurysms, 105, *105*

Aortic graft, infected, 253–265
  aortic stump management in, 262
  aortobifemoral, 257–259, *257–259*
  bacteriology in, 254
  diagnosis of, *255,* 255–256
  enteric fistula in, 260–262, *261, 262*
  etiology of, 253–254
  in situ revascularization in, 259–260, *260*
  localized, 262–263, *263*
  management of, 256
  presentation and symptoms of, 254–255
  prevention of, 263–264
  reconstruction materials of, 256–257
  polytetrafluoroethylene, 59
  position of, 55
Aortic sepsis, 174
Aortitis, 105
Aortobifemoral graft infection, 257–259, *257–259*
Aortoenteric fistula, diagnosis of, 255, 256
  iliac-iliac anastomosis in, 262, *262*
  in aortofemoral bypass, 167
  in axillofemoral bypass, 174
  secondary, 260–262, *261, 262*
Aortofemoral bypass (AFB), 160–168
  medical management of, 164
  results of, 164–168, 165t, 166t
  technical details of, 161t, 161–163, 163t
Aortography, in graft infections, 256
  in thoracoabdominal aortic aneurysm, 106, *108*
Aortoiliac disease, 29
Aortoiliac endarterectomy, 168–169
Aortoiliac graft, angioscopy in, 226, *226*
Aortoiliac occlusive disease, reconstruction in, 157. *See also*
      Aortoiliac reconstruction.
Aortoiliac reconstruction, 157–185
  bypass in, aortofemoral, 160–168. *See also* Aortofemoral
      bypass.
    axillofemoral, 174t, 174–178, 177t
    femorofemoral, 171–174, 172t
    iliofemoral, 169–171, 170t
  endarterectomy in, 168–169
  endovascular, 243–251. *See also* Endovascular aortoiliac
      reconstruction.
  presentation in, 157–158, *158*
  workup in, 158–160, 159t
Aorto-superficial femoral artery stented graft, 247–248, *249*
APG (air plethysmography), 9
  in venous dysfunction, 378–379, 379t
APS. *See* Antiphospholipid syndrome (APS).
aPTT (activated partial thromboplastin time), 394–397, 396t, 397t
Argatroban, 348t
Arteria magna syndrome, 71
Arteria radicularis magna, 116–117
Arterial access, in endovascular aortoiliac reconstruction, 244, *245–246*
Arterial autografts, 257
Arterial bifurcation, *233*
Arterial dilation, 244, *245–246*
Arterial occlusion, 296–298, *297*
Arterial prostheses, bioresorbable, 63–64
Arterial system hemodynamics, 3–9
  pressure measurements in, 4–7
  velocity in, 7–9
Arterial thromboemboli, 35

Arterial thrombosis, 338, 338t
Arterial wall dissection, 237
Arteriectasis, 71
Arteriography, hemodynamics in, 6
  in aortic aneurysms, 74–76, 77
  in aortoiliac reconstruction, 159, 160
  in axillofemoral bypass, 175
  in femoropopliteal bypass, 191
  in infected infrainguinal grafts, 269
  in lower extremity ischemia, 208
  in percutaneous intraarterial thrombolysis, 281
  in peripheral arterial occlusive disease, 34
  in popliteal artery aneurysms, 125, *126*
Arteriomegaly, 71
  in popliteal artery aneurysms, 125
Arteriorrhaphy, 129
Arteriosclerotic occlusive disease, 157–185. *See also* Aortoiliac
    reconstruction.
Arteriovenous fistula, 191
Artery(ies). *See names of specific artery*; Arterial *entries*.
Aspiration, needle, 256
Aspirin, after vascular surgery, 48
  as antiplatelet agent, 348, *349*
  in fibrinolytic therapy, 350t, 351
  in free-tissue transfer, 212
  in hypercoagulability, 49t, 50
  in iliac angioplasty, 220
  in peripheral arterial occlusive disease, 38–39
  in venous thrombolysis, 324
  warfarin versus, 391
AT III (antithrombin III), 49
  deficiency of, 45, 47
Atheroembolism, 32
Atherogenesis, 26–28
Atherosclerosis, 4, 13–23
  cholesterol in, 15–16, 18t
  in peripheral arterial occlusive disease, 26
  in thoracoabdominal aortic aneurysm, 105, *108*
  lipids in, 13–15, 14t, *15, 16*
  regression of, 16–22, 19t, *20, 21*, 21t
Atrial-femoral bypass, 117
Auscultation, 31
Autogenous graft, in aortic graft infection, 257
  in femoral artery aneurysm, 138
  in femoropopliteal bypass, 189
  in popliteal artery aneurysm, 130
Autologous transfusion, 164
AXF (axillofemoral bypass), in aortoiliac reconstruction,
    174t, 174–178, 177t
  in infected aortic graft, 257, *257*
Axial reflux, 378
Axillary artery anastomosis, 178
Axillary artery thrombosis, 178
Axillary vein transfer, 421, 422t
Axillofemoral bypass (AXF), in aortoiliac reconstruction,
    174t, 174–178, 177t
  in infected aortic graft, 257, *257*
Axillofemoral graft position, 55

Bacteremia, 253–254
Bacteria, gram-negative and gram-positive, 253–254, 268
  in graft infections, 268
Balloon angioplasty, 221, 237
Balloon expandable stent, 220
Balloon thromboembolectomy, 227

Balloon ultrasound imaging catheter, 237
Bat plasminogen activator, 342–343
Benadryl, 364
Bentson guidewire, 282
Bernoulli's theorem, 72–73
Beta blockers, 35
Beta-carotene, 40
Bifurcation, arterial, *233*
  stent graft, 83
BioMedicus pump, 111, *111,* 112, *112*
Bioresorbable arterial prostheses, 63–64
Bird's nest filter, 412, 412t
Bitistatin, 350t, 351
Bleeding. *See* Hemorrhage.
Blood and blood components, 109
Blood cultures, 255
Blood pressure, 4–7
  in peripheral arterial occlusive disease, 30
Blood supply, spinal cord, 116
Blood transfusion in aortofemoral bypass, 164
Blue toe syndrome, 158–159
B-mode ultrasonography, in abdominal aortic aneurysms, 74, *74*
  in atherosclerosis, 21, 22
  in deep venous thrombosis, 387, 388
Bowel injury, 82
Bowel repair, 262, *262*
Brachial false aneurysm, *306*
Brodie-Trendelenburg test, 378
Buerger's disease, 4, 35, 37
Burst therapy, 303
Bypass, aortofemoral, 160–168. *See also* Aortofemoral bypass.
  atrial-femoral, 117
  axillofemoral, in aortoiliac reconstruction, 174t, 174–178,
      177t
    in infected aortic graft, 257, *257*
  crural, 422
  femoral-to-tibial artery, 210
  femorofemoral, 171–174, 172t
  femoropopliteal, 187–194. *See also* Femoropopliteal bypass
      (FPB).
  iliofemoral, 169–171, 170t
  in acute arterial occlusion, 296, 297
  in situ vein, 227, *228*
  in venous obstruction, 419
  infrapopliteal artery, 195–200, *197–199. See also*
      Infrapopliteal artery bypass.
  of Palma, 381
  plantar artery, 200–202, *201–203*
  tibiotibial artery, 205

Calcification, medial, 4
Calcium channel blockers (CCBs), 42
Calf muscle pump, 9–11
Cannula, Pruitt perfusion, 111
Capacitance system, 9
Carcinoma, 79
Cardiac catheterization, 225
Cardiac system, complications of, in aortic aneurysm repair,
    114t
  in aortofemoral bypass, 164–165
  in femorofemoral bypass, 174
  in iliofemoral bypass, 170–171
  dysfunction of, 360
  evaluation of, in aortic aneurysms, 78
  in thoracoabdominal aortic aneurysm, 106–108

Cardiovascular disease, 13–15, 14t, *15, 16*
Carotid artery, in velocity measurement, 7–8
    internal, tortuous, 72
    stenosis of, 72
Catheter, balloon ultrasound imaging, 237
    Cook French endhole infusion, 283–285
    EDM infusion, 287
    Fogarty, in thoracoabdominal aortic aneurysm, 111
        in thromboembolectomy, 226
    French. *See* French catheter.
    in arterial thrombolysis, 302–304, *303*
    in percutaneous intraarterial thrombolysis, *279,* 279–281,
        280, 281
    in thrombolytic therapy, 133
    in venous thrombolysis, 322, 323
    intravascular ultrasound, 229–231, *230,* 232, 233
    McNamara, 289
    Mewissen infusion, 287
    multisidehole, 3302
    single-endhole, 303
    Tracker II, 290, *290*
Catheter-directed venous thrombolysis, 322
    role of, 325–326, *326–327*
    technical considerations for, 327–328
Catheter embolectomy, 413–414
Catheterization, cardiac, 225
CCBs (calcium channel blockers), 42
Cefazolin, 264
Cefoxitin, 59
Cellular adaptation, in ischemic muscle, 28–29
Cephalosporin, 268
Cephazolin (Ancef), 268
Cerebrospinal fluid, 118, 118t, 119
    drainage of, 113, 114
    pressure of, 117
Cerebrovascular disease, 78, *108*
Cerebrovascular insufficiency, 78
CGS 13080, 350t, 351
Check mechanisms, 377
Cholelithiasis, 79
Cholesterol, in cardiovascular disease, 13–14, *15*
    risk reduction of, 15–16, 18t
    in peripheral arterial occlusive disease, 26
    intermittent claudication and, 37
Cholesterol Lowering Atherosclerosis Study, 17
Chronic obstructive pulmonary disease (COPD),
    108
Cigarette smoking, aneurysms and, 72
    in aortoiliac occlusive disease, 158
    intermittent claudication and, 37
Cigarette-paper facies, 30
Circular arteriorrhaphy, 129
Circulation, 36
Clamps, 190, *197*
Claudication, intermittent, femoropopliteal bypass in, 187,
    188–189
    in peripheral arterial occlusive disease, 29, 34–35
    venous, 30
Clinical study design, 151–152
Coagulation, 304
Coaxial infusion system, in iliac occlusions, 285, *287*
    in intraarterial thrombolysis, *279,* 279–281, *280*
Colestipol, 19, 19t
Colitis, 167
Collateral reflux, 421

Colon, carcinoma of, 79
    ischemia of, 83
Color ultrasonography, in abdominal aortic aneurysms, 74,
        75
    in aortoiliac reconstruction, 160
    in peripheral arterial occlusive disease, 34
Common femoral artery, *271*
Common iliac artery stenosis, 220
Common iliac occlusions, 283–285, *283–285*
Compartment syndrome, 360
Compression, extravascular, 35
    intermittent leg, 391–392
    pneumatic leg, 389, 393
Compression stockings, 392
Computerized three-dimensional image reconstruction,
        231–232, *232*
Computerized tomography (CT), in aneurysms, abdominal
        aortic, 74, *76,* 234–236, *235, 236*
    juxtarenal and pararenal, 92, *92, 93*
    popliteal artery, 125
    thoracoabdominal aortic, 106, *107*
    in aortic graft infection, 255
    in endovascular grafting, 148–151
    in infrainguinal graft infection, 269
    in intravascular graft assessment, 238
Computerized two-dimensional images, 231–232, *232*
Concomitant visceral lesions, 98t, 98–100, 99t
Congenital hypercoagulable states, 45–46
Conray 60, 281
Continuous-wave (CW) Doppler, in blood pressure
        measurement, 4–5
    in velocity measurement, 7–9
    in venous dysfunction, 378, 379, 379t
    in venous stasis, 380
Contralateral catheter, 283, *283–285*
Contrast arteriography, 75–76, 77
Contrast-mixed blood extravasation, 363
Cook French endhole infusion catheter, 283–285
Cook rendition of SOS wire, 283
COPD (chronic obstructive pulmonary disease), *108*
Corethane-Dacron graft, 62–63
Corkscrew collaterals, 35
Coronary angioplasty, 78
Coronary Drug Project, 15
Coronary heart disease, 13, 14t
Coumadin, 49t, 50
Cragg infusion guidewire, 283, 290, *290*
Crawford's type IV thoracoabdominal aneurysm, 87
    spinal cord ischemia, 98
Crural bypass, 422
Cryoprecipitate, in hemorrhage, 304
    in thoracoabdominal aortic aneurysm, 109
CT. *See* Computerized tomography (CT).
Cultures, 255
Cutaneous stigmata, of venous dysfunction, 378
CW Doppler. *See* Continuous-wave (CW) Doppler.
CY216 Fraxiparine. *See* Heparin.
Cystic adventitial disease, 35
Cytokines, 27

Dacron graft, 53–57, *54, 61*
    in aortic aneurysm repair, 111
    in aortofemoral bypass, 161, 166
    in axillofemoral bypass, 175, 176
    in femoral artery aneurysm repair, 137, 138

Dacron graft, *continued*
  in femorofemoral bypass, 172
  in iliofemoral bypass, 170
  in popliteal artery aneurysm repair, 130
  in valve reconstruction, 421, 422t
Dade-C, 398
Dazoxiben, 350t, 351
D-Dimer, in urokinase study, 312, *315,* 317
  in venous thromboembolism, 386
Deep venous occlusion, 378
Deep venous thrombosis (DVT), 385–408
  clinical features of, 386
  diagnosis of, 386–388
  differential diagnosis of, 386, 386t
  fibrinolytic therapy in, 338t, 338–339
  hemodynamics in, 9–10, 11
  iliofemoral, 321
  in pregnancy, 393–394
  laboratory features of, 386
  laboratory monitoring of, 398–399
  management of, 321
  pathogenesis of, 385
  prevention of, 389t, 389–393, 393t
  pulmonary embolism and, 388–389
  symptoms, location, and etiology of, 325t
  treatment of, 394–401, 396t, 397t
Degeneration, in aortic aneurysm disease, 72–73
  in thoracoabdominal aortic aneurysm, 104–105, *105*
Denucleation, 62
Dependent rubor, 32
Derra clamps, 190
Dextran, heparin versus, 391
  in femoropopliteal bypass, 190
  in fractured hip, 393
  in hip replacement, 393
  in hypercoagulability, 49t, 50
  in neurosurgery, 393
Dextrose, 106t
DHA (docasahexanoic acid), 39
Diabetes, 4
  femoropopliteal bypass in, 191
  intermittent claudication and, 37
  soft tissue defects in, 207, 208, *209*
  type II, 4, 5
Diagnosis-related groups, 367
Diaphragm, in venous flow, 9
Dilatation, aneurysmal, 71
  arterial, 244, *245–246*
  Dacron graft, 56
Disappearing pulse syndrome, 159
Dissecting aneurysm, 71
Dissection, aortic, aneurysmal dilatation from, 71
  in throacoabdominal aneurysms, 105, *105*
  arterial wall, 237
Distal anastomosis, in aortofemoral bypass, 163
Distal aortic perfusion, 118, 118t, 119
Distal cuff, 142–143
Distal embolization, after aneurysm repair, 83
  thrombolysis and, 304
Distal limb ischemia, 166–167
Distal tibial wounds, 208, *211, 212*
Distal vascular disease, 214–215
DMP728 in fibrinolytic therapy, 350t, 351
Docasahexanoic acid (DHA), 39
Dolichomegaarteries, 71

Doppler imaging, continuous-wave. *See* Continuous-wave
    (CW) Doppler.
  in aortoiliac occlusive disease, 159
  in deep venous thrombosis, 387–388, 400
  in femoropopliteal bypass, 191, 192
  in peripheral arterial occlusive disease, 31, 34
  in velocity measurement, 7–9
  in venous stasis, 380
Dressing, in graft preservation, 273
Duplex imaging, in abdominal aortic aneurysms, 74, *75*
  in aortoiliac reconstruction, 160
  in endovascular grafting, 149–151
  in valvular incompetence, 418–419
  in venous dysfunction, 378, 379, 379t
  in venous stasis, 380
DVT. *See* Deep venous thrombosis (DVT).
Dysfibrinogenemia, 45–46

Echistatin, 350t, 351
Ectasia, 71
Edema, from venous reflux, 420
EDM catheter, in combined iliac occlusions, 278, 287
  in venous thrombolysis, 322
EDRF (endothelium-dependent relaxing factor), 28
EE anastomosis. *See* End-to-end (EE) anastomosis.
Ehlers-Danlos syndrome, 105
Eichelter sieve, 410
Eicosapentanoic acid, 39
Ejaculation
  retrograde
    after aneurysm repair, 82
    in aortofemoral bypass, 168
    in aortoiliac endarterectomy, 169
Elastic supports, 379
Elephant trunk technique, in aneurysm repair, 113–114, *115*
ELISA (enzyme-linked immunosorbent assay), 386
Embolectomy, angioscopic, 225–227, *226*
  pulmonary catheter, 413–414
Embolism, in axillofemoral bypass, 178
  pulmonary, 388–389
Embolization, distal, after aneurysm repair, 83
    thrombolysis and, 304
  in popliteal artery aneurysms, 124, 124t
  secondary, 304
  to plantar arteries, *291–292*
Eminase. *See* Anistreplase (Eminase).
Endarterectomy, aortoiliac, 168–169
Endhole catheter, in common iliac occlusions, 283–285,
    286
  in thrombolysis, 279, *283,* 283–285
Endoaneurysmorrhaphy, 137–138
  in femoral artery aneurysms, 137
  in popliteal artery aneurysms, 128–129
  obliterative, 128
Endogenous nitric oxide, 42
Endoluminal repair, of aortic aneurysms, 83
Endoluminal stents, 328
Endoscopy, 256
Endothelium, in peripheral arterial occlusive disease, 28
  in seeding of prosthetic grafts, 62
Endothelium-dependent relaxing factor (EDRF), 28
Endovascular aneurysm repair, 141–153
  clinical systems in, 145–148, *147–150*
  follow-up in, 149–151
  future directions in, 151–152

Endovascular aneurysm repair, *continued*
  history of, 143–145
  morphology and design considerations in, 141–143, 142t
  preoperative assessment in, 148–149, *151*
Endovascular aortoiliac reconstruction, 243–251
  cases of, 246–248, *247–249*
  discussion of, 248–250
  technique of, *244,* 244–246, *245–246*
Endovascular imaging, 223–241
  angiography in, 223
  angioscopy in, 223–229. *See also* Angioscopy.
  ultrasonography in, 229–239. *See also* Ultrasonography.
Endovascular stent, 144–145, 243–246, *244–246*
End-to-end (EE) anastomosis, in aortofemoral bypass, 162
  in femoral artery aneurysm, 137
  in popliteal artery aneurysms, 129, 130
End-to-side (ES) anastomosis, in aortofemoral bypass, 162
  in lower extremity ischemia, 208
Enoxaparin. *See* Heparin (Enoxaparin).
Enteric fistula, prosthetic, 260–262.*261, 262*
Enzyme-linked immunosorbent assay (ELISA), 386
EPA (eicosapentanoic acid), 39
Epidural anesthesia, in aortic aneurysm repair, 78–79
  in aortofemoral bypass, 164
  in femorofemoral bypass, 171
Epsilon amino caproic acid, 304
Equipment, angioscopy, 224
Ergot preparation, 37
ES (end-to-side) anastomosis, in aortofemoral bypass, 162
  in lower extremity ischemia, 208
Escherichia coli, 254, 268
Estrogens, coronary heart disease and, 13, 14t
  in aortoiliac occlusive disease, 158
  venous function and, 377–378
European Consensus Document on Critical Leg Ischemia,
    41
Excision, in peripheral arterial graft infection, 269–270
  of infected occluded grafts, 270–271, *271*
  revascularization after, 271–272, *272*
Exercise, in arterial disease, 5–6
  in peripheral arterial occlusive disease, 38
  ischemic muscle and, 28–29
Expanded polytetrafluoroethylene grafts, 57
External valvuloplasty, 421, 422t
Extrapopliteal aneurysms, 121–122, *123*
Extravasation, of contrast-mixed blood, 363
Extravascular compression, 35
Extremity, lower. *See* Limb *entries.*

Failing graft, 202–204
False aneurysm, anastomotic, 167
  femoral, *306*
  paraanastomotic, 94
Familial Atherosclerosis Treatment Study (FATS), 17, 19t
Familial occurrence, of abdominal aneurysms, 72
FATS (Familial Atherosclerosis Treatment Study), 17, 19t
FDPs (fibrinogen degradation products), in intraoperative
    urokinase study, 312, *315,* 316–317
  in venous thromboembolism, 386
Femoral artery, anastomosis to, *271*
  angiography of, 221
  superficial. *See* Superficial femoral artery (SFA).
Femoral artery aneurysm, 135–138, 136t
Femoral artery lesion, 225
Femoral artery stented graft, 247–248, *249*

Femoral false aneurysm, *306*
Femoral vein thrombectomy, 227
Femoral-popliteal-tibial thromboembolectomy, 226
Femoral-to-popliteal bypass, Dacron grafts for, 55
  free-tissue transfer in, 210
  polytetrafluoroethylene grafts for, 59
Femoral-to-tibial artery bypass, 210
Femorofemoral bypass (FFB), 171–174, 172t
Femoropopliteal aneurysm, 72
Femoropopliteal bypass (FPB), 187–194
  autogenous versus prosthetic, 189
  clinical presentation of, 187–188
  Dacron graft for, 55
  history of, 187
  in lower extremity ischemia, 210
  in popliteal artery aneurysm, 130, *131*
  in situ versus reversed, 189–190
  indications for, 188–189
  operative graft assessment in, 192
  postoperative graft surveillance in, 192–193
  PTFE graft for, 59
  results of, 188
  surgical technique of, 190–192
FFB (femorofemoral bypass), 171–174, 172t
Fiberoptic gastrointestinal endoscopy, 256
Fibrin, 312, *313*
Fibrinogen, glycoprotein IIb/IIIa and, 349, *350,* 350–351
  in intraoperative urokinase study, 312, *314,* 316
  in venous thrombolysis, 323
  proteolysis of, 312, *313*
Fibrinogen degradation products (FDPs), in intraoperative
    urokinase study, 312, *315,* 316–317
  in venous thromboembolism, 386
Fibrinolytic therapy, 337–357
  anticoagulants in, 347–348, 348t
  antiplatelet agents in, 348–351, *349, 350,* 350t
  plasmin inhibitor in, 346
  plasminogen activators in, 339–343, *340,* 341t
  plasminogen in, 343–344, *345*
  problems with, 337–339, 338t, *339*
  transport in, 346–347
  ultrasound in, 344–346, *346*
Fibrinopeptide A, 386
Fibrinopeptide B-β 15-42, 312, *316,* 317
Filter, in venal caval interruption, *411,* 411–413
Fingers, in peripheral arterial occlusive disease, 30
Fistula, anastomotic prosthetic enteric, 261, *261*
  aortoenteric. *See* Aortoenteric fistula.
  arteriovenous, 191
  lymph, 167
  prosthetic enteric, 260–262.*261, 262*
Flap, in femoropopliteal bypass, 191
  in lower extremity ischemia, 210–214
Fluid overload, 229
Fluoroscopy, 269
Foam cells, 26–27
Fogarty catheter, in thoracoabdominal aortic aneurysm
    repair, 111
  in thromboembolectomy, 226
Foot muscle flaps, 213
Foot wounds, 208, *209*
Forearm flap, 213
Forward-looking intravascular ultrasound, 232–233, *233*
FPB. *See* Femoropopliteal bypass (FPB).
Fractured hip, 393

Fragmin. *See* Heparin.
Framingham Study, 13
Fraxiparine. *See* Heparin.
Free radical scavengers, 117
Free-tissue transfer, 207–217
   amputation versus reconstruction in, 215–216
   free-flap selection in, 210–214
   in nonreconstructable distal vascular disease, 214–215
   independent ambulation in, 214
   morbidity and mortality in, 214
   patient selection in, 207
   soft tissue defect in, 207–208, *209–212*
   timing of, 208
   vascular reconstruction in, 208–210
French catheter, in arterial thrombolysis, 302
   in iliac occlusions, 283–285, *286,* 287
   in infrapopliteal artery occlusions, 290
   in percutaneous intraarterial thrombolysis, 279–282,
      279–285
   in popliteal artery occlusion, 289
   in venous thrombolysis, 322
French micropuncture sets, 283
French paradox, 40
Fresh-frozen plasma, in hemorrhage, 304
   in hypercoagulability, 49t, 50
   in thoracoabdominal aortic aneurysm repair, 109

Gangrene, 124, 124t, 125
Gastrointestinal endoscopy, 256
GCSF (granulocyte colony stimulating factor), 26
Gelatin-cast boots, 379
Gel-phase plasminogen, 298
Gemfibrozil, 16
Gene therapy, 42
General anesthesia. *See* Anesthesia.
Genitourinary complications, following aortofemoral bypass,
   168
Gentamycin, 268
Giant cell aortitis, 105
Gianturco stents, 144, 145, 146–147
Glidewire, 282
Glycoprotein IIb/IIIa (GPIIb/IIIa), 348–349, *350,* 350–351
GPIIb/IIIa (glycoprotein IIb/IIIa), 348–349, *350,* 350–351
Graduated compression stockings, 392
Graft, 53–68
   aortic. *See* Aortic graft.
   aortofemoral bypass, 164
   aortoiliac, 226, *226*
   aorto-superficial femoral artery stented, 247–248, *249*
   autogenous, in femoral artery aneurysm repair, 138
      in femoropopliteal bypass, 189
      in popliteal artery aneurysm repair, 130
   Dacron. *See* Dacron graft.
   failure of, 202–204
   in aortic aneurysm repair, 83
   in aortoiliac reconstruction, 245–246, *246*
   in endovascular aneurysms, 141–153. *See also*
      Endovascular aneurysm repair.
   in popliteal artery aneurysm, 129–133, 132t
   infection of. *See* Graft infection.
   infrainguinal, 48
   polytetrafluoroethylene. *See* Polytetrafluoroethylene
      (PTFE) graft.
   prosthetic. See *Prosthetic graft.*
   saphenous vein, 48

Graft infection, after aneurysm repair, 83
   aortic, 253–265. *See also* Aortic graft.
   infrainguinal, 267–274. *See also* Infrainguinal graft.
Gram-negative and gram-positive bacteria, 254, 268
Granulocyte colony stimulating factor (GCSF), 26
Greenfield filter, *411,* 411–412, 412t, 413
Groin incision, 267
Growth factors, 27
Guidewire, Bentson, 282
   Cragg, 290, *290*
   in percutaneous intraarterial thrombolysis, *281, 282,*
      283–285, *284, 285*
   in venous thrombolysis, 322, 323
   Katzen, 287, 289
   SOS, 283, *291–292*
   thrombolysis, 322
GUSTO trial, of plasminogen activators, 343
Gynecologic surgery, 392–393

Heart. *See* Cardiac system.
Helsinki Heart Study design, 16
Hematoma, 362, 363
Hemodynamics, 3–12
   arterial, 3–9. *See also* Arterial system hemodynamics.
   venous, 9–11
Hemorrhage, after aneurysm repair, 82
   after aortic aneurysm repair, 114t, 116
   fibrinolytic therapy and, 338t, 339
   thrombolytic therapy and, 304
   with infected arterial grafts, 269
   with local intraarterial thrombolysis, 362, 363
Hemorrheologic therapy, 39–40
Heparin (Enoxaparin, Fragmin, Fraxiparine), 390–391
   complications of, 220
   continuous intravenous, 400, 401
   in abdominal thoracic surgery, 392–393
   in acute ischemia, 292
   in aortofemoral bypass, 162
   in deep venous thrombosis, 394–397, 396t, 397t
      indications for, 410
      monitoring of, 399
   in femorofemoral bypass, 171
   in femoropopliteal bypass, 190
   in fibrinolytic therapy, 348t
   in fractured hip, 393
   in free-tissue transfer, 212
   in gynecologic surgery, 392–393
   in hip replacement, 393
   in hypercoagulability, 49t, 50
   in neurosurgery, 393
   in popliteal artery aneurysms, 133
   in pregnancy, 393
   in rethrombolysis prevention, 362–363
   in thrombolytic therapy, 312
   in venous thromboembolism, in moderate risk patients,
      394
      prevention of, 389
   in venous thrombolysis, 323
   in venous thrombosis, 400–401
   recombinant tissue plasminogen activator and, 343, 347
   warfarin and, 394, 398
Heparin-induced platelet activation (HIPA), 48, 49t, 50
Heparinoid ORG 10172, 50
Heredity, in venous stasis disease, 378
Hernia, inguinal, 79

Hexabrix, 281
High-density lipoprotein, 13–14, *15*
High-dose isolated limb perfusion, 310, *311–312*
Hip fracture and replacement, 393
HIPA (heparin-induced platelet activation), 48, 49t, 50
Hirudin, 347–348, 348t
    polytetrafluoroethylene grafts and, 60
Hirugen, 347, 348t
Hirulog, 347, 348t
Histamine blocker, in aortography, 106t
    in urokinase-induced reaction, 327
Hollier's method, of cerebrospinal fluid drainage, 117
Homocystinemia, 35
Homologous arterial grafts, 130
Hormones, 377–378
Horseshoe hook catheter, in iliac occlusions, 285, *286*
    in percutaneous intraarterial thrombolysis, 281–282, *282*
Horseshoe kidneys, 80
Hospitalization, for free-tissue transfer, 214
Host defenses, 254
Hunter balloon, 410
Husni bypass, 422
Hydration, in angiography, 160
    in aortography, 106t
Hydrocortisone, 364
Hydrodynamic reflux, 377
Hydrostatic pressure, 377
Hydrostatic reflux, 377
Hypercholesterolemia, 28
Hypercoagulable syndromes, 45–52
    acquired, 46t, 46–47
    congenital, 45–46
    laboratory tests in, 48, 48t
    management of, 48–50, 49t
    primary, 45, 46t
    secondary, 45, 46t
    vascular surgery and, 47–48, 48t
Hypertension, aneurysms and, 72
    intermittent claudication and, 37–38
    venous, 375
Hypoperfusion, 29
Hypoplastic aorta syndrome, 35
Hypoplastic aortoiliac system, 157, 158, *158*
Hypoxia, tissue, 29

IFB (iliofemoral bypass), 169–171, 170t
Ileus, 82
Iliac angiography, 220–221
Iliac artery, aneurysm of, 72
        graft repair and, 143
    in aortoiliac reconstruction, 157. *See also* Aortoiliac
        reconstruction.
    in femoral artery aneurysm repair, 137
    in popliteal artery aneurysm repair, 130
    occlusion of, arteriogram of, 247–248, *249*
        percutaneous intraarterial thrombolysis in, 283–287,
        283–287
        stenting of, 220
    stenosis of, 220
    tortuosity of, 143
    transfemoral thromboembolectomy of, 226
Iliac vein thrombectomy, 227
Iliac-iliac anastomosis, 262, *262*
Iliofemoral bypass (IFB), 169–171, 170t
Iliofemoral deep venous thrombosis, 321

Iliofemoral occlusion, 247–248, *249*
Iloprost, in fibrinolytic therapy, 351
    in hypercoagulability, 49t
    in ischemia, 42
IMA (inferior mesenteric artery), in aortic aneurysm repair,
        80
    in aortofemoral bypass, 162, 163, 163t
Imaging. *See specific type, e.g.,* Magnetic resonance imaging
        (MRI).
Immune-mediated acquired hypercoagulability, 46
Immunoglobulin G scans, 269
Impedance plethysmography (IPG), 387, 388, 400
Impotence, after aneurysm repair, 82
    after aortofemoral bypass, 168
In situ femoropopliteal bypass, 189
    postoperative surveillance of, 192–193
    technique of, 191–192
In situ revascularization, 259–260, *260*
In situ thrombosis, 220
In situ vein bypass, 227, *228*
Incision, graft infections and, 267
    in aortic aneurysm repair, 78, 79
    in aortofemoral bypass, 161, 161t, 162
    in axillofemoral bypass, 175
    in infrapopliteal bypass, *197–199*
    in plantar artery bypass, 201
    in thoracoabdominal aortic aneurysm repair, 109–111,
        110
Indium-labeled scans, 269
Infarction, myocardial. *See* Myocardial infarction.
Infection, bypass, aortofemoral, 167
        axillofemoral, 178
        femorofemoral, 174
    graft. *See* Graft infection.
    gram-negative and gram-positive bacteria in, 254, 268
    in paraanastomotic false aneurysms, 94
Inferior mesenteric artery (IMA), in aortic aneurysm repair,
        80
    in aortofemoral bypass, 162, 163, 163t
    reimplantation of, 163, 163t
Inferior vena cava obstruction, 418, *418*
Inflamed skin flaps, 191
Inflammatory abdominal aortic aneurysm, 81–82
Infrainguinal graft, infected, 267–274
        diagnosis of, 268–269
        etiology of, 267–268
        management of, 269–273, *271, 272*
    laboratory tests in, 48
    occlusion of, 288, *289*
Infrapopliteal artery, angiography of, 221
    in percutaneous intraarterial thrombolysis, 290, *291–292*
Infrapopliteal artery bypass, 195–200, *197–199*
    angiography in, 196
    patient evaluation in, 195–196
    results of, 196–200, *200*
Infrarenal aortic aneurysm, 71–85
    complications of, 82–83
    definitions in, 71
    diagnosis of, 74–76, *74–77*
    history of, 71
    incidence of, 72
    pathogenesis of, 72–73
    preoperative evaluation of, 78
    surgical repair of, 78–82
    treatment of, 76–78

Infusion catheter, in iliac occlusions, 283–285, 287
  in percutaneous intraarterial thrombolysis, 283, *283*, *284*, *285*
Infusion guidewire, in combined iliac occlusions, 287
  in plantar artery embolization, *291–292*
  in popliteal artery occlusion, 289
  loop in, 290, *290*
Infusion pumps, 290
Infusion system, *279*, 279–281, *280*, 285
  in iliac occlusions, 287, *287*
  in percutaneous intraarterial thrombolysis, 278–281, *279*, *280*, *281*
Inguinal hernia, 79
Injury, after aneurysm repair, 82
INR (international normalized ratio), 398–399
INTACT trial study on calcium channel blockers, 42
Intermittent claudication, femoropopliteal bypass in, 187, 188–189
  in aortoiliac occlusive disease, 159
  in peripheral arterial occlusive disease, 29, 34–35
Intermittent leg compression, 391–392, 393
Internal valvuloplasty, 420–421, 422t
International normalized ratio (INR), 398–399
Interventional angiography, 219–222
Intraarterial thrombolysis, 359–365
  complications of, 362–364
  patient selection in, 359–362, 360t
Intracranial bleeding, local intraarterial thrombolysis and, 361
  thrombolytic therapy and, 304
Intraluminal ultrasound, 229
Intraluminal venal caval interruption devices, 410–413, *411*
Intraoperative angioscopy, 225
Intraoperative thrombolytic therapy, 307–317
  clinical application of, 308–310, *309*, *311–312*
  randomized study of, 310–317, *313–316*
Intravascular ultrasonography (IVUS), 229–239, *230*
  angiography versus, 234–236, *235*, *236*
  catheter design in, 229–231, *230*
  clinical utility of, *234*, 234–239, *235*, *236*, *238*
  forward-looking, 232–233, *233*
  in arterial wall dissections, 237
  three-dimensional, 231–232, *232*, 234–237, *235–236*
  two-dimensional, 231–232, *232*, 234–236, *235–236*
IPG (impedance plethysmography), 387, 388, 400
Ischemia, in colitis, 167
  limb. See Limb ischemia.
  microcirculatory disturbances in, 29
  muscle, 28–29
  myocardial, 82
  of colon, 83
  percutaneous intraarterial thrombolysis in, 277
  spinal cord, 97
  treatment of, 41–42
  urokinase and heparin in, 292
ISIS-2 clinical trial, of antiplatelet agents, 348
Isradipine, 42
IVUS. See Intravascular ultrasonography (IVUS).

Juxtarenal aneurysm, definition of, 87, *88–90*
  diagnosis of, 92–94, *92–95*
  etiology of, 91
  incidence of, 87–90
  results of, 97–98
  rupture of, 97t
  treatment of, 94–97

Katzen infusion system, 278, 287, 289
Ketanserin, 40
Kidney. *See also* Renal *entries.*
  horseshoe, 80
Kistner technique, in valve reconstruction, 422t
  in venous reconstruction, 381
Kistrin, 350t, 351
Klebsiella, 254
Knee surgery, 393

Laboratory evaluation, of aortoiliac occlusive disease, 159–160
  of deep venous thrombosis, 386, 398–399
  of infected aortic grafts, 255
  of peripheral arterial occlusive disease, 32–34
Lacing, 303
Lactide-glycolide copolymeric bioresorbable prostheses, 63
Latex agglutination, 386
Latissimus dorsi muscle, 213
Law of Laplace, 72–73
LDL. *See* Low-density lipoprotein (LDL).
Leather valvulotome, 190
Left atrial-femoral bypass, 117
Left ventricular thrombi (LVT), 362
Leriche syndrome, 29, 158
Lesions, of external iliac artery, 220
  of superficial femoral artery, 225, *225*
Leukocyte scans, radionucleotide-labeled, 256
Leukocyte-labeled scintigraphy, 94
LGM filter, 412t, 412–413
Lidocaine, 322
Lifestyle Heart Study, 17
Ligation, of iliac artery, 137
  of popliteal artery aneurysms, 125–127
Light reflection rheography (LRR), 378–379, 379t
Limb compression, 379–380
  for deep venous thrombosis, 391–392
  for hip replacement, 393
  for neurosurgery, 393
  for venous thromboembolism, 389
Limb graft infection, 262–263, *263*
Limb ischemia, 41
  acute, 277
  endovascular aortoiliac revascularization for, 246–248, *247–249*
  femoropopliteal bypass in, 188
  free-tissue transfer in, 207–217. *See also* Free-tissue transfer.
  in aortofemoral bypass, 166–167
  in axillofemoral bypass, 175
  severity of, classification of, 296
Limb perfusion, 310, *311–312*
Limb salvage, 134
Lipid Research Clinics Coronary Primary Prevention Trial (LRC-CPPT), 15–16
Lipids, 17, 18t
Lipodermatosclerosis, 378
Lipoproteins, 13–23. *See also* Atherosclerosis.
Local anesthesia, 171. *See also* Anesthesia.
Local intraarterial thrombolysis, 359–365
  complications of, 362–364
  patient selection in, 359–362, 360t
Localized graft limb infection, 262–263, *263*
Logiparin. *See* Heparin.
Lomoparin, 391

Lovastatin, 19, 19t
Low-density lipoprotein (LDL), 20, 21t
    in atherosclerosis, 40–41
    in cardiovascular disease, 13–14
    in peripheral arterial occlusive disease, 26
Lower extremity *See* Limb *entries.*
LRC-CPPT (Lipid Research Clinics Coronary Primary
        Prevention Trial), 15–16
LRR (light reflection rheography), 378–379, 379t
Lumbar sympathectomy, 128–129
Lupus anticoagulant, 46–47
LVT (left ventricular thrombi), 362
Lymph fistula, in groin, 167
Lymphocytes, T, 27
Lys-plasminogen with urokinase, 344 < sp >

Macrophages, 27–28
Magnetic resonance arteriography (MRA), 74–75
Magnetic resonance imaging (MRI), of abdominal aortic
        aneurysms, 74–75
    of aortic graft infection, 255
    of endovascular grafting, 149, *151*
    of graft deployment, 238
    of infrainguinal graft infection, 269
    of juxtarenal and pararenal aneurysms, 92–93
    of thoracoabdominal aortic aneurysm, 106, *107*
Magnetic resonance phlebography, 379, 379t
Malleolar wounds, 208, *211, 212*
Manchester comparative reagent, 398
Mannitol, 106t
Marfan syndrome, 105
Markers, of thrombin and plasmin-mediated proteolysis, of
        fibrinogen and fibrin, 312, *313*
    radiodense, 281, *281*
MARS (Monitored Atherosclerosis Regression Study),
        19–20
Martorell's sign, 35
Maximum venous outflow, 9
McNamara catheter, in percutaneous intraarterial
        thrombolysis, 283, *283, 284*
    in popliteal artery occlusion, 289
McNamara infusion system, in iliac occlusions, 285, 287,
        287
    in percutaneous intraarterial thrombolysis, 278, *279,*
        279–281, *280*
MCP (monocyte chemotactic protein), 26
Mechanical transducers, 230, *230*
Medicare insurance, 367
Menopause, 158
Meperidine hydrochloride, 327
Mercury, 220
Mercury strain gauge plethysmography (MSG), 378–379,
        379t
Mesenteric angina, 8
Mesenteric artery, in aortic aneurysm repair, 80
    in aortofemoral bypass, 162, 163, 163t
Mesenteric circulation, 8
Methylene blue, 190, 191
Methylxanthines, 380
Mewissen infusion system, 278, 287
Microanastomosis, 208, 211–212
Microcirculatory disturbances, 29
Micropuncture sets, 283
MIDAS trial of Isradipine, 42
Midline abdominal incision, 78, 79

Mills valvulotome, 227, *228*
MoAB 7E3 (monoclonal antibody 7E3), 349–350, 350t
Mobin-Uddin umbrella, 410
Mönckeberg's sclerosis, 4
Monitored Atherosclerosis Regression Study (MARS),
        19–20
Monitoring, of coagulation, 304
    of deep venous thrombosis, 398–399
    of thoracoabdominal aortic aneurysm repair, 108–109,
        114
Monoclonal antibody, as adjunct to fibrinolytic therapy,
        349–350, 350t
    plasminogen activators and, 342
    to α_2-antiplasmin inhibitor, 346
Monocyte adhesion, 26–27
Monocyte chemotactic protein (MCP), 26
Montreal Heart Institute study, on calcium channel blockers,
        42
Morbidity, in free-tissue transfer, 214
Mortality, in acute lower limb ischemia, 277
    in aortic graft infection, 253
    in aortofemoral bypass, 164–165
    in aortoiliac endarterectomy, 169
    in axillofemoral bypass, 176
    in femorofemoral bypass, 172
    in free-tissue transfer, 214
    in iliofemoral bypass, 170, 170t
    in peripheral arterial graft infection, 270
    in thrombolysis versus surgery, 358
Moser balloon, 410
Mosquito clamp, *197*
Motarjeme catheter, 285
MRA (magnetic resonance arteriography), 74–75
MRFIT (Multiple Risk Factor Intervention Trial), 14t,
        14–15
MRI. *See* Magnetic resonance imaging (MRI).
MSG (mercury strain gauge plethysmography), 378–379,
        379t
Multiple Risk Factor Intervention Trial (MRFIT), 14t,
        14–15
Multisidehole catheters, 3302
Muscle flaps, 210–214
Muscle necrosis, 360
MVO (maximum venous outflow), 9
Mycotic aortic aneurysm, 174
Myocardial infarction, acute, 361
    after aneurysm repair, 82
    hemorrhage in, 361
    regional thrombolysis and, 362, 363
Myocardial ischemia, 82

NaCl (sodium chloride), 322–323
National Cholesterol Education Program, 13
Neck, aneurysm, 141–143
Necrosis, in thoracoabdominal aortic aneurysms, 105
    muscle, 360
Needle aspiration, 256
Nerve compression, 124, 124t
Neurogenic claudication, 159
Neurologic deficit, in thoracoabdominal aortic aneurysm,
        incidence of, 103–104
    postoperative, 114t, 116–119, 117t, *118,* 118t
Neuropathy, 4
Neurosurgery, 393
Niacin, 19, 19t

Nicotinic acid, 19, 19t
Nitinol filter, 412t, 413
Nitrates, organic, 351
Nitric oxide (NO), antioxidants and, 41
    in peripheral arterial occlusive disease, 28, 42
Nitroglycerine, 220
NO (nitric oxide), antioxidants and, 41
    in peripheral arterial occlusive disease, 28
Nutrition, 32
Nylon grafts, 130
Nylon sutures, 212

Obliterative endoaneurysmorrhaphy, 128
Occlusion, angioplasty in, 220
    aortoiliac, 157. *See also* Aortoiliac reconstruction.
    arteriosclerotic, 157–185. *See also* Aortoiliac
        reconstruction.
    deep venous, 378
    endovascular aortoiliac reconstruction for, 243–251. *See
        also* Endovascular aortoiliac reconstruction.
    iliac, 283–287, *283–287*
    of femoral and popliteal artery, 221
    of infected peripheral arterial graft, 270–271, *271*
    of inferior vena cava, 418, *418*
    of infrainguinal graft, 288, *289*
    of suprainguinal graft, *287,* 287–288
    peripheral arterial. *See* Peripheral arterial occlusive disease.
    plethysmography in, 418
    venous, surgery for, 419, 420–422
Omentum, 213
Omni-Tract self-retaining retractor, 109
Oxypentoxifylline, 380

PAD. *See* Peripheral arterial occlusive disease (PAD).
PAF (platelet activating factor), 27
Pain, in severe venous reflux, 420
    in venous dysfunction, 375–377
Pallor, 32
Palma, venous bypass of, 381
Palmaz stent, 220
    in iliofemoral occlusion, 248, *249*
    in venous thrombolysis, 323, 324, *326, 328*
Palpation, 31
Pancreatitis, 83
Papaverine, in femoropopliteal bypass, 190
    in iliac angioplasty, 220
    in neurologic deficit, 117
Paraanastomotic aneurysm, definition of, 87, *88–90*
    diagnosis of, 93–94
    etiology of, 91
    false, 94
    incidence of, 90–91
    results of, 98t, 98–100, 99t
    rupture of, 97t, 99, 99t
    treatment of, 94–97
Paraplegia, after aneurysm repair, 82
    in thoracoabdominal aortic aneurysm repair, 117, 117t
Paraprosthetic enteric fistula, 260–261, *261*
Pararenal aneurysm, definition of, 87, *88–90*
    diagnosis of, 92–94, *92–95*
    etiology of, 91
    incidence of, 87–90
    results of, 97–98
    rupture of, 97t
    treatment of, 94–97

Partial thromboplastin time (PTT), 323
Pate clip, 410
Patency, of aortofemoral bypass graft, 165t, 165–166
    of aortoiliac endarterectomy, 169
    of axillofemoral bypass graft, 176
    of femorofemoral bypass graft, 172t, 172–174
    of femoropopliteal bypass graft, 188, 193
    of iliofemoral bypass graft, 170, 170t
    of infrapopliteal bypass graft, 196–198
    of polytetrafluoroethylene graft, 189
    of popliteal artery aneurysm repair, 130–133, 132t
Patient selection, for thrombolysis, 359–362, 360t
PDGF (platelet-derived growth factor), 27
Pearson chi-square test, 118t, 119
Penicillin, 59
Pentoxifylline, 39–40
Percutaneous angioscopy, 224–225, *225*
Percutaneous intraarterial thrombolysis (PIAT), 277–293
    antegrade approach to, 282–283
    arteriography in, 281
    contralateral access in, 281–282, *282*
    in femoral occlusions, 288
    in iliac occlusions, 283–287, *283–287*
    in infrainguinal graft occlusions, 288, *289*
    in suprainguinal graft occlusions, *287,* 287–288
    infrapopliteal artery in, 290, *291–292*
    popliteal artery in, 288–290, *290*
    pumps and connections in, 290–292
Percutaneous transluminal coronary angioplasty (PTCA), 78
Perforator bypass, 422
Perfusion, limb, 310, *311–312*
    renal, 97
    tissue, 32
Perigraft fluid, 255, *255*
Perioperative blood, 109
Peripheral arterial graft infections, 267–268
Peripheral arterial occlusive disease (PAD), 25–44
    cellular adaptation in, 28–29
    clinical evaluation of, 29–32, 31t
    history of, 25–26
    laboratory studies in, 32–34
    management of, 34–42
        antioxidant therapy in, 40–41
        antiplatelet treatment in, 38–39
        arteriography in, 34
        circulation assessment in, 36
        exercise rehabilitation in, 38
        future therapy in, 42
        general assessment in, 36–37
        hemorrheologic therapy in, 39–40
        ischemia treatment in, 41–42
        premature, 34–35
        revascularization in, 34
        risk factor modification in, 37–38
        vasodilator therapy in, 40
    microcirculatory disturbances in, 29
    pathophysiology of, 26–28
    thrombolysis in, 295–320. *See also* Thrombolysis.
Peripheral arteries, 8
Peripheral neuropathy, 4
Perthes test, 378
PGE_1 (prostaglandin E_1), 41, 351
PGI_2 (prostacyclin), 41
Phased-array transducers, *230,* 230–231
Phenindione, 397

Phlebography, 379, 379t
Phleborrhaphy, 129
Photoplethysmography (PPG), 378–379, 379t
PIAT. *See* Percutaneous intraarterial thrombolysis (PIAT).
Pigtail catheter, 281
Plantar artery bypass, 200–202, *201–203*
Plantar artery embolization, *291–292*
Plaque, atherosclerotic, 17, 18t
Plasma, fresh-frozen, 304
 in hypercoagulability, 49t, 50
 in thoracoabdominal aortic aneurysm repair, 109
Plasmin, in thrombolysis, 295–296
 properties of, 298t
Plasmin inhibitor, 346
Plasmin-mediated proteolysis, 312, *313*
Plasminogen, domainal structures of, *340*
 gel-phase, 298
 in arterial thrombolysis, 301, *301*
 in fibrinolytic therapy, 343–344, *345*
 in intraoperative urokinase study, 312, *313, 316*
 properties of, 298t
 transport of, 300
Plasminogen activators, development of, 341t
 in fibrinolytic therapy, 339–343, *340,* 341t, 342–343
 in thrombolysis, 298
 inhibitors of, 298t
 transport of, 300
Plasminogen streptokinase activator complex, economics of,
     367–368
 pharmacology of, 299
 properties of, 298t
Platelet activating factor (PAF), 27
Platelet-derived growth factor (PDGF), 27
Plethysmography, air, 9
 in venous dysfunction, 378–379, 379t
 occlusion, 418
Pneumatic leg compression, 389, 391–392, 393
Polypropylene sutures, in aortoiliac endarterectomy, 169
 in femoropopliteal bypass, 190, 191
 in infrapopliteal bypass, 196
Polytetrafluoroethylene (PTFE) graft, 57–61, *58, 60*
 in aortofemoral bypass, 161, 166
 in axillofemoral bypass, 175, 176
 in femoral artery aneurysm repair, 137
 in femorofemoral bypass, 172, 174
 in femoropopliteal bypass, 189
 in iliofemoral bypass, 170
 in postthrombotic obstruction, 422
  infected, replacement of, 272
 occlusion of, *289*
 seeding and sodding of, 62
Popliteal artery, angiography of, 221
 in percutaneous intraarterial thrombolysis, 288–290, *290*
Popliteal artery aneurysm, 72, 121–135, 122t, 123t
 bilateral, 121–122, 122t, 125
 complications associated with, 124, 124t
 contralateral, 121, 122t, 125
 diagnosis of, 125, *126*
 enlargement of, 135
 history of, 124t, 124–125
 pathogenesis of, 122–124
 surgery for, 125–130, *131*
  results of, 130–135, 132t, 134t
Popliteal artery entrapment syndrome, 35
POSCH trial, 17

Postmenopausal estrogen, 13, 14t
Postoperative graft surveillance, 192–193
Postoperative monitoring, 114
Postphlebitic state, 375
Postthrombotic state, 375
Postthrombotic syndrome, collateral reflux in, 421
 valvular incompetence in, 417, 420
PPACK, 348, 348t
PPG (photoplethysmography), 378–379, 379t
Pregnancy, deep venous thrombosis in, 393–394
 varicosities in, 377
Premature menopause, 158
Premature peripheral arterial occlusive disease, 34–35
Preoperative assessment, 148–149, *151*
Pressure stockings, 394
Progesterone, 377–378
Prolene sutures, 111, 112, 113
Prostacyclin (PGI$_2$), 41
Prostaglandin derivatives, 41
Prostaglandin E$_1$ (PGE$_1$), 41, 351
Prostanoid analogues, 42
Prosthesis, bioresorbable, 63–64
Prosthetic enteric fistula, 261, *261*
Prosthetic graft, 53–68. *See also* Graft.
 angioscopic examination of, *226,* 226–227
 Dacron in, 53–57, *54,* 61
 extravasation of contrast-mixed blood through, 363
 for femoropopliteal bypass, 189
 polytetrafluoroethylene in, 57–61, *58, 60*
 seeding and sodding of, 62, *63*
 thrombosis in, 48
Protein C, in congenital hypercoagulability, 45
 in fibrinolytic therapy, 348, 348t
 in hypercoagulability, 49
Protein S, in congenital hypercoagulability, 45
 in hypercoagulability, 49
Proteus, 254, 268
Prothrombin fragment 1.2, 386
Prothrombin time (PT), 398
Pro-urokinase, 298t
Pruitt perfusion cannula, 111
Pseudoaneurysm(s), Dacron grafts and, 56
 in axillofemoral bypass, 178
Pseudoclaudication, 29
 in aortoiliac occlusive disease, 159
Pseudomonas, 254, 268, 273
PT (prothrombin time), 398
PTCA (percutaneous transluminal coronary angioplasty), 78
PTFE. *See* Polytetrafluoroethylene (PTFE) graft.
PTT (partial thromboplastin time), 323
Pulmonary catheter embolectomy, 413–414
Pulmonary embolism, deep venous thrombosis and,
     388–389
 vena caval interruption and, 409–415. *See also* Vena caval
     interruption.
Pulmonary system, in aortic aneurysms, 78
 in thoracoabdominal aortic aneurysm repair, 114t,
     114–116
Pulse, 31
Pulse volume recordings (PVRs), in aortoilliac
     reconstruction, 159, 160
 in peripheral arterial occlusive disease, 33
Pulsed Doppler, 7–9
Pulse-spray technique, in arterial thrombolysis, 303
 in percutaneous intraarterial thrombolysis, 279, *279*

Pump, BioMedicus, 111, *111,* 112, *112*
    in percutaneous intraarterial thrombolysis, 290–292
    Travenol IVAC infusion, 290
Puncture-site hematoma, 363
PVRs (pulse volume recordings), in aortoilliac
    reconstruction, 159, 160
    in peripheral arterial occlusive disease, 33

Rabbit brain thromboplastin, 398
Radial forearm flap, 213
Radicular arteries, 116–117
Radiodense markers, 281, *281*
Radiography, 105, *106*
    contrast agent in, 233
Radiologic contrast phlebography, 379, 379t
Radionucleotide-labeled leukocyte scans, 256
Rapid red cell agglutination assay (SIMPLI-RED test),
    386
Real-time B-mode ultrasound, 387
Recombinant tissue plasminogen activator (rt-PA), allergic
        reaction with, 363
    comparison of, 331–336
    costs of, 367–368, 368t
    hemorrhage with, 361
    heparin and, 347
    heparin versus, 343
    in fibrinolytic therapy, 344
    in high-dose isolated limb perfusion, 310
    in venous thrombolysis, 326
    intraoperative, 309
    pharmacology of, 299
    properties of, 298t
    surgery versus, 358
    urokinase versus, 343, 363
Reconstruction, aortoiliac. *See* Aortoiliac reconstruction.
    computerized three-dimensional image, 231–232, *232*
    endoaneurysmorrhaphy in, for femoral artery aneurysms,
        137
        for popliteal artery aneurysms, 128
    in venous stasis disease, 381
Rectus abdominis, 213, 214
Reflux, axial, 378
    collateral, 421
    hydrodynamic, 377
    hydrostatic, 377
    superficial, 380–381
    venous, 419–422, 422t
Rehabilitation, exercise in, 38
Renal artery, 8
Renal carcinoma, 79
Renal failure, after aneurysm repair, 82
    in limb ischemia status, 360
    in thoracoabdominal aortic aneurysm repair, 114t, 116
    thrombolytic therapy and, 363
Renal insufficiency, *108*
Renal perfusion, 97
Renal system, in aortic aneurysms, 78
    in juxtarenal and pararenal aneurysms, 97
Reoperation of bypasses, 204
Reperfusion syndrome, 360
Respiratory system, 9
Restorative endoaneurysmorrhaphy, in femoral artery
        aneurysm repair, 137
    in popliteal aneurysms, 128
Reticular varicosities, 376t

Retrograde ejaculation, after aneurysm repair, 82
    in aortofemoral bypass, 168
    in aortoiliac endarterectomy, 169
Retroperitoneal approach, to aortic aneurysms, 78, 94, 96
    to aortofemoral bypass, 161, 161t, 162
    to localized graft infection, 263, *263*
Retroperitoneal hematoma, 362, 363
Revascularization, after graft excision, 271–272, *272*
    in graft infections, 259–260, *260*
    in peripheral arterial occlusive disease, 34
Reversed femoropopliteal bypass, 189
Ridrogel, 350t, 351
Ringer's lactate, 116
Ring-reinforced polytetrafluoroethylene graft, 59
Rochester trial of thrombolysis versus surgery, 369
Rotating-mirror devices, *230,* 230–231
Rotating-transducer, *230,* 230–231
rt-PA. *See* Recombinant tissue plasminogen activator (rt-PA).
Rubor, 32
Rummel tourniquet, 111

Saline, in angioscopy, 225
    in intravascular ultrasound, 233
Saphenous vein graft, for popliteal artery aneurysm, 129,
        130, *131*
    in femoropopliteal bypass, 190, 192
    thrombosis in, 48
Scapular flap, 213
Scimitar sign, 35
Scintigraphy, 94, 256
Sclerosis, Mönckeberg's, 4
scu-PA (single-chain urokinase-like plasminogen activator),
        340, 340–344
Seeding, of vascular prosthetic grafts, 62, *63*
Segmental pressure measurements, 33
Seldinger technique, 160, 219
Self-expanding stents, 144–145
Semirigid Velcro support, 379
Sepsis, aortic, 174
    thrombolytic therapy and, 363
    with peripheral arterial grafts, 269, 270
Serum cholesterol, 26
Sexual dysfunction, after aneurysm repair, 82
    in aortofemoral bypass, 168
    in aortoiliac endarterectomy, 169
SFA. *See* Superficial femoral artery (SFA).
Shepherd's hook catheter, 282, 283, *283*
Silastic loops, *197*
Simon nitinol filter, 412t, 413
Simplastin, 398
SIMPLI-RED test (rapid red cell agglutination assay), 386
Single-chain urokinase-like plasminogen activator (scu-PA),
        340, 340–344
Single-endhole catheter, 303
Sinogram, 256, 269
SK. *See* Streptokinase (SK).
Skin flap inflammation, 191
Smoking, aneurysms and, 72
    aortoiliac occlusive disease and, 158
    intermittent claudication and, 37
Smooth muscle cells, 27
Society for Vascular Surgery/International Society for
        Cardiovascular Surgery, 296
Sodding, of vascular prosthetic grafts, 62, *63*
Sodium bicarbonate, 106t, 109

Sodium chloride (NaCl), 322–323
Sodium nitroprusside, 109
Soluble-phase plasminogen, 298
SOS wire, Cook rendition of, 283
   in plantar artery embolization, *291–292*
   in venous thrombolysis, 322
Spinal anesthesia, 171
Spinal cord, blood supply to, 116
Spinal cord ischemia, 97–98
SQ 30741, 350t, 351
Stainless steel Greenfield filter, 412, 412t, 413
Staphylococcus aureus, 254, 268, 273
Staphylococcus epidermidis, 254, 268, 272
Staphylokinase, 342
Stenosis, of carotid arteries, 72
   of common iliac artery, angioplasty in, 220
   of superficial femoral artery and popliteal artery, 221
   velocity measurement in, 7–8
Stent, endovascular, 144–145, 243–246, *244–246*
   Gianturco, 146–147
   in aortic aneurysm repair, 83
   in iliac occlusions, 220
   in venous thrombolysis, 323–324, 325, *326,* 328
   intravascular ultrasound assessment of, 237, 238
   Palmaz. *See* Palmaz stent.
Steroids, after vascular surgery, 48
   in aortography, 106t
   in neurologic deficit, 117
STILE (surgery versus thrombolysis for ischemia of lower
     extremity) trial, 306–307
   of thrombolysis versus surgery, 369
Stockings, compression, graduated, 392
   pressure, 394
   support, 379–380
Stool guaiac examination, 255
Stopcock in percutaneous intraarterial thrombolysis, *280,*
   281
Streptase. *See* Streptokinase (SK).
Streptococcus faecalis, 268
Streptococcus viridans, 268
Streptokinase activator complex, economics of, 367–368
   pharmacology of, 299
Streptokinase (SK), allergic reaction with, 363
   as antiplatelet agent, clinical trial of, 348, *349*
   comparative costs of, 367–368, 368t
   comparison of, 331–336
   hemorrhage with, 361
   high-dose, 343
   in acute lower limb ischemia, 277, 278
   in arterial thrombolysis, 300–301, 301t
   in fibrinolytic therapy, 339
   in peripheral arterial occlusion, 304–306
   in popliteal artery aneurysms, 133
   in thrombolysis, 295–296, 401
   in venous thrombolysis, 326
   intraoperative, 308–309
   pharmacology of, 299
   plasminogen with, 344
   properties of, 298t
   surgery versus, 369t
   tissue plasminogen activator combined with, 343
   transport of, 300
Stump, aortic, 262
Sub-total excision, 270–271, *271*
Sulatroban, 350t, 351

Superficial femoral artery (SFA), endovascular aortoiliac
     reconstruction with, 246–247, *247, 248*
   in aortofemoral bypass, 163
   in graft infection, 263, *263*
   occlusion of, 288, 289
   percutaneous angioscopy of, 225
Superficial reflux, 380–381
Support stockings, 379–380
Suprainguinal graft occlusion, *287,* 287–288
Suprarenal aneurysm, 87
Surgery, angioscopy in, 225
   for deep venous thrombosis, 392–393
   for femoral artery aneurysms, 136–138
   for popliteal artery aneurysms, 125–130, *131*
   for venous stasis disease, 380t, 380–381
   for venous thrombolysis, 321–322
   hypercoagulability and, 47–48, 48t
   thrombolysis versus, 307, 307t, 369, 370t
Surgery versus thrombolysis for ischemia of lower extremity
     (STILE) trial, 306–307, 369
Sutures, in free-tissue transfer, 212
   in thoracoabdominal aortic aneurysm repair, 111, 112
   polypropylene, in aortoiliac endarterectomy, 169
      in femoropopliteal bypass, 190, 191
      in infrapopliteal bypass, 196
Swelling, from venous reflux, 420
Sympathectomy, lumbar, 128–129
Syphilis, 122
Systolic pressure measurements, 33

T lymphocytes, 27
Takayasu's syndrome, 105
TAP (tick anticoagulant peptide), 348, 348t
Taylor patch, 59
Teeth, in peripheral arterial occlusive disease, 30
Teflon graft, 57–61, *58, 60*
   in popliteal artery aneurysms, 130
Telangiectasias, 375, 376t. *See also* Venous stasis disease.
Terumo glidewire, 322
TFPI (tissue factor pathway inhibitor), 348, 348t
Thigh pressure, 160
Thigh-ankle pressure, 160
Thoracic surgery, 392–393
Thoracoabdominal aneurysm, classification of, 103–104, *104*
   complications of, 114t, 114–119, 117t, *118,* 118t
   Crawford's type IV, 87, 103–120
   etiology of, 104–105, *105*
   history of, 104
   repair of anesthetic monitoring in, 108–109
      operative technique in, 109–114, *110–115*
      perioperative blood use in, 109
      postoperative monitoring in, 114
   spinal cord ischemia and, 98
   symptoms and signs of, 105–108, 106t, *106–108*
Thoracoabdominal incision, 94, 96
Thoracoretroperitoneal approach, 96
Three-dimensional ultrasound scan, in abdominal aortic
     aneurysms, 234–236, *235, 236*
   in arterial wall dissections, 237
   in image reconstruction, 231–232, *232*
Three-way stopcock, *280,* 281
Thrombectomy, 225–227, *226*
Thrombin inhibitors, 347, 348t
Thrombin proteolysis, 312, *313*
Thrombin-antithrombin complexes, 386

Thromboangiitis obliterans, 35
Thromboembolectomy, balloon, 227
  in acute arterial occlusion, 296, 298
  intraoperative thrombolysis with, 308
Thromboembolism, arterial, 35
  venous, 385–408. *See also* Deep venous thrombosis (DVT).
Thrombolysis, 295–320
  agents in, 298t, 298–299. *See also* Thrombolytic agents.
  history of, 295–296
  in arterial occlusion, 296–298, *297*
  in ischemia, 41
  in popliteal artery aneurysm repair, 133–134, 134t
  indications for and contraindications to, 360t, 361
  intraarterial, local, 359–365. *See also* Local intraarterial
    thrombolysis.
    percutaneous, 277–293. *See also* Percutaneous
      intraarterial thrombolysis (PIAT).
  intraoperative, 307–310, *309, 311–312*
    randomized study of, 310–317, *313–316*
  results of, 304–307, *306*, 307t
  technique of, 300–304, *301,* 301t, *303,* 304t, *305*
  transport phenomena in, 299–300
  venous, 321–330. *See also* Venous thrombolysis.
Thrombolysis or peripheral arterial surgery (TOPAS) trial, 369
Thrombolytic agents, comparison of, 331–336
  in peripheral arterial occlusive disease, 367–371
    comparisons of, 369–370, 370t
    costs versus charges in, 367
    economics of, 367–369, 368t, 369t
  in venous thrombolysis, 326–327
  nonrandomized trials of, 332–333
  pharmacology of, 298t, 298–299
  randomized trials of, 333–334
Thromboplastin, 398
Thrombosis, after aneurysm repair, 83
  bypass, 204
  Dacron grafts and, 56
  deep venous. *See* Deep venous thrombosis (DVT).
  fibrinolytic therapy in, 338, 338t
  in angioplasty, 220
  in aortofemoral bypass, 166, 167–168
  in aortoiliac endarterectomy, 169
  in axillofemoral bypass, 178
  in femorofemoral bypass, 174
  in popliteal artery aneurysms, 124t, 124–125
  in vascular surgery, 47–48
Thromboxane A_2 receptor antagonists, 351
Thromboxane synthase inhibitors, 351
Thrombus, aneurysm, 143
Tibial pulse, 25
Tibial wounds, 208, *211, 212*
Tibiotibial artery bypass, 205
Tick anticoagulant peptide (TAP), 348, 348t
Ticlopidine, 39
Tissue factor pathway inhibitor (TFPI), 348, 348t
Tissue hypoxia, 29
Tissue perfusion, 32
Tissue plasminogen activator (t-PA), accelerated, 343
  domainal structures of, *340*
  in fibrinolytic therapy, 339, 340, 341–342
  plasmin inhibitor and, 346
  scu-PA combined with, 343
  streptokinase combined with, 343
  urokinase versus, 343
Titanium Greenfield filter, 412, 412t, 413

Tobacco, aneurysms and, 72
  in aortoiliac occlusive disease, 158
  intermittent claudication and, 37
Toe systolic blood pressure (TSBP), 5
  in ischemia, 41
  in peripheral arterial occlusive disease, 33
TOPAS (thrombolysis or peripheral arterial surgery) trial,
  369
Tortuosity, carotid, 72
  iliac, 143
Touhy-Borst adapter, *280,* 283, *284*
t-PA. *See* Tissue plasminogen activator (t-PA).
Tracker II catheter, 290, *290*
Transabdominal approach, to abdominal aortic aneurysms,
  94–96
Transducer, ultrasound, *230,* 230–231
Transfemoral Seldinger approach, to aortoiliac
  reconstruction, 160
Transfemoral thromboembolectomy, 226
Transfusion, for aortofemoral bypass, 164
Transluminal stented graft, *244*
Transperitoneal midline incision, 161, 161t, 162
Transplantation, 129–130
Transport, in fibrinolytic therapy, 346–347
  in thrombolytic therapy, 299–300
Transvenous venal caval interruption devices, 410–413, *411*
Transverse abdominal incision, 78
Trash foot syndrome, 166–167
Travenol IVAC infusion pumps, 290
TSBP. *See* Toe systolic blood pressure (TSBP).
Two-dimensional ultrasound scan, 231–232, *232*
  in abdominal aortic aneurysm, 234–236, *235, 236*

UK. *See* Urokinase (UK).
Ulcers, in peripheral arterial occlusive disease, 32
  ischemic, 41, 42
Ultrasonography, 229–239
  angioscopy with, 229
  clinical utility of, *234–236,* 234–239
  device development and imaging configurations in,
    229–233, *230, 232, 233*
  in abdominal aortic aneurysms, 74, *74,* 75
  in aortoiliac occlusive disease, 159, 160
  in atherosclerosis, 21, 22
  in deep venous thrombosis, 387–388, 400
  in endovascular grafting, 149–151
  in fibrinolytic therapy, 344–346, *346*
  in infected infrainguinal grafts, 269
  in peripheral arterial occlusive disease, 34
  in popliteal artery aneurysms, 125, *126*
  in volume flow measurement, 6
  intravascular. *See* Intravascular ultrasonography (IVUS).
  techniques of, 233
Ureter injury, 82
Urokinase (UK), allergy to, 326–327
  comparative costs of, 367–368, 368t
  comparison of, 331–336
  complications with, 364
  in arterial thrombolysis, 302–304, *305*
  in femoropopliteal graft occlusion, *289*
  in fibrinolytic therapy, 339
  in high-dose isolated limb perfusion, 310, *311–312*
  in ischemia, 292
  in lower limb ischemia, 277, *278*
  in percutaneous intraarterial thrombolysis, *286*

Urokinase (UK), allergy to, *continued*
  in peripheral arterial occlusion, 304–306
  in plantar artery embolization, *292*
  in venous thrombolysis, 322–323, *324,* 326, 328
  intraoperative, 308–309, *309*
  lys-plasminogen with, 344
  pharmacology of, 299
  plasminogen with, 344
  properties of, 298t
  randomized study of, 310–317, *313–316*
  rt-PA versus, 343, 363
  scu-PA combined with, 343
  surgery versus, 369, 369t
  thrombolysis versus, 370, 370t
  t-PA versus, 343

Valve closure times, 419
Valvular incompetence, 417–424
  grading of, 418, 419t
  pathology of, 420, *421*
  surgery in, 419–423, 422t
Valvuloplasty, 420–421, 422t
Valvulotome, Leather, 190
  Mills, 227, *228*
Valvulotomy, 227, *228*
Van Bemmelen measurement, of valve closure, 419
Vancomycin, 268
Varicose veins, 375, 376t. *See also* Venous stasis disease.
  reticular, 376t
Vascular endothelial growth factor (VEGF), 42
Vascular graft, 53–68. *See also* Prosthetic graft.
Vascular reconstruction, 208–210
Vascular surgery, 47–48, 48t
Vascular system, in aortofemoral bypass, 166t, 166–168
  in diabetes, 4
Vasodilator therapy, 40
VEGF (vascular endothelial growth factor), 42
Velcro support, 379
Velocity, in arterial hemodynamics, 7–9
Vena caval anomalies, 79–80
Vena caval interruption, 409–415
  in pulmonary catheter embolectomy, 413–414
  transvenous/intraluminal devices for, 410–413, *411*
Venatech filter, 412t, 412–413
Venography, in deep venous thrombosis, 388
  venous obstruction and, 418, *418*
Venous autograft, 257
Venous claudication, 30, 419
Venous compression, 124
Venous dysfunction. *See* Venous stasis disease.
Venous filling index (VFI), 10
Venous hemodynamics, 9–11
Venous hypertension. *See* Venous stasis disease.
Venous insufficiency, chronic, 375
  treatment of, 379–380

Venous pressure, dynamic, 379t
  in venous stasis disease, 377
Venous reconstruction, in valvular incompetence, 417–424.
    See also Valvular incompetence.
  in venous stasis disease, 381
Venous reflux, 419–420
  surgical technique in, 420–422, 422t
Venous stasis disease, 375–383
  cutaneous stigmata in, 378
  diagnostic evaluation in, 378–379, 379t
  heredity in, 378
  hormonal influence in, 377–378
  operative intervention in, 380t, 380–381
  reconstruction in, 381
  signs and symptoms of, 375–377, *376*
  treatment options for, 379–380
Venous thromboembolism. *See* Deep venous thrombosis
    (DVT).
Venous thrombolysis, 321–330
  anticoagulation therapy in, 321
  catheter-directed, 322
    role of, 325–326, *326–327*
    technical considerations for, 327–328
  complications of, 328
  endoluminal stents in, 328
  procedure of, 322–324, *323–324*
  results of, 324, 325t
  surgical therapy in, 321–322
  thrombolytic agents in, 322, 326–327
VFI (venous filling index), 10
Video angioscopy, 224
Visceral lesions, concomitant, 98t, 98–100, 99t
Vitamin C, 40
Vitamin E, 40
Vitamin K, 397–398
Volume flow, in arterial hemodynamics, 6–7

Walking, 38
Wallstent, 144
  in angioplasty, 220
  in venous thrombolysis, 324, 328
Warfarin, in deep venous thrombosis, 391, 394, 399
  in oral anticoagulant therapy, 397–398
  in venous thromboembolism, 399–400
  in venous thrombolysis, 324
  prothrombin time of, 398
Wet-to-dry soaks, in graft preservation, 273
  in ischemic ulcerations, 41
White blood cell scans, 269
White blood cell trapping, 378

Xanthelasmas, 30
Xanthomas, 30
X-ray, of thoracoabdominal aortic aneurysm, 105,
    106

ISBN 0-7216-4749-9

90038